HUMAN ANATOMY

Regional and Applied
(General, Head, Neck and Brain)

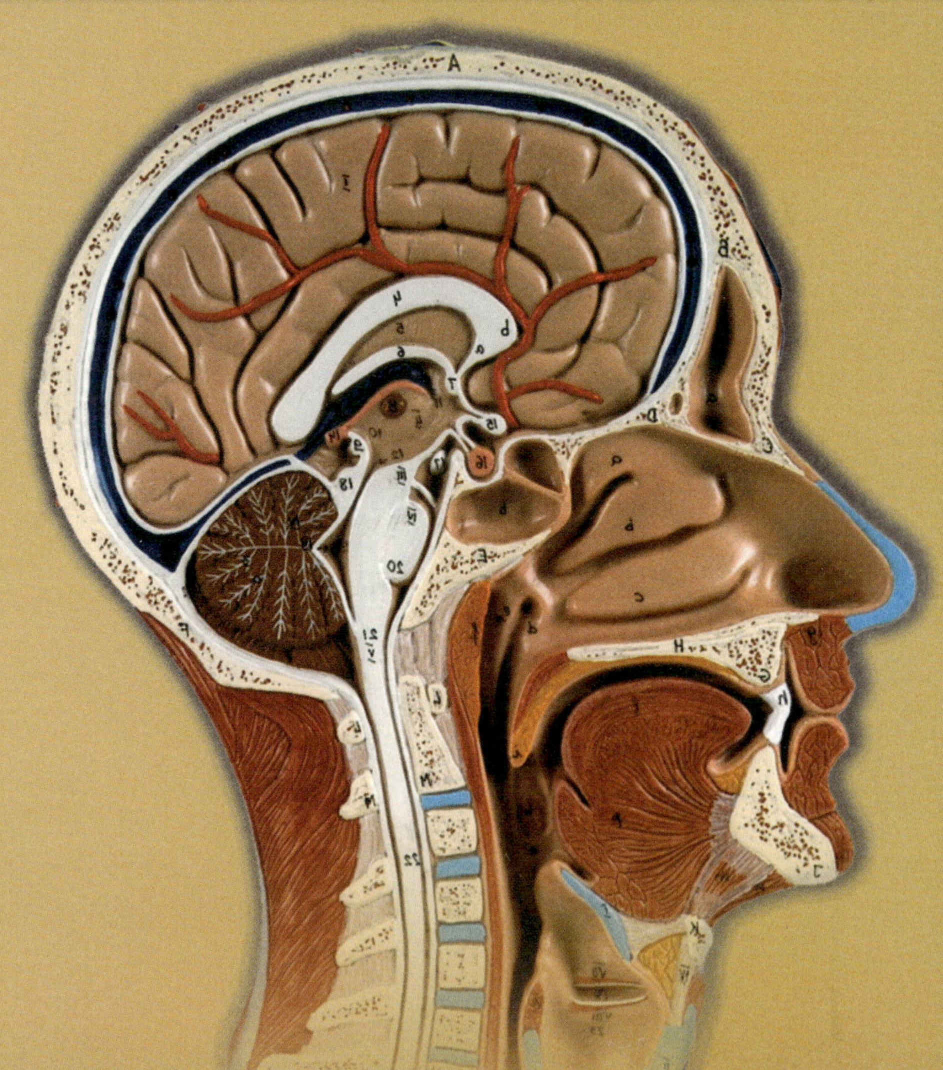

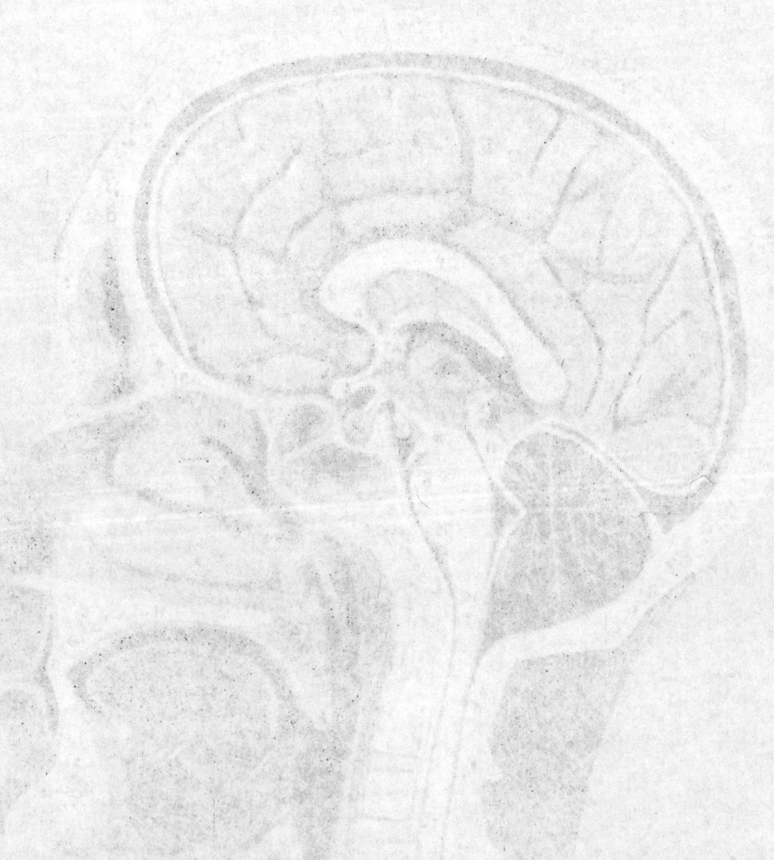

HUMAN ANATOMY

Regional and Applied
(General, Head, Neck and Brain)

Dr. Rama Shankhdhar

M.B.B.S., M.S., FICS (Human Anatomy – KGMC, Lucknow)
Dip. GO (Kolkata)

Professor and Head Department of Anatomy
BBDCODS, BBDU, Lucknow, Uttar Pradesh

Former:

Lecturer Department of Anatomy
BRD Medical College, Gorakhpur, Uttar Pradesh

Associate Professor Anatomy
L.N. Medical College, Bhopal, Madhya Pradesh

Ex Prof. & Head Anatomy Department
Chandra Dental College and Hospital, Barabanki, Uttar Pradesh

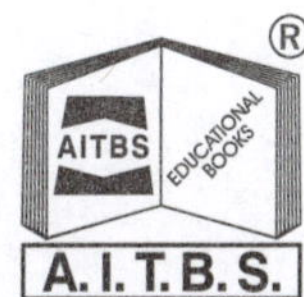

AITBS PUBLISHERS, INDIA

MEDICAL PUBLISHERS

J-5/6, Krishan Nagar, Delhi-110051 (INDIA)
Phone: 011-49067602, 40167052; Fax: 011-22009074
E-mail: aitbsindia@gmail.com & aitbsindia@hotmail.com
Website: www.aitbspublishersindia.com

First Edition : 2011
Second Edition : 2022-23

ISBN: 978-81-7473-446-4

Published by:
Virender Kumar Arya for
AITBS Publishers, India
MEDICAL PUBLISHERS
J-5/6 Krishan Nagar, Delhi-110051 (INDIA)
Phone: 011-49067602, 40167052; Fax: 011-22009074
E-mail: aitbsindia@gmail.com & aitbsindia@hotmail.com

Printed by AITBS, Delhi

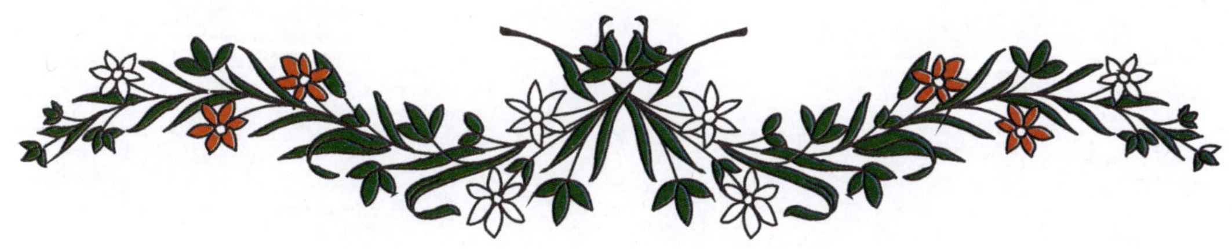

This Books is Dedicated to
My Beloved Family

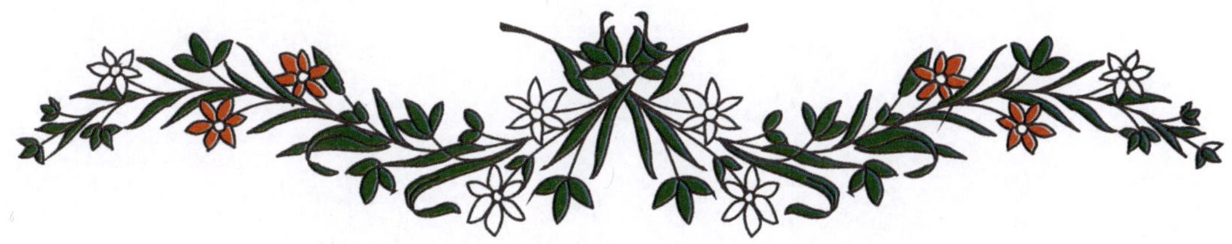

Foreword

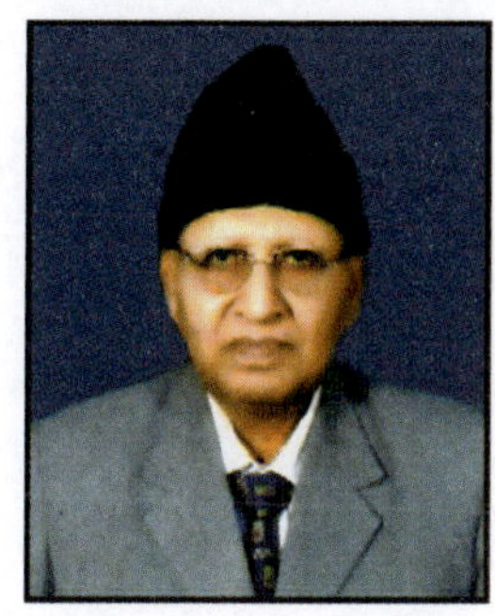

It gives me great pleasure to focus on the book **"Human Anatomy – Regional and Applied"** by **Dr. Rama Shankhdhar**. I have carefully gone through the manuscript and in my considered opinion it reads well, documents essential anatomy required by the undergraduate medical students. The book opens with General Anatomy which, at the outset introduces desirable historical background and anatomical nomenclature. Easily reproducible line diagrams are pleasantly explanatory and enrich the text. The chapter dealing with 'Skin and Fasciae' deserves special mention as it embodies clinically pertinent information, not ordinarily emphasized by text-books of Anatomy available in our country. For example, structural-functional correlations have been admirably dealt with. Histomorphology and applied anatomy comprise the hallmark of this useful book. Regional anatomy of the Head and Neck has been comprehensively addressed to and will be useful for the postgraduate entrance examinations too. Over and above gross anatomy, essentials of embryology, histology and applied anatomy of the salivary glands, ear and teeth standout prominently in this text. Tables have been judiciously used to highlight relations, origins insertion and branches of nerves and arteries in various regions of this book which will be adored by the students while revising the entire syllabus before professional examinations. Unequivocally, I recommend this book to the undergraduate students of medicine and surgery and dentistry. Those preparing for PGME may find it very useful too.

(Late) Prof. Dr. Mahdi Hasan
M.B.B.S., M.S. (Honours), Ph.D., D.Sc., F.A.M.S., F.I.C.S., F.N.A.Sc., F.N.A.
Recipient of Dr. B.C. Roy National Award
Hony. Guest Faculty, Department of Anatomy, C.S.M. Medical University, Lucknow (India)
Formerly President – Anatomical Society of India
Formerly Member – Medical Council of India
Principal, Dean & Chief Medical Superintendent
Professor & Chairman, Department of Anatomy, J.N. Medical College, Aligarh

Preface

I am very glad to present this upgraded latest edition of **"Human Anatomy"**. First of all, I would like to thank my Lord Almighty, who has showered me with blessings to complete this task.

This book of **"Human Anatomy"** will provide as complete, comprehensive, up-to-date, readable and informative textbook. General anatomy which is the foundation of understanding the medical science is included in the beginning. It is written in a clear, coinse and simple way to help the students in preparing for examinations.

I would like to express my gratitude to the Chairman, Dr. C.P. Chaudhary, M.D.S., President and Mr. V.K. Sharma, Secreatary of Chandra Dental College & Hospital, Safedabd, Barabanki for encouraging academic work but also providing peaceful environment to achieve it and their co-operation and hospitality.

During my tenure of teaching I feel that the students are finding difficulty in making diagrams and remembering the subject of anatomy. All the time, I was thinking how can I help them and make the subject easy and interesting, so that they can grasp more and succeed in examination. Every year they are getting photocopy of my diagrams and lectures. For the benefit of my students I thought I should work little more and present my work in the form of a book. All the diagrams in the book have been made by me after through study.

All important details have been covered adequately. Every care has been taken to ensure the accuracy and correctness of each illustration. Though this book is essentially for undergraduate students, can be useful for various postgraduate entrance examinations and as a basic knowledge guide for postgraduate students.

This book is made interesting by making emphasis on the clinical importance of what student studies in the anatomy classroom in the form of applied anatomy is included in the subject.

It gives me extreme pleasure to acknowledge the support, assistance and co-operation rendered by all those who were closely involved in the making of this book. I hope the students will be more benefited by reading this book.

Dr. Rama Shankhdhar

Acknowledgement

At the outset, I want to acknowledge my respected Parents and Guru's, without their ambition, support and blessings, I could not achieve the heights, where I am today.

The most important person in my life always ready to extend his helping hand and taking me out from the jargon of darkness is none except Prof. Ramakant, MS, FICS, FLCS, Head of the Department of Surgery (Gen.), CSMMU, President of Teachers' Association, U.P. Chapter of A.S.I., UPMA and so many other societies, without his support it was not possible for me to do this work successfully. My children Mr. Bobby working in HDN & Seoul Times as Asian Correspondent, recipient of many national & international awards and Dr. Pooja, MS, DNB-SR in Endocrinology, SGPGIMS, Lucknow always loved and supported me. I am obliged for their patience and acceptance of lost evenings and week ends.

I am also grateful to the staff and students of the Chandra Dental College and Hospital, especially Dr. Kamlakant, Assistant Professor who extended their help in the form of respect, support and love. Without their support it was again a difficult task.

I highly appreciate the aptitude of Mr. Arohi Srivastava for his precious time for composing and organizing my work in the form of a book.

I am also thankful and obliged by those whose name must have been forgotten by me in giving their support in any form, please pardon me for that and accept my thanks and regards.

Last, but not the least, my special thanks to Virender Kumar Arya, AITBS Publishers, India for untiring efforts in direction of bringing out this book on time.

Dr. Rama Shankhdhar

Contents

Foreword vii

Preface ix

Acknowledgement xi

PART 1: GENERAL ANATOMY

1. Introduction 3-8
2. Cell and Its Components 9-10
3. Tissues 11-14
4. Muscular System 15-18
5. Nervous System 19-22
6. Cardiovascular System 23-27
7. Skeletal System 28-33
8. Skin and Fasciae 34-39

Review of General Anatomy 40-41

PART 2: HEAD AND NECK

9. Skull 45-73
10. Scalp 74-77
11. Face 78-86

12. Bony Landmarks of the Back 87-95
13. Orbit and Eyeball 96-112
14. Neck 113-122
15. Subdivision of Anterior Triangle of Neck 123-128
16. Parotid Gland 129-134
17. Submandibular Gland 135-139
18. Temporal and Infra Temporal Fossa 140-149
19. Temporo Mandibular Joint 150-152
20. The Pterygo Palatine Fossa 153-156
21. Teeth 157-160
22. The Palate 161-163
23. Tongue 164-168
24. Lymphatic Drainage of Head and Neck 169-170
25. Waldeyer's Ring 171-173
26. Nose and Para Nasal Air Sinuses 174-181
27. Pre-Vertebral Region and Root of Neck 182-192
28. Carotid Arteries, Internal Jugular Vein and Cervical Sympathetic Trunk 193-203
29. Thyroid Gland 204-210
30. The Pharynx 211-216
31. Larynx 217-223
32. Trachea and Oesophagus 224-227
33. Ear 228-241
34. Cranial Cavity 242-256
35. Cranial Nerves 257-273
Review of Head and Neck 274-276

PART 3: BRAIN

36. Brain ____ 279-289
37. Mid Brain (Mesencephalon) ____ 290-292
38. Cerebellum ____ 293-295
39. Pons ____ 296-298
40. Medulla Oblongata ____ 299-301
41. Spinal Cord ____ 302-306
Review of Brain ____ 307-308

National Board Type Questions ____ 309-317

Index ____ 318-325

PART 1

GENERAL ANATOMY

THE CHAPTERS ARE:

1. Introduction to Anatomy
2. Cell and Its Components
3. Tissues
4. Muscular System
5. Nervous System
6. Cardiovascular System
7. Skeletal System
8. Skin and Fasciae

Chapter 1

Introduction to Anatomy

INTRODUCTION

Human anatomy is a wide field of study, which deals with the structural organization of the human body. It is the lifeline and forms firm foundation of the whole art of medical science and introduces different varieties of medical terminology. Anatomy forms the basis of the practice of medicine, leads the physician towards an understanding of a patient's disease when he or she is carrying out a physical examination or using the most advanced imaging techniques. The ability to interpret a clinical observation correctly is therefore, the end point of a sound anatomical understanding.

Observation and visualization are the primary techniques a student should use to learn anatomy. Although the language of anatomy is important, the network of information needed to visualize the position of physical structures in a patient goes far beyond simple memorization.

HISTORY OF ANATOMY

1. Greek Period (B.C.)

Hippocrates of Cos (Circa 400 B.C.)

The father of Medicine is considered as one of the founders of Anatomy. Parts of his collection are the earliest anatomical description.

Herophilus (Circa 300 B.C.) is the **"Father of Anatomy"**. He was a Greek Physician, who first dissected the human body. He distinguished cerebrum from cerebellum, nerves from tendons, arteries from veins and motor from sensory nerves. Herophilus was a very successful teacher and wrote a book on Anatomy.

2. Roman Period (A.D.)

Galen (Circa 130–200 A.D.)

"Prince of Physician" Practiced medicine at Rome. He demonstrated and wrote on Anatomy. His teachings were followed and considered as the infallible authority on the subject for nearly 15 centuries.

3. Fourteenth Century

Mundinus (1276–1326)

The "Restorer of Anatomy" was an Italian anatomist and Professor of Anatomy at Bologna. He wrote a book "Anathomia" which was the standard anatomical text for over a century. He taught anatomy by dissection for which his text was used as a guide.

4. Fifteenth Century

Leonardo da vinci of Italy (1452–1519)

The originator of cross-sectional anatomy, was of the greatest geniuses. He was the first to describe the moderator band of the right ventricle. The most admirable of his work are the drawings of the things he observed with perfection and fidelity. His 60 note books containing 500 diagrams were published in 1898.

5. Sixteenth Century

Vesalius (1514–1564)

The "Reformer of Anatomy" was German in origin by birth and found an Italian University favourable for his work. He was professor of Anatomy at Padna. He was regarded as founder of Modern Anatomy because he taught that anatomy could be learned only by dissections. He opposed and corrected the erroneous concepts of Galen and fought against his authority, thus reviving anatomy after a dead lock of about 15 centuries. His great anatomical treatise "De Febricia – Human Corporis", written in 7 volumes, revoluntionized the teaching of Anatomy and remained as authoritative text for two centuries.

6. Seventeenth Century

Willium Harvey (1578–1657)

Discovered the circulation of blood and published it as "*Anatomical Exercise on the Motion of the Heart and Blood in Animals*". He also published a book on embryology. Other events of this century are:

(a) First recorded human dissection in 1638 in Massachusetts.

(b) Foundation of microscopic anatomy by Malpighi.

(c) Introduction of alcohol as a preservative.

7. Eighteenth Century

Willium Hunter (1718–1783)

Was a London Anatomist and Obstetrician. He introduced embalming with the help of Harveys Discovery and founded with his younger brother *John Hunter* the famous Hunterian museum.

8. Nineteenth Century

In Edinburgh (1826) and Maryland (1833)

Dissection by medical students was made compulsory.

Warbunton Anatomy Act 1932, was passed in England under which the unclaimed bodies were made available for dissection. The 'act' was passed in America (Massachusetts) in 1831. Formalin was used as a fixative in 1890s, X-ray was discovered by Roentgen in 1895. Various endoscopes were devised between 1819 and 1899.

The anatomical societies were founded in Germany (1886), Britain (1887) and America (1888).

Anatomists of this century were – Astley Cooper (1768-1841), Cuvier (1769-1832), Meckel (1724-1774) and Henry Gray (1827-1861). The author of Gray's Anatomy.

The term anatomy is derived from a Greek word – "Anatome" – meaning cutting up (Ana = structure, tome = cutting up). In Latin – Greek Anatome means "dissection".

Dissection is merely a technique where as anatomy is a wide field of study by using the technique of dissection.

Anatomy describes the theatre in which action takes place – means – anatomy is to physiology as Geography is to History.

In ancient days anatomy was studied mainly by dissection. But now-a-days scope of modern anatomy has become very wide and now it is studied by all possible methods which clarify and enlarge the boundaries of anatomical knowledge.

SUBDIVISIONS OF ANATOMY

It depends on the different methods by which we study the structure of human body, helping us in reaching correct diagnosis in patients and treating their diseases, for example:

1. Cadaveric Anatomy

Study is done on dead bodies – cadavers – by dissecting different parts of human body with the help of naked eye called "Gross Anatomy" or Macroscopic Anatomy. This can be done by one of the two approaches:

A. **Regional anatomy:** Body is studied in parts means regions like upper limb, lower limb, thorax, abdomen, head and neck and brian.

B. **Systemic anatomy:** Body is studied system wise, for example:

- We study all bones of the body – called skeletal system – under heading of osteology.
- Study of muscular system – Myology.
- Study of vascular system – Angiology.
- Study of articulatory system – Arthrology or Syndesmology.
- Study of nervous system – Neurology.
- Pulmonology.
- Study of digestive system – Gastrology.
- Study of urogenital system – Urology, Gynaecology.
- Study of endocrine system – Splanchnology.
- Locomotor system – includes – osteology, arthrology and myology.

2. Living Anatomy

Study is done on living human being by using different techniques, for example:

(a) **Inspection:** It is done with the help of eyes, here, we inspect whole human being – in form of facial expression, gait and posture etc.

(b) **Palpation:** It is done with the help of palm and fingers – we feel the lump, its consistency and tenderness.

(c) **Percussion:** It is done with the help of fingers to know the different type of sounds produced in different situations, e.g., cystic, solid lesion etc.

(d) **Auscultation:** It is done with the help of stethoscope – we listen different types of respiratory, heart and bowel sounds.

(e) **Endoscopy:** It is done with help of endoscopes, e.g., bronchoscopy, gastroscopy, sigmoidoscopy, cystoscopy etc.

(f) **Radiography:** We take the help of X-rays – plain and contrast.

(g) **Electromyography:** We study the electrical waves produced by action of tissues, e.g., E.C.G., E.E.G. etc.

3. Embryology or Developmental Anatomy

Here, we study prenatal and postnatal developmental changes in an individual. The developmental history is called ontogeny. The evolutionary history on the other hand is called phylogeny.

4. Histology (Microscopic Anatomy)

We study the different tissues and their structure with the help of microscope.

5. Surface Anatomy (Topograhic Anatomy)

It is the study of deeper part of the body in relation to the skin surface. It is helpful in clinical practice and surgical operations.

6. Radiographic Anatomy

It is the study of deeper organs by plain and contrast radiography.

7. Comparative Anatomy

It is the study of anatomy of the other animals and compare them to explain the changes in the form, structure and function of different parts of the human body.

8. Physical Anthropology

It deals with the external features and measurements of different races and groups of people and with the study of the prehistoric remains.

9. Applied Anatomy (Clinical Anatomy)

It deals with the application of the anatomical knowledge to the medical and surgical practice.

10. Experimental Anatomy

It is the study of the factors, which influence and determine the form, structure and function of different parts of the body.

ANATOMICAL NOMENCLATURE

Galen (2nd century) wrote his book in Greek, and Vesalius (16th century) did it in Latin. Most of the anatomical terms, therefore are either in Greek or Latin.

In 1895, the German Anatomical Society held a meeting in Basle and approved a list of about 5000 terms known as *Basle Nomina Anatomica* (BNA).

The following six rules were laid down to be followed strictly:

1. Each part shall have only one name.
2. Each term shall be in Latin.
3. Each term shall be as short and simple as possible.
4. The terms shall be merely memory signs.
5. Related terms shall be similar, e.g., Femoral Artery, Femoral Vein and Femoral Nerve.
6. Adjectives shall be arranged as opposites, e.g., Major and Minor, Superior and Inferior, Anterior and Posterior, Lateral and Medial etc.

The drafts on Nomina Histologica and Nomina Embryologica prepared by the subcommittee of the International Anatomical Nomenclature Committee (IANC) was approved in a plenary session of the

Eleventh International Congress of Anatomists held, in Leningrad in 1970.

DESCRIPTIVE TERMS

1. **Terms used for describing the position of the body:**

Anatomical Position: In this position:

(a) Body is erect.

(b) Eyes look straight to the front.

(c) Upper limbs hang by the side of the trunk with the palm directed forwards.

(d) Lower limbs are parallel with the toes pointing forwards.

All the structures are described presuming the body in anatomical position, although during study the body may be placed in any position.

(i) **Supine position:** Lying down position with the face directed upwards.

(ii) **Prone position:** Lying down position with the face directed downwards.

(iii) **Lithotomy position:** Lying supine with the buttocks at the edge of the table, hips and knees fully flexed and the feet strapped in position.

2. **Anatomical Planes:**

(a) **Median or midsagittal plane:** Divides the body into right and left equal halves.

(b) **Sagittal plane:** Any plane paralled to the median plane.

(c) **Coronal plane:** It is a vertical plane at right angles to the median plane.

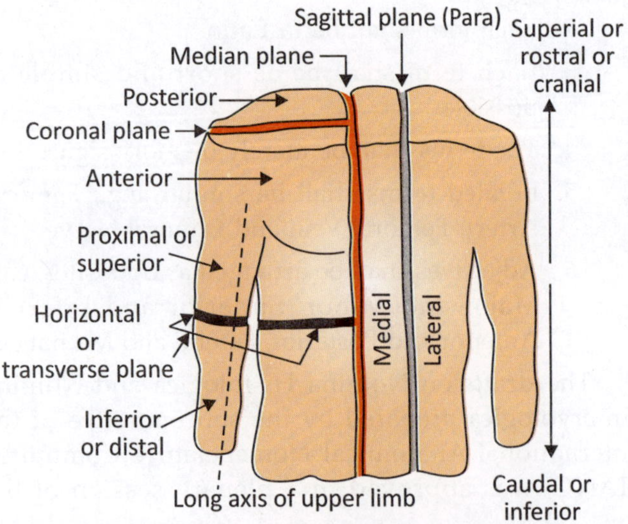

Fig. 1.1: *The three planes in the body*

(d) **Transverse plane:** A plane at right angles to a vertical plane, or at right angles to the longitudinal axis of any part.

(e) **Horizontal plane:** A plane parallel to the ground or transverse plane. It is at right angles to both sagittal and coronal planes.

(f) **Oblique plane:** Any plane other than the aforementioned planes.

3. **Terms of relations commonly used in gross anatomy:**

(a) **Anterior:** Towards the front.

(b) **Posterior:** Towards the back.

(c) **Superior:** Towards the head.

(d) **Inferior:** Towards the feet.

(e) **Medial:** Towards the median plane.

(f) **Lateral:** Away from the median plane.

4. **Terms used in embryology and comparative anatomy, sometimes in gross anatomy:**

(a) **Ventral:** Towards belly (Anterior).

(b) **Dorsal:** Towards back (Posterior).

(c) **Cranial or Rostral:** Towards head (Superior).

(d) **Caudal:** Towards tail.

5. **Special terms for limbs:**

(a) **Proximal:** Nearer to the trunk.

(b) **Distal:** Away from the trunk.

(c) **Radial:** Outer border of upper limb.

(d) **Ulnar:** Inner border of upper limb.

(e) **Fibular:** Outer border of lower limb.

(f) **Tibial:** Inner border of lower limb.

(g) **Preaxial border:** Outer border in the upper limb and inner border in lower limb.

(h) **Postaxial border:** Inner border in the upper limb and outer border in lower limb.

(i) **Flexor surface:** Anterior surface in the upper limb and posterior surface in the lower limb.

(j) **Extensor surface:** Posterior surface in the upper limb and anterior surface in the lower limb.

(k) **Palmar:** Pertaining towards the palm of the hand.

(l) **Plantar:** Pertaining to the sole of the foot.

6. **Certain other terms:**

(a) **Terms used for hollow organs:**

1. Interior or inner.
2. Exterior or outer.

3. Invagination or inward protrusion.
4. Evagination or outward protrusion.

(b) **Terms used for solid organs:**

(i) **Superficial:** Towards the surface.

(ii) **Deep:** Inner to the surface.

(c) **Terms used to indicate the side:**

(i) **Ipsilateral** to the same side.

(ii) **Contralateral** of the opposite side.

7. Terms used for describing muscles:

(a) **Origin:** Relatively fixed end of a muscle during its contraction.

(b) **Insertion:** Moving end of a muscle during its contraction.

(c) **Belly:** Fleshy contractile part of a muscle.

(d) **Tendon:** Fibrous, cord-like, non-contractile part of a muscle.

(e) **Aponeurosis:** Fibrous, flattened sheat of a muscle replacing tendon.

(f) **Raphe:** A fibrous band made up of inter-digitating fibres of the tendon or aponeurosis. It is slightly stretchable.

(g) **Ligaments:** They are fibrous, inelastic bands which connect two segments of a joint.

8. Terms used for describing movements:

(a) **Flexion:** Approximation of flexor surfaces in which the angle of the joint is reduced.

(b) **Extension:** Approximation of extensor surfaces, in which angle of the joint is increased.

(c) **Adduction:** Movement towards the central axis.

(d) **Abduction:** Movement away from the central axis.

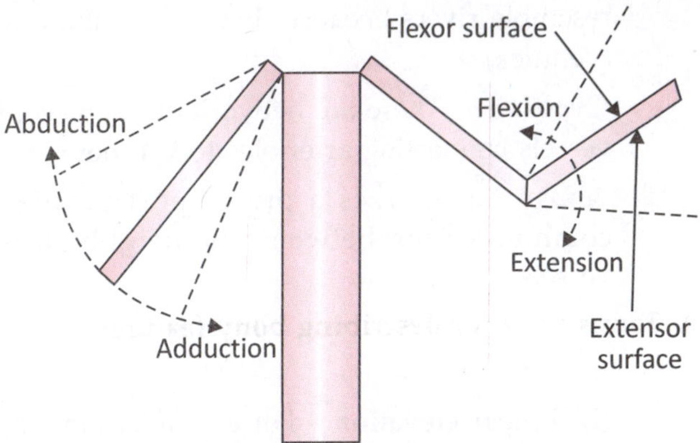

Fig. 1.2: *Angular movements*

(e) **Medial rotation:** Inward rotation.

(f) **Lateral rotation:** Outward rotation.

(g) **Circumduction:** Combination of various foregoing movements.

(h) **Pronation:** Rotation of the forearm so that the palm is turned backwards.

(i) **Supination:** Rotation of the forearm so that the palm is turned forwards.

(j) **Protraction:** Forward protrusion.

(k) **Retraction:** Movement reverse of protrusion, i.e., backward retraction.

9. Terms used for describing vessels:

(a) **Arteries:** Carry oxygenated blood away from heart with the exception of pulmonary and umbilical arteries, which carry deoxygenated blood. Arteries resembles trees because they have branches (Arterioles).

(b) **Veins:** Carry deoxygenated blood towards heart with the exception of pulmonary and umbilical veins – carry oxygenated blood. Veins

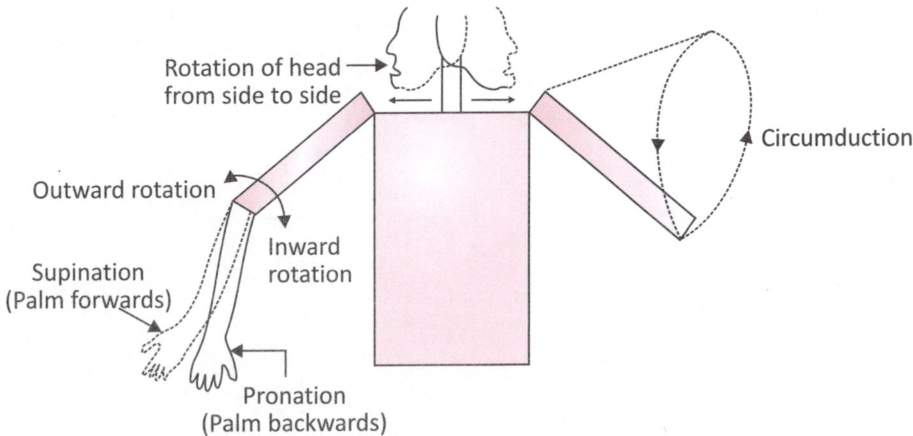

Fig. 1.3: *Rotatory movements*

resemble rivers because they have tributaries (venules).

(c) Capillaries: These are network of microscopic vessels connecting arterioles to venules.

(d) Anastomosis: It is a pre or post-capillary communication between the neighbouring vessels.

10. Terms used for describing bony features:

(a) Elevations:

(i) **Linear elevation** – For example: Line, lip, ridge or crest.

(ii) **Sharp elevations** – For example: Spine, styloid process, cornu etc.

(iii) **Rounded or irregular elevations** – For example: Tubercle, tuberosity, epicondyle, malleolus or trochanter etc.

(b) Depressions: For example: Pit, impression, fovea, fossa, groove, sulcus or notch etc.

(c) Openings: For example: Foramen, canal, hiatus etc.

(d) Cavities: For example: Sinus, cell or antrum etc.

(e) Smooth articular areas: For example: Facet, condyle, head, capitulum or trochlea.

ARRANGEMENT OF STRUCTURES IN THE BODY: FROM WITHIN OUTWARDS

1. Bony framework of the body.
2. Muscles are attached to bones.
3. Blood vessels, nerves and lymphatics form neurovascular bundles which run in between the muscles, along the fascial planes.
4. Thoracic and abdominal cavities contain several internal organs – called viscera.
5. **Whole body has three general coverings:**
   (a) Skin
   (b) Superficial fascia
   (c) Deep fascia.

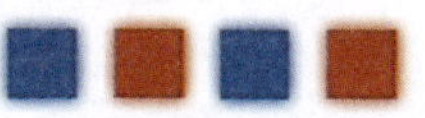

Cell and its Components

UNIT OF LIFE IS CELL

Cell forms the basic structural unit of all tissues and organs of the body.

Organs constitute the various systems of the body according to the functional, survival and propogative needs of the body.

STRUCTURE OF CELL

1. **Cell membrane:** It is semipermeable to Na^+, K^+, Ca^{++}, Cl^+ and made-up of 3 layers outer and inner layer is formed by protein and intermediate layer is made-up of phospholipid.
   - This maintains the shape of the cell.
   - Lipid soluble substances pass through cell membrane.
   - Amino acids, proteins and nucleic precursor's pass via channels in the membrane and various receptors are present.
2. **Cytoplasm:** Is present between cell membrane and nucleus. It consists of:
   (a) Organelles – in the form of ribosomes:
   - Mitochondria
   - Golgi apparatus
   - Endoplasmic reticulum (smooth ribosomes and rough ribosomes)
   - Phagosome
   - Lysosomes (hydrolytic enzymes present)
   - Centrioles and microtubules (responsible for cell division)
   - Filaments and fibres.

   (b) Inclusion substances:
   - Glycoproteins

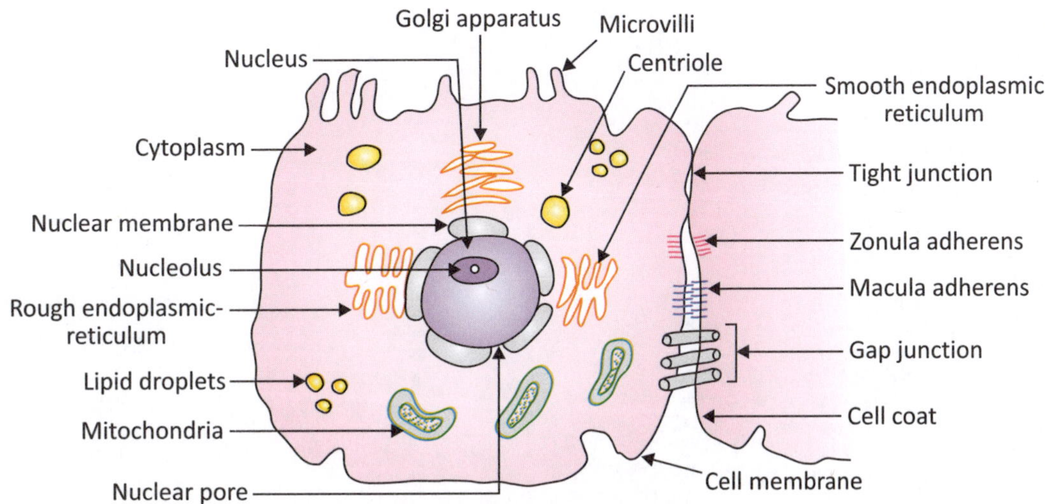

Fig. 2.1: ***Structure of Cell (E.M.)***

- Pigments
- Fat globules.

3. Nucleus: Is present in all cells except R.B.C.

- Round or ellipsoid mass covered by nuclear membrane – having pores
- Its location depends on cell type
- In leucocytes present in center
- Near the base – in tall columnar cells
- Near periphery – in skeletal muscle.

It consists of:

- Nuclear membrane derived from rough endoplasmic reticulum
- Chromatin threads in a resting cell or chromosomes in dividing cell
- Nucleolus – a dense mass cell
- Nuclear sap.

Sex chromatin or barr bodies: In a normal female – a plano convex body, made up of (xx) hetrochromatin is found beneath the nuclear membrane in a cell, known as barr body.

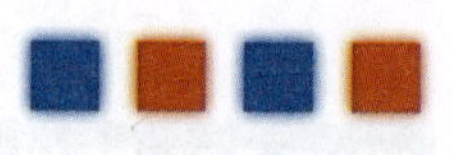

Tissues

INTRODUCTION

Tissues are made-up of groups of cells with similar functions.

TYPES OF TISSUES

A. **Epithelial tissue.**
B. **Connective tissue.**
C. **Muscular tissue:** It is a contractile tissue which brings about movements.
D. **Nervous tissue:** The tissue which has taken special properties of sensitivity, conductivity and responsiveness excitable or non-excitable.

A. EPITHELIAL TISSUE

Forms epithelium lines the body cavities, tubes and covers the outer surface of the body.

Classified: As shape of cells, number of cells, layers and cell surface modifications.

I. Simple Epithelium:

(a) Simple squamous epithelium: Meant for exchange of substances found in:

- Blood vessels
- Alveoli
- Peritoneum
- Pleura

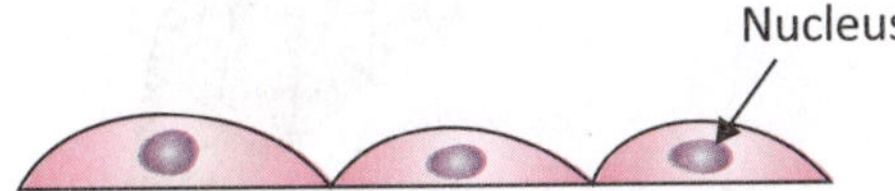

Fig. 3.1: *Simple squamous epithelium*

- Single layer of flat cells lying on the basement – membrane.

(b) Simple cuboidal epithelium

- Cuboidal in shape
- **Found in ducts:** For example:
  - Thyroid
  - Ducts of G.I.T.
  - Salivary glands
  - Single layer of cells.

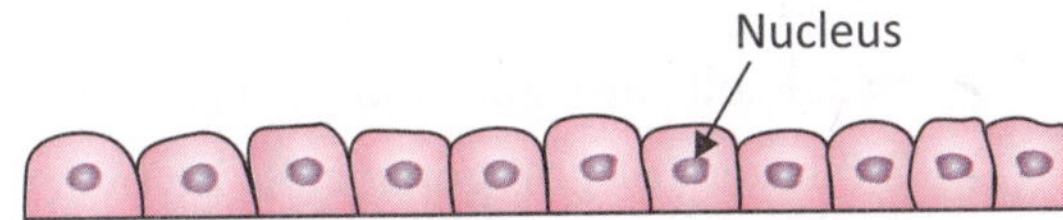

Fig. 3.2: *Simple cuboidal epithelium*

(c) Simple columnar epithelium

- Found on secretary and absorptive surfaces
- For example uterus
- Uterine tubes
- Tympanic cavity
- G.I.T.
- Gall bladder
- Ependyma of spinal cord
- Cells are shaped like column
- Single layer of cells
- Height being more than width.

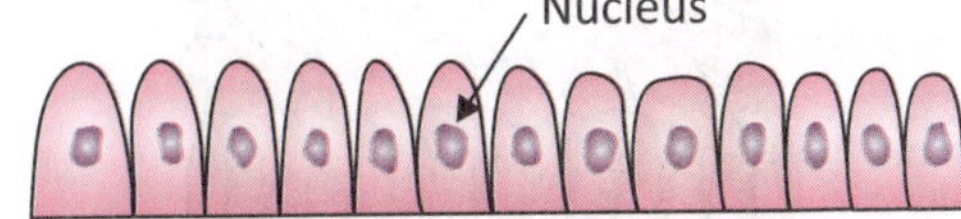

Fig. 3.3: *Simple columnar epithelium*

These three types of epithelium are variety of Simple Epithelium – I.

II. Pseudostratified Epithelium: Cells are of different heights. Found in:

- Respiratory tract and male genital system
- For example: Trachea
- Bronchi
- Ductus deferens
- Male urethra etc.
- Single layered
- Tall columnar
- Level of nucleus is different in different cells
- Gives a false appearance of stratification.

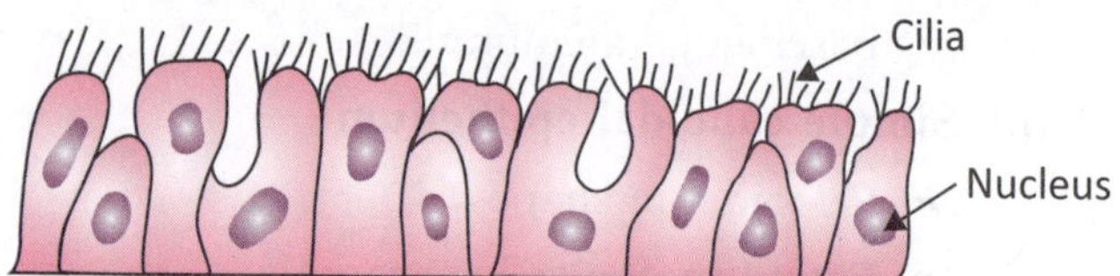

Fig. 3.4: *Pseudostratified ciliated columnar epithelium*

III. Stratified Epithelium

(a) Stratified squamous epithelium

- More than one layer of cells are present – 5-6 layers
- Basal cells are columnar cells
- 2-3 layers of polygonal cells lie over it
- Superficial cells are flat squamous
- Protective in nature.

Found at:

- Oral cavity
- Pharynx
- Tongue
- Tonsil
- Oesophagus
- Conjunctiva and
- Cornea etc.

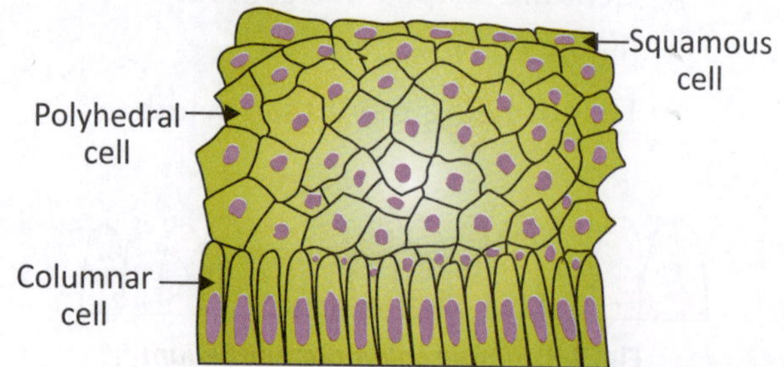

Fig. 3.5: *Stratified squamous epithelium*

(b) Keratinized stratified squamous epithelium:

Characterised by layer of keratin over superficial cells.

Found at:

- Skin
- It protects the exposed parts of body.

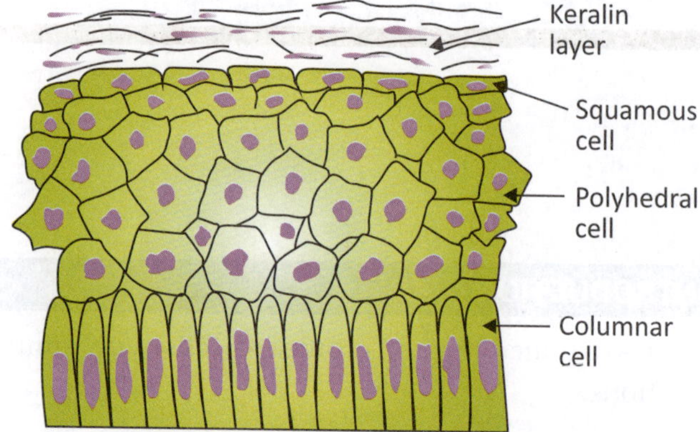

Fig. 3.6: *Keratinized stratified squamous epithelium*

C. Stratified cuboidal epithelium: Two layers of cuboidal cells.

Found in:

- Large ducts, e.g., ducts of sweat glands and mammary gland.
- Ovarian follicles etc.

D. Transitional epithelium:

- Transition of cells from basal to superficial layer – 5 6 layers.
- Basal cells – columnar cells become polygonal above.
- Superficial cells are umbrella shape.

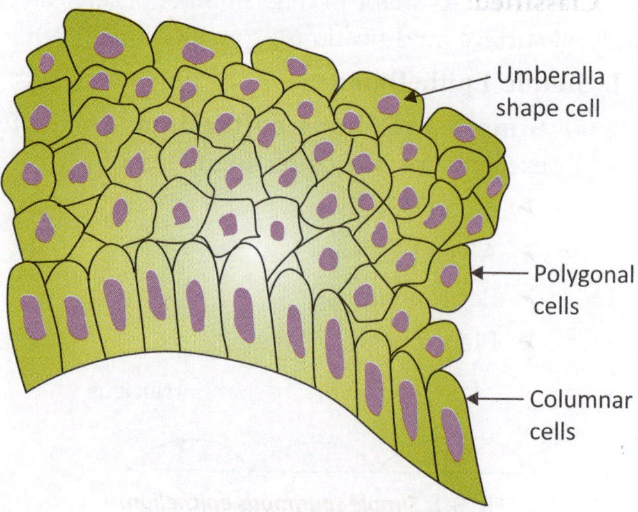

Fig. 3.7: *Transitional epithelium*

Found in:

- Urinary tract
- Renal pelvis
- Ureter
- Bladder
- Urethra etc.

E. **Stratified columnar epithelium:** Two layers of columnar cells.

Found at:

- Conjunctival fornix
- Anal mucous membrane etc.

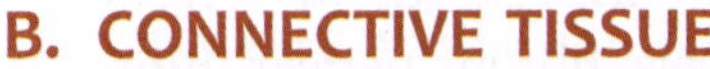

B. CONNECTIVE TISSUE

Connects different tissues and facilitates passage of nerves and vascular bundles in different tissues.

Made up of:

- Cells
- Fibres and matrix

Cells

Two types of cells

A. Resident Cells:

I. **Fibroblast:** Large spindle shaped cells with irregular process – they produce collagen and elastic fibres.

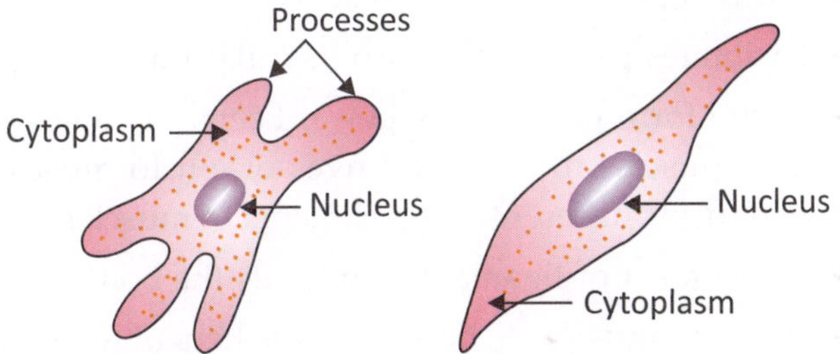

Fig. 3.8: *Fibroblast and Fibrocyte*

II. **Fibrocyte:** Fibrocyte are mature fibroblasts they are spindle shaped with centrally placed nucleus.

III. **Adipocytes:**

- Nucleus is at peripherally placed
- Cytoplasm contains lipids.
- In obese state – fat cells get enlarged.

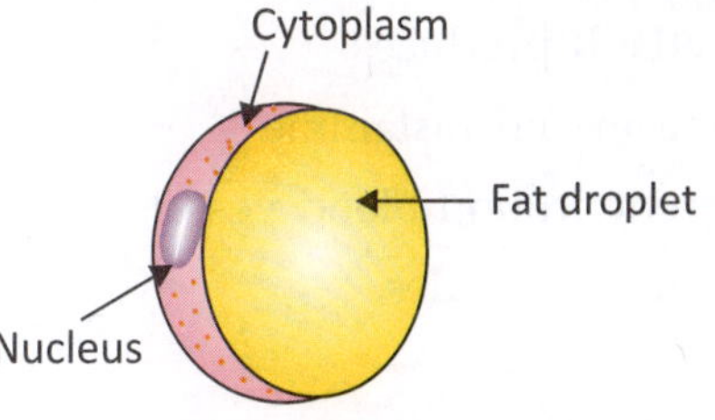

Fig. 3.9: *Adipocytes*

IV. **Mesenchymal Stem Cell:**

- Derived from mesenchyme are capable to differentiate into mature cells of connective tissue during growth and development.
- They are pluripotent cells.
- Have multiple process.
- They are phagocytose foreign bodies.

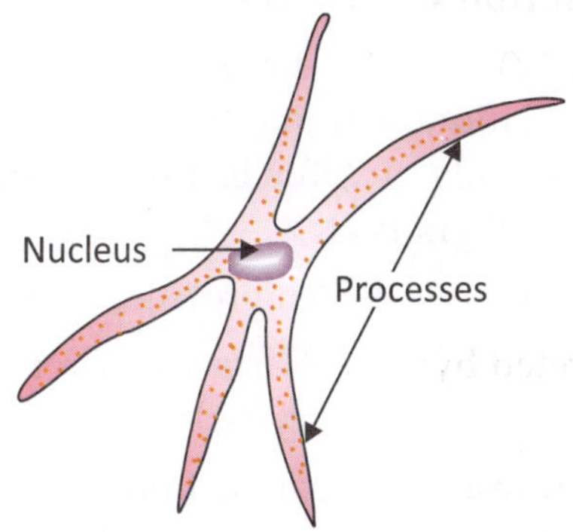

Fig. 3.10: *Mesenchymal Stem Cell*

B. Migrant Cells:

- Macrophages
- Plasma cells
- Mast cells
- Pigment cells
- Lymphocytes
- Monocytes.

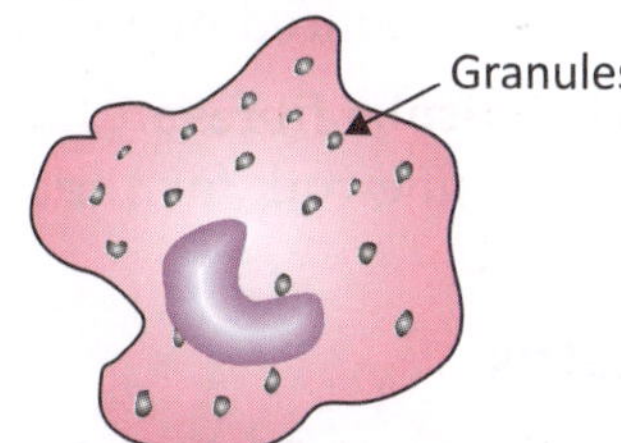

Fig. 3.11: *Macrophages*

Plasma cells: It produces:

- Antibodies.
- Characteristic cart wheel appearance of nucleus.

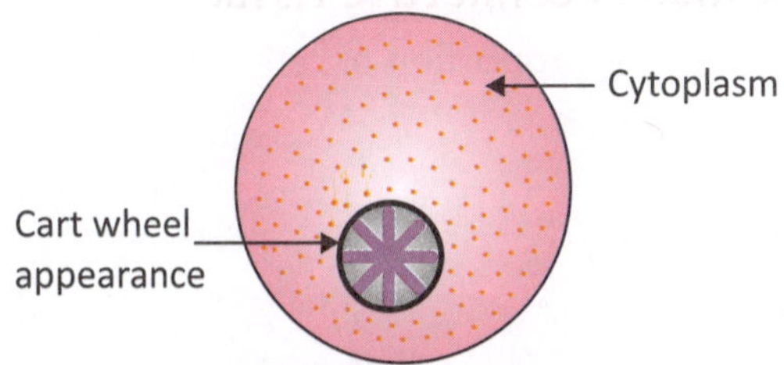

Fig. 3.12: *Plasma Cells*

Mast cells: It produces:

- Heparin and histamine
- Present around blood vessels
- Contain granules.

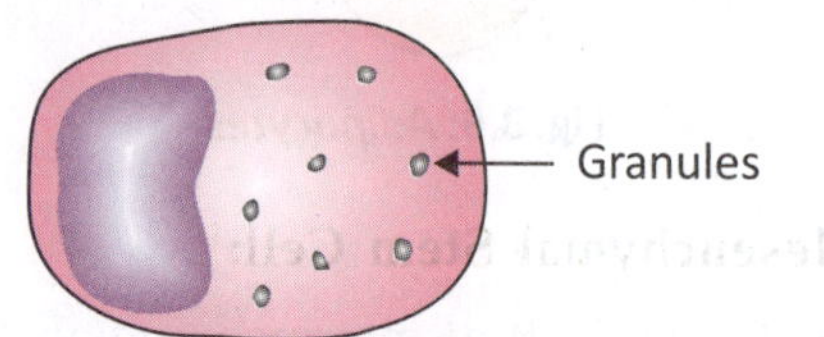

Fig. 3.13: *Mast Cells*

Fibres

Fibres are present in matrix of connective tissue. They are of three types:

(a) Collagen fibres: Thick bundle of colourless fibres

- They branched and rebranched and take part information of framework of certain organs and glands etc., for example, lymphnodes, spleen, thymus etc.
- Made-up of collagen protein
- **Secreted by:** Fibroblasts, chondroblasts, osteocytes and chondrocytes.

(b) Elastic fibres: Run as single fibres.

- Branch and anastomose with each other.
- Broken ends of these fibres – recoil.
- Produced by fibroblasts.

(c) Reticular fibres are fine collagen fibres, which form a framework for various tissues.

Matrix

Matrix or ground substance made-up of carbohydrate and protein.

Mucopolysaccharides and adhesive glycoproteins are present in the matrix.

Classification of Connective Tissue

Based on relative proportion of cells, fibres and matrix in connective tissue.

(a) Irregular connective tissue:

- Loose areolar connective tissue, thin collagen and elastin fibres.
- Dense irregular connective tissue.
- Adipose tissue – found in breast, mesentry, bone marrow etc. contains fat cells.

(b) Regular connective tissue: Fibres are regularly oriented.

- Collagen fibres are present in bundles and run in one direction, also known as white fibrous tissue.
- Present in tendons, ligaments and aponeurosis.

Fascia: Collagen fibres interlace in various directions, e.g., deep fascia, aponeurosis, fibrous pericardium.

Specialized form of Connective Tissue

At certain places it forms a framework for the organs e.g., lymph nodes, spleen, liver, bones and cartilages.

According to the need of the body stem cells of the connective tissue changes its form and takes part in the formation of blood cells, muscular and nervous tissue.

Example: Cartilage, bone, blood, muscular and nervous tissue.

Functions of Connective Tissue

- Binds together various structures.
- Facilitates passage of neuro vascular bundle.
- In the form of deep fascia – it keeps the tendons and muscles in position, gives origin to muscles and forms different compartments of muscles.
- In the form of ligaments – it binds the bones.
- Attaches muscles to bone with the help of tendons.
- Facilitates venous return in lower limb with the help of deep fascia.
- Helps in wound repair – due to presence of fibroblasts.
- Apponeurosis is a regular dense connective tissue.

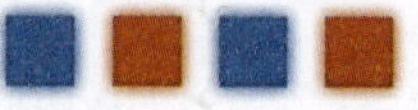

CHAPTER 4

Muscular System

INTRODUCTION

Muscle is a contractile tissue and primarily designed for movements.

L – Musculus = muscle

- It resembles a mouse with their tendons representing the tail.
- All muscles are developed from mesoderm, except – arrector pilorum, muscles of iris and myoepithelial cells of salivary, sweat and lacrimal glands which are derived from ectoderm.

TYPES OF MUSCLES

Muscles has three types:

I. Skeletal muscles

II. Smooth muscles

III. Cardiac muscles.

I. Skeletal Muscles (Striped, striated, somatic and voluntary muscles)

1. Most abundant, found attached to skeleton.
2. Exhibit cross-striations under microscope.
3. Supplied by somatic nerves (cerebro spinal) and are under voluntary control.
4. Respond quick to stimuli, being capable of rapid contractions and get fatigued easily.
5. Help in adjusting the individual to external environment.
6. Are under highest nervous control of cerebral cortex.

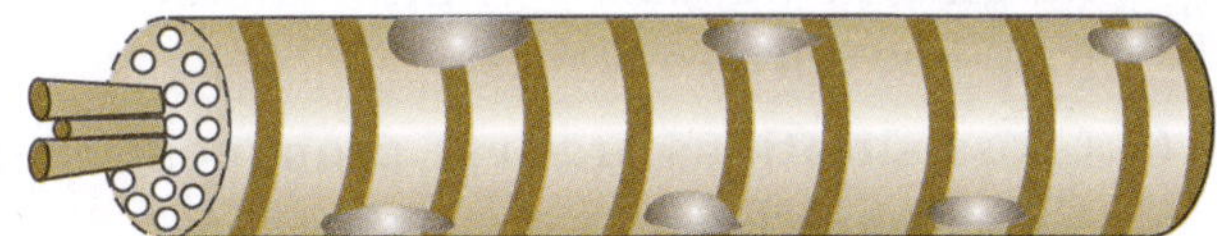

Fig. 4.1: *Skeletal muscle cell*

7. Each muscle fibre is multinucleated cylindrical cell, containing groups of myofibrils made up of myosin, actin, and trapomyosin – myofilaments – are actual centractile elements.

   Example: Muscles of limbs and body wall.

II. Smooth Muscles (Plain, unstriped, non-straited, visceral and involuntary muscles)

1. These muscles often surround the viscera.
2. Do not exhibit cross-striations under microscope.
3. Supplied by autonomic nerves and are not under voluntary control (sympathetic).
4. Respond slowly to stimuli, being capable of sustained contraction and do not fatigue easily.
5. Provide motor power for digestion, circulation, secretion and excretion.
6. Less dependent on nervous control, capable of contracting spontaneously, automatically and often rhythmically.

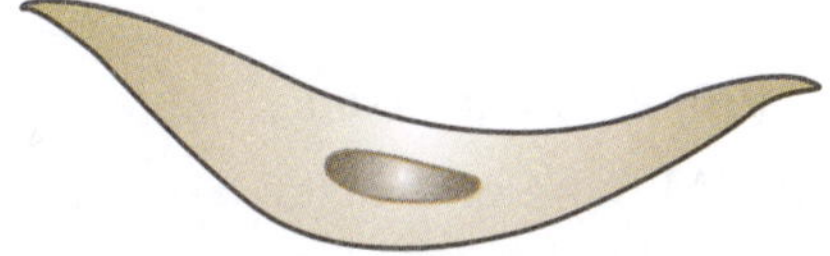

Fig. 4.2: *Smooth muscle cell*

7. Each muscle fibre is an elongated, spindle shaped cell, with a single nucleus placed

centrally. Myofibrils show longitudinal striations, e.g., muscles of blood vessels and G.I.T., G.U.T., arrectorpili muscles of skin.

III. Cardiac Muscle

1. It forms myocardium of the heart.
2. Intermediate in structure, being striated and involuntary.
3. Meant for automatic and rhythmic contractions.
4. Each muscle fibre has a centrally placed single nucleus.
5. Fibres branch and anastomose with neighbouring fibres at intercalated discs (opposed cell membranes).
6. Cross-striations are less prominent than skeletal muscles.

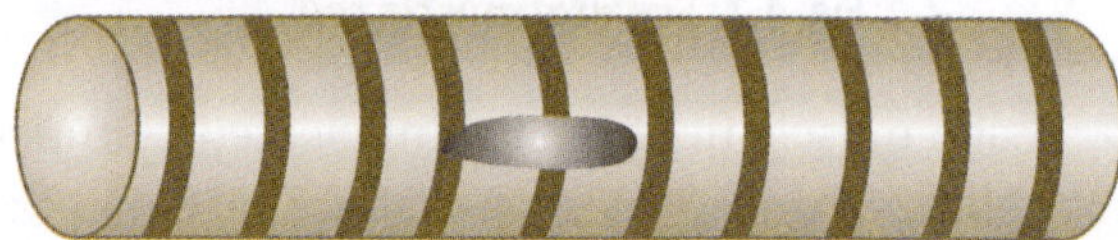

Fig. 4.3: ***Heart muscle cell***

Myoepithelial Cells are basic muscular cell belongs to smooth muscle type.

Myoepithelial cells are present at bases of secretary acini of sweat gland and help in expulsion of secretion from acini.

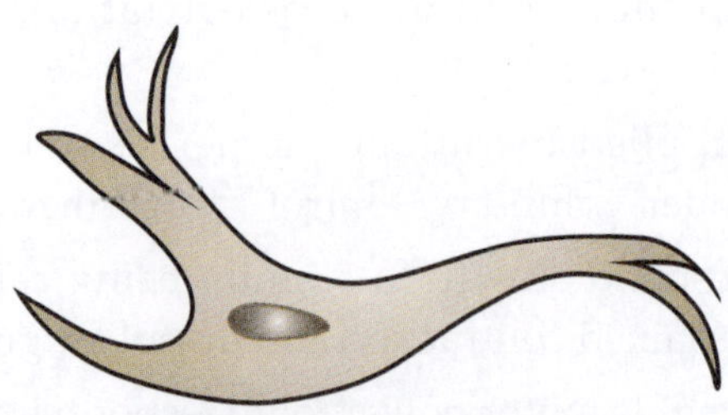

Fig. 4.4: ***Myoepithelial cell***

PARTS OF A MUSCLE

Two ends:

- Origin – Proximal and fixed.
- Insertion – Moving and distal.

Two parts:

- Fleshy part – contractile – belly.
- Fibrous part – non-contractile – tendon, aponeurosis etc.

STRUCTURE OF SKELETAL MUSCLE

1. **Contractile tissue** – Myofibrils
   - Dark band
   - Light band.

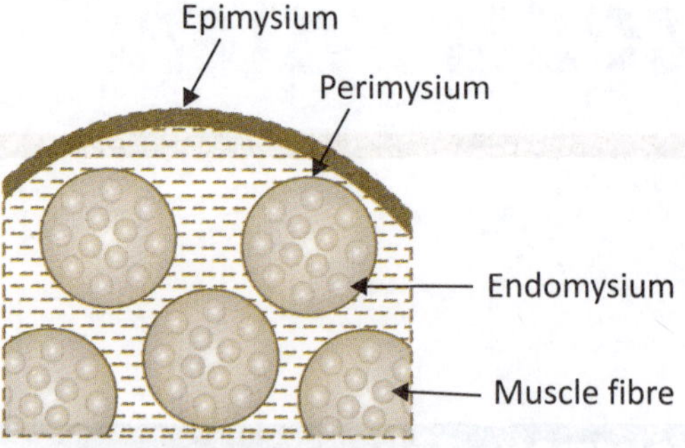

Fig. 4.5: ***Skeletal muscle structure***

2. **Supporting tissue**
   - Endomysium
   - Perimysium
   - Epimysium.

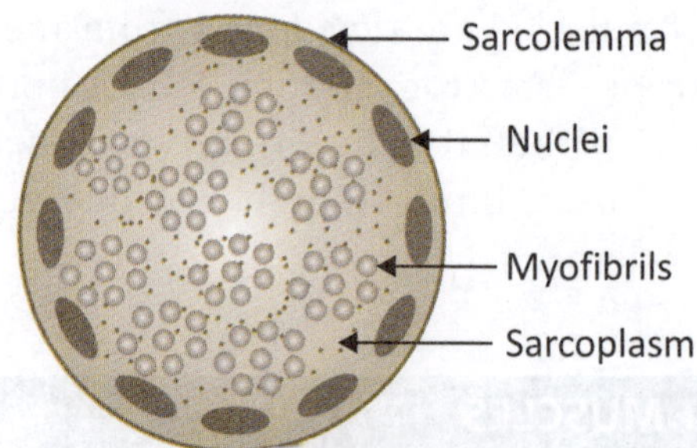

Fig. 4.6: ***Muscle fibre***

FASCICULAR ARCHITECTURE OF MUSCLE

Arrangement of muscle fibres varies according to direction, force and range of movement at a joint.

A. Parallel – Fasciculi

- Thyrohyoid
- Sternohyoid
- Biceps, digastric etc.

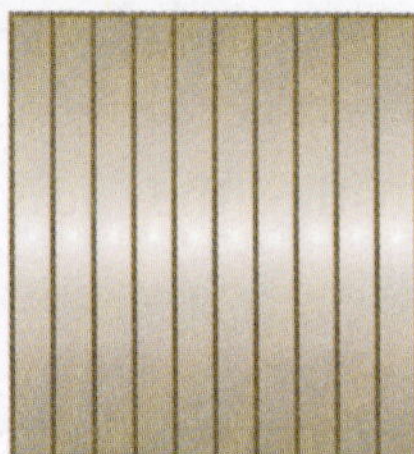

Fig. 4.7: ***Quadrilateral***

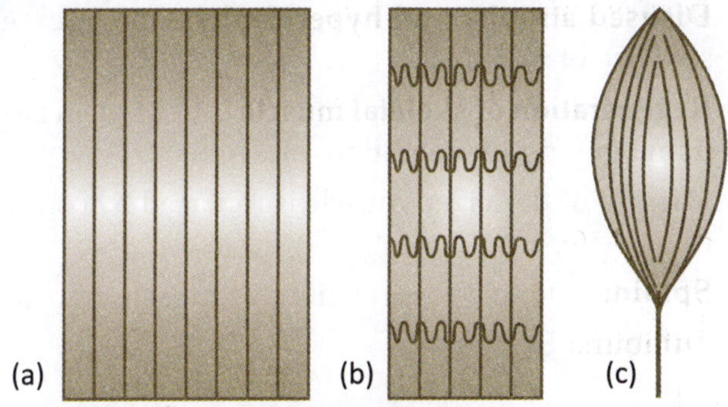

Fig. 4.8: *(a) Strap like, (b) Strap like with tendinous intersections, (c) Fusiform*

B. Oblique – Fasciculi

- Temporalis
- Flexor pollicis longus
- Rectus femoris
- Deltoid
- Tibialis anterior

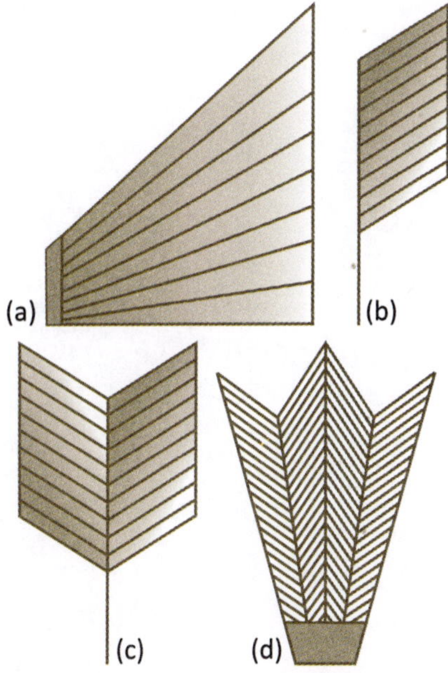

Fig. 4.9: *(a) Triangular, (b) Unipennate, (c) Bipennate, (d) Multipennate*

C. Spiral or Twisted Fasciculi

- Masseter

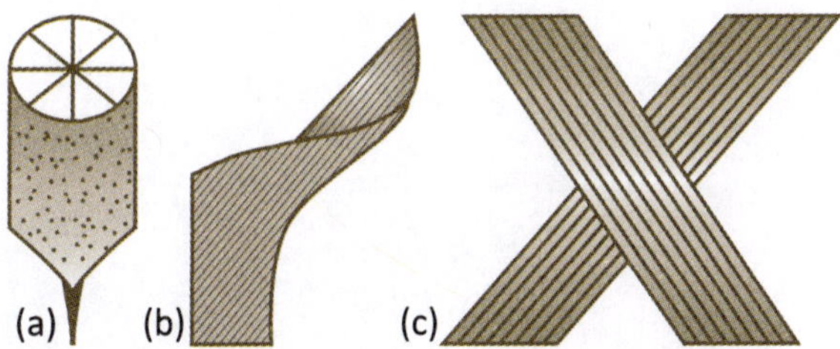

Fig. 4.10: *(a) Circumpennate, (b) Twisted, (c) Cruciate*

- Sternocleidomastoid (Cruciate)
- Trapezius

NOMENCLATURE OF MUSCLES

Depends on number of ways, for example:

1. According to shape, e.g., Trapezius, rhomboideus etc.
2. According to number of heads of origin, e.g., Biceps, quadriceps, triceps, digastric.
3. According to gross structure, e.g., Semitendinosus, semi-membranosus etc.
4. According to location, e.g., Temporalis, supraspinatous, intercostals etc.
5. According to attachments, e.g., Stylohyoid, cricothyroid etc.
6. According to function, e.g., Adductor longus, flexor-carpi ulnaris etc.
7. According to direction of fibres, e.g., Rectus abdominis, obliquus abdominis, transversus etc.

BLOOD SUPPLY OF SKELETAL MUSCLES

Derived from neighbouring arteries. Arteries, veins and nerves pierce the muscle at a point known as neurovascular hilum.

Lymphatics: Accompany blood vessels and drain into neighbouring lymph nodes.

Nerve supply:

Motor nerve – 60%

Sensory fibres – 40%

ACTIONS OF MUSCLES

When a muscle contracts it shortens by 1/3 (30%) of its belly length and brings about a movement.

(a) Prime movers: Bring about desired movement (Agonists).

(b) Antagonists: (Opponents) – Oppose the prime movers.

(c) Fixators: Which stabilize the proximal joints of a limb so that desired movement at the distal joint may occur on a fixed base.

(d) Synergists: When prime movers cross more than one joint, the undesired actions at the proximal joints are prevented by certain muscles known as synergists.

APPLIED ANATOMY

1. **Paralysis:** Loss of motor power is paralysis.
2. **Muscular spasm** are quite painful and localized spasm caused by a muscle pull generalized spasm – occurs in tetanus and epilepsy.
3. **Disused atrophy and hypertrophy:** Due to excessive use of muscles.
4. **Regeneration of skeletal muscle** is limited, in large damage – no regeneration.

   Missing or damaged muscle is replaced by connective tissue.
5. **Sprain:** Due to overstretching of muscle fibres.
6. **Tumours:** Sarcoma.

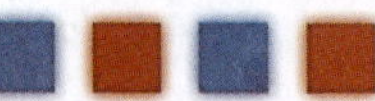

CHAPTER 5

Nervous System

INTRODUCTION

The Nervous System is chief controlling and coordinating system of the body.

- It controls and regulates all activities weather voluntary or involuntary and adjusts the individual to the given surroundings.
- It is based on special properties of sensitivity, conductivity and responsiveness.

PARTS OF NERVOUS SYSTEM

1. **Central nervous system:** Brain and spinal cord.
2. **Peripheral nervous system:** It has two parts:
   (a) **Cerebrospinal part (Somatic):** This comprises of:
   - 12 pairs of cranial nerves and 31 pairs of spinal nerves.
   - Exteroceptors.

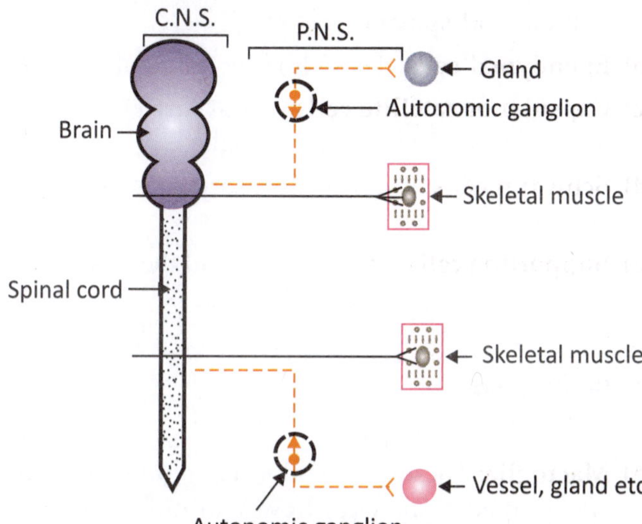

Fig. 5.1: ***Parts of nervous system***

   (b) **Autonomic nervous system (visceral):** This has two constituents:
   - Sympathetic nervous system.
   - Parasympathetic nervous system.

Nervous Tissue

Develops from neuro-ectoderm and mesoderm.

NEURON

It is the main structural and functional unit of nervous system (ectodermal in origin). This consists of:

(a) **Soma or cell body:** Having a central nucleus and nissl's granules in its cytoplasm.

(b) **Neurites or processes:**
- Long – Axons
- Short – Dendrites
- Cell bodies of the neurons form grey matter and nuclei in the CNS, and ganglia in PNS.
- Cell proceses (axons) form tracts in CNS and nerves in PNS.

TYPES OF NEURONS

I. According to number of their processes these are called:

1. Unipolar, e.g., Mesencephalic nucleus.
2. Bipolar, e.g., Spiral and vestibular ganglia.
3. Pseudounipolar, e.g., Sensory ganglia.
4. Multipolar, e.g., Most common type.

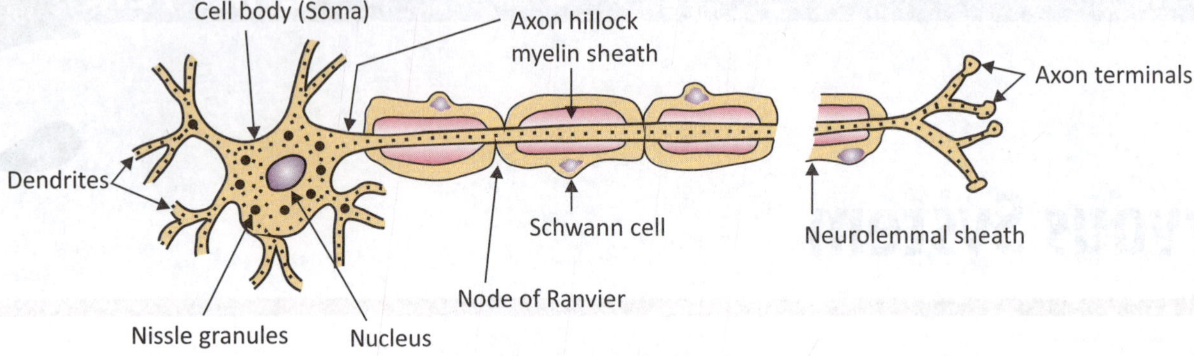

Fig. 5.2: ***Structure of a neuron***

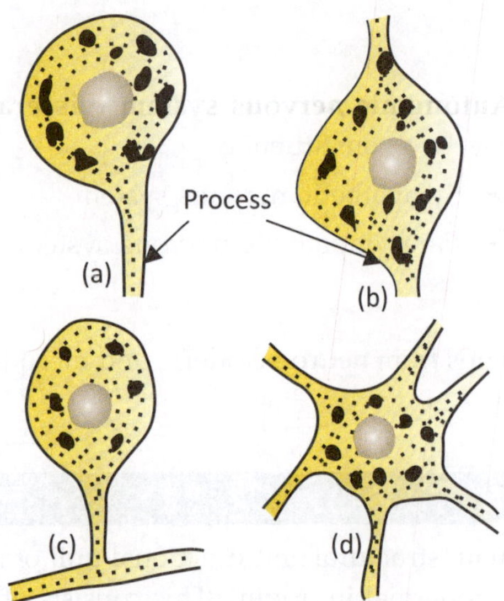

Fig. 5.3: ***(a) Unipolar, (b) Bipolar, (c) Pseudounipolar, (d) Multipolar***

II. According to length of Axon:

(a) **Golgi type I:** Neurons with a long axon.

(b) **Golgi type II:** Neurons (microneurons) with a short or no axon.

Dynamic polarity: It is present in the processes of neurons.

- Impulse flows towards soma in the Dendrites and away in the axons.
- In microneurons – which has no neurons, the impulse can flow in either direction through their dendrites.

SYNAPSE

Neurons form long chains along which impulses are conducted in different directions.

- Junction between neurons is called synapse.
- Contact is by contiguity and not by continuity.
- Impulse is transmitted by specific neuro-transmitters like – acetylcholine, catecholamine (nor-adrenaline and dopavarine), serotonin, histamine, glycine, and certain polypeptides).

TYPES OF SYNAPSE

1. Axo-dendritic
2. Somato-dendritic
3. Somato-somatic
4. Axo-axonic
5. Somato-axonic
6. Dendro-dendritic.

The synapse may be inhibitory or excitatory.

NEUROGLIA

Neuroglia are non-excitable supporting cells in nervous system. These are:

(a) **Neuroglial cells:** These are found in parenchyma of brain and spinal cord.

(b) **Ependymal cells:** These line the internal cavities.

(c) **Capsular or satellite cells:** These surround nerves of sensory and autonomic ganglia.

(d) **Schwann cells:** From sheaths for axons of peripheral nerves.

(e) **Supporting cells:** Several types and these ensheath motor and sensory nerve terminals.

Nuroglial Cells

They are of two types:

(a) **Macroglia:** These are ectodermal in origin and are star shaped astrocytes, (fewer in number) oligodendrocytes and glioblasts (stem cells).

(b) Microglia: Mesodermal in origin and are much smaller but more numerous than neurons.

These are phagocytic in nature and are derived from circulating monocytes.

Functions of Glial and Ependymal Cells

1. Provide mechanical support to nervous tissue.
2. Act as insulator between nerves and prevents spreading of impulses in unwanted directions.
3. Phagocytosis – remove cell debris and foreign body.
4. Can repair damaged areas of nervous tissue.
5. Stores neurotransmitters.
6. Maintains a suitable metabolic and ionic environment for neurons.
7. Oligodendrocytes – These are myelinated tracts.
8. Ependymal cells – Help in exchange of materials between brain and C.S.F.
9. Glial cells provide nutrition to nerve cells.

BLOOD BRAIN BARRIER

- Barrier exists at the capillary level between blood and nerve cells and is formed by:
  - (a) Capillary endothelium without fenestration.
  - (b) Basement membrane of endothelium.
  - (c) End feet of astrocytes covering the capillary walls.
- Barrier permits a selective passage of blood contents to the nervous tissue.

REFLEX ARC

Is the basic functional unit of nervous system. This is made up of:

- (a) Receptor, e.g., skin.
- (b) A sensory or afferent neuron.
- (c) A motor or efferent neuron.
- (d) An effector, e.g., muscle.

Nerves are solid white cords.

- Nerve fibre is an axon with its coverings.
- Fibres are supported and bound together by connective tissue sheaths at different levels.
- Whole trunk is ensheathed by Epineurium.
- Each fasciculus is covered by Perineurium.
- Each nerve fibre is covered by a delicate Endoneurium.
- Toughness of the nerve is due to its fibrous sheaths.

Spinal Nerves: These are 31 pairs of spinal nerves. These are as follows:

- Cervical – 8
- Thoracic – 12
- Lumbar – 5
- Sacral – 5
- Coccygeal – 1

Dermatome: It is the area of skin supplied by a single segment of spinal cord.

Formation, course and branches of a typical spinal nerve.

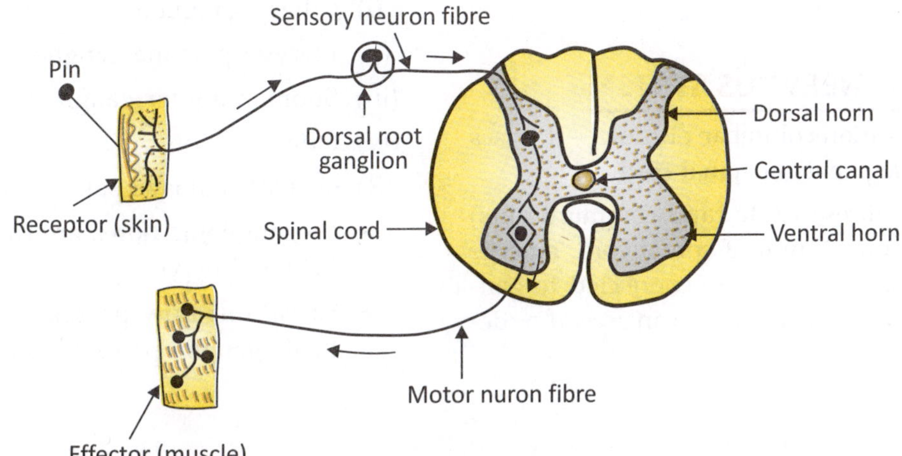

Fig. 5.4: *Components of reflex arc (Arrows indicate the direction of conduction of the impulse)*

Blood and Nerve Supply of Peripheral Nerves:

- Supplied by vessels – called vasa – nervosum.
- Supplied by nerves – called nervi nervorum.

Functional components of a spinal nerve – are three

1. **Somatic component:**
   - Somatic efferents innervate skeletal muscle.
   - Somatic afferents – convey impulses to *CNS* from skin, fascia, muscle and joints etc.
2. **Visceral component:** Constitutes autonomic nervous system
   - Efferents, sympathetic and parasympathetic.
   - Afferents, innervate, viscera and glands.
3. **Meningeal branch:** Receives grey rami communicantis and supplies duramater of spinal cord.

I. AUTONOMIC NERVOUS SYSTEM (ANS)

A.N.S. is divided into two parts:

1. Sympathetic
2. Parasympathetic
   - It controls involuntary activities of body like – Sweating, salivation, peristalsis etc.
   - It differs from CNS in having:
     (a) Preganglionic fibres arising from CNS.
     (b) Ganglia for relay of preganglionic fibres.
     (c) Post-ganglionic fibres arising from ganglia to supply effectors – smooth muscles and glands.

II. SYMPATHETIC NERVOUS SYSTEM

1. Also known as thoracolumbar outflow – it arises from T_1 to L_2 segments of spinal cord.
2. Preganglionic fibres (white rami communicants) arise from lateral column of spinal cord, emerge through ventral rami and are connected to ganglia of sympathetic chain. Fibres can ascend or descend down.
3. Post-ganglionic fibres (grey rami) run for some distance and supply the organ.
4. These are total of 22-23 sympathetic ganglia in each sympathetic chain. When T_1 ganglion does not fuse with lower cervical sympathetic ganglion – there will be 23 sympathetic ganglion. When T_1 fuses with lower cervical ganglion it becomes 22 in number. Subsidiary ganglia are also present, e.g., celiac, mesenteric etc.
5. Ganglia lie on sympathetic trunk (mostly).

   Structure of sympathetic ganglia: Consists of

   (a) Outer connective tissue capsule – contains fibres, fibroblasts, blood capillaries and satellite cells.

   (b) Ganglion cells – multipolar neurons.

III. PARASYMPATHETIC NERVOUS SYSTEM (PNS)

- Also known as cranio-sacral outflow.
- Preganglionic fibres are carried by – III, VII, IX, X cranial nerves.

  Cranial Part: Parasympathetic nuclei are present in brain are:

  1. Edinger-Westphal nucleus
  2. Superior salivatory nucleus
  3. Inferier salivatory nucleus
  4. Dorsal nucleus of vagus (X).
- **Cranial out flow passes through four small para sympathetic ganglia:**

  (i) Ciliary ganglion
  (ii) Pterygo palatine ganglion
  (iii) Submandibular ganglion
  (iv) Otic ganglion.

  Sacral Part (Parasympathetic system)

  - Preganglionic fibres are carried by S_2, S_3 and S_4 spinal nerves.
  - Sacral out flow passes through parasympathetic ganglia present near organs.

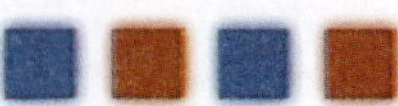

CHAPTER 6

Cardiovascular System

INTRODUCTION

- It is the transport system of the body, through which nutrients are conveyed to the tissues for utilization and metabolites (waste products) are conveyed to appropriate places for excretion.
- Conveying medium is liquid – blood flows in blood vessels
- Central pumping organ, i.e., heart maintains circulation of blood into tissues.

COMPONENTS OF CARDIOVASCULAR SYSTEM

Cardiovascular System Components are:

1. **Heart:** Is a four chambered muscular organ which pumps blood into tissues of body.
   - Receiving chamber is atrium.
   - Pumping chamber is ventricle.
2. **Arteries:** Distributing channels
   - Carry blood away from heart.
   - Branch-like trees in the course.
   - Large arteries rich in elastic tissue.
   - Medium arteries rich in muscular tissue.
   - Arterioles are minute branches visible to naked eyes.
3. **Veins** are draining channels
   - These bring back blood to heart from tissues.
   - Like rivers – veins are formed by tributaries.
   - Venules – are small veins – join and form larger veins.

Capillaries are network of microscopic vessels:

- Connects arterioles with venules
- Causes free exchange of nutrients and metabolites across their walls between blood and tissue fluid.

Capillaries are replaced by sinusoids in certain organ, e.g., liver, spleen, uterus etc.

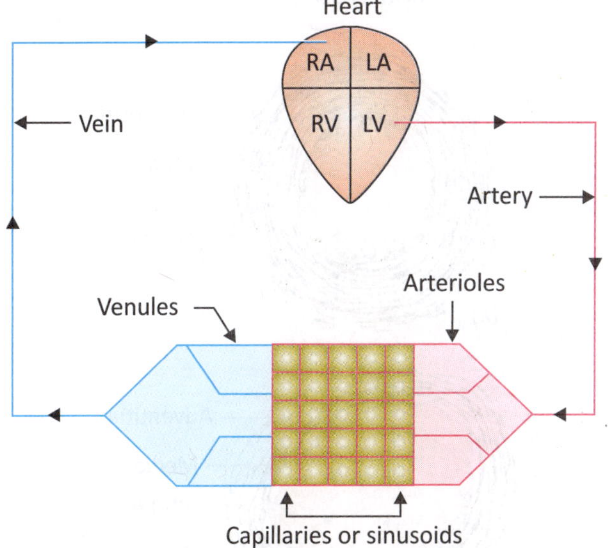

Fig. 6.1: *Components of Cardiovascular System*

FUNCTIONAL CLASSIFICATION OF BLOOD VESSELS

Functional Classification of Blood Vessels are:

(a) **Distributing vessels** are large arteries, e.g., aorta and its branches.

(b) **Resistance vessels** are arterioles with muscular wall and precapillary sphincter. These controls flow of blood into tissues.

(c) **Exchange vessels** are capillaries, sinusoids and post capillary venules.

(d) **Capacitance vessels or (reservoir):** Large venules and veins – convey blood back to heart.

(e) **Shunts:** Including various types of anastomoses.

STRUCTURE OF BLOOD VESSELS

Three coats are present in all blood vessels except capillaries and sinusoids.

1. **Tunica intima:** This is inner most layer made-up of endothelium supported by fibrous connective tissue.
2. **Tunica media:** It consists of smooth muscle – fibres and extends from internal elastic lamina to external elastic lamina. Thickness – depends on type and function of vessel.
3. **Tunica adventitia:** Outer most layer made-up of fibrous connective tissue contains nerve and blood supply for blood vessel.

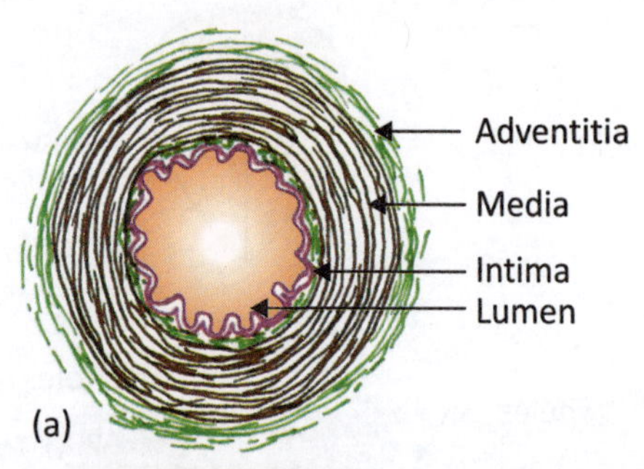

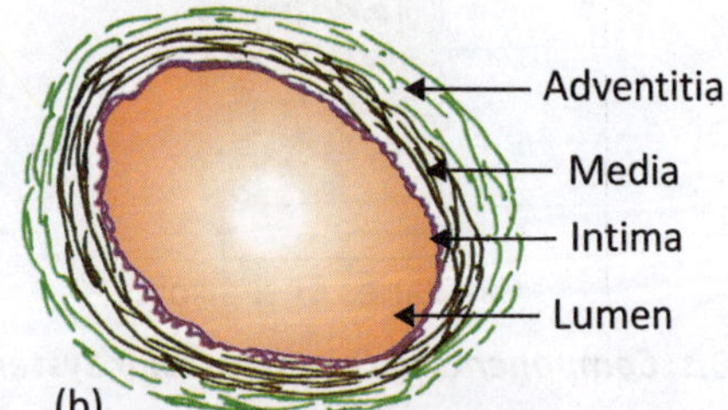

Fig. 6.2: ***(a) Transverse section of artery, (b) Transverse section of vein***

Capillary Structure (*Capillus = hair*)

- Microscopic endothelial tubes without smooth muscle cell – single layer of endothelial cells.
- Basal lamina of glycoprotein which surrounds endothelial cells and splits at places and encloses pericytes.
- Pericapillary layer of connective tissue cells and fibres.
- Average diameter is 6 to 8 microns – just sufficient to permit R.B.C. to pass through it in 'single file'.
- Size varies from organ to organ, largest – 20 microns in skin and bone marrow.

Blood supply of blood vessels is by vasa vasorum which forms dense capillary network in tunica adventitia and supply outer part of tunica media and adventitia.

Intima and inner part of media is nourished directly by diffusion from luminal blood.

- Minute veins accompany arteries and drain the blood from outer part of vessel.
- Lymphatics are also present in adventitia.

NERVE SUPPLY OF BLOOD VESSELS

- Nerve accompany arteries and are called nervivascularis.
- Sympathetic fibres are vasoconstrictor in function.
- Few sensory fibres are present in outer and inner coats of vessels.

Sinusoids: Replace capillaries in certain organs like liver, spleen, bone marrow etc.

Characteristics: Sinusoids are large, irregular, vascular spaces, closely surrounded by parenchyma of the organ.

- Walls are thinner and may be incomplete, lined by endothelium in which phagocytic cells (R.E.C.) are often distributed.
- Adventitia is absent.
- Basal lamina is replaced by thin layer of reticular fibres.
- May connect arteries with venules in spleen, bone marrow or venule with venule (liver).

Anastomoses: A pre-capillary or post-capillary communication between the neighbouring vessels is called anastomosis.

Circulation through anastomosis is called collateral circulation.

Types:

(a) Arterial anastomosis – communication between branches of arteries.

(b) Venous anastomosis – communication between veins.

(c) Arterio venous anastomosis (shunt) communication between artery and vein.

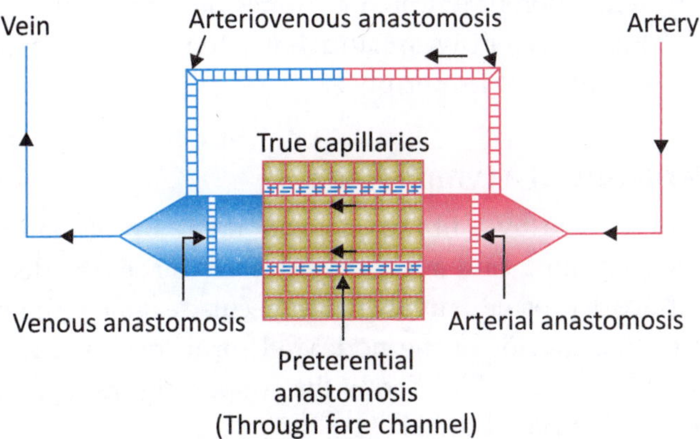

Fig. 6.3: *Different types of anastomoses*

END ARTERIES

Arteries which do not anastomose with other arteries are called end arteries, e.g., central artery of retina, central branches of cerebral arteries.

Applied Importance

Occlusion of an end artery causes sudden serious nutritional disturbances resulting in death of tissue supplied by it, e.g., occlusion of central artery of retina – results in permanent blindness.

Types of Circulation of Blood:

A. **Systemic circulation (greater)**: Blood flows from left ventricle, through various parts of the body – to the right atrium, i.e., from left to right side of heart.

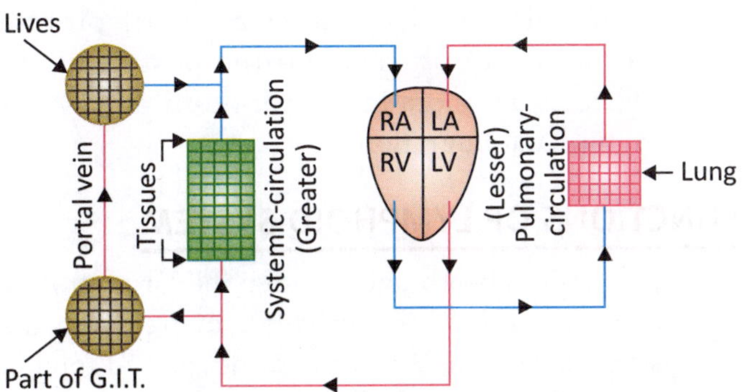

Fig. 6.4: *Types of blood circulation*

B. **Pulmonary circulation:** Blood flows from right ventricle, through the lungs, to the left atrium, i.e., from right to the left side of heart.

C. **Portal circulation:** It is a part of systemic circulation, characteristics of it:

   (i) Blood passes through two sets of capillaries before draining into a systemic vein.

   (ii) Vein draining first set of capillary network is known as portal vein – it branches like an artery to form second set of capillaries or sinusoids.

COMPONENTS OF CARDIO VASCULAR SYSTEM (CVS)

Applied Importance

Normal BP – 120/80 mm Hg ± 10.

1. **Pulse pressure:** Difference between systolic and diastolic pressure is pulse pressure.
2. **Haemorrhage**
   - Bleeding – from rupture of blood vessels.
   - Venous – or arterial haemorrhage.
3. **Vascular catastrophies**
   - Thrombosis
   - Embolism
   - Haemorrhage.
4. **Arteriosclerosis** in old age – arteries become stiff.
5. **Arteritis and phlebitis:** Due to inflammation.

Applied Anatomy of CVS

Blood Pressure:

It is the arterial pressure exerted by blood on the arterial walls.

- Maximum pressure during ventricular systole is systolic pressure.
- Minimum pressure during ventricular diastole is diastolic pressure.
- Systolic pressure generated by force of contraction of heart.
- Diastolic pressure is due to peripheral resistance.

LYMPHATIC SYSTEM

Comprises

- Lymph vessels
- Lymph nodes
- Lymphocytes.

Relationship of lymph system to blood system

Lymph is a tissue fluid – 10-20% absorbed by lymphatics which begins blindly in the tissue spaces.

Lymph is filtered in lymph nodes and finally drains into venous blood.

Lymph is clear, colourless but lymph from small intestine is milky white – due to absorption of fat. Milky lymph is called Chyle.

LYMPH NODES

Lymph nodes are small nodules of lymphoid tissue present in the course of smaller lymphatics. Lymph passes through one or more lymph nodes before reaching the larger lymph trunks.

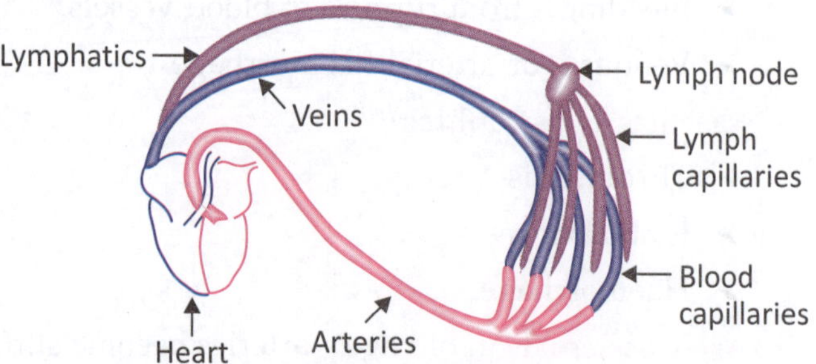

Fig. 6.5: ***Relationship of lymph system to the blood system***

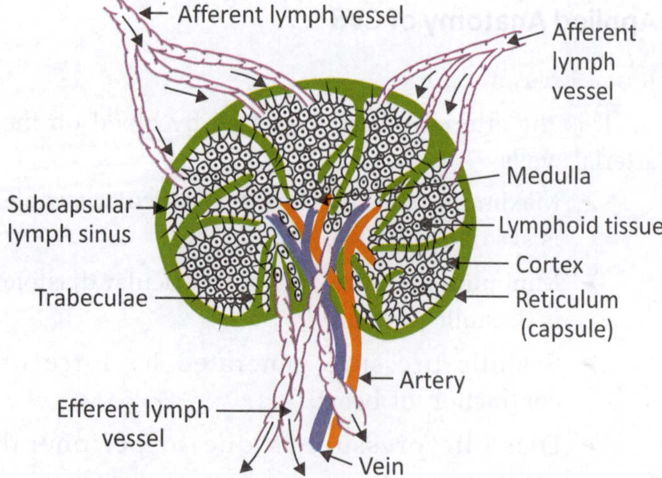

Fig. 6.6: ***Microscopic structure of a lymph node***

- Superficial nodes are arranged along the veins and the deep nodes along the arteries.
- Each lymph node has a slight depression on one side called hilum. Artery enters the node and vein with efferent lymphatics comes out of it, at the hilum. Afferent lymphatics enter the node at different parts of its periphery.

Structure of a Lymph Node

It is covered by a fibrous capsule made up of mainly collagen fibres and a few elastin fibres. From the deep surface of capsule a number of trabeculae extend radially into the interior of the node and form mesh work of reticulin fibres which forms the supporting framework for the lymphoid tissue.

The subcapsular sinus lies beneath the capsule and surrounds the node except at the hilum. Afferent lymphatics open into the sinus, which gives rise to numerous cortical sinuses running towards medulla, where they unite with each other and form larger medullary sinus, which join together to form the efferent lymphatics draining the lymph node. Sinuses are lined by endothelial cells.

- **Cortex:** It is the outer part of the node situated beneath the subcapsular sinus, being absent at hilum. It is made-up of lymphatic follicles and is traversed by fibrous trabeculae. Cortex is more densely cellular than the medulla.
- **Medulla:** It is the central part of the lymph node made-up of an interlacement of the trabeculae. The interstitial spaces contain loosely packed lymphocytes, plasma cells and macrophages.
- **Blood vessels:** The artery enters the hilum and divides into straight branches which run in the trabeculae. The capillaries are more profuse around the follicles and the post-capillary venules are more in the para-cortical zone for lymphatic migration.

FUNCTIONS OF LYMPHOID SYSTEM

1. Lymphatics absorb and remove the large protein molecules and other particulate matter from the tissue spaces. Thus, the cellular debris and foreign particles (dust particles inhaled into the lungs, bacteria and other micro-organisms) are conveyed to the regional lymph nodes. Lymphatics also help in transportation of fat from the gut.

2. Lymph nodes serve a number of functions:

(a) They act as filters for the lymph which percolates slowly through the intricate network of its spaces. Thus, the foreign particles are prevented from entering the blood stream.

(b) The foreign particles are engulfed by the macrophages in the sinuses.

(c) Antigens are also trapped by the phagocytes.

(d) Mature B-lymphocytes (plasma cells are capable of producing antibodies) and mature T-lymphocytes are produced in the node.

(e) Humoral antibodies are freely produced by the lymph nodes.

3. Production and maturation of B- and T-lymphocytes is the main function of lymphoid tissue.

Applied Anatomy

1. Lymphangitis and lymphadinitis.
2. Elephantiasis – due to filarial infection.
3. Lymphatics provide the most convenient route of spread of the cancer cells.

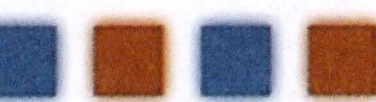

CHAPTER 7

Skeletal System

Skeleton is formed by

- Bones
- Cartilages
- Joints

BONES

- Osteon – G – Bones contains
- 1/3 – C.T. (Connective tissue)
- 2/3 – Calcium salts

  Total bones in the body = 206
- It forms structural framework of the body.
- It is bilaterally, symmetrical and divided into:

I. **Axial Skeleton:** This is formed by bones of head, vertebral column, ribs and sternum.

Skull – is made up of 22 + 6 bones

Vertebrae – Total 33 (26)

(Typically, an adult vertebral column consists of 26 vertebrae, when we include coccygeal and sacral vertebrae, the total numbers of vertebrae becomes 33.)

Ribs – 12 pairs

- Sternum and xiphoid process – 1
- Hyoid bone – 1

Total bones = 80

II. **Appendicular Skeleton:** Formed by bones of extremities:

- **Bones of upper limb:**
  - Clavicle – 2
  - Scapula – 2
  - Humerus – 2
  - Ulna – 2
  - Radius – 2
  - Carpels – 16
  - Meta carpels – 10
  - Phalanges – 28

  Total = 64
- **Bones of lower limb:**
  - Hip bone – 2
  - Femure – 2
  - Fibula – 2
  - Tibia – 2
  - Patella – 2
  - Tarsals – 14
  - Metatarsals – 10
  - Phalanges – 28

  Total = 62

Total bones = 64 + 62 = 126

Functions:

1. Bones give shape and support to the body and resist all forms of stress.
2. Provide surface for attachment of ligaments, muscles and tendons.
3. Serve as levers for muscular action.
4. Protect vital organs and manufacture blood cells.
5. Bones store 97% of body calcium and phosphorus.
6. Reticulo endothelial cells are – phagocytic and take part in immune responses of the body.
7. Large para nasal sinuses – affect the timber of voice.

CLASSIFICATIONS OF BONES

1. According to Ossification:

(a) Membranous bones, e.g., Bones of skull.

(b) Cartilaginous, e.g., Bones of limbs.

(c) Membrano – cartilaginous bone, e.g., Mandible, clavicle, occipital.

2. According to Position in the Body (Regional):

(a) *Axial bones* – skull, ribs, sternum, vertebrae.

(b) *Appendicular bones* – upper limb, lower limb bones.

3. According to Structure:

(a) Compact bone.

(b) Cancellous bone or spongy.

4. According to Shape:

(a) Long bones

(b) Short bones

(c) Flat bones – e.g., ribs.

(d) Irregular bones, e.g., Vertebra, hip bone, sphenoid and maxilla.

(e) Pneumatic bone, e.g., Maxilla, sphenoid and ethmoid.

(f) Sesamoid bone, e.g., Patella, pisiform, fabella.

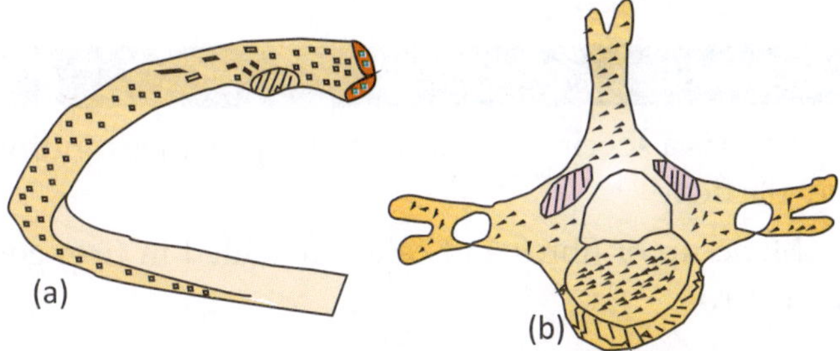

Fig. 7.1: *(a) Flat bone-rib, (b) Irregular bone vertebra*

Parts of a Long Bone are:

1. **Diaphysis:** The shaft of long bone ossifies by primary center.
2. **Epiphysis:** The ends of a long bones ossify by secondary centres.
3. **Epiphyseal plate of cartilage** is responsible for growth of long bones by proliferation of cells in it.
4. **Metaphysis:** Characteristic features are:

   (a) Most actively growing end of long bone.

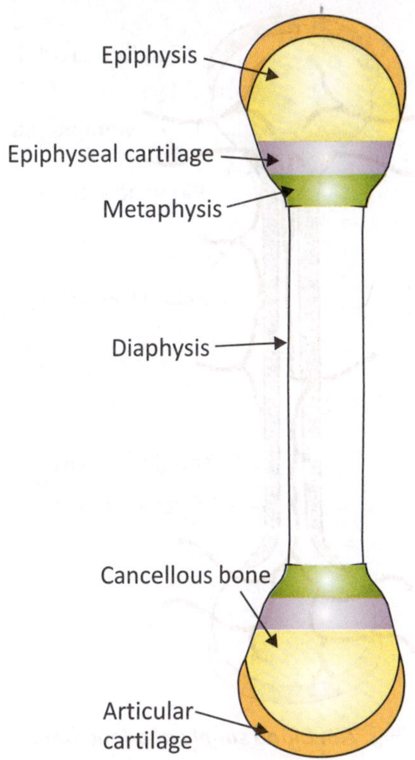

Fig. 7.2: *Parts of long bone*

   (b) Has rich blood supply, nutrient artery form pin like capillary loops in metaphysis – circulating microorganism, entangled at the curve.

   (c) Muscles, capsule and ligaments are attached close to it.

Growing End of a Long Bone

To the elbow I go, from the knee I flee – means in upper limb bones growing end of humers is upper end for ulna and radius growing end is lower end, while in lower limb growing end of femur is lower end and in tibia and fibula upper end is the growing end.

BLOOD SUPPLY OF BONES

1. Nutrient artery – supply inner 2/3 of cortex and bone marrow.
2. Metaphyseal artery.
3. Epiphyseal arteries.
4. Periosteal arteries – supplies outer 1/3 of cortex.
5. Nutrient artery – enters through volkman's canal.

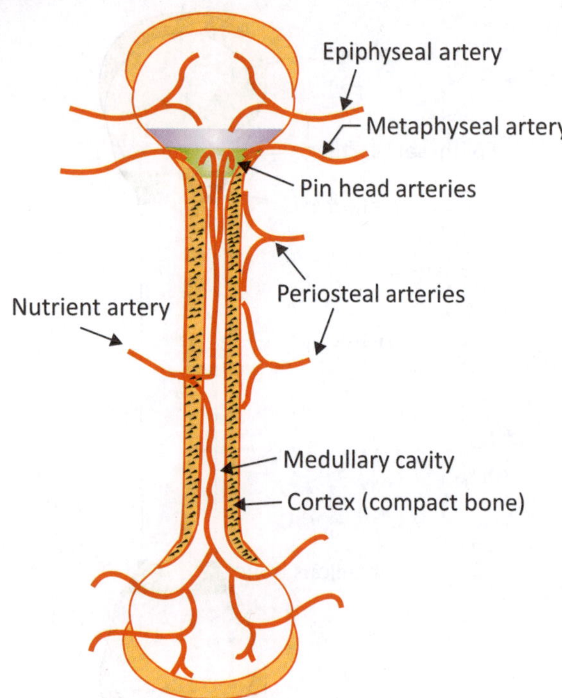

Fig. 7.3: *Blood supply of a long bone*

NERVE SUPPLY OF BONES

- Nerves accompany blood vessels and are sympathetic and vasomotor in function.
- Sensory supply is distributed to periosteum.

Ossification is of two types – membranous and cartilaginous.

Membranous ossification: Mesenchymal cells differentiate into osteoblasts alongwith network of collagen fibres and form membrane, e.g., bones of vault of skull.

Cartilaginous ossification: Cartilage dies and formation of bone occurs, e.g., long bones of limbs, vertebrae etc.

Composition of bone: It is made of 40% organic component in form of collagen fibres with osteoblasts, osteoclasts and osteocytes.

Inorganic components is 60% and comprises of calcium salts, phosphates, small amount of magnesium and sodium carbonate.

FACTORS AFFECTING BONE GROWTH

1. **Vitamin A:** Controls activity, distribution and co-ordination of osteoblasts and osteoclasts.
   - High concentration of Vitamin A – causes – resorption of bone.
   - Deficiency of Vitamin A – causes – slow destruction of bones.
2. **Vitamin C:** Helps in formation of intercellular matrix.
   - Deficiency of vitamic C leads to decreased production of trabeculae which causes separation of epiphysis.
3. **Vitamin D:** Is essential for absorption of calcium and phosphorus from intestine.
   - Deficiency – calcification of osteoid matrix is interfeared.
   - Causes – interfered which leads to osteomalacia and rickets.
4. **Hormonal:** Pituitary – growth hormone affects growth of bones.
   - Parathyroid – Parathormone – causes resorption of Ca^{++} from bones.
   - Thyrocalcitonin (Thyroid) – helps in deposition of Ca^{++}.
   - Sex hormones – cause early fusion of epiphysis.
5. **Mechanical factors:** Tensile forces help in bone formation. Compression forces – favour bone resorption. In paralysed or immobile limb – local osteoporosis occurs.

CARTILAGE

Cartilage is a specialized tissue which provides rigidity and elasticity.

Made-up of fibres and cells embedded in firm gel like matrix.

STRUCTURE

1. Cells – are chondroblasts and chondrocytes.
2. Intercelluar substance.
3. Fibres – are collagen and elastic fibres.

CHARACTERISTIC FEATURE OF CARTILAGE

1. It is avascular – it receives its nutrition through diffusion from nearest capillaries. These are no lymphatics here.
2. It has no nerves so it is insensitive.
3. It is surrounded by perichondrium.
4. It grows by interstitial method of growth.

5. When it calcifies – chondrocytes die – because they are deprived of nutrition by diffusion.
6. It has low antigenicity due to lack of lymphatics.

TYPES OF CARTILAGE

I. Hyaline Cartilage: Bluish, opalescent tissue:

- Widely distributed in body.
- Surrounded by dense irregular connective tissue layer, i.e., perichondrium – outer fibrous and inner cellular layers.
- Cells are arranged in groups of two or more (2-6) with straight outlines where they come in contact with one another.
- Matrix is homogenous, fibres are not visible as refrective index of fibres and matrix is same.

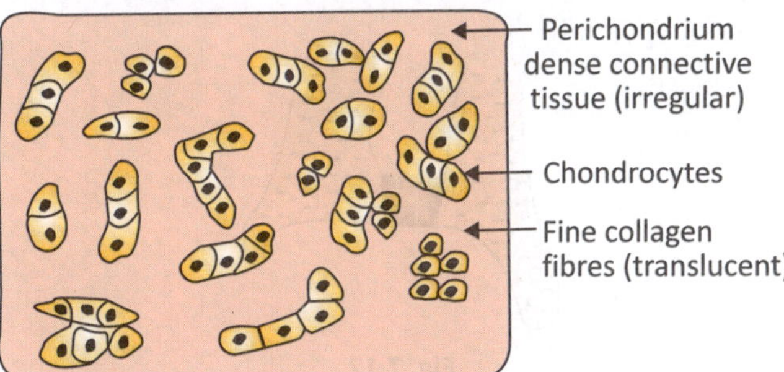

Fig. 7.4: ***Structure of hyaline cartridge***

Distribution of Hyaline Cartilage:

- Articular cartilage
- Thyroid cartilage
- Cricoid cartilage
- Tracheal rings
- Costal cartilages
- Bronchial and nasal cartilages
- Lower part of arytenoids, cartilage of larynx.

II. Elastic Cartilage:

- Matrix is traversed by yellow elastic fibres which anastomose and branch in all directions.
- Extra cellular matrix is metachromatic due to high concentration of glycosaminoglycons.
- Perichondrium is present.
- Cells are present singly or in groups of 2-3.

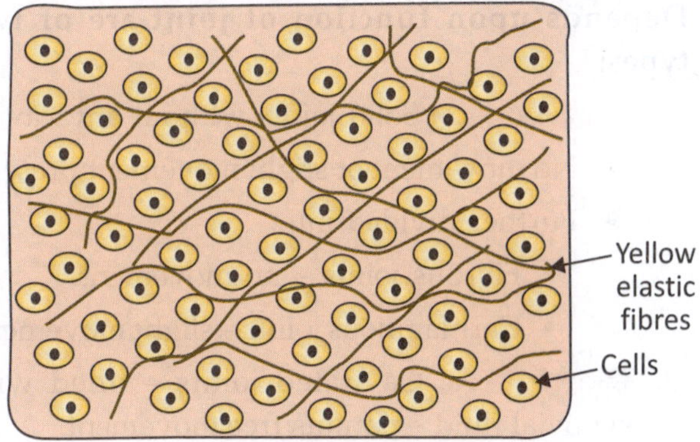

Fig. 7.5: ***Elastic cartilage***

Distribution: Pinna of external ear, auditory tube.

- Epiglottis, corniculate and cuniform cartilage, apex of arytenoids cartilage.
- External auditory meatus.

III. White Fibro Cartilage:

- Perichondrium is absent.
- Many regularly arranged collagen fibres, look like a tendon.
- Less cellular, chondrocytes are scattered sparsely all over.

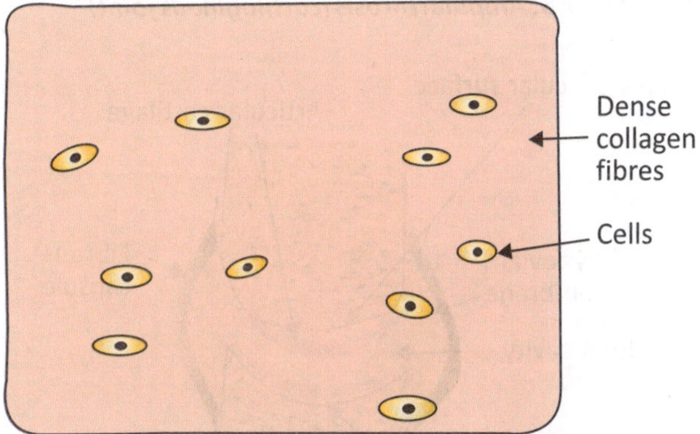

Fig. 7.6: ***Structure of fibro cartilage***

JOINTS

Junction between two or more bones.

- Responsible for movement.
- Growth or transmission of forces.

CLASSIFICATION OF JOINTS

A. Depends upon function of joint are of two types:

1. **Synarthroses:** Solid joints without any cavity.
   - No movement or slight movement present.
   - Further divided into:
     - Fibrous joints – no movement.
     - Cartilaginous joints – slight movement.
2. **Diarthroses:** Cavitated joints – filled with synovial fluid – permits free movement.

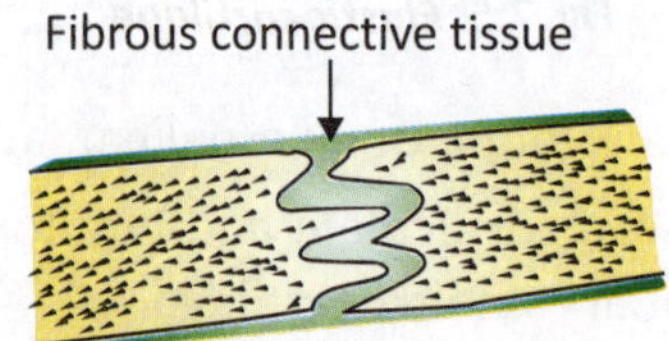

Fig. 7.7: *Synarthroses (fibrous joint)*

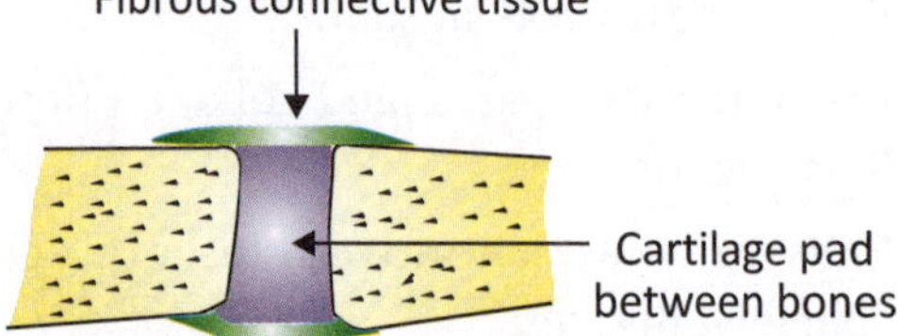

Fig. 7.8: *Amphiarthrosis (cartilaginous joint)*

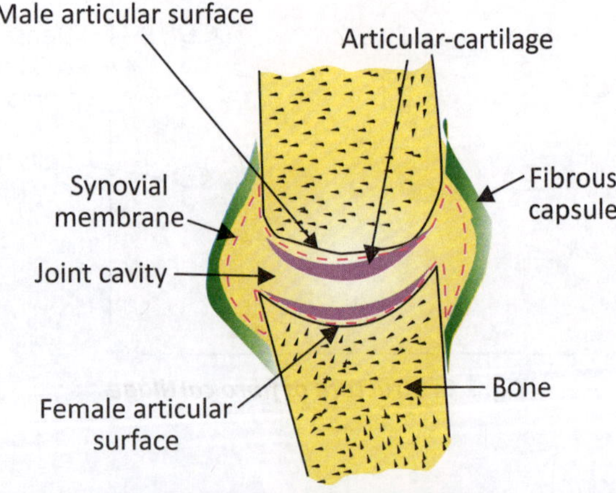

Fig. 7.9: *Diathroses (synovial joint)*

B. Structural classification:

1. **Fibrous joints:**
   (a) Sutures present in skull bones.
   (b) Syndesmosis – Inferior tibio fibular joint.
   (c) Gomphosis – Peg and socket joint.

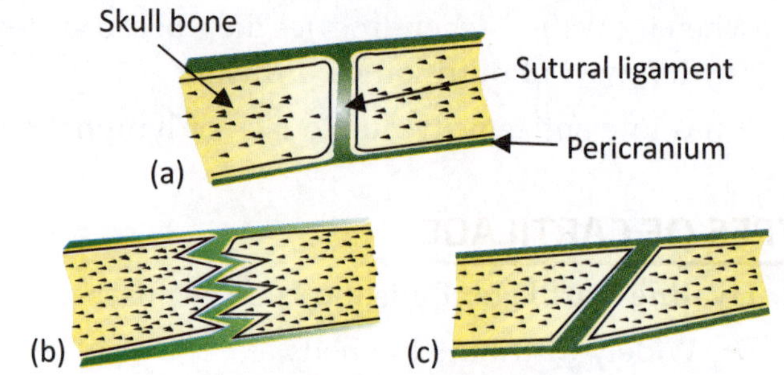

Fig. 7.10: *(a) Plane suture, (b) Serrate suture, (c) Squamous suture*

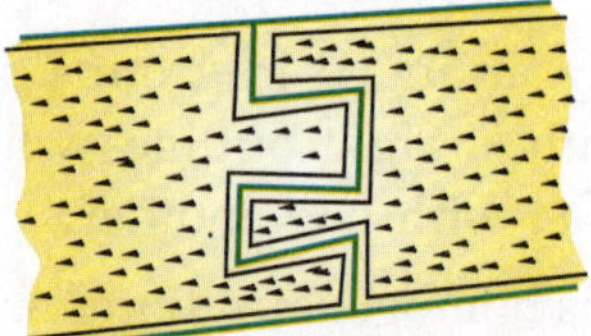

Fig. 7.11: *Denticulate suture*

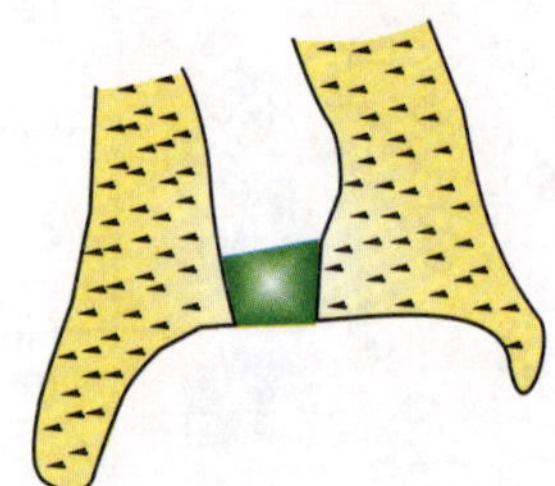

Fig. 7.12

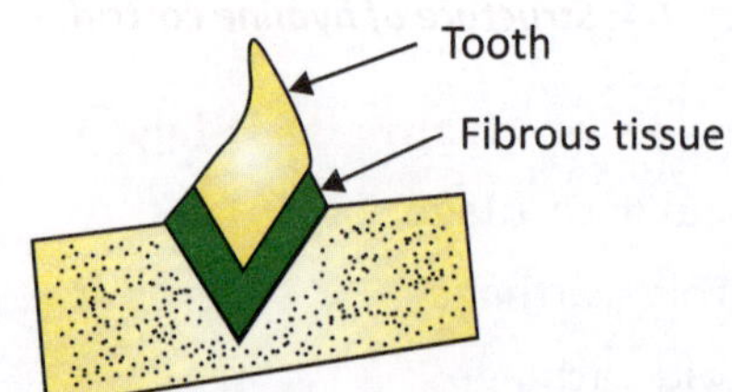

Fig. 7.13: *Gomphosis (peg and socket joint)*

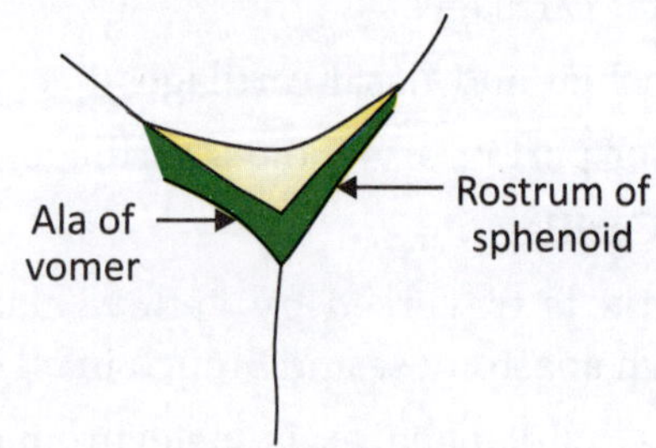

Fig. 7.14: *Schindylesis (wedge and groove suture)*

2. **Cartilaginous joints:**
   - Primary cartilaginous joint or synchondrosis.
   - Secondary cartilaginous joint or symphysis.

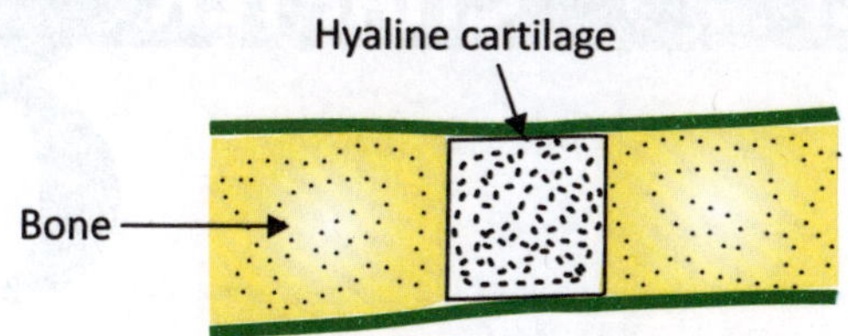

Fig. 7.15: *Synchondrosis (Primary cartilaginous joint)*

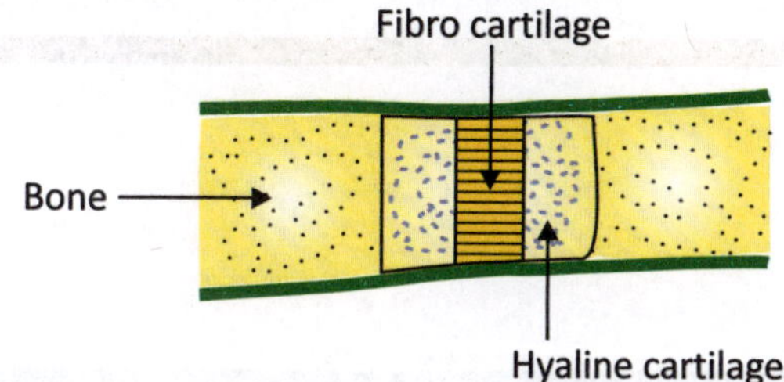

Fig. 7.16: *Symphysis (Secondary cartilaginous joint)*

3. **Synovial joints:**
   - (a) Ball and socket joint
   - (b) Saddle joint
   - (c) Condylar joint
   - (d) Ellipsoid joint
   - (e) Hinge joint
   - (f) Pivot joint
   - (g) Plane joint.

C. Regional Classification:

1. Skull type – immovable
2. Vertebral type – slightly movable
3. Limb type – freely movable.

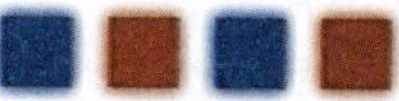

CHAPTER 8

Skin and Fasciae

Synonyms of skin are – cutis (L), derma (G) – integument.

Example: Cutaneous, dermatology, dermatomes etc.

DEFINITION

Skin is the general covering of the entire external surface of the body.

It is continuous with the mucous membrane at the orifices of the body.

SURFACE AREA

- In an adult total surface area of skin is 1.5 to 2 sq. meters.
- Area involved in cases of burns can be assessed by following:

RULE OF NINE

- Head and neck – 9%
- Each upper limb – 9%
- Front of the trunk – 18%
- Back of the trunk (including buttocks) – 18%
- Each lower limb – 18%
- Perineum – 1%

Dubois Formula: For calculation of skin surface area of a person.

Surface area in sq. cm = weight in kg × height in cm. × 71.84

$$A = W \times H \times 71.84$$

PIGMENTATION OF SKIN

Five pigments present at different levels and places of skin – which gives colour to it – are:

1. **Melanin:** Brown in colour and present in germinative zone of the epidermis.
2. **Melanoid:** Resembles melanin, present diffusely throughout the epidermis.
3. **Carotene:** Yellow to orange in colour, present in stratum corneum and fat cells of dermis and superficial fascia.
4. **Haemoglobin:** Purple.
5. **Oxyhaemoglobin:** Red, present in cutaneous vessels.
   - Pigment vary with race, age and part of body
   - Colour of skin depends on – pigments and vascularity of dermis
   - Thickness of keratin
   - Colour is red – where keratin is thin, e.g., lips
   - Colour is white – where keratin is thick, e.g., palms and soles

THICKNESS OF SKIN

Varies from about 0.5-3 mm.

STRUCTURE OF SKIN

Skin structure is composed of two layers:

- Epidermis and
- Dermis.

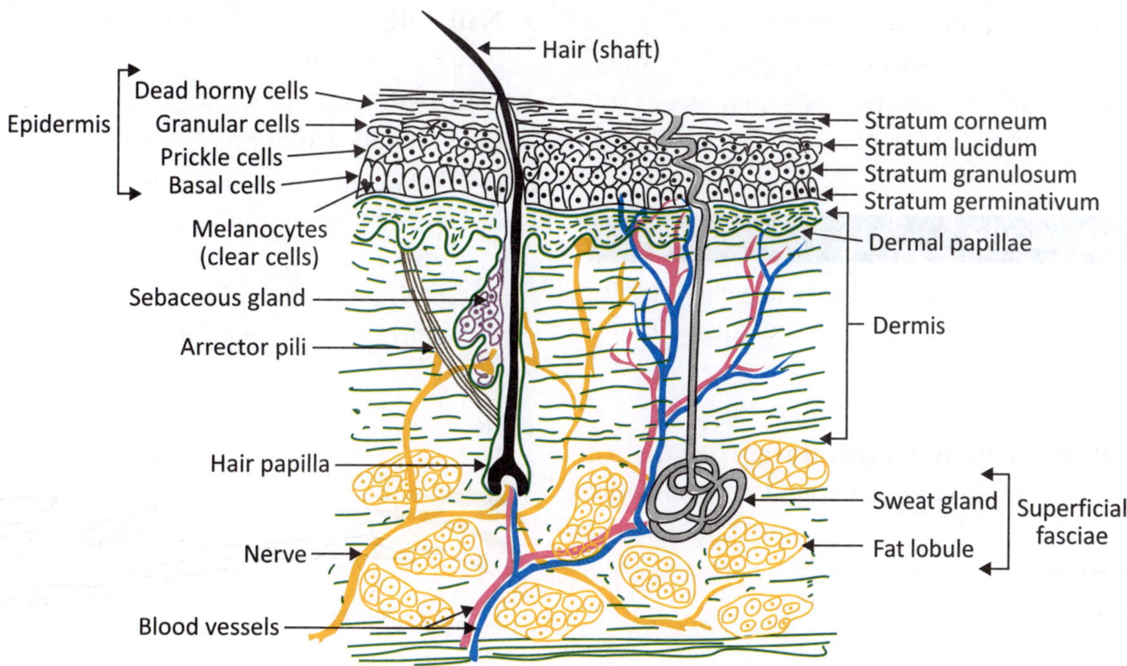

Fig. 8.1: ***Structure of skin (thick)***

I. Epidermis: It is superficial, avascular layer of stratified squamous keratinized epithelium.

- Ectodermal in origin.
- Gives rise to appendages of skin, e.g., hair, nails, sweat gland and sebaceous gland.

It has:

Superficial – cornified zone:

- Stratum corneum
- Stratum lucidum
- Stratum granulosum.

Deep – germinative zone:

- Stratum spinosum (polyhedral cells).
- Stratum basale (columnar cells).
- Cells of basal layer – proliferate and pass towards surface to replace cornified cells lost due to wear and tear.
- Basal cells also contains – melanocytes. These synthesis the pigment melanin.
- It synthesize – melanin.

II. Dermis: It is deep and vascular layer which is derived from mesoderm.

- This is made-up of connective tissue – with variable elastic fibres mixed with blood vessels, lymphatics and nerves.
- Connective tissue is arranged into a superficial papillary layer and deep reticular layer (white fibrous tissue in parallel bundles).
- Direction of bundles – constitute cleavage lines (Langer's line) longitudinal in limbs and horizontal on trunk and neck.
- In old age elastic fibres atrophy and skin becomes wrinkled.
- Over stretching of skin – leads to rupture of fibres and scar formation which form white streaks on skin. For example: Linea gravida.

SURFACE IRREGULARITIES OF THE SKIN

1. **Tension lines:** Form a network of linear – furrows – which divide the surface into polygonal areas.
   - Correspond to variations in the pattern of fibres in dermis.
2. **Flexure lines (skin creases or skin joints):** Skin folds during flexion – skin is thin and firmly bound to deep fascia, e.g., skin of soles, palms and digits.
3. **Papillary ridges** (Friction ridges)
   - Confined to palms, soles and their digits – form narrow ridges separated by fine parallel grooves arranged in curved arrays.

- They correspond to dermal papillae.
- Helps in finger prints recognition – loops, whorls and arch controlled – genetically by multifactorial inheritance.

FUNCTIONS OF SKIN

- **Protection** from mechanical injuries, bacterial infections, heat and cold, wet and drought, acid and alkali and rays of Sun.
- **Sensory** to touch, pain and temperature.
- **Regulation of body temperature:** Heat is lost through evaporation of sweat and conserved by fat and hair.
- **Absorption** of oily substances.
- **Secretion** of sweat and sebum.
- **Excretion** of excess of water, salts and waste products through sweat.
- **Regulation of pH** by excretion of acid in sweat.
- **Synthesis** of Vitamin D from ergosterol by action of ultraviolet rays of Sun.
- **Storage** of chlorides.
- **Reparative:** Cuts and wounds heals quickly.

SKIN APPENDAGES

Skin appendages are:

- Nails
- Hairs
- Sweat glands
- Sebaceous glands.

NAILS

Nails are hardened keratin plates on the dorsal surface of fingers.

Parts of Nail

- **Root:** is proximal hidden part, buried into nail groove and is overlapped by nail fold of skin.
- **Free border:** Distal free part of nail.
- **Body:** Exposed part of nail adherent to underlying skin. Proximal part of body has a white opaque crescent – called Lunule.
- **Nail wall:** Lateral border of nail body is overlapped by a fold of skin.
- **Nail bed:** germinative zone and corium beneath the root and body of nail is nail bed
  - Germinative zone beneath the root and lunule is thick and proliferative is responsible for growth of nail.
  - Rest of the nail bed is thin (sterile matrix) over which growing nail glides.

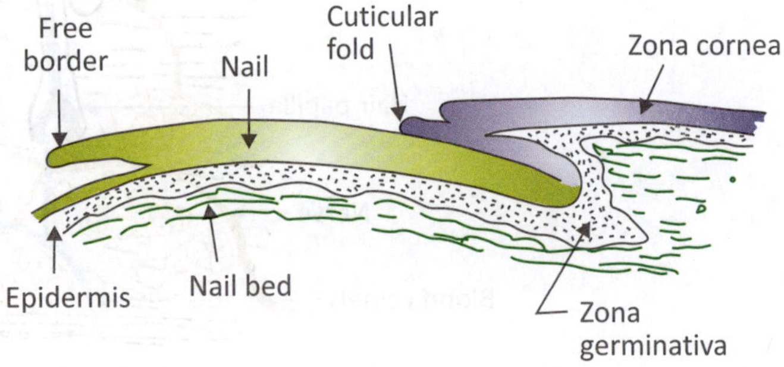

Fig. 8.2: ***L.S. nail***

Applied

1. **In anaemia:** Nails are pale, white thin, brittle and spoon shaped (Koilonychias).
2. **Clubbing:** Hypertrophy of nail bed occurs in chronic suppurative disease, e.g., lung abscess, osteomyelitis, bronchiectasis.
3. **Cyanosis:** Nails become blue due to lack of oxygen.
   - Average growth of nail is about 0.1 mm per day or 3 mm per month
   - Growth is faster in summer than winter
   - Growth is faster in fingers than toes.
   - Whole nail grows in 90-129 days.
4. **In fungal infections of nail:** Course of treatment should be for 3-4 months.

HAIR

Hair are keratinous filaments derived from invaginations of the germinative layer of epidermis into dermis.

- Help in conservation of body heat.
- Distributed all over the body except – palms, soles, dorsal surface of distal phalanges, umblicus etc.

➤ Length, thickness and colour of hair – vary in different, parts of body and in different individuals.

Parts of Hair

1. Root is implanted part
2. Shaft is projecting part.

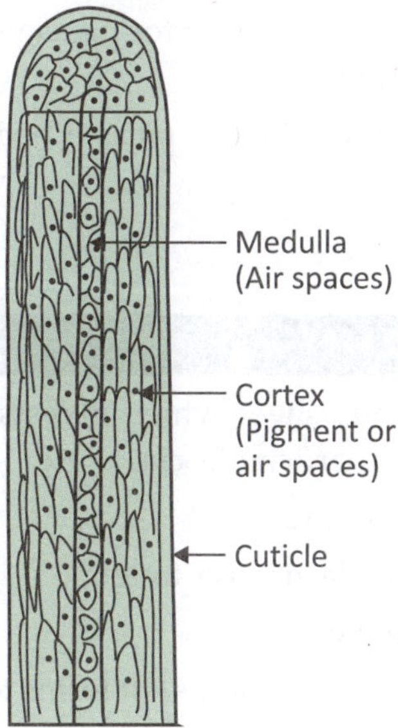

Fig. 8.3: *Parts of a hair*

Hair Follicle

It is formed by expanded proximal end of root which is invaginated by a tuft of neurovascular connective tissue and its sheath.

Hair grows by proliferation of cells capping the papilla.

Arrectores pilorum – smooth muscle fibres connect the hair follicles to dermal papilla. Contraction leads to erection of hair and squeezes out sebum.

Shaft of hair is made-up of medulla, cortex and cuticle.

SWEAT GLANDS (SUDORIFEROUS)

Sweat glands are distributed all over the body except – lips, glans penis, nail bed etc.

Types of Sweat Glands

1. Eccrine glands
2. Apocirne glands

1. **Eccrine Glands:** Abundant and present in every part of skin. It has a single tube (duct), deep part is coiled called body of the gland which lies in deeper part of skin or in subcutaneous tissue.
   - ➤ Produce – thin watery secretion.
   - ➤ Help in regulation of body temperature by evaporation of sweat.
   - ➤ Supplied by sympathetic nerves.
   - ➤ Excreting body salts.
2. **Apocrine Glands:** Confined to axilla, eyelids, nipple and areola of breast, perianal region and external genitalia.
   - ➤ Glands are larger and produce thicker secretion having a characteristic odour (chemical signals or pheromones).
   - ➤ On an average – 1 liter sweat is secreted per day.
   - ➤ Through lungs – 400 ml of water lost.
   - ➤ In faeces – 100 ml of water lost.
   - ➤ Total water loss per day from a person is about 1500 ml.
   - ➤ In summer – increase sweating – water loss 3-10 liters/day.
   - ➤ Regeneration of skin – occurs if sweat glands are intact.
   - ➤ Skin is dry in – dhatura poisoning, heat stroke, diabetics.
   - ➤ Sweating – in coma, shock, hypoglycaemic coma, M.I. (Myocardial Ischaemia)

SEBACEOUS GLANDS

Produce oily secretion widely distributed all over dermis of skin except – palms and soles, abundant – in scalp and face, around apertures of ear, nose, mouth and anus.

SUPERFICIAL FASCIA

Subcuteneous tissue or hypodermis or tela subcutanea or panniculus adiposus

- ➤ It is a general coating beneath the skin.
- ➤ Made up of loose areolar tissue with varying amount of fat (adipose tissue).

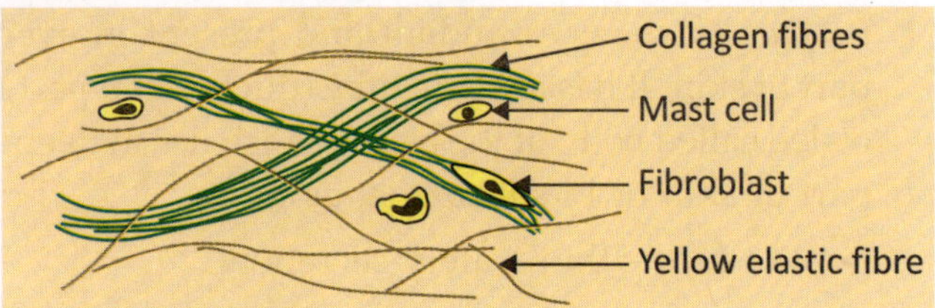

Fig. 8.4: *Areolar connective tissue*

Distribution of fat in this fascia:

1. Fat is abundant in gluteal region, lumbar region, anterior abdominal wall lower part, mammary gland etc.
2. In females – fat is more and evenly distributed.
3. Fat is absent in eyelids, external ear, penis and scrotum.
4. Subcutaneous layer of fat is called panniculus – adiposus.
5. Fat fills hollow spaces, e.g., orbits, axilla, ischio rectal fossa.
6. Fat is present around kidneys and supports it.

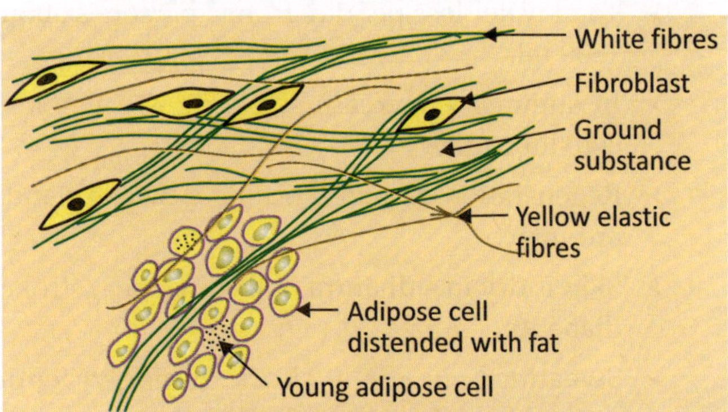

Fig. 8.5: *Connective tissue from dermis and subcutaneous layer*

Types of fat:

- Yellow – most of fat is yellow.
- Brown fat – found in hibernating animals.

Important Features:

1. Most distinct in lower part of anterior abdominal wall etc.
2. It is very thin on dorsal aspect of hand and feet, sides of neck and face etc.
3. Very dense in scalp, palms and soles.
4. It contains:
   (a) Muscles in face, neck and scrotum
   (b) Mammary gland
   (c) Lymph nodes
   (d) Cutaneous nerves and vessels
   (e) Sweat glands.

FUNCTIONS OF SUPERFICIAL FASCIA

- Facilitates movements of skin.
- It serves as soft medium for passage of vessels and nerves to skin.
- Conserves body heat – fat is a bad conductor of heat.

DEEP FASCIA

- It is a fibrous sheet which invests the body beneath the superficial fascia.
- It is devoid of fat.
- Usually – inelastic and tough.

Distributions:

1. Best defined in limbs – it forms tough and tight sleeves.
2. Ill defined on trunk and face.

Important Features:

1. Extensions of deep fascia form – intermuscular septa – divides the muscle into compartments.
2. Thickenings – form – retinacula – are retention bands around wrist and ankle joints.
   - Palmar and planter aponeurosis for protection.
3. Interruptions in deep fascia on subcutaneous bones.

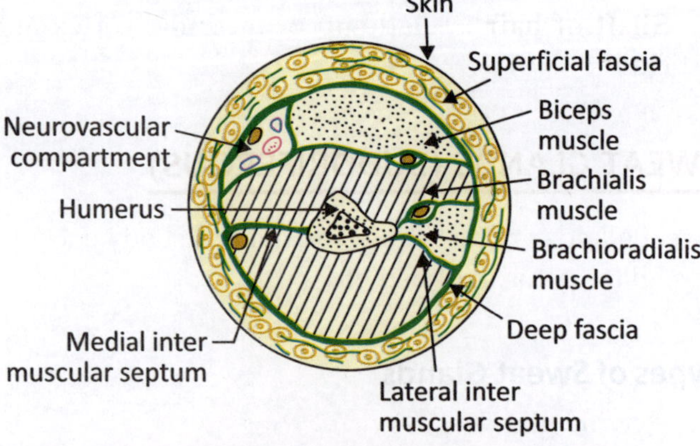

Fig. 8.6: *Cross-section of an arm showing arrangement of superficial and deep fascia*

4. Deep fascia forms sheaths around large arteries and veins, e.g., carotid sheath, axillary sheath etc.
5. Forms capsule, synovial membrane and bursae in relation to joints.
6. Forms tendon sheath and bursae where tendon cross over a joint – prevents wear and tear of tendon.

FUNCTIONS OF DEEP FASCIA

- It keeps underlying structures in position and preserves the surface contour of limbs.
- Provides extra surface for muscular attachment.
- Helps in venous and lymphatic return.
- Retinacula – acts as pully and prevent the loss of power.
- Assists muscles in their action by degree of tension and pressure it exerts upon their surfaces.

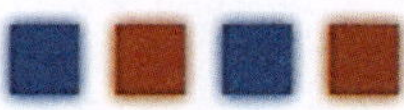

Review of General Anatomy

1. **Define lithotomy position?**

Ans.: Refer pg no. 6, chapter 1.

2. **Name the types of bones in the body?**

Ans.: Refer pg no. 29, chapter 7.

3. **What is anatomical position and its importance?**

Ans.: **Anatomical position:** Body is erect, the eyes, face forward and arms are kept by the side with palms facing forward. The legs are kept together with feet directed forwards.

Importance of anatomical position: All structures of our body are described in relation to this position, irrespective to anybody posture in space.

4. **Give examples of pneumatic bones.**

Ans.: Maxilla, sphenoid and ethmoid.

5. **Give examples of sesamoid bone?**

Ans.: Patella, pisiform, fabella.

6. **Enumerate different types of epithelium.**

Ans.: Refer pg no. 11-13, chapter 3.

7. **Where do you find simple squamous epithelium?**

Ans.: Refer pg no. 11, chapter 3.

8. **Enumerate the sites where simple cuboidal epithelium is present?**

Ans.: Refer pg no. 11, chapter 3.

9. **Enumerate the sites where simple columnar epithelium is present?**

Ans.: Refer pg no. 11, chapter 3.

10. **Enumerate the sites where stratified cuboidal epithelium is present?**

Ans.: Refer pg no. 12, chapter 3.

11. **Where do you find stratified columnar epithelium?**

Ans.: Refer pg no. 13, chapter 3.

12. **Where do you find transitional epithelium?**

Ans.: Refer pg no. 12, chapter 3.

13. **What is collateral circulation?**

Ans.: Refer pg no. 24, chapter 6.

14. **How many spinal nerves are there in the body?**

Ans.: Refer pg no. 19, chapter 5.

15. **Enumerate the different layers of epidermis of skin?**

Ans.: Refer pg no. 35, chapter 8.

16. **What is the largest round cell in the human body?**

Ans.: Ovum its size is 120-140 μ.

17. **Enumerate the endocrine glands in the body?**

Ans.: **Important endocrine glands in the body are:**

1. Pituitary gland (hypophysis-cerebri)
2. Pineal gland (epiphysis cerebri)
3. Thyroid glands
4. Parathyroid glands
5. Adrenals
6. Islets of Langerhans (pancreas)
7. Ovaries, in females
8. Testes, in males
9. Placenta, during pregnancy

18. Define anthropometry?

Ans.: It is the study of variations in the dimensions and bodily proportions of various bones in different races and of variations with age and sex in a single race.

19. What is a dermatome?

Ans.: Refer pg no. 21, chapter 5.

20. What are end arteries? Enumerate them?

Ans.: Refer pg no. 25, chapter 6.

21. Define neuron?

Ans.: Refer pg no. 19, chapter 5.

22. Explain Bones?

Ans.: Refer pg no. 28-30, chapter 7.

23. What are characteristic feature, different types of cartilage and their distribution?

Ans.: Refer pg no. 29-30, chapter 7.

24. Explain types and parts of muscle?

Ans.: Refer pg no. 15-16, chapter 4.

25. Explain classification of joints?

Ans.: Refer pg no. 32-33, chapter 7.

SELF ASSESSMENT QUESTIONS

1. What is anatomical position and its importance.
2. Define lithotomy position.
3. Enumerate different types of epithelium and where they are present.
4. Enumerate cells present in connective tissue along with their functions.
5. Define different types of bones present in body with examples.
6. Define different types of cartilages and their characteristic features and distribution.
7. Define characteristic features of different types of muscles.
8. Define different types of joints with their characteristics features.
9. What is neuron and its function.
10. Different types of cells found in nervous system and their functions.

PART 2

HEAD AND NECK

THE CHAPTERS ARE:

9. Skull
10. Scalp
11. Face
12. Bony Landmarks of the Back
13. Orbit and Eyeball
14. Neck
15. Subdivisions of Anterior Triangle of Neck
16. Parotid Gland
17. Submandibular Gland
18. Temporal and Infra Temporal Fossa
19. Temporo Mandibular Joint
20. The Pterygo Palatine Fossa
21. Teeth
22. The Palate
23. Tongue
24. Lymphatic Drainage of Head and Neck
25. Waldeyer's Ring
26. Nose and Para Nasal Air Sinuses
27. Pre-vertebral Region and Root of Neck
28. Carotid Arteries, Internal Jugular Vein and Cervical Sympathetic Trunk
29. Thyroid Gland
30. The Pharynx
31. Larynx
32. Trachea and Oesophagus
33. Ear
34. Cranial Cavity
35. Cranial Nerves

CHAPTER 9

Skull

SKULL

Forms the skeleton of head and includes the mandible. The skull without mandible is called cranium.

It has a large cranial cavity inside containing brain with its meninges, blood vessels and cranial nerves.

Skull is made-up of 22 bones + 6 ear ossicles and is divided into:

(a) **Neurocranium or calvaria:** Consists of 8 bones:
   (i) **Paired bones:** Parietal and temporal.
   (ii) **Unpaired bones:** Frontal, occipital, sphenoid and ethmoid.

(b) **Facial skeleton:** Consists of 14 bones:
   (i) **Paired bones:** Maxilla, zygomatic, nasal, lacrimal, palatine and inferior nasal concha.
   (ii) **Unpaired bones:** Mandible and vomer.

ANATOMICAL POSITION OF SKULL

1. Orbital cavities are directed forwards.
2. Lower margins of the orbits and upper margins of external acoustic meatuses should be in the same horizontal plane (Frankfurt's plane).

EXTERNAL FEATURES OF THE SKULL

It is studied in five different views:

1. Superior view or norma verticalis
2. Posterior view or norma occipitalis
3. Anterior view or norma frontalis
4. Lateral view or norma lateralis
5. Inferior view or norma basalis

NORMA VERTICALIS

Skull appears oval and wider posteriorly than anteriorly. Four bones participating in it's formation – frontal anteriorly, two parietals – one on each side and one occipital bone posteriorly.

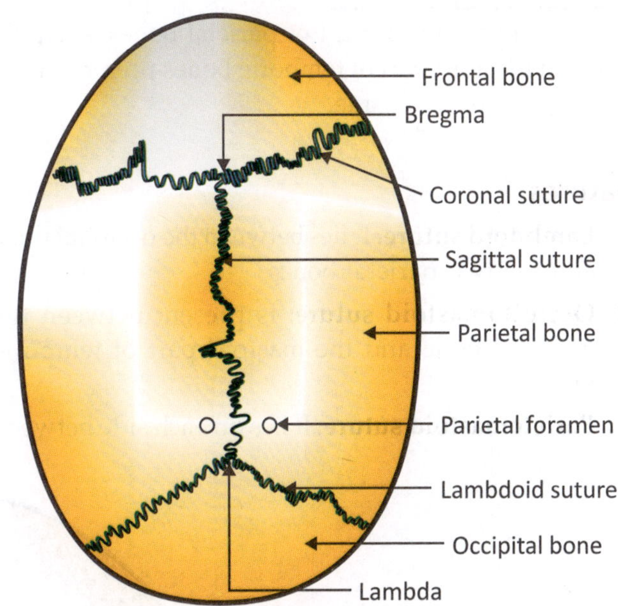

Fig. 9.1: *Norma verticalis*

These bones are united by three sutures:

(a) **Coronal suture:** Lies between the frontal and the two parietal bones.
(b) **Sagittal suture:** Lies between the two parietal bones.
(c) **Lambdoid suture:** Lies between the two parietal bones and occipital bone.

Metopic suture: This is present in 3 to 8% cases and is seen between the two halves of the frontal bones.

Other features are:

(a) **Bregma:** It is the point at which coronal and sagittal sutures meet.

(b) **Parietal eminence:** It is the area of maximum convexity of parietal bone.

(c) **Vertex:** It is the highest point of the skull and lies near the middle of the sagittal suture.

(d) **Parietal foramen:** A small foramen is present on each parietal bone near the sagittal suture about 3 cm in front of lambda.

(e) **Temporal lines:** Begin at the posterior border of zygomatic process of the frontal bone and arch backwards and upwards over the parietal bone and further divides into superior and inferior temporal lines. Superior line fades backwards but inferior continues downwards and forwards to become continuous with the supramastoid crest.

NORMA OCCIPITALIS

It consists of posterior part of parietal bones, occipital bone and mastoid part of temporal bones present infero laterally, one on each side.

Features

1. **Lambdoid suture:** It lies between the occipital bone and the two parietal bones.
2. **Occipitomastoid suture:** Is present between the occipital bone and the mastoid part of temporal bone.
3. **Parietomastoid suture:** It lies on each side between parietal bone and the mastoid part of temporal bone.
4. **Lambda:** Is the point at which sagittal and lambdoid sutures meet.
5. **External occipital protuberance:** It is the median bony projection, midway between the lambda and foramen magnum.
6. **Inion:** It is the most prominent point of external occipital protuberance.
7. **Superior nuchal lines:** These are curved bony ridges passing laterally on each side from external occipital protuberance.
8. **Highest nuchal lines:** In some cases a curved, faint bony ridge is seen 1 cm above the superior nuchal lines.
9. **External occipital crest:** It is a median vertical ridge passing downwards from the external occipital protuberance to the posterior margin of foramen magnum.
10. **Inferior nuchal lines:** These are curved bony ridges passing laterally on each side from the middle of external occipital crest.

NORMA FRONTALIS

It is the front view of skull – oval in shape, wider above and narrow below. Bones forming this view are:

1. **Frontal bone:** Forms forehead.
2. **Right and left nasal bones:** Forms bridge of nose.
3. **Right and left maxillae:** Form upper jaw.

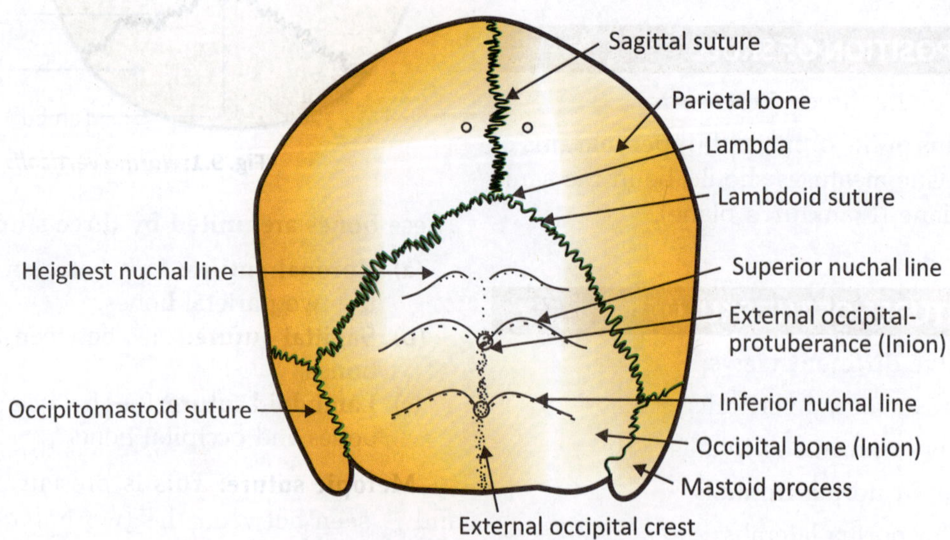

Fig. 9.2: ***Norma occipitalis***

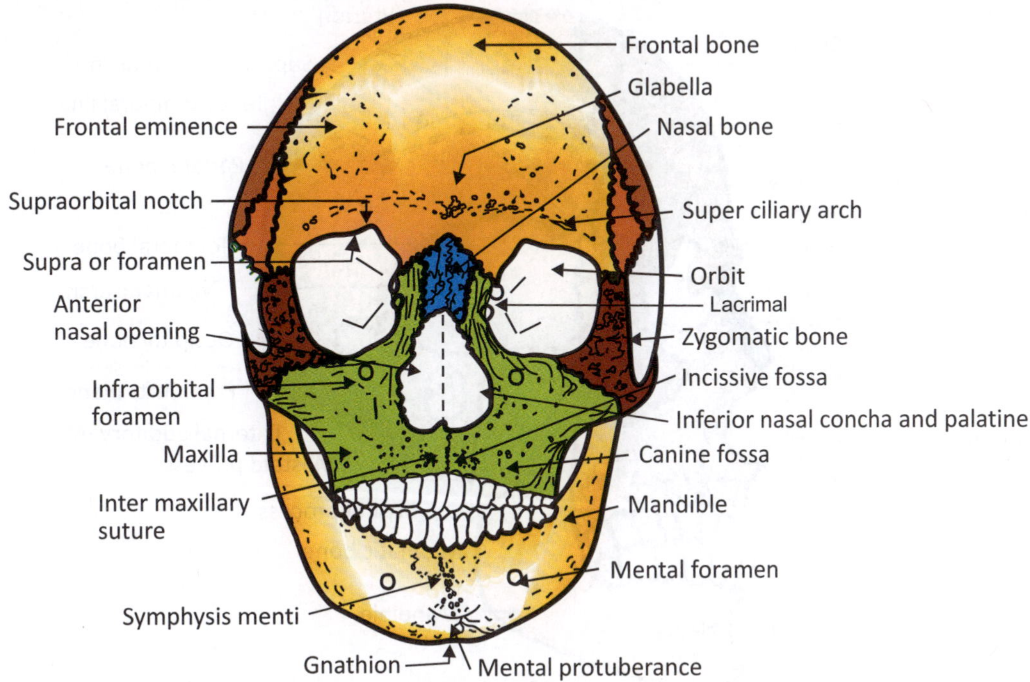

Fig. 9.3: ***Norma frontalis***

4. **Right and left zygomatic bones:** Form cheek prominences.
5. **Mandible:** Forms lower jaw.

Characteristic Features

Characteristic features are divided into:

A. In the median region:

1. **Glabella:** Is a median elevation between the super ciliary arches above the nasion.
2. **Nasion:** Is the meeting point of internasal and frontonasal sutures.
3. **Anterior nasal spine:** It is a sharp bony projection in the median plane below the anterior nasal aperture.
4. **Symphysis menti:** Is a median ridge joining the two halves of the mandible.
5. **Mental protuberance:** Lower end of symphysis menti ends in a triangular elevation called mental protuberance.
6. **Gnathion:** Is the middle point at the base of mandible.

B. In the lateral region: From above down-wards:

1. **Frontal prominence:** Is a rounded elevation above the super ciliary arch.
2. **Three foramen lying in same vertical plane:**
   (a) Supra orbital notch or foramen
   (b) Infra orbital foramen
   (c) Mental foramen.
3. **Oblique line on body of mandible:** Extending from below the lower end of anterior border of ramus of mandible to the mental tubercle.

NORMA LATERALIS

Lateral aspect of skull shows following features:

1. **Above:** Bones from anterior to posterior are nasal, frontal, parietal and occipital.
2. **In middle:** Bones are maxilla, zygomatic, sphenoid and temporal.
3. **Below:** Body and ramus of mandible.

Sutures: They are:

1. Coronal suture.
2. Parieto – squamosal suture – between parietal and squamous part of temporal bone.
3. Parieto mastoid suture – between parietal and mastoid part of temporal bone.
4. Occipitomastoid suture – between occipital and mastoid part of temporal bone.
5. Lambdoid suture.

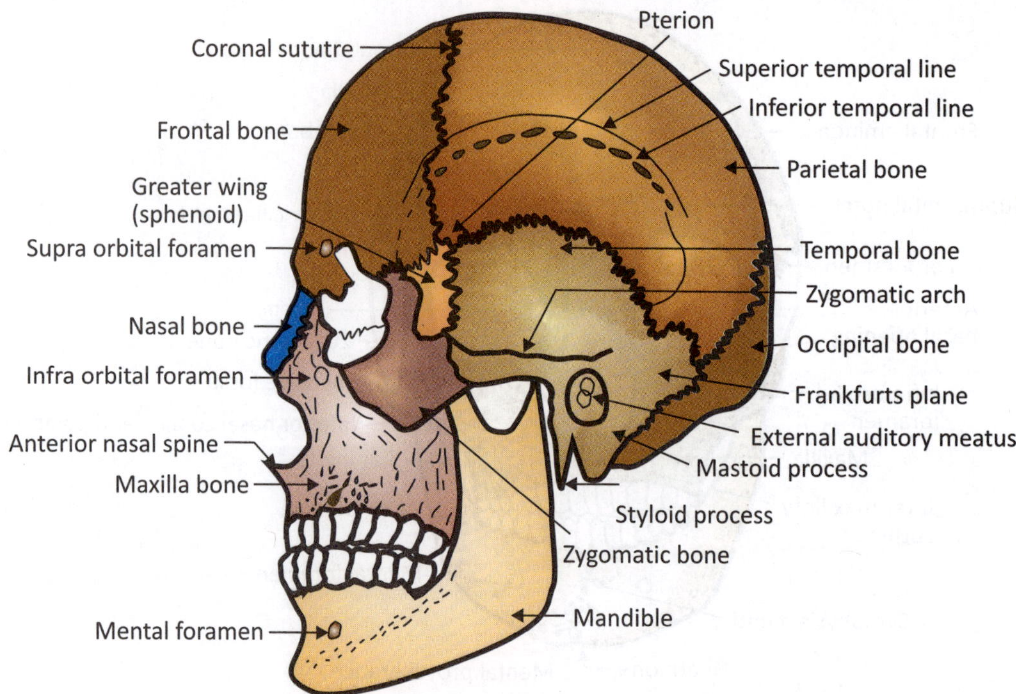

Fig. 9.4: ***Norma lateralis***

Characteristic Features

Characteristic features are:

1. **Temporal lines:** Superior and inferior temporal lines.
2. **Zygomatic arch:** Is formed by union of temporal process zygomatic bone and zygomatic process of temporal bone.
3. **External acoustic meatus:** Lies just below the posterior root of zygoma.
4. **Suprameatal triangle of Macewen:** Is a small triangular depression lies postero-superior to external auditory meatus, bounded by:
   - Superiorly – Supramastoid crest.
   - Anteriorly – Postero superior margin of external acoustic meatus.
   - Posteriorly – A vertical line passing through posterior margin of meatus.
   - Aditus-ad-antrum lies 12 mm deep to this triangle in adults.
5. **Mastoid process:** Behind the meatus part of temporal bone projecting downwards.
6. **Asterion** is the meeting point of parietomastoid, occipitomastoid and lambdoid sutures. In infant it is the site of postero lateral fontanelle.
7. **Styloid process:** A thin long bony process projecting downwards, medially and forwards from the temporal bone. Its base is ensheathed by the tympanic plate of temporal bone.
8. **Temporal fossa:** Is the depressed area bounded above by temporal line and below by zygomatic arch laterally and infratemporal crest of sphenoid medially.
9. **Pterion:** Lies in the anterior part of the temporal fossa, where four bones meet at an 'H' shaped suture – frontal, parietal, temporal and greater wing of sphenoid. It is situated 4 cm above the mid-point of the zygomatic arch. Internally it is related to middle meningeal vessels.
10. **Infra temporal fossa:** Lies on the side of the skull below the zygomatic arch, bounded by lateral pterygoid plate medially and by ramus of mandible laterally.

NORMA BASALIS

Inferior aspect of skull externally studied by dividing it into three parts – anterior, middle and posterior part.

1. **Anterior Part:** Formed by alveolar arch and hard palate. Features are:
   (a) **Alveolar arch:** Formed by maxilla, bears sockets for roots of upper teeth.

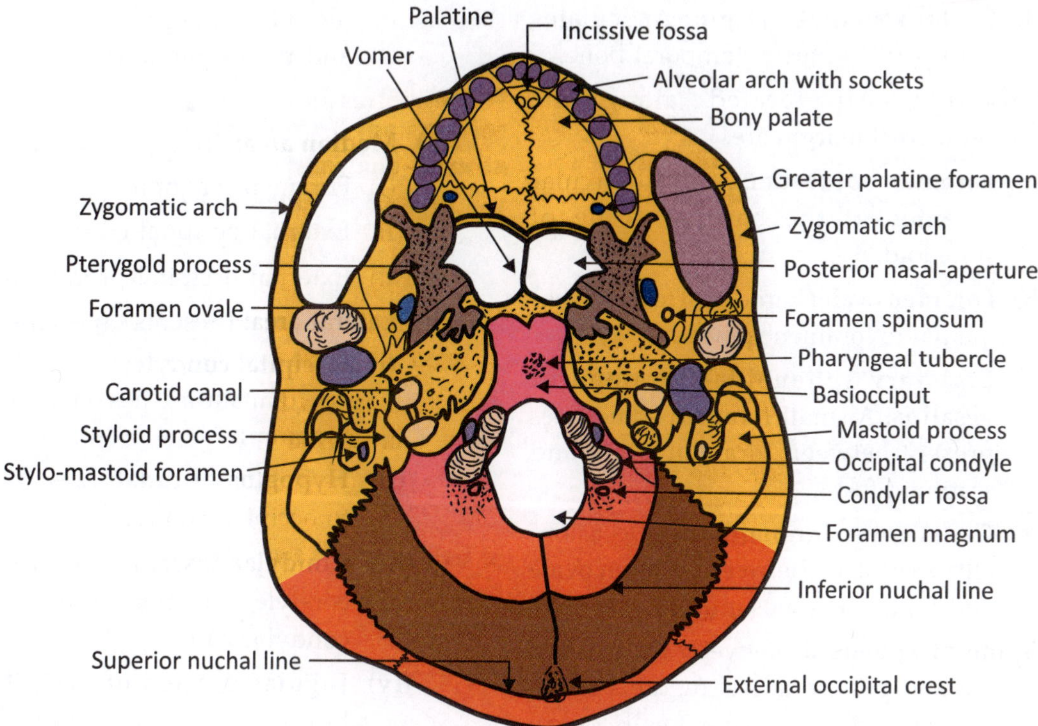

Fig. 9.5: *Norma basalis externa*

(b) Hard palate: Is formed by palatine process of maxilla – anterior 3/4th and by horizontal plates of palatine bones – posterior 1/4th. It has following features:

- **(i) Incissive fossa:** Present anteriorly in the median plane behind the incisor teeth. Two (right and left) incissive foramina pierce the wall of the fossa.
- **(ii) Greater palatine foramen:** One on each side, lies postero laterally, medial to last molar tooth.
- **(iii) Lesser palatine foramina:** Usually two in number lies behind the greater palatine foramen.
- **(iv) Posterior nasal spine:** A conical bony projection in the median plane on the sharp free posterior border of hard palate.

2. **Features in the Middle Part:** It lies behind the hard palate upto a line passing through the anterior margin of foramen magnum transversely.

(a) Median area presents:

- **(i) Posterior border of vomer** separating two posterior nasal apertures.
- **(ii) A broad bar of bone:** Formed by fusion of body of sphenoid and basilar part of occipital bone. In the centre of basiocciput a bony elevation is seen called pharyngeal tubercle.

(b) Lateral area presents:

- **(i) Pterygoid process:** Projecting downwards from sphenoid bone behind last molar tooth. It divides into medial and lateral pterygoid plates, separated by pterygoid fossa. Each plate has a posterior free border. Upper end of posterior border of medial pterygoid plate encloses a triangular boat shaped depression called scaphoid fossa, lower end bears a hook-like process called pterygoid hamulus.
- **(ii) Infra temporal surface of greater wing of sphenoid** lies lateral to pterygoid process and presents with four margins and four foramina.

Margins are:

- **(a) Anterior margin:** Forms posterior margin of inferior orbital fissure.
- **(b) Anterolateral margin:** Forms infratemporal crest.
- **(c) Posterolateral margin:** Articulates with the squamous part of temporal bone.

(d) **Postero medial margin:** Articulates with petrous part of temporal bone.

Foramina: All located along the posteromedial margin are:

(a) **Foramen spinosum:** A small circular foramen at the base of spine of sphenoid.

(b) **Foramen ovale:** Large oval foramen lies medial to foramen spinosum.

(c) **Emissary sphenoidal foramen of vesalius:** A small foramen sometimes present between foramen ovale and scaphoid fossa.

(d) **Canaliculus innominatus:** Occasionally present lies between foramen ovale and foramen spinosum.

(iii) **Spine of sphenoid:** Between the postero medial and postero lateral margins of the greater wing of sphenoid a small conical bony projection is present called spine of sphenoid. Two nerves are related to it – auriculo temporal nerve lies laterally and chorda tympani nerve lies medial to spine.

(iv) **Sulcus tubae** is a groove between postero lateral margin of greater wing and petrous temporal bone. It lodges cartilaginous part of the auditory tube.

(v) **Inferior surface of petrous temporal bone:** Is triangular in shape. The apex is directed medially and anteriorly, forms the posterior part of foramen lacerum on articulating with sphenoid. In this part opening of carotid canal is seen.

(vi) **Tympanic part of temporal bone:** It lies lateral to petrous part and joins with squamous part above at squamotympanic suture.

(vii) **Squamous part of temporal bone:** Mandibular fossa is present behind the anterior root of zygomatic process and the squamous part contributes to articular part of fossa.

(viii) **Tegmen tympani** is a thin plate of bone, arises from anterior surface of petrous temporal part – divide the squamotympanic suture into two parts – petrotympanic and petrosquamous.

3. Features in the Posterior Part:

(a) **Median area:** Presents from before backwards:

(i) Foramen magnum

(ii) External occipital crest

(iii) External occipital protuberance.

(b) **Lateral area:** Presents on each side:

(i) **Occipital condyle:** It is oval having convex articular surface lies on the side of foramen magnum.

(ii) **Hypoglossal canal:** Lies anterosuperiorly to occipital condyle.

(iii) **Condylar fossa:** Lies behind the occipital condyle, sometimes it has a canal – called condylar canal.

(iv) **Jugular process of occipital bone:** Lies lateral to occipital condyle and forms posterior boundary of jugular foramen.

(v) Squamous part of occipital bone.

(vi) **Jugular foramen:** It is a large elongated foramen at posterior end of petro occipital suture. Its anterior wall is hollowed out to form jugular fossa.

(vii) **Petrous temporal bone:** Shows tympanic canaliculus lies between jugular fossa and carotid canal.

(viii) **Styloid process:** Projecting downwards between petrous and tympanic part is the posterior aspect.

(ix) **Stylomastoid foramen:** Situated between styloid and mastoid process of temporal bone.

(x) **Mastoid process:** Projecting downwards laterally from temporal bone.

FUNCTIONS OF SKULL

1. It protects the brain and meninges.
2. Lodges eye, ear, nose and tongue (organs of special senses).
3. It lodges masticatory apparatus and upper digestive tracts.
4. Upper part of respiratory system is found within it.

Cranial Capacity: It gives an idea about the approximate volume of the brain.

- Average capacity in normal adult – 1350 – 1400 cc.
- In female 10% less than male.
- Microcephalic – capacity below – 1350 cc.
- Megacephalic – capactiy above – 1450 cc.
- The normal skull is mesocephalic.

NEONATAL SKULL

Neonatal skull has the following parts:

1. Vault
2. Face
3. Base.

The vault of the foetal skull is formed by a pair of frontal, a pair of parietal, occipital, a pair of temporal and greater wings of sphenoid bone. There are membrane filled areas in between these bones – called fontenelles. At the time of birth six fontenelles are present. The two frontal bones are separated by the metopic suture.

ANTERIOR FONTANELLE

It is lozenge shaped, situated at the junction of coronal and sagittal sutures. It is the junction of four bones – a pair of frontal and parietal bones. The pulsation of the cerebral arteries can be felt on the surface of the fontenelle.

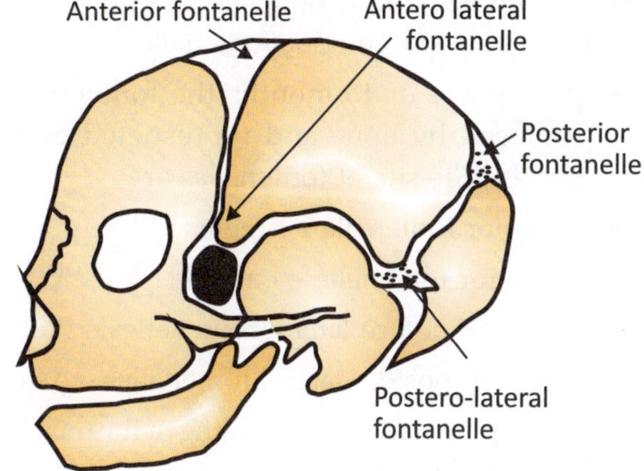

Fig. 9.6: *Fontanelles of skull*

Table 9.1: *Differences between Male and Female Skull*

Character	Male	Female
1. Size	Large and thick	Smaller and thin walled
2. Architecture	Rough	Smooth
3. Zygomatic arch	Well developed	Not well developed
4. Frontal eminence	Ill defined	Large
5. Parietal eminence	Ill defined	Large
6. External occipital protuberance	Well developed	Not very well developed protuberance
7. Glabella	Prominent	Less prominent
8. Forehead	Steep	Vertical and round
9. Orbit	Square smaller than female borders are rounded	Round and larger than male
10. Supra orbital ridge	Well developed	Less prominent
11. Mastoid process	Large and well developed	Small
12. Occipital condyle	Large and well developed	Small
13. Digastric groove	Very deep	Shallow
14. Nasal opening	Narrow and in a higher level	Broad and in a lower than female level than male
15. Palate	Large, broad and 'U' shaped	Small and somewhat parabolic
16. Teeth	Larger in size	Small

Clinical Importance

1. Vertex presentation of foetal head can be diagnosed during pregnancy.
2. Intra cranial pressure can be juged by palpating this fontenelle. Child is well nourished or not, can be diagnosed.
3. Age of the child can be determined – above or below two years.
4. Blood samples can be obtained from the superior sagittal sinus via anterior fontenelle.
   - By the age of 18 months the fontenelles are replaced by bone and represneted by bony points. The site of fontenelles are:
   - Anterior fontenelle – Bregma ⎤ Median Fontenelle
   - Posterior fontenelle – Lambda ⎦
   - A pair of antero lateral fontenelles – Pterion.
   - A pair of postero lateral fontenelles – Asterion.
   - The fontenelles help moulding of the foetal head during childbirth.
   - The mandible is bifid and united by fibrous tissue, angle of mandible is obtuse. The coronoid process extends to a higher level than condylar process.
   - The mastoid process is not devleoped at the time of birth but mastoid air sinus is well developed. Facial nerve is superficial and liable to be injured during forcep's delivery.
   - Styloid process is cartilagenous and zygomatic process is not articulating with the zygomatic bone.

MANDIBLE

- It is the bone of lower jaw, develops from mesoderm of first pharyngeal arch.
- It is the thickest and strongest bone of the face.
- It takes part in the formation of temporo mandibular joint.

Parts: It has two parts:

I. Body and

II. Ramus.

BODY OF THE MANDIBLE

Two halves of the body meets in the midline and form symphysis menti.

- Body has two surfaces – external and internal surface.
- **Two borders:**
  1. Alveolar border or superior border.
  2. Base or inferior border.

External Surface of Mandible

Shows following features:

1. **Mental foramen:** Lies in between upper and lower borders at the level of second premolar tooth, directed upwards and backwards. Mental nerve and vessels passes through this foramen.
   - In old age due to wear and tear of the alveolar – border, mental foramen moves upwards.
2. **Symphysis menti:** It is the line of fussion of two halves of the foetal mandible, seen as a faint ridge on the upper part of the body in the midline.
3. **Mental protuberance:** Lies below the symphysis menti, in the form of a triangular prominence, forms chin lateral to the protuberance an elevation called mental tubercle is present.
4. **External oblique line:** It extends from the mental tubercle, ill defined anteriorly and well defined posteriorly. It joins anterior border of ramus posteriorly.
5. **Incissive fossa:** It is a small depressed area below the incisor teeth.

Attachments on the External Surface of Body

1. Incissive fossa gives origin to mentalis muscle and deepest part of the orbicularis oris.
2. Oblique line gives origin to depressor labii inferioris, depressor anguli oris and buccinator muscle from anterior to posterior.
3. The lower border or base gives insertion to platysma and investing layer of deep fascia neck is attached to it.
4. Mental vessels and nerve are emerging out from the mental foramen onto the face.

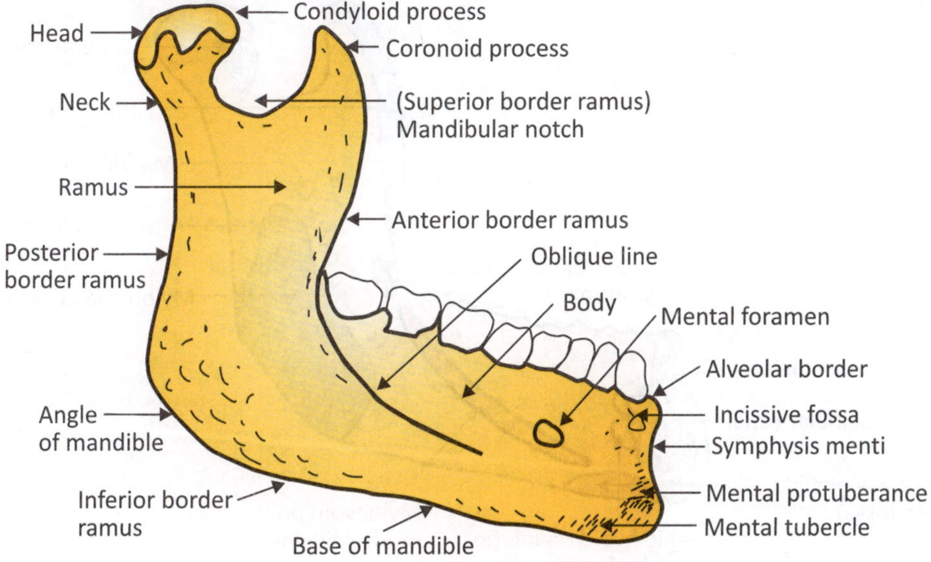

Fig. 9.7: ***External surface of mandible***

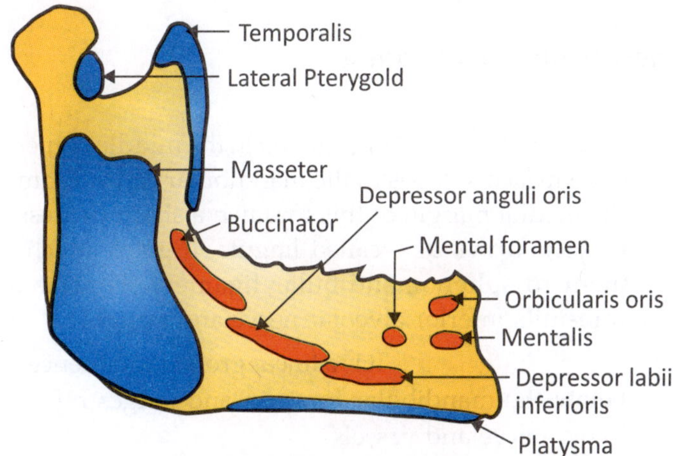

Fig. 9.8: ***Attachments of lateral view of mandible***

Internal Surface of Body of Mandible

Features are

1. **Genial tubercles:** A pair of tubercles are present in the midline of mandible internally. They are a pair of superior genial tubercles and a pair of inferior genial tubercles.
2. **Mylohyoid line:** Begins below the third molar tooth. It is oblique, runs forwards and faids away near the anterior end. It divides the inner surface into two areas. Upper one is the sublingual fossa and lower one is submandibular fossa.
3. **Mylohyoid groove:** It lies below the posterior end of mylohyoid line.

Characteristic Features

1. Superior genial tubercles give origin to genioglossus muscle.
2. Inferior genial tubercle gives origin to geniohyoid.
3. Submandibular fossa lodges submandibular salivary gland, submandibular lymph nodes and facial artery.
4. Mylohyoid line gives attachment to deep cervical fascia and mylohyoid muscles arises from it.
5. Sublingual fossa lodges – sublingual salivary gland.
6. Lingual nerve makes a groove just below the third molar tooth.
7. The pterygo mandibular raphe is attached behind the posterior end of mylohyoid line. It also gives origin to superior constrictor muscle of pharynx.
8. Mylohyoid groove lodges nerve and artery to mylohyoid muscle.
9. Alveolar border has sockets for the teeth of the lower jaw and lodging them.

Lower Border of the Mandible

It is thick and round, shows:

1. **Digastric fossa:** It is a shallow depression lies lateral to the midline. Anterior belly of digastric muscle originate from it.
2. Platysma inserted on the lower border and investing layer of deep cervical fascia is attached to it.

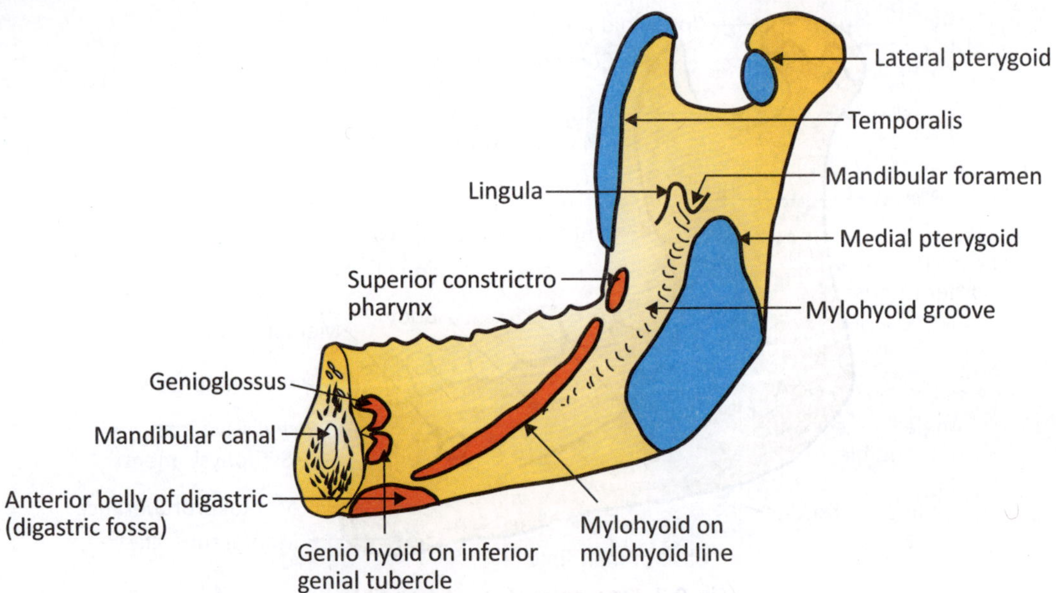

Fig. 9.9: *Attachments on medial aspect of mandible*

RAMUS OF THE MANDIBLE

It is quadrangular shaped, lies posteriorly. All muscles of mastication are attached to it. Ramus has four borders and two surfaces.

Borders are:

1. **Anterior border:** This is sharp and continuous with the anterior border of coronoid process. On this border temporalis muscle is inserted.
2. **Posterior border:** This is thicker, superiorly it is continued as condyloid process and inferiorly it forms the angle of mandible by joining with the inferior border. On this border stylomandibular ligament is attached, which is formed by the thickening in the deep cervical fascia.
3. **Superior border:** It is concave and sharp, forms mandibular notch. Through the notch masseteric nerve and vessels are passing. Coronoid and condyloid processes are projecting upwards from this border.
4. **Inferior border:** Is blunt, posteriorly it forms angle of mandible by joining with posterior border, anteriorly it is continuous with the base of mandible. It is related to facial artery and vein. Marginal mandibular branch of facial nerve runs along this border.

Lateral Surface of Ramus

Is rough gives insertion to masseter muscle.

Medial Surface of Ramus

Features are:

1. **Mandibular foramen:** Situated in the middle of medial surface, it leads to the mandibular canal. From the medial margin of this foramen a sharp process projects upwards – called lingula. It gives attachment to sphenomandibular ligament. Foramen transmits inferior alveolar nerve and vessels.
2. **Mylohyoid groove:** It is a linear groove commences below the mandibular foramen and lodges mylohyoid nerve and vessels.
3. Inner surface of ramus anterior to the angle is rough and gives insertion to medial pterygoid muscle.

PROCESSES OF MANDIBLE

Processes of mandible are coronoid and condyloid process – projecting upwards from ramus.

1. **Coronoid process:** It is sharp and pointed, triangular in shape, lies anterior to mandibular notch. It gives insertion to temporalis muscle.
2. **Condyloid process:** Upward continuation of upper border of ramus, forms posterior boundary of mandibular notch. The upper end of the process is the head of the mandible, which articulates with the mandibular fossa of temporal bone and forms T.M.J., below the head and neck of mandible is situated, gives attachment to capsular ligament of the joint. On the anterior surface of the neck, a pit or

depression lies called pterygoid fovea gives insertion to lateral pterygoid muscle. The lateral surface of the neck gives attachment to temporomandibular ligament (lateral ligament). Medial surface of the neck is related to maxillary artery and auriculo temporal nerve.

The head of the mandible is broader transversely. The lateral aspect of head shows a rounded tubercle.

Mandibular Canal

Found within the mandible. It extends between mandibular foramen and mental foramen. Terminally it divides into mental and incissive canals. Inferior alveolar nerve and vessels are passing through it.

Ossification

It is the second bone to ossify in the body. It is formed from Meckel's cartilage, later develop in membrane bone. Each half of the lower jaw is ossifies from a single centre, appears by the 6th neck of intra uterine life. The center appears on the membrane covering the anterior half of the Meckel's cartilage, anterior to the mental foramen. The condyloid and a part of coronoid process are formed from the Meckel's cartilage.

Table 9.2: *Age Changes in Mandible*

Changes	In children	In adults	In old age
Mandible	Two halves fuse during	Single bone 1st year of life	Single bone
Mental foramen	Near the lower border	Midway between upper	Close to alveolar border and lower border
Angle	Is abtuse, 140° or more	Angle – reduces to	It is obtuse – about 140° about 110°-120°

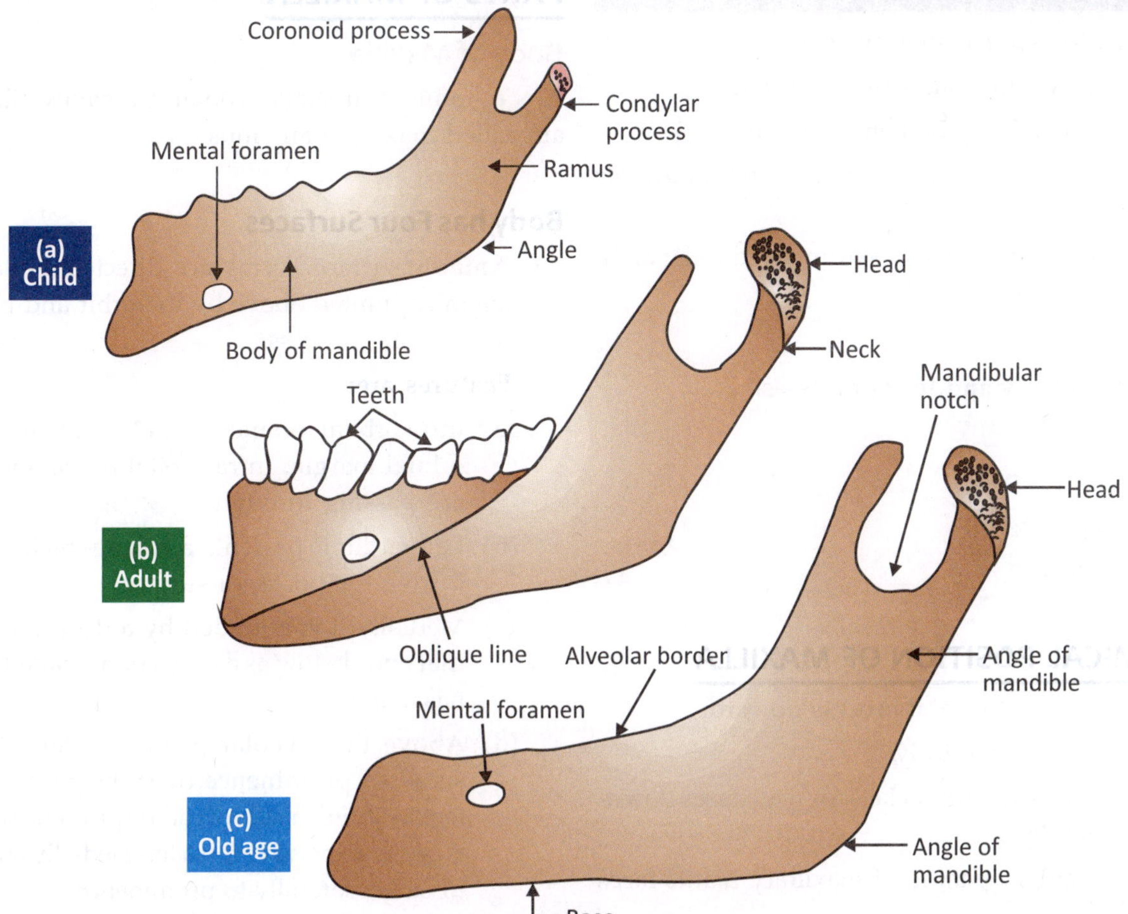

Fig. 9.10: *Age changes in the mandible*

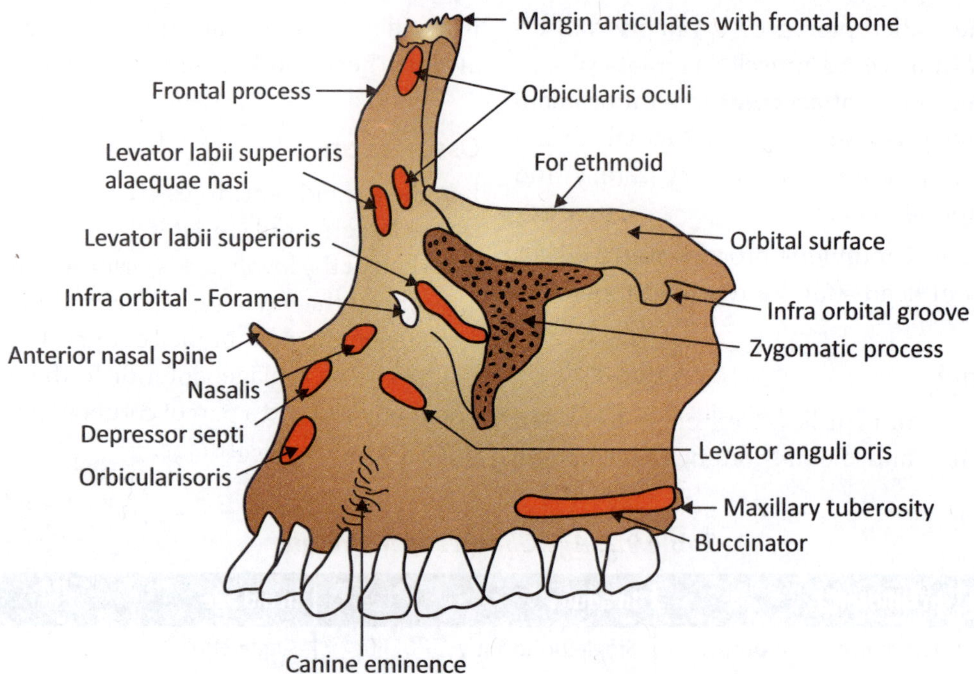

Fig. 9.11: *Lateral aspect of maxilla*

MAXILLAE

- The maxilla is a irregular pyramidal shaped bone.
- There are two maxillae – right and left.
- They together form the bone of the upper jaw.
- It is a pneumatic bone – means – containing air sinus.
- Embryologically it develops from mandibular arch.

Parts

It has a central body and four processes:

1. Frontal process
2. Zygomatic process
3. Alveolar process
4. Palatine process.

ANATOMICAL POSITION OF MAXILLA

1. Keep the longest frontal process upwards.
2. Nasal notch is anteriorly.
3. Alveolar process with sockets for teeth faces downwards laterally.
4. Large irregular opening of maxillary hiatus faces medially.

PARTS OF MAXILLA

Body of Maxilla

It is pyramidal in shape, contains a cavity filled with air, called maxillary air sinus.

Body has Four Surfaces

1. **Anterior surface:** Forms face, directed forwards and laterally, limited above by the orbit and below by the alveolar process.

   Features are:

   (a) Infra orbital foramen – lies 1 cm below the infra orbital margin. Infra orbital nerve and vessels are passing through it.

   (b) Lateral limit presents a ridge which separates it from the posterior surface.

   (c) Medially it is bounded by a deep nasal notch that ends below as a projection – called anterior nasal spine.

   (d) Above the alveolar process anterior surface shows a prominence over the root of canine teeth. On either side of canine prominence a fossa is present. Incissive fossa lies medially and canine fossa lies laterally to prominence.

2. **Posterior surface:** It forms the anterior wall of infra temporal fossa that's why it is also called as infratemporal surface. It is convex and facing posterolaterally.

   Features are:

   (a) Maxillary tuberosity is roughened impression above the third molar tooth. Medially it articulates with the pyramidal process of palatine bone. Laterally it gives origin to superficial head of medial pterygoid muscle.

   (b) There are 2-3 openings present on this surface above the tuberosity – transmits posterior superior alveolar nerve and vessels.

   (c) Upper posterior part is smooth and bounds the pterygo palatine fossa. It has a groove to lodge maxillary nerve.

3. **Superior surface:** It forms the floor of the orbit. It has three borders:

   (a) Anterior border separates the superior surface from the anterior surface and forms the lower margin of orbital opening.

   (b) Posterior border separates the superior surface from the infra temporal surface and forms the inferior boundary of the inferior orbital fissure.

   (c) Medial border separates the superior surface from the medial surface. It has a notch anteriorly situated, articulates with the lacrimal bone and forms naso lacrimal canal, lodges naso lacrimal duct:

   - Posterior to the lacrimal notches this border articulates with lacrimal bone and orbital process of labyrinthine part of the ethmoidal bone and orbital process of the palatine bone.
   - The infra orbital groove is present on this surface, leads to infra orbital canal. Infraorbital nerve and vessels are passing through it.
   - Superior surface forms the roof of the maxillary sinus.

4. **Medial surface:** It forms the lateral wall of the nose. Features are –

   (a) Maxillary Hiatus: Is a large opening of maxillary air sinus. The opening is reduced by the following bones:

   - From above – Ethmoid bone
   - From below – Inferior nasal concha
   - From anterior – Lacrimal bone
   - From posterior – Palatine bone.

   (b) Naso lacrimal groove: Lies anterior to the maxillary hiatus, converted into a canal by lacrimal bone and inferior nasal concha.

   (c) Conchal crest is rough impression, lies anterior to naso lacrimal groove, articulates with inferior nasal concha.

   (d) Greater palatine canal is formed between the medial surface of maxilla and perpendicular plate of palatine bone behind the hiatus. It transmits – anterior, middle and posterior palatine nerves and greater palatine vessels.

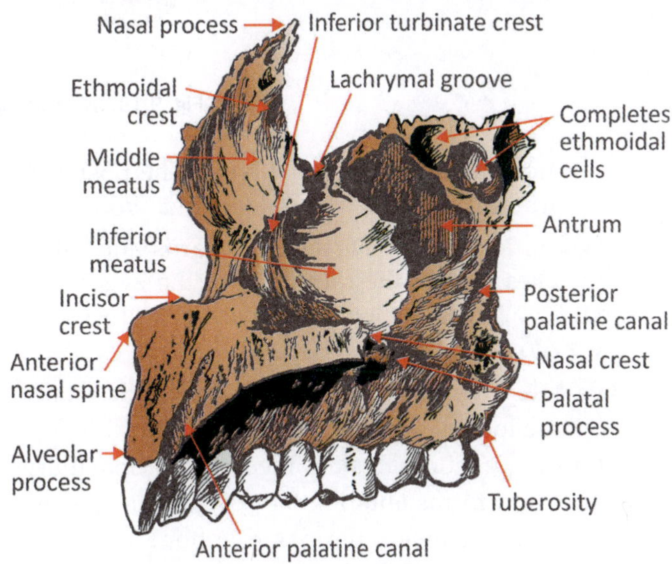

Fig. 9.12: *Medial surface of maxilla*

Processes of Maxilla

1. **Frontal process:** It is a long pointed process projecting upwards. It has two surfaces and two borders.

   (a) Lateral surface: Is large, having anterior lacrimal crest, behind the crest is a lacrimal groove, lodges lacrimal sac. Crest gives attachment to:

   - Medial palpebral ligament
   - Lacrimal fascia
   - Orbicularis oculi
   - Levator labii superioris.

   (b) Medial surface: Bounds the lateral wall of nasal cavity. Superiorly it articulates with the frontal bone at the nasal notch. Anterior border

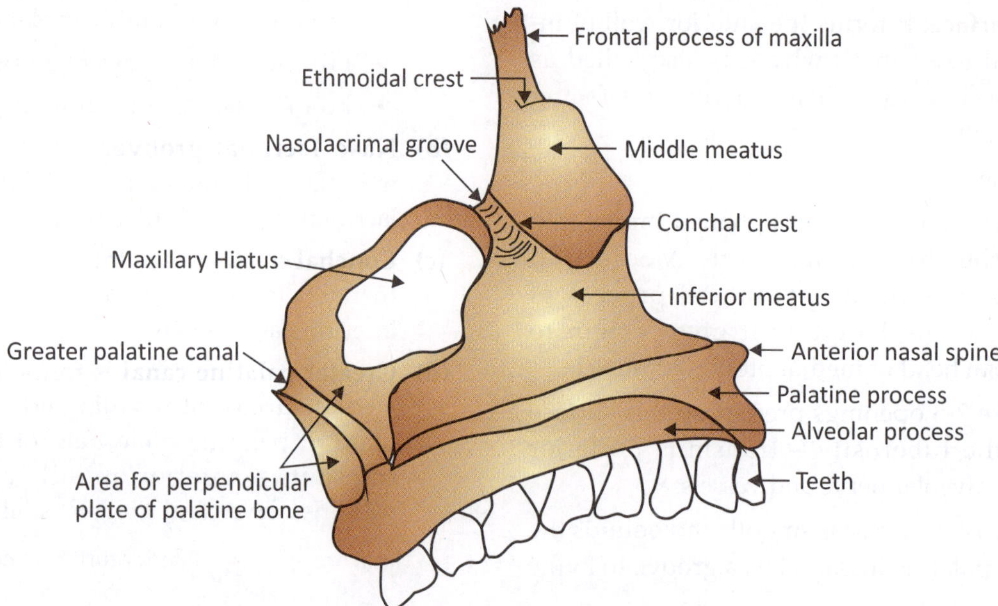

Fig. 9.13: *Medial aspect of left maxilla*

articulates with the nasal bone. The posterior border articulates with the lacrimal bone.

2. **Zygomatic process:** Directed upwards and laterally, takes part in the formation of the zygomatic arch by articulating with the maxillary process of the zygomatic bone.
3. **Palatine process:** Projects like a shelf, horizontally from the medial surface of the body of maxilla. Palatine process of both sides meet at inter maxillary suture and forms anterior 3/4th of the hard palate. Posteriorly it meets the palatine bone at palato maxillary suture and completes hard palate.

   Anteriorly at the junction between the two maxillae the incissive fossa is situated. On the lateral wall of the fossa, the incissive canal lies, transmits the greater palatine artery and naso palatine nerve towards the nasal cavity.

   The upper surface of the medial border of the palatine process, shows a raised elevation called nasal crest, which articulates with the vomer. The anterior end of the nasal crest is known as incisor crest. Anteriorly it becomes the anterior nasal spine.
4. **Alveolar process:** Lies in the lower part of the body of maxilla antero laterally. It has sockets for the teeth of the upper jaw.

Ossification: Maxilla ossifies in membrane from three centres. One centre for maxilla proper, appears above the canine fossa at 6th week of intrauterine life. The centres appear for premaxilla, one above the incisive fossa at 7th week of intrauterine life. The second centre appears at the ventral margin of nasal septum during 8th week of intrauterine life and soon fuses with the palatal process of maxilla around 10th week.

FRONTAL BONE

This is a membrane bone, forms forehead and lodges frontal air sinus, i.e., pneumatic bone.

Parts

Three parts:

1. Squamous part
2. Orbital plates are on either sides
3. Nasal part.

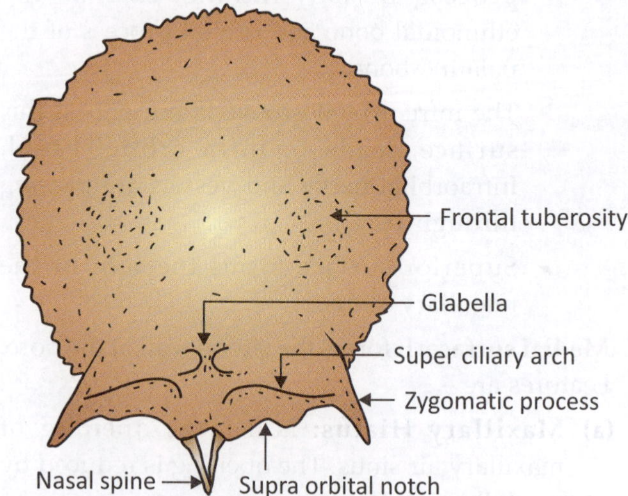

Fig. 9.14: *Frontal bone anterior view*

1. **Squamous Part:** Squamous part has following surfaces – external, internal and right and left temporal surfaces.

Surfaces of Squamous Part of Frontal Bone:

(a) **External surface:** It is smooth and convex. Inferiorly it is limited by nasal notch and supra orbital borders, superiorly limited by coronal suture. Laterally superior temporal lines bounds this surface. Features are:

- **Frontal tuberosities:** Situated on either sides of the midline – site of maximum convexity.
- **Super ciliary arches:** Lies above the supra orbital margin.
- **Supra orbital margin:** It separates the squamous part from the orbital plate. It is rounded medially and sharp laterally. It has – supra orbital notch lies between lateral 2/3 and medial 1/3 of the supra orbital border. Through this notch supra orbital nerve and vessels are passing. Sometimes this notch in converted into a foramen – called supra orbital foraman.
- **Glabella:** It is a smooth elevation in the midline in between two super ciliary arches.

(b) **Internal surface:** It is concave, lodges frontal lobe of cerebrum. Features are:

- Median frontal crest is a bony elevation in midline gives attachment to falx cerebri.

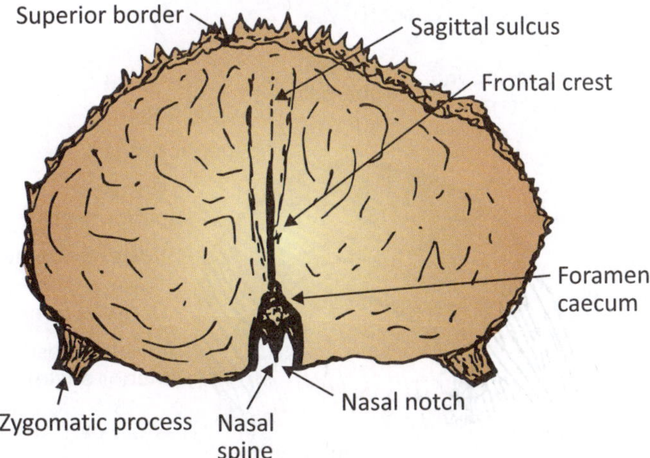

Fig. 9.15: ***Frontal bone – Internal surface***

- Foramen caecum – Lies in between frontal crest and crista galli of ethmoid bone. An emissary vein passes through it from nose to superior sagittal sinus in early childhood, later on it obliterates.
- Median sagittal sulcus lodging superior sagittal sinus.
- Impression caused by frontal gyri, sulci and meningeal vessels.
- Pits on either sides of the median sagittal sulcus to lodge the arachnoid granulations and villi of the superior sagittal sinus.

(c) **Right and left temoporal surfaces:** It forms the anterior part of the temporal fossa. Superior temporal lines separate this surface from the external surface. Temporal fascia and temporalis muscle is attached to the lines.

- **Posterior:** Frontal bone articulates with parietal bones at coronal suture. Junction between two parietal and frontal bone is called **Bregma.**
- Nasion is the junction of two nasal bones with the frontal bone.
- **Frontal air sinuses:** These are situated within the frontal bone separated by a thin septum. Lies deep to glabella and super ciliary arches making the bone pneumatic bone.

2. **Orbital Plates:** Lower surface forms the roof of the orbit, while upper surface forms the floor of the anterior cranial fossa.

- Medial aspect of the lower surface has a spine called trochlear spine, a fibro cartilaginous ring is attached that forms a pulley for the superior oblique muscle.
- The lateral aspect of the orbital surface has a depression called lacrimal fossa – lodges lacrimal gland.

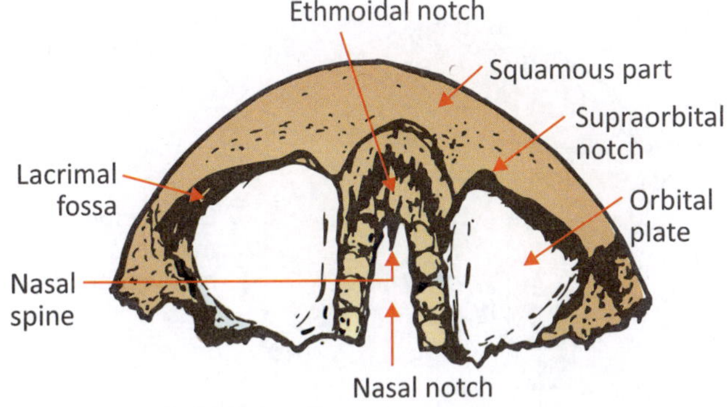

Fig. 9.16: ***Frontal Bone – Orbital Plates and Nasal Notch***

Ethmoidal notch: It is a "U" shaped gap present in between the two orbital plates. There are anterior and posterior ethmoidal notches – which are converted into foramina by the ethmoid bone. Through these foramina anterior and posterior ethmoidal nerves and vessels are passing.

- Cranial surface is marked by impressions of sulci and gyri of frontal lobe of cerebrum.
- Posterior border articulates with the lesser wing of sphenoid bone.

3. **Nasal Part:** It is situated below to glabella. It shows a triangular nasal notch, which articulates with the nasal bone, frontal process of maxilla and lacrimal bone.

   Nasal spine is a midline projection from the nasal notch. Behind the nasal spine nasal grooves are present, forms the nasal cavity.

Metopic suture: It is a midline suture present in the foetal frontal bone. It represents the line of fusion between two halves. Rarely it may be present in the adult crossing the midline of squamous part of the bone.

Ossification: Two primary centres appears by 8th week of intrauterine life near the super ciliary arch. They unite at the age of 2-8 years. The secondary centres rarely develop at the nasal part of the bone by 10th year.

PARIETAL BONES

There are two parietal bones present on the top of skull, develops from membrane. Each bone comes in contact – to all the lobes of cerebral hemisphere.

- **It has two surfaces:**
  (a) External surfaces
  (b) Internal surfaces.

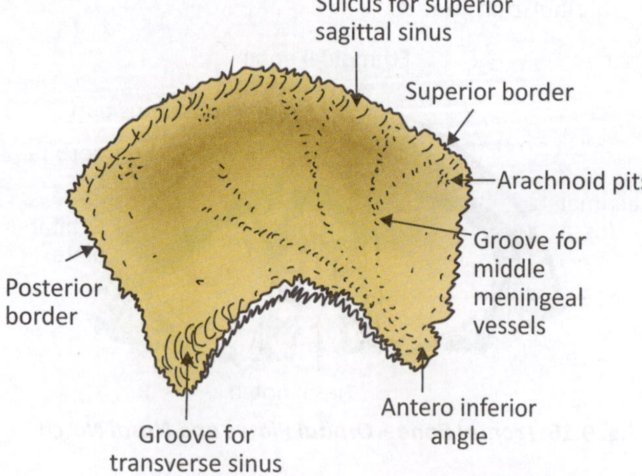

Fig. 9.17: *Parietal bone – internal surface*

- **Four borders:**
  (a) Anterior borders
  (b) Posterior borders
  (c) Superior borders
  (d) Inferior borders.
- **Four angles:**
  (a) Antero-superior angle
  (b) Antero inferior angle
  (c) Postero superior angle
  (d) Postero inferior angles.

Surfaces of the Parietal Bone

External Surface:

It is convex, shows:

- **Parietal tuberosity:** Lies near the centre of the bone – it is the site of maximum convexity.
- **Vertex:** It forms the maximum prominent point on the top of skull.
- **Temporal lines:** They are two superior and inferior temporal lines – gives attachment to temporal fascia and temporalis muscle.
- **Parietal emissary foramen:** It lies anterior to posterior border but lateral to the superior border. An emissary vein passes through it, connecting the superior sagittal sinus with the veins of the scalp.

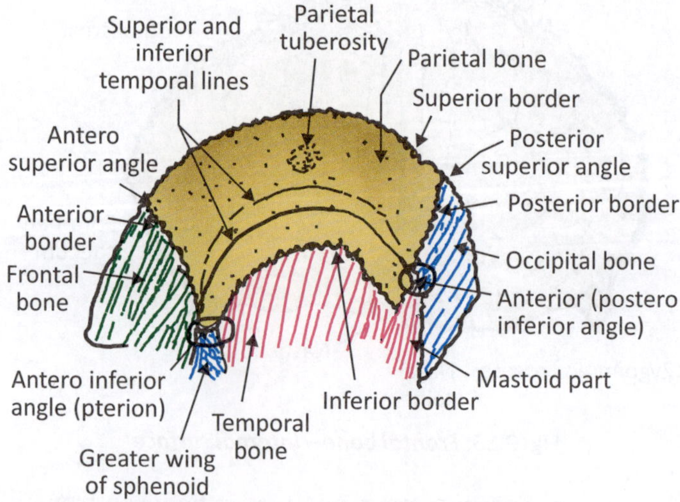

Fig. 9.18: *External surface of parietal bone*

Internal Surface:

It is concave and is grooved by the anterior and posterior branches of middle meningeal vessels.

- Along the superior border – groove for superior sagittal sinus is present. Along this groove depressions or pits lie, lodging arachnoid granulations.
- Inner aspect of postero inferior angle has a groove for the transverse sinus.

Borders of the Parietal Bone

Anterior Border:

It is thick and serrated, articulates with the frontal bone and forms coronal suture.

Posterior Border:

Also thick and serrated, articulates with squamous part of occipital bone and form lambdoid suture.

- **Lambda** is the meeting point of two parietal and occipital bone, i.e., junction of sagittal and lambdoid suture. In the foetal skull it is represented as the posterior fontenelle.

Superior Border:

It is thick and serrated articulates with the parietal bone of opposite side at the sagittal suture.

Inferior Border:

Is concave and divided into three parts. The anterior part articulates with the greater wing of sphenoid at pterion.

- Intermediate part articulates with the squamous part of the temporal bone.
- Posterior part is the thickest part articulates with the mastoid part of temporal bone.

Angles of the Parietal Bone

Antero-superior angle: Lies where sagittal and coronal sutures meet, and forms bregma. In foetus it forms anterior fontenelle.

Antero inferior angle: Joins at pterion – This represents antero lateral fontenelle of the foetus. At this point following features are seen:

- Anterior branch of middle meningeal artery.
- Lateral sulcus of cerebrum divides into three parts.
- Motor speech area lies.

Postero superior angle: Represents lambda and posterior fontenelle of the foetus.

Postero inferior angle: Takes part in formation of asterion. It is the meeting point of parietal, occipital and temporal bones. In foetus it forms postero lateral fontenelle.

Ossification: Two primary centers appear at 7th week of intra uterine life. One is situated above the parietal tuberosity and another lies on the tuberosity. Both centers fuse and ossification spreads.

OCCIPITAL BONE

It is unpaired skull bone, lies posteriorly. It bounds the posterior cranial fossa and has a large foramen called foramen magnum.

Parts of the Bone

1. Squamous part
2. Condylar part
3. Basilar part.

1. **Squamous part** is situated above and posterior to foramen magnum. It is the largest part, has a convex posterior surface and concave anterior surface (inner).

   External occipital protuberance (inion): An elevation lies in the middle of external surface. Deep to it lies confluence of sinuses. The trapezius muscle and ligamentum nuchae is attached to it.

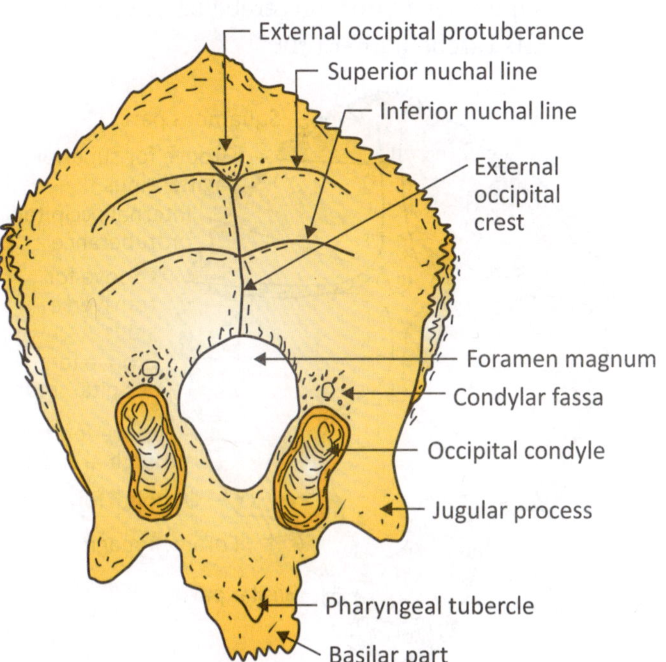

Fig. 9.19: *Occipital bone – external surface*

Highest nuchal line: Runs laterally on either sides of the inion, commences from external occipital protuberance.

Superior nuchal line: On either side of external occipital protuberance, a curved line situated called superior nuchal line lies just below the highest nuchal line. It separates the scalp from the back of neck and gives attachment to trapezius and occipital belly of the occipito frontalis muscle.

External occipital crest: It extends from the external occipital protuberance to the posterior border of the foramen magnum, lies in the midline. It gives attachment to the ligamentum nuchae.

Inferior nuchal line: Extends from the middle of the occipital crest, runs below the superior nuchal line, gives insertion to rectus capitis posterior minor.

The medial part of the interval between superior and inferior nuchal lines – semispinalis capitis is inserted. Lateral part of this area gives insertion for obliquus capitis superior.

Inner surface of squamous part: Main features are:

- Internal occipital protuberance – centrally placed.
- From here cruciform shaped lines (sulcus) radiate superiorly, inferiorly and transversely, lodging superior sagittal sinus above right and left transverse sinus and occipital sinus from below. Margins give attachment to falx cerebri superiorly, tentorium cerebelli transversely and falx cerebelli inferiorly.

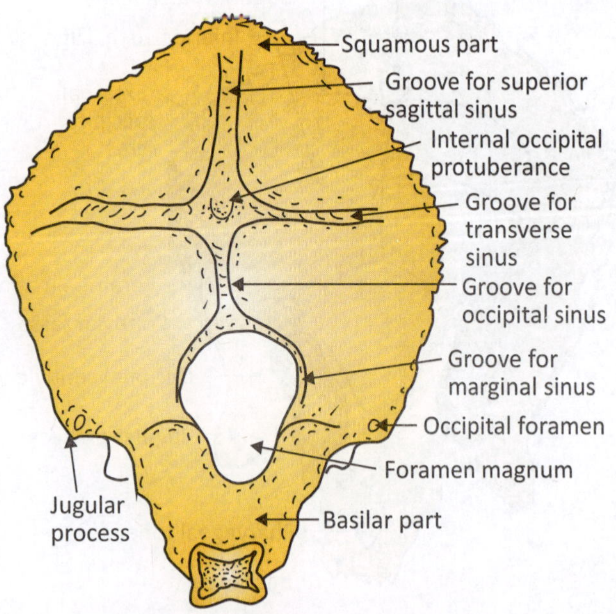

Fig. 9.20: *Occipital bone – inner surface*

Internal occipital crest is the lower vertical part from internal occipital protuberance to the posterior margin of the foramen magnum it forms a triangular depression called vermian fossa. It gives attachment to falx cerebelli and lodges occipital sinus.

Angles of the squamous part: Superior angle joins lambda, the lateral angles meet the mastoid part of the temporal bone and postero inferior angle of parietal bone at asterion.

Borders of the squamous part: Lambdoid border joins with the posterior border of parietal bone and forms lambdoid suture, mastoid border articulates with the mastoid part of the temporal bone.

2. **Condylar part:** Lies lateral to occipital condyles. Each part shows superior and inferior surfaces.

Features: On inferior surface of condylar part are –

(a) Occipital condyle
(b) Condylar fossa
(c) Condylar canal
(d) Hypoglossal canal
(e) Jugular process.

(a) **Occipital condyles:** These are oval or kidney shaped structure situated below the foramen magnum.

(b) **Condylar fossa:** It is a depression situated behind the occipital condyles, occasionally condylar canal opens into this fossa.

(c) **Condylar canal:** Not always present. When present it transmits an emissary vein connecting sigmoid sinus and sub occipital plexus of veins.

(d) **Hypoglossal canal:** Lies at the junction of basilar part and occipital condyle. It transmits:

- Hypoglossal nerve.
- Meningeal branch of ascending pharyngeal artery.
- Emissary vein – connecting basilar plexus of veins with the pharyngeal venous plexus.

(e) **Jugular process:** It lies lateral to occipital condyle, quadrangular shaped bar of bone.

- The upper and anterior part of the jugular process is grooved by the sigmoid sinus called jugular notch. Notch is converted into a foramen by petrous part of temporal bone – called jugular foramen. It transmits – sigmoid sinus, inferior petrosal sinus, glossopharyngeal (IX), vagus (X) and (XIth) accessory cranial nerves, an emissary vein and meningeal branch of occipital artery.

- Superior surface of condylar part – shows a smooth elevation called jugular tubercle which is grooved by IXth, Xth and XIth cranial nerves.

Foramen magnum: Oval shaped largest foramen, bounded anteriorly by basilar part of occipital bone, posteriorly by squamous part and laterally by condylar part of occipital bone.

Communication: It communicates posterior cranial fossa with the vertebral canal.

Structures passing: Foramen is divided into anterior and posterior compartments by the attachment of alar ligaments.

Anterior compartment transmits:

1. Apical ligament
2. Upper part of cruciate ligament
3. Membrana tectoria.

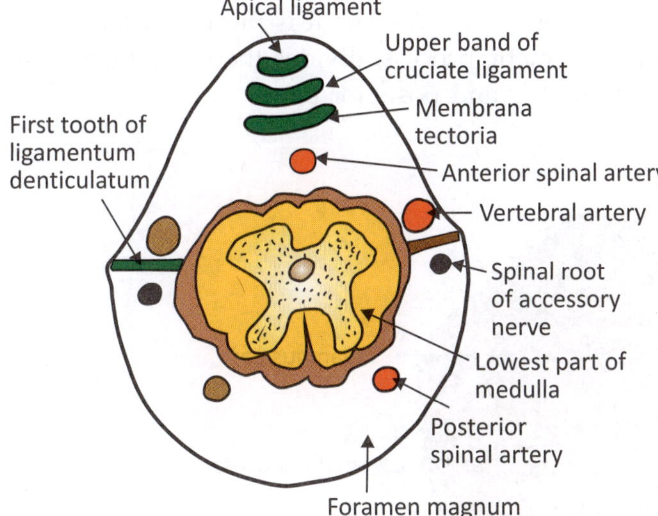

Fig. 9.21: *Structures passing through foramen magnum*

Posterior compartment transmits:

1. Lower part of medulla oblongata to become spinal cord.
2. Meninges and cerebro spinal fluid.
3. Tonsil of cerebellum.
4. Right and left vertebral arteries.
5. Anterior (one) and two posterior spinal arteries.
6. Spinal root of accessory nerve.
7. Sympathetic plexus around the blood vessels.
8. Veins accompanying the arteries.
9. First teeth of ligamentum denticulatum: Along the anterior border of foramen magnum the anterior atlanto occipital membrane is attached and along the posterior border – posterior atlanto occipital membrane is attached.

3. Basilar part: Extends forwards and upwards from the foramen magnum. It is thick and narrow anteriorly articulates with the body of sphenoid to form spheno occipital synchondroses.

Superior surface (Clivus): It is concave, related to pons and medulla. Vertebral arteries, basilar artery and basilar plexus of veins are present on clivus.

- The upper surface gives attachment to the ligaments entering the cranium through foramen magnum are:
  (a) Membrana tectoria
  (b) Superior band of cruciate ligament
  (c) Apical ligament.
- The lower surface of basilar part shows pharyngeal tubercle, gives attachment to median pharyngeal raphe and superior constrictor of pharynx.

VARIATIONS

1. **Sulural bones** are wormian bones may be present along the lambdoid suture.
2. **Occipitalisation:** Fusion of atlas with the occipital condyles.

Ossification is of two types: Membranous and cartilaginous type.

(a) Primary centre of ossification appears above the external occipital protuberance at 8th week of intra uterine life in membrane.

(b) Below the external occipital protuberance cartilagenous type of ossification:

- Two centres for squamous part appears at 7th week.
- Two centres for occipital condyle appears at 8th week.
- One centre for basilar part appears at 6th week.

(c) Occipital condyles unite with the lower squamous part by 2nd year.

(d) The basilar part unites with the occipital condyles by 6th year.

TEMPORAL BONE

Paired bones, situated along the lower part of the lateral wall of the cranium. It contains the hearing and vestibular organs and takes part in the formation of temparo mandibular joint.

PARTS OF TEMPORAL BONE

It has five parts:

1. Squamous part
2. Petrous part
3. Mastoid part
4. Tympanic part
5. Styloid part.

1. Squamous Part

It is the upper expanded part, forms lateral wall of the cranium. It has two surfaces – medial and lateral surfaces, two borders – superior and inferior borders, one process, i.e., zygomatic process and a mandibular fossa.

Lateral surface: Is smooth and slightly convex, takes part in formation of temporal fossa. This surface is grooved by middle temporal vessels. External auditory meatus is also present. Antero superior to the meatus – a ridge called – supra mastoid crest is seen.

Supra meatal triangle: It is a small depression, lies above the external auditory meatus. In the floor of the triangle, supra meatal spine is situated. Deep to the triangle mastoid antrum lies.

Zygomatic process: It is a finger like process passes forwards, above and in front of external auditory meatus. It articulates with the temporal process of zygomatic bone and forms zygomatic arch, which separates temporal and infra temporal fossae.

Tubercle of the root of zygoma: Lies at the junction of anterior and posterior parts of the zygomatic process. It gives attachment to the temporo mandibular ligament.

Articular tubercle: This elevation lies along the inferior surface of the posterior part of the zygomatic arch, anterior to the mandibular fossa.

Mandibular fossa is a shallow depression lies between the squamous and tympanic parts, lies behind the articular tubercle. Anterior part of this fossa articulates with the head of the mandible to form temporo mandibular joint.

Post glenoid tubercle: It is present at the root of the zygomatic process, divides the mandibular fossa into anterior and posterior parts.

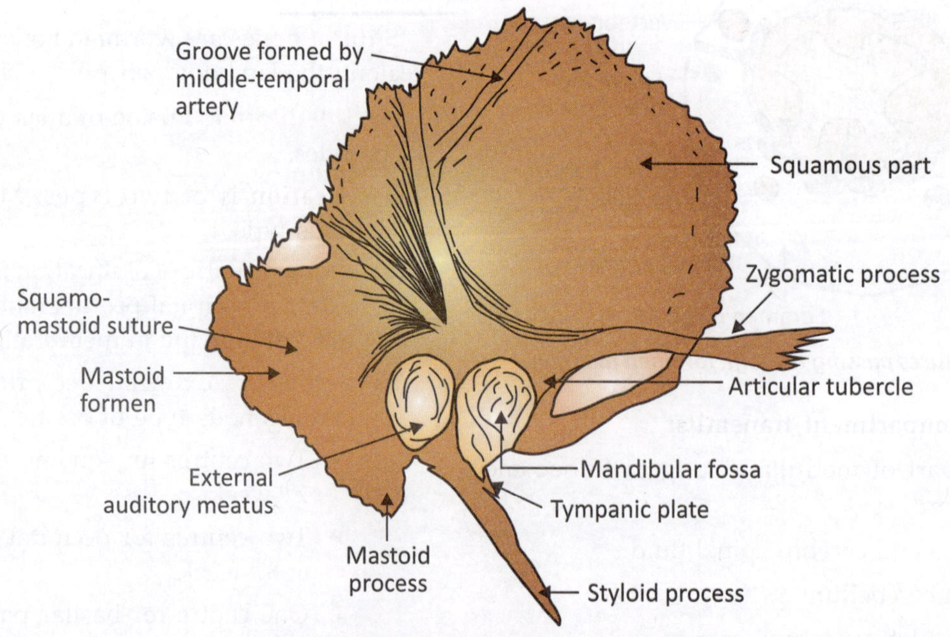

Fig. 9.22: *Right temporal bone – lateral view*

Squamo tympanic fissure: Lies in the medial part of the mandibular fossa. It is divided into two parts by tegmen tympani – petro tympanic and petro squamous portions. To the petro tympanic fissure the anterior ligament of malleus is attached and it transmits – chorda tympani nerve and anterior tympanic branch of the maxillary artery to supply middle ear.

Muscles attached:

- Temporalis muscle originate from lateral surface of squamous part of temporal bone.
- Temporal fascia is attached upper border of zygomatic arch and lower border and inner surface of the arch gives origin to masseter muscle.

Inner surface of the squmous part – It is related to the temporal lobe of cerebrum, is slightly concave and grooved by middle meningeal vessels. At the junction of petrous and squamous part – petrosquamous suture is present.

Upper border of squamous part articulates with the lower border of parietal bone at squamosal suture. Anteriorly it articulates with the greater wing of sphenoid bone. Squamous part is thin and translucent near mandibular fossa.

2. Petrous Part

It is stony hard, i.e., hardest part of the bone in the body, pyramidal in shape, sandwitched between sphenoid and occipital bone. It has a base, apex, three surfaces and three borders.

- **Base:** Lies laterally, united with mastoid and squamous part of the bone.
- **Apex** is directed antero medially and forms foramen lacerum when it comes in contact with sphenoid and basilar part of occipital bone.
- Upper opening of carotid canal lies at the apex of the bone.

Surfaces

These are anterior, posterior and inferior surface.

I. Features of the anterior surface:

(a) **Trigeminal impression** is a small depression at the apex lodging trigeminal ganglion in its cave.

(b) **Arcuate eminence** is an elevation overlying the superior semi circular canal of the internal ear.

(c) **Facial nerve canal:** Lies deep to postero lateral aspect of the arculate eminence.

(d) **Tegmen tympani** is a thin plate of bone lies lateral to arcuate eminence. It forms roof of the middle ear and mastoid antrum, auditory tube and tensor tympani canal.

(e) **Grooves on the anterior surface:** They are one for greater petrosal nerve situated laterlly.

II. Posterior surface: It lies behind the superior border of petrous temporal bone, related to cerebellum. It is flat and triangular forms anterior wall of posterior cranial fossa, related to three dural venous sinuses. Superior petrosal sinus lies above, inferior petrosal sinus lies below and sigmoid sinus lies below and behind. Features on this surface are:

(a) **Internal auditory meatus:** Lies in the middle of this surface, transmits facial and auditory nerves with labyrinthine vessels.

(b) **Opening of aqueduct of vestibule:** Like a vertical slit lies postero inferior to internal auditory meatus, directed medially. It lodges saccus and ductus endo lymphaticus part of internal ear.

(c) **Subarcuate fossa** is a shallow depression lies postero superior to internal acoustic meatus, directed laterally overlies the superior semicircular canal. It gives attachment to a process of duramater.

III. Inferior surface of petrous temporal bone: It is triangular, near the apex it gives origin to levator veli palatini muscle. Behind the apex – cartilaginous part of the auditory tube is attached to it.

(a) **Opening of carotid canal (Inferior opening):** Lies just posterior to bony part of the auditory tube. It transmits – internal carotid artery with its sympathetic nerve plexus and venous plexus.

(b) **Jugular fossa:** It is situated posterior to the carotid canal opening, lodges superior bulb of internal jugular vein and it forms the floor of the middle ear.

(c) **Impression of glossopharyngeal ganglion:** Lies medial to carotid canal and anterior to jugular fossa.

(d) **Tympanic canaliculus:** It is situated between the carotid canal and jugular fossa. It transmits tympanic branch of glossopharyngeal nerve (Jacobson's nerve) to middle ear.

(e) **Opening for mastoid canaliculus:** Lies in the triangular depression for glosso-pharyngeal ganglion, it leads to the cochlear canaliculus to lodge aqueduct of cochlear and cochlear vein – drains into subarachnoid space.

Jugular Surface: It articulates with the jugular process of the occipital bone and forms jugular foramen.

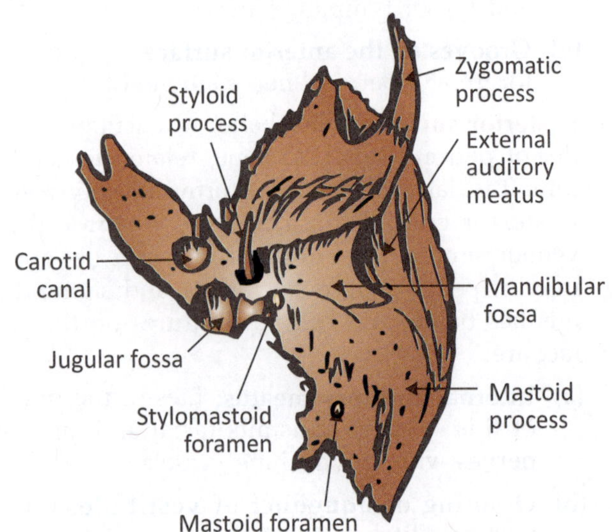

Fig. 9.23: *Inferior surface of temporal bone*

Borders of Petrous Part

(a) **Superior border:** It is grooved by superior petrosal sinus and separates anterior and posterior surface. It gives attachment to the tentorium cerebelli. The medial end of this border is crossed by the sensory and motor roots of the trigeminal nerve, while tip is crossed by abducent nerve deep to petro clinoid ligament of Gruber (Canal of Dorollo).

(b) **Posterior border:** Medially it articulates with the basilar part of the occipital bone and is grooved by inferior petrosal sinus. Lateral part forms jugular foramen.

(c) **Anterior border:** Lies in the floor of middle cranial fossa, it articulates with the greater wing of sphenoid medially and laterally with the squamous part of the temporal bone.

At the petro squamosal suture two canals open into the middle ear. Upper canal is for the tensor tympani muscle and lower canal is for Eustachian tube. Both canals are separated by a septum.

3. Mastoid Part

It is situated postero inferiorly. It has:

- Two surfaces – external and internal surface.
- Two borders – superior and posterior border.
- Prolongation of the external surface is called mastoid process.

Surfaces of the mastoid part:

A. **External surface:** It is rough and convex gives insertion to – sternomastoid, splenius capitis and longissimus capitis from above downwards.

Mastoid foramen: Lies near the occipito mastoid suture. It transmits meningeal branch of maxillary artery and an emissary vein connecting sigmoid sinus and posterior auricular vein.

Mastoid notch is present along the medial surface of mastoid process gives origin to posterior belly of digastric. Groove for occipital artery lies medial to the notch.

B. **Internal surface:** Forms posterior cranial fossa, and is grooved by sigmoid sinus.

Border of the mastoid part:

A. **Superior border of the mastoid part:** It is thick and serrated articulates with the inferior border of the parietal bone at the mastoid angle.

B. **Posterior border:** Thick and serrated articulates with the squamous part of the occipital bone.

Mastoid air cells and mastoid antrum are present in the mastoid part. They communicate with the middle ear through aditus. When air cells are not developed mastoid proces is solid and sclerotic.

4. Tympanic part

It is present below the squamous part, anterior to the mastoid part and forms squamo tympanic fissure and tympano mastoid suture.

It has two surfaces – anterior and posterior surfaces, three borders – lateral, superior and inferior border.

Inferior surface: It forms non-articualar part of the mandibular fossa and lodges glenoid part of parotid gland.

Posterior surface: It forms major boundary of external auditory meatus – floor, anterior wall and part of posterior wall.

Tympanic sulcus or sulcus of Riveni: Lies along the medial aspect of external auditory meatus, deficient superiorly and gives attachment to the tympanic membrane.

Superior border: Squamo tympanic fissure is present. Tegmen tympani turns downwards and divide it into petro tympanic and petro squamous fissures.

Inferior border: Enters the inferior surface of petrous part and forms opening of carotid canal and it ends into an expansion to the styloid process enclosing it forming the sheath.

Lateral border: Forms the opening of external auditory meatus and gives attachment to the cartilagenous part of the meatus.

5. Styloid Part or Process

It is about 2.5 cm long, directed downwards and forwards, from the petrous part of the temporal bone. It develops from second pharyngeal arch.

Muscles attached: These are styloglossus, stylohyoid and stylopharyngeus takes origin from it.

Ligament attached: These are stylohyoid and stylomandibular ligament.

- Muscles and ligaments attached to styloid process together they form – styloid apparatus.
- The lateral surface of styloid process is crossed by facial nerve, while medially it is related to carotid sheath with its contents. Posteriorly stylomastoid foramen lies – it transmits – facial nerve and stylomastoid branch of posterior auricular artery.

Ossification: Squamous and tympanic part are ossified from membrane – primary centre appear at 8th and 12th week of intra uterine life.

- Petrous part, mastoid part and styloid process are ossified from cartilage. About 14 centres appear at 20th week of intra uterine life in petrous and mastoid part and fuses with squamous and styloid part during first year.
- Styloid process has two centers – one in the upper part appears just before birth and one for the lower part appears by 2nd year.

SPHENOID BONE

It resembles a bat or butterfly with outstretched wings. It takes part in the formation of orbit, middle cranial fossa, infra temporal, temporal and pterygopalatine fossae. It is a pneumatic bone – containing sphenoidal air sinus in its body.

PARTS OF THE SPHENOID BONE

It has:

1. A centrally placed body
2. A pair of greater wings
3. A pair of lesser wings
4. A pair of pterygoid processes.

Body: Contains a pair of sphenoidal air sinuses separated by a septum. It shows following surfaces –

1. Superior Surface

Shows a small bony projection from the anterior part which articulates with the cribriform plate of ethmoid bone – it is called **ethmoidal spine.**

Jugum sphenoidale is smooth lies behind the ethmoidal spine, laterally limited by the olfactory grooves lodging oflfa ctory tract.

Sulcus chiasmaticus is a transverse groove lies behind the jugum sphenoidale, laterally it ends to the optic canal. Optic chiasma lies postero superior to the sulcus.

Tuberculum sellae: It is an oval elevation situated in between chiasmatic sulcus and sella turcica.

Sella turcica: It is a deep depression behind the tuberculum sellae. It lodges hypophysis cerebri. The upper surface of sella is covered by the diaphragma sellae.

- Dorsum sellae limited above and laterally by posterior clinoid process – forms posterior boundary of fossa.
- Posterior clinoid process gives attachments to the attached border of tentorium cerebelli.

Petrosal processes are the lateral parts of the dorsum sellae – articulates with the apex of petrous temporal bone.

Clivus: It is the downward sloping posterior surface of dorsum sellae. It articulates with the basilar part of occipital bone. Pons is related to clivus.

Inferior surface of body is also called nasal surface – it forms the part of the roof of the nasal cavity. In the midline a bony process called rostrum – articulates with the vomer, in the nasal septum.

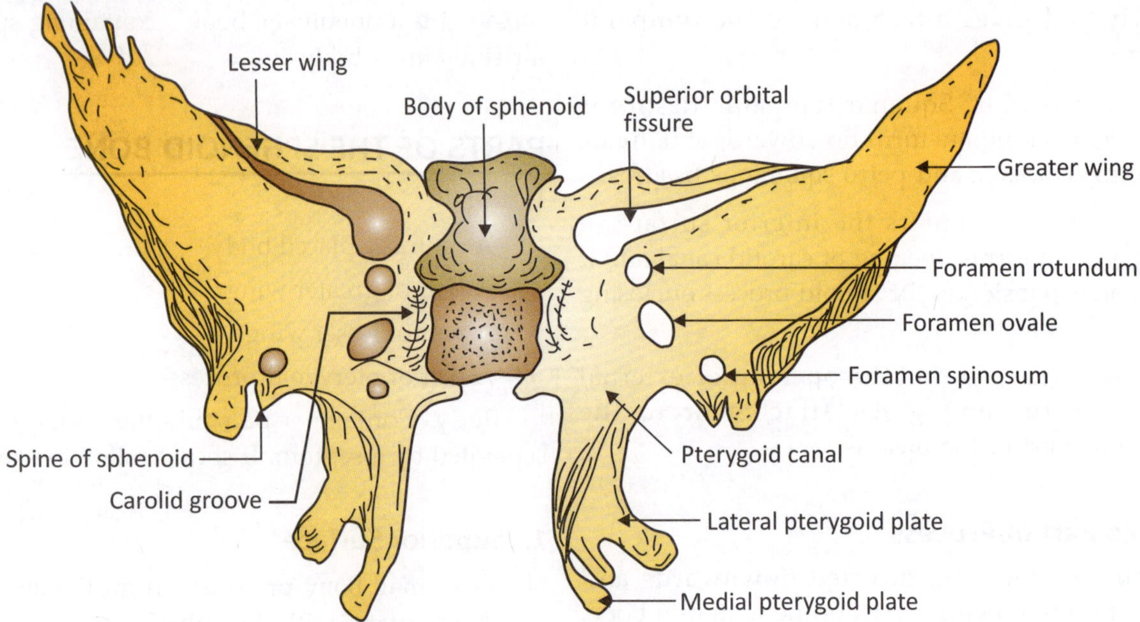

Fig. 9.24: *Sphenoid bone – postero superior view*

Anterior surface of body: Sphenoidal crest is present in the midline – articulates with the perpendicular plate of the ethmoid bone and vomer.

Lateral surface of the body: Fuses with the pterygoid process and greater wing of sphenoid bone. Carotid sulcus is present lodging internal carotid artery and cavernous sinus.

2. Greater Wing of Sphenoid

Arise from body, directed upwards and laterally. Posteriorly it articulates with the petrous and squamous part of the temporal bone. It has three surfaces – superior, inferior and lateral surface.

Superior surface forms the floor of the middle cranial fossa and has foramina – rotundum, foramen ovale and foramen spinosum.

Foramen rotundum is directed forwards and opens into pterygo palatine fossa – it transmits maxillary nerve.

Foramen ovale: is oval, large foramen communicates middle cranial fossa to infra temporal fossa. It transmits:

(a) Sensory and motor roots of mandibular nerve
(b) Accessory middle meningeal artery
(c) Lesser superficial petrosal nerve
(d) Emissary vein – communicating cavernous sinus and pterygoid venous plexus.

Foramen spinosum: It communicates middle cranial fossa and infra temporal fossa and transmits middle meningeal vessels and nervi spinosus.

Foramen of vesalius: Not always present. It transmits an emissary vein connecting cavernous sinus and pterygoid venous plexus, when present.

Lateral surface of greater wing is divided into temporal and infra temporal surfaces by the infra temporal crest. Temporal surface gives origin to temporalis muscle and takes part in the formation of the temporal fossa.

Infra temporal surface: Forms the roof of the infra temporal fossa and inferior openings of the foramina are present. Spine of the sphenoid is present gives attachment to the spheno mandibular ligament and is related to chorda tympani nerve medially and auriculotemporal nerve laterally.

Infra temporal crest – gives origin to lateral pterygoid muscle.

Orbital surface of the greater wing: Forms a part of lateral wall of the orbit and is quadrangular shaped. Medial border bounds the superior orbital fissure inferiorly. In the middle of this border a tubercle is situated – gives attachment to the common tendinous ring. Below the fissure this orbital surface is pierced by the foramen rotundum.

Pterion: It is the meeting point of greater wing of sphenoid, parietal bone, frontal and temporal bones. It is deeply related to middle meningeal vessels.

Foramen lacerum is situated behind the greater wing of sphenoid but lies anterior to the apex of petrous temporal bone.

3. Lesser Wing of Sphenoid

Arises from the body and is triangular in shape, forms a part of floor of anterior cranial fossa and roof of the orbit. Superior orbital fissure lies below it. Superior surface is related to frontal lobe and inferior surface gives origin to levator palpebrae superioris and superior oblique muscles.

- Spheno parietal sinus (venous) is related to its posterior border. Medially this border projects to form the anterior clinoid process.
- Medial end of the lesser wing divides and encloses the optic canal – which transmits – optic nerve with meninges and ophthalmic artery with its sympathetic plexus.

Superior orbital fissure: Communicates orbit and middle cranial fossa. It is triangular in shape situated at the apex of the orbit.

Boundaries:

- **Superior** – Lesser wing of sphenoid.
- **Inferior** – Greater wing of sphenoid.
- **Medial** – Body of sphenoid.
- **Lateral** – Frontal bone.

Structures passing through superior orbital fissure: Common tendinous ring divides this fissure into three parts:

A. **Lateral part:** It transmits from lateral to medial:
   (a) Recurrent branch of lacrimal artery
   (b) Lacrimal nerve
   (c) Frontal nerve
   (d) Trochlear nerve
   (e) Superior ophthalmic vein.

B. **Intermediate part:** within the tendinous ring – transmits:
   (a) Upper division of oculomtor nerve.
   (b) Nasociliary nerve.
   (c) Lower division of oculomotor nerve.
   (d) Abducent nerve.

C. **Medial part:** Transmits inferior ophthalmic vein.

4. Pterygoid Process

It arises where the greater wing meets the body of sphenoid. It has medial and lateral pterygoid plates – separated by pterygoid fossa postero inferiorly. Anteriorly both plates fuse in its upper part and forms posterior boundary of pterygo palatine fossa.

Scaphoid fossa is shallow depression lies at the upper end of medial pterygoid plate – gives origin to levator veli palatini muscle.

Lateral pterygoid plate: Forms medial boundary of infra temporal fossa. Its lateral surface gives origin to lateral pterygoid muscle and medial surface gives origin to medial pterygoid muscle. The upper part of the anterior border forms posterior boundary of pterygo maxillary fissure.

Medial pterygoid plate is larger, its lower end forms pterygoid hamulus, gives origin to superior constrictor muscle of the pharynx and pterygo mandibular raphe is attached to it. Medial pterygoid forms lateral wall of posterior nasal opening. Pharyngo basilar fascia is attached to its posterior border.

The upper part of medial pterygoid plate forms the vaginal process – articulates with the sphenoidal process of palatine bone and with vomer. Between vaginal process and sphenoidal process of palatine bone a palato vaginal canal lies which transmits pharyngeal branches of pterygo palatine ganglion and maxillary artery.

Sphenoidal concha: A pair of curved thin plates are situated along the anterior aspect of the floor of sphenoidal sinus. It has a vertical portion situated anteriorly and a horizontal portion situated posteriorly.

Anterior vertical portion of both sides meet in the midline and forms sphenoidal crest.

Posterior horizontal portion is triangular forms roof of the nose and bounds spheno palatine foramen.

Ossification: The tuberculum sellae divides the developing sphenoid into pre-sphenoidal and post-sphenoidal parts. Two parts remain separate upto 7-8 months of intra uterine life.

- **Pre-sphenoidal part forms:** Tuberculum sellae and lesser wings sphenoidal concha.
- **Post-sphenoidal part forms:** Pterygoid process, greater wing of sphenoid, sellaturcica and dorsum sellae.

ETHMOID BONE

It lies between two orbital cavities, cuboidal in shape.

It takes part in the formation of – orbit, anterior cranial fossa, roof, lateral wall and septum of nose.

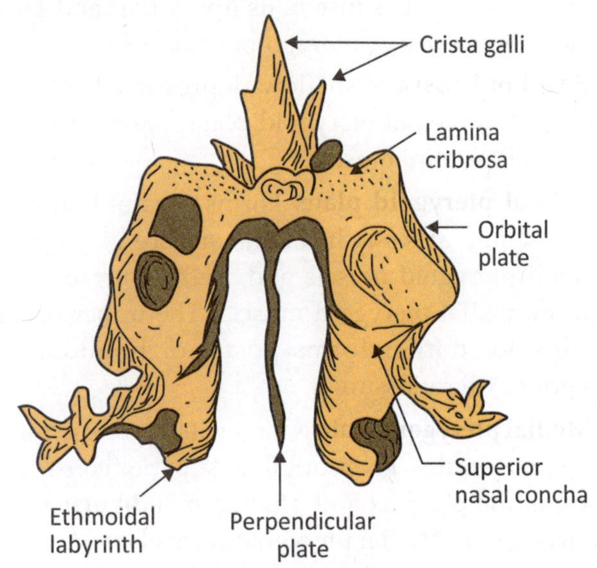

Fig. 9.25: ***Ethmoid bone***

PARTS OF ETHMOID BONE

It has three parts: Cribriform plate, perpendicular plate and labyrinthine part.

At the time of birth bone has three pieces: median plate, right and left labyrinths.

Cribriform Plate

It is sieve like, horizontal, fragile plate – forms part of floor of anterior cranial fossa and roof of nose.

It has two surfaces – superior and inferior surface and four borders – anterior, posterior, right and left lateral borders.

Superior surface: Shows an upward projection called crista galli, situated in the midline, gives attachment to falx cerebri. Anterior to crista galli lies a foramen called foramen caecum and lateral to it sieve like cribriform plate lies. Olfactory nerve passes through the openings.

- **Lateral to crista galli:** A slit is present lodging duramater, lateral to slit anterior and posterior ethmoidal foramen is situated which transmits anterior and posterior ethmoidal nerve and vessels.

Inferior surface: Forms roof of the nose. From the middle of this surface perpendicular plate projects downwards and forms bony part of nasal septum.

Perpendicular Plate

It is quadrangular in shape. Anterior border articulates with the frontal and nasal bones. Posterior border articulate with sphenoid bone above and vomer bone below. Upper border articulates with cribriform plate and lower border is attached to septal cartilage.

Labyrinthine Part

It contains ethmoidal air sinuses. It has superior, inferior, posterior, medial and lateral surfaces.

Superior surface: Contains air cells. These air cells are complete by articulating with orbital plate of frontal bone.

Inferior surface: It is articulating anteriorly with the body of maxilla and orbital process of palatine bone posteriorly.

Anterior surface: Articulates with frontal process of maxilla and lacrimal bone.

Posterior surface: Large air cells present. They are closed by sphenoidal concha and orbital process of the palatine bone. The labyrinthine part forms superior and middle concha of noses.

Medial surface: Forms lateral wall of the nose.

Lateral surface: It is very thin, covers the middle and posterior ethmoidal air cells and takes part in formation of medial wall of the orbit.

ETHMOIDAL AIR CELLS

These are anterior, middle and posterior. Anterior cells opens into anterior part of hiatus semilunasis present in the middle meatus of nose. Middle cells form bulla ethmoidalis and opens on its surface. The posterior ethmoidal cells drian into superior meatus present in the lateral wall of nose.

- From the anterior end of the labyrinth – a process is projecting downwards – called uncinate process. Deep to it hiatus semi lunaris is situated.

Ossification is by three primary centres. Two centres appear at 16-28 weeks of intra uterine life for labyrinth and one for perpendicular plate appears near crista galli around first year.

- During second year ossification completes and labyrinth unites with perpendicular plate of ethmoid bone.

ZYGOMATIC BONE

It forms the bony prominence of the cheek. Shape is irregular. It takes part in the formation of lateral wall and floor of the orbit. Also forms the anterior wall of temporal and infra temporal fossa.

Parts: It has three surfaces – lateral, medial and orbital surface and five borders – antero superior, antero inferior, postero superior, postero inferior and postero medial border.

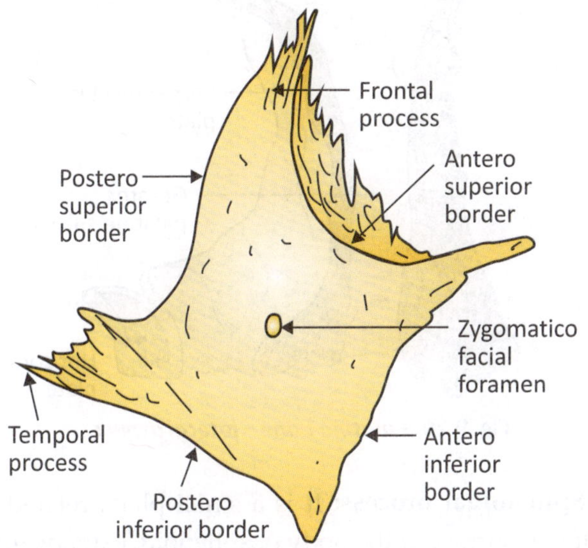

Fig. 9.26: *Zygomatic bone – lateral surface*

Process: These are frontal and temporal process, articulate with frontal and temporal bone.

Lateral surface: It is convex and prominent, shows zygomatico facial foramen which transmits zygomatico nerve and vessels.

Muscles attached are Origin of masseter near postero inferior border.

Zygomaticus minor: Originates inferior to the zygomatico facial foramen.

Zygomaticus major: Originates from the lateral surface behind the origin of zygomaticus minor.

Levator Labii Superioris

Medial surface: Forms temporal and infra temporal fossae. Anterior part of this surface is rough and articulates with the zygomatic process of maxilla. This surface also shows zygomatico temporal foramen which transmits zygomatico temporal nerve and vessels.

Superior surface: Forms floor and lateral wall of orbit. It has a foramen called zygomatico orbital foramen leads to zygomatico temporal and zygomatico facial foramen.

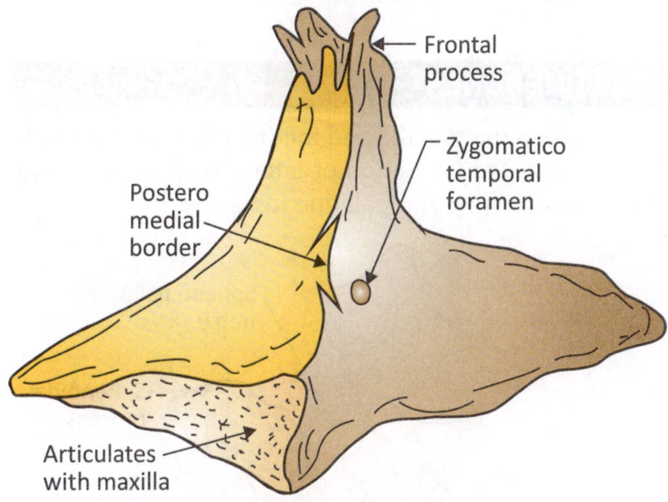

Fig. 9.27: *Zygomatic bone – medial surface*

Orbital border: It is non-articular, concave, gives attachment to the orbital septum.

Maxillary border: Articulates with maxilla, is also called as postero inferior border.

Temporal border (postero superior border): It is sharp gives attachment to temporal fascia.

Posteromedial border: Upper part articulates with the greater wing of sphenoid and lower par articulates with the orbital surface of maxilla. Middle part is non articular, forms inferior orbital fissure.

Postero inferior border: It is non-articular, masseter muscle originates.

Frontal process has three surfaces: anterior, posterior and lateral surface, anterior surface takes part in formation of orbit. Close to the orbital border Whitnall's tubercle lies. It gives attachment to:

- Lateral check ligament
- Suspensory litament of lockwood
- Lateral palpebral ligament
- Aponeurosis of the levator palpebrae superioris

Frontal process has three borders: Anterior, posterior and medial border. Anterior border forms orbital margin, posterior border gives attachment to temporal fascia, while medial border joins the greater wing of sphenoid.

Temporal process: Upper part articulates with the zygomatic process of temporal bone, lower part gives origin to masseter muscle.

Ossification: One center appears for the body of the bone at 8th week of intra uterine life and ossification spreads on all sides.

PALATINE BONE

Lies between the maxilla and medial pterygoid plate. It takes part in the formation of lateral wall of nose and medial wall of pterygo palatine fossa.

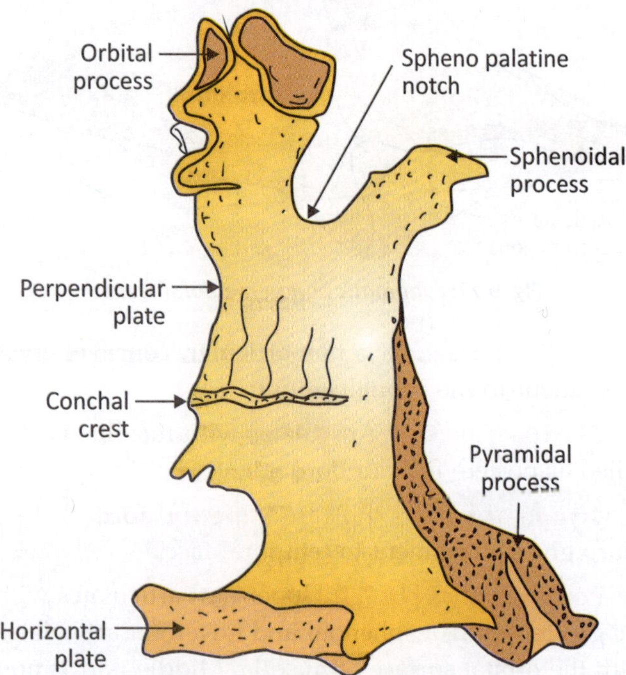

Fig. 9.28: *Palatine bone – medial aspect*

Perpendicular plate has medial and lateral surface. Lateral surface shows a groove called greater palatine groove, it is converted into a canal by articulating with the maxilla. This canal transmits greater palatine nerves and vessels.

Processes of palatine bone: They are pyramidal, orbital and sphenoidal process.

Pyramidal process: It lies in between posterior border of maxilla and medial and lateral pterygoid plates of the sphenoid bone. It gives origin to medial pterygoid muscle. Inferior surface has lesser palatine foramen – transmits lesser palatine nerves and vessels.

Orbital process: Lies along the upper part of perpendicular plate separated by a notch from the sphenoidal process. It is called spheno palatine notch. Orbital process lies in the floor of the orbit posteriorly, maxillary nerve grooves the lower part of this surface. It articulates with maxilla, sphenoidal concha and labyringh of the ethmoidal bone.

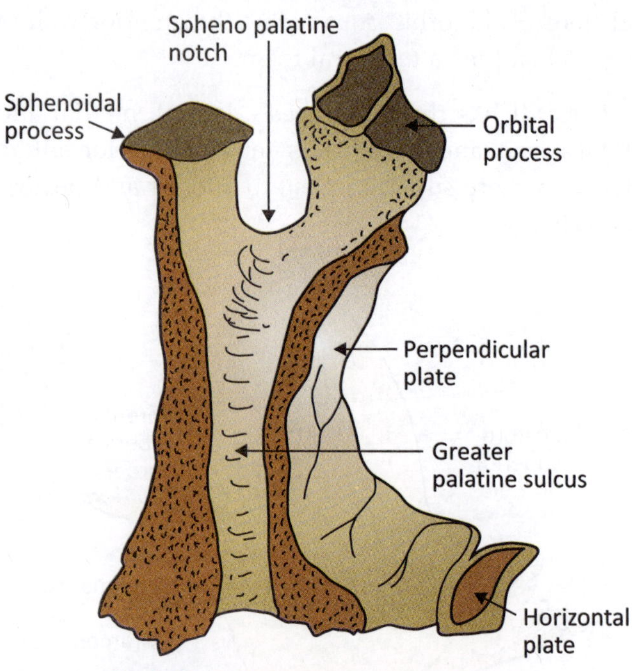

Fig. 9.29: *Palatine bone – lateral aspect*

Sphenoidal process: It is a small plate, related to the lower surface of the body of sphenoid, extends upto ala of vomer.

Horizontal plate: It meets its fellow of opposite side and forms posterior 1/3 of hard palate. At the meeting point it forms nasal crest which articulates with vomer and projects back in the midline to form posterior nasal spine.

- The anterior border of the horizontal plate meets the posterior border of palatine process of maxilla at palato maxillary suture.
- The posterior border is sharp and concave.

Ossification: One center of ossification appears by 8th week of intra uterine life on the perpendicular plate. Ossification spreads to the other parts of bone.

VOMER BONE

It is unpaired bone, lies in the midline of the nose and forms nasal septum, dividing the nose into two cavities. It has two surfaces right and left, grooved by nasopalatine nerves and vessels.

- Superior border divides into two wings called alae.
- Inferior border articulates with perpendicular plate of ethmoid bone above and septal cartilage below.

Ossification: Two centers appear by 8th week of intra uterine life, one on either side. At puberty these plates fuse.

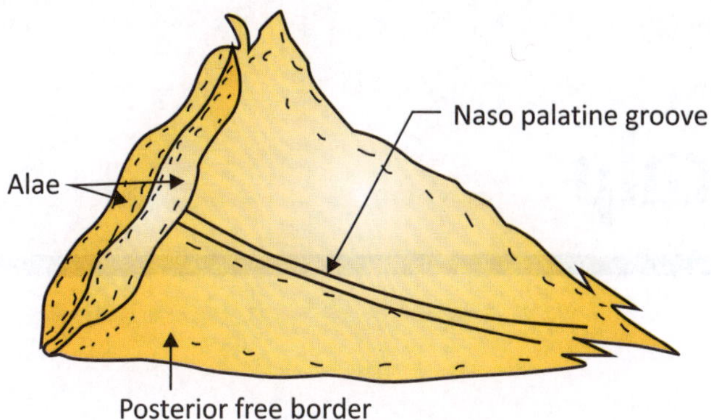

Fig. 9.30: *Vomer bone*

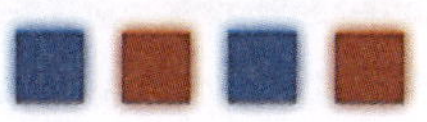

CHAPTER 10

Scalp

DEFINITION

Soft tissue covering the top of skull is called **scalp**.

Extent:

- **Anteriorly:** Up to supra orbital border.
- **Posteriorly:** Up to external occipital protuberance and superior nuchal line.
- **Laterally:** Up to superior temporal lines.

LAYERS OF THE SCALP

1. **S for – Skin:** This is thick and dense. It is intimately connected to subcutaneous tissue containing hair and plenty of sebaceous glands, thus, sebaceous cysts are common in scalp.
2. **C for – Connective tissue:** Dense with fibrous septa dividing into compartments called locules containing blood vessels, nerves and fat lobules. It is non-elastic, hence collection of fluid in this layer is highly painful. Vessels are firmly attached to fascia, so wounds of scalp causes severe bleeding.
3. **A for – Aponeurosis** of occipito frontalis muscle.
4. **L for – Loose areolar tissue:** Loosely connects above three layers with the pericranium, missary veins lies in it.
5. **P for – Pericranium:** Outer covering of skull bones.

NERVE SUPPLY OF SCALP

Scalp is divided into 4 quadrants. Each quadrant has 4 sensory nerves and 1 motor nerve.

Anterior quadrant: Sensory nerves are branches of trigeminal nerve:

1. Supra trochlear nerve (V_1).
2. Supra orbital nerve (V_1).
3. Auriculo temporal nerve (V_3).
4. Zygomatico temporal nerve (V_2).

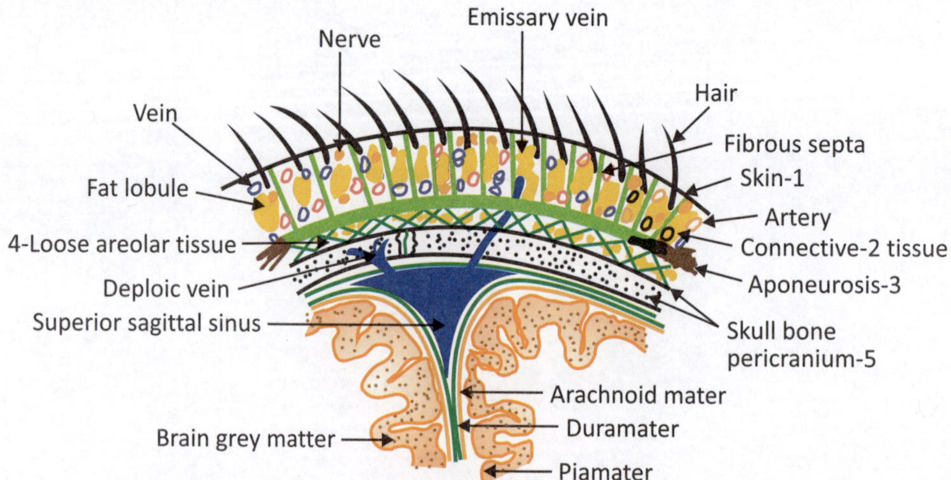

Fig. 10.1: *Structure of the scalp - layers*

5. Temporal branch of facial nerve (VII) motor nerve.

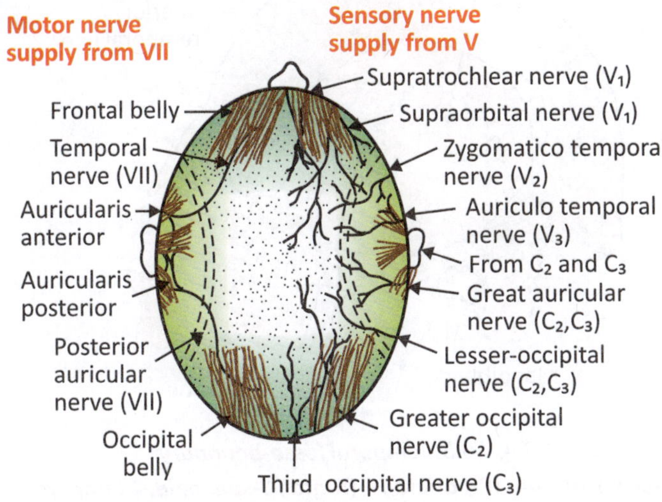

Fig. 10.2: *Muscles and nerves of scalp*

Posterior quadrant: Motor nerve – Posterior auricular branch of facial nerve.

Sensory nerve: These are branches of cervical plexus.

1. Great Auricular Nerve $C_{2'3}$
2. Lesser Occipital Nerve C_2
3. Greater Occipital Nerve C_2
4. Third Occipital Nerve C_3.

BLOOD SUPPLY OF SCALP

Arterial supply: In scalp branches of internal and external carotid arteries anastomoes with each other.

Branches of external carotid-artery are:

1. Superficial temporal artery.
2. Posterior auricular artery.
3. Occipital artery.

Branches of internal carotid-artery are:

1. Supra trochlear artery.
2. Supra orbital artery.

VENOUS DRAINAGE

1. Supratrochlear and supra orbital veins unite at the medial angle of eye and form anterior facial vein.
2. Superficial temporal vein joins maxillary vein and form retro mandibular vein in the parotid gland.
3. Posterior auricular vein unites with posterior division of retromandubular vein to form external-Jugular vein.
4. Occipital vein ends in sub occipital venous-plexus and drains into internal jugular vein.

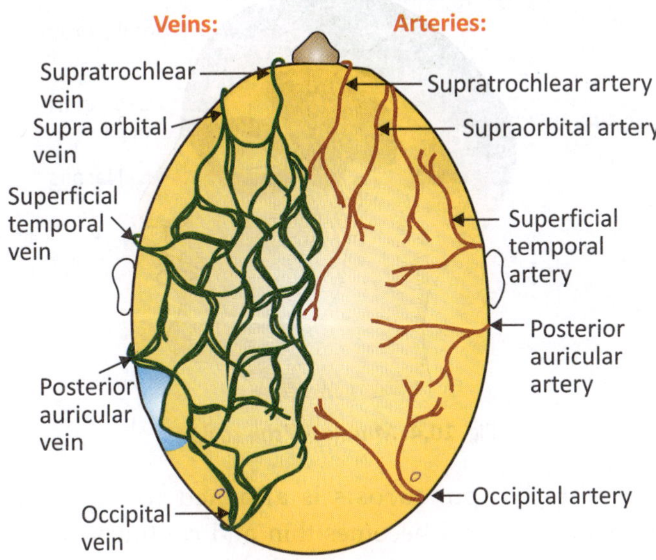

Fig. 10.3: *Blood vessels of scalp*

Clinical Applications

1. Due to rich blood supply large wounds of the scalp bleed profusely but heals quickly.
2. All the vessels converge from periphery of the scalp to the centre so incisions for skin flaps are made in center and reflected towards periphery- preserving blood supply.
3. Midline area has poor blood supply–loss of hair begins in this region (alopacia or balding).
4. Scalp is the commonest site for sebaceous cysts.

LYMPHATIC DRAINAGE OF SCALP

1. Anterior part drains into submandibular lymph nodes.
2. Lateral part drains into parotid group of lymph nodes.
3. Posterior part drains into-occipital lymph nodes (mastoid group).

Occipitao-frontalis muscle: Consists of

1. Central galea aponeurotica or epicranial-aponeurosis.

2. Two frontal bellies on front.
3. Two occipital bellies on back.

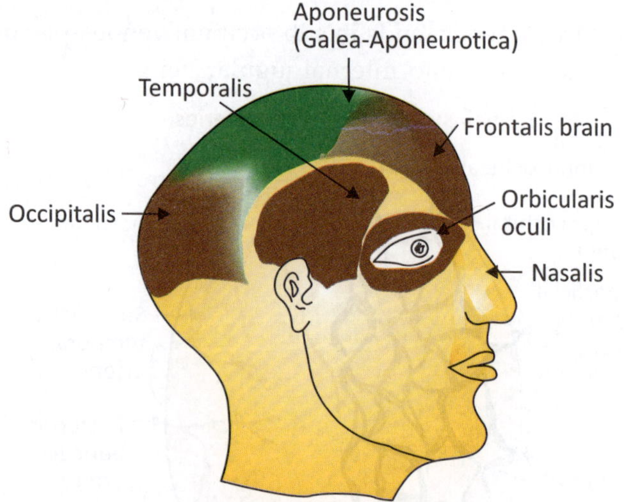

Fig. 10.4: *Muscles of the scalp*

Laterally aponeurosis is attached to superior temporal lines and becomes thin and continued over temporal fascia to gain attachment on zygomatic arch.

Frontal bellies: Arise from front of aponeurorsis unite along their medial edges to get attached or inserted to the upper part of orbicularis oculi and skin of eye brows. It has no bony attachment.

Occipital bellies: Arise from lateral halves of superior nuchal lines and inserted on the posterior border of epicranial aponeuroris and do not join one another.

Action: Frontal bellies elevate eyebrows and produce transverse wrinkles on forehead as in surprise.

Occipital bellies: Anchor aponeurois due to their bony attachment.

Nerve supply: Branches of facial nerve (VII) temporal branch and posterior auricular branch.

TEMPORAL FOSSA

- Temple is the area between temporal lines and the zygomatic arch.
- It is a shallow depression.

Bones taking part are:

1. Squamous part of temporal bone.
2. Greater wing of sphenoid.
3. Lower part of frontal.
4. Parietal bones.

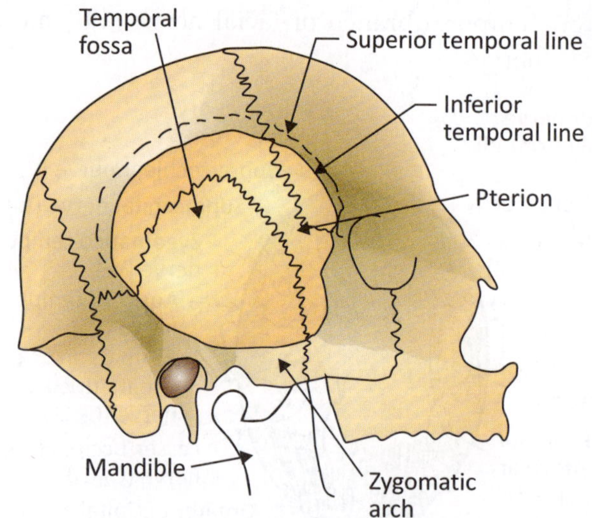

Fig. 10.5: *Temporal fossa-boundary*
Norma lateralis (P-parietal, F-frontal, S-sphenoid, T-temporal)

Bones articulate at 'H' suture called pterion.

Layers in temporal region: Six layers

1. Skin.
2. Cutaneous tissue.
3. Expansion of epicranial aponeurosis from which auricularis anterior and superior muscles arise.

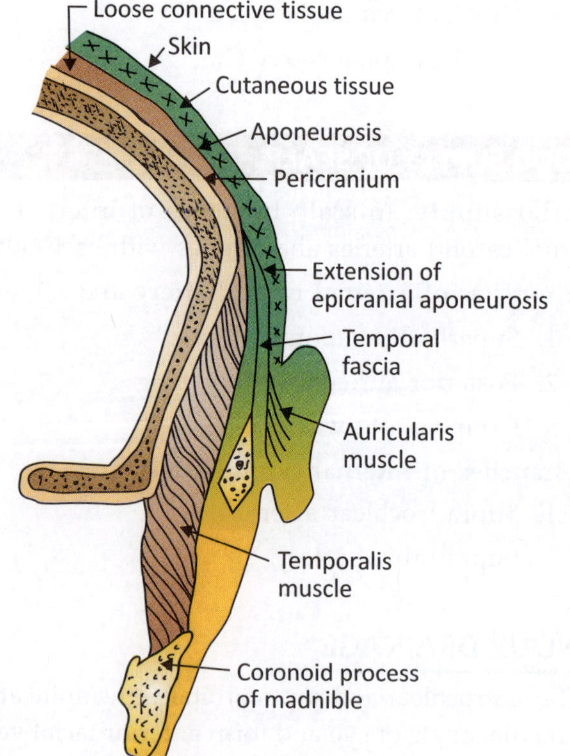

Fig. 10.6: *Layers in temporal region*

4. Temporal fascia-attached above to superior temporal line and below to zygomatic arch. It is a rugged membrane on which – superficial temporal vessels and auriculo temporal nerve lies and it is perforated by middle tempral artery and vein.
5. Temporalis muscle is one of the muscle of mastication and is fanshaped
   - Muscle arise from temporal fossa and fascia-converges towards coronoid process of mandible for insertion.

     Supplied by — Two deep temporal nerve and vessels.

     Nerve — Is branch of mandibular nerve.

     Action — Retraction and elevation of mandible.
6. Pericranium.

APPLIED ANATOMY OF SCALP

1. **Sebaceous cyst** is a retention cyst due to collection of sebum as a result of obstruction of sebaceous duct. Secondary infection may sets in.
2. **Dermoid cyst** is a congenital cyst develops in midline.
3. **Cephal haematoma:** Blood collected in subperiosteal space.
4. **Osteomyelitis** of skull bones.
5. **Avulsion of scalp:** During scalp injury at the level of loose areolar tissue-scalp separates (avulsed).
6. **In frontal sinusitis:** Pain is referred up to vertex along the supratrochlear, and supraorbital nerves.
7. **Caput Succedanum:** Heeping up of scalp in foetus occurs during labour due to over lapping of skull bones and collection of fluid in the loose areolar tissue due to forces of labour and poor venous and lymphatic return.
8. **Loose areolar tissue** is dangerous layer of scalp because emissary veins lies in this layer. Extra cranial infection can spread intra canially due to presence of emissary veins or *vice-versa.*
9. **Scalp wound bleed profusely:** Due to dense connective tissue septa attached to wall of blood vessels which prevents retraction of blood vessels.
10. **Scalp wounds-heal quickly:** Due to rich vascularity.
11. **In head injury:** Blood easily tracks down anteriorly over eyelids-resulting in black eye.

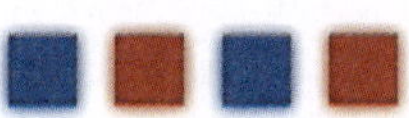

CHAPTER 11

Face

BOUNDARIES

- **Superiorly:** Upto hair line.
- **Inferiorly:** Upto chin and base of mandible.
- **Sides:** Upto auricle.

Note: Forehead is common in face and scalp.

SKIN

1. It is very vascular.
   Wounds → Bleed profosely → Heals rapidly.
2. Skin is rich in sebaceous and sweat glands oily skin → acne in adults.
3. Laxity of skin → rapid spread of oedema.
   Renal oedema → first appears on eyelids and face.
4. Fixity of skin to underlying cartilage boils in nose and ear → acutely painful.
5. Skin is thick and elastic.

Note: All facial muscles → inserted in skin so wounds of face → gape.

Superficial fascia: Contains

1. Facial muscles.
2. Vessels and nerves.
3. Fat (absent in eyelids) present in cheek as buccal pad of fat – helps in sucking in infants.

Deep fascia: Absent on face and present on parotid as parotid fascia and on buccinator as → bucco-pharyngeal fascia.

FACIAL MUSCLES

Facial muscles are subcutaneous muscles and helps in different facial expressions. Hence, they are called as muscles of facial expression.

Embryologically: It develops from mesoderm of second branchial arch and supplied by facial nerve.

Insertion: All facial muscles inserted into skin.

These facial muscles are arranged around the openings of the face. The main functions of these muscles will be either to open or close these openings. While doing these movements the facial expression results as a biproduct.

Muscles are Grouped as

A. **Muscle of Scalp:** Occipito-frontalis (muscle of surprise).

B. **Muscles of Auricle:**
   (a) Auricularis anterior
   (b) Auricularis superior
   (c) Auricularis posterior.

C. **Muscles of Eyelids:**
   (a) Orbicularis-oculi – sphincter
   (b) Corrugator supercilli (Frowning)
   (c) Levator palpebrae superioris (extra ocular muscle – supplied by 3rd cranial nerve – is dilator).

D. **Muscles of Nose:**
   (a) Procerus muscle causes frowning with corrugator supercilli.
   (b) Compressor naris is sphincter – compresses the nose.

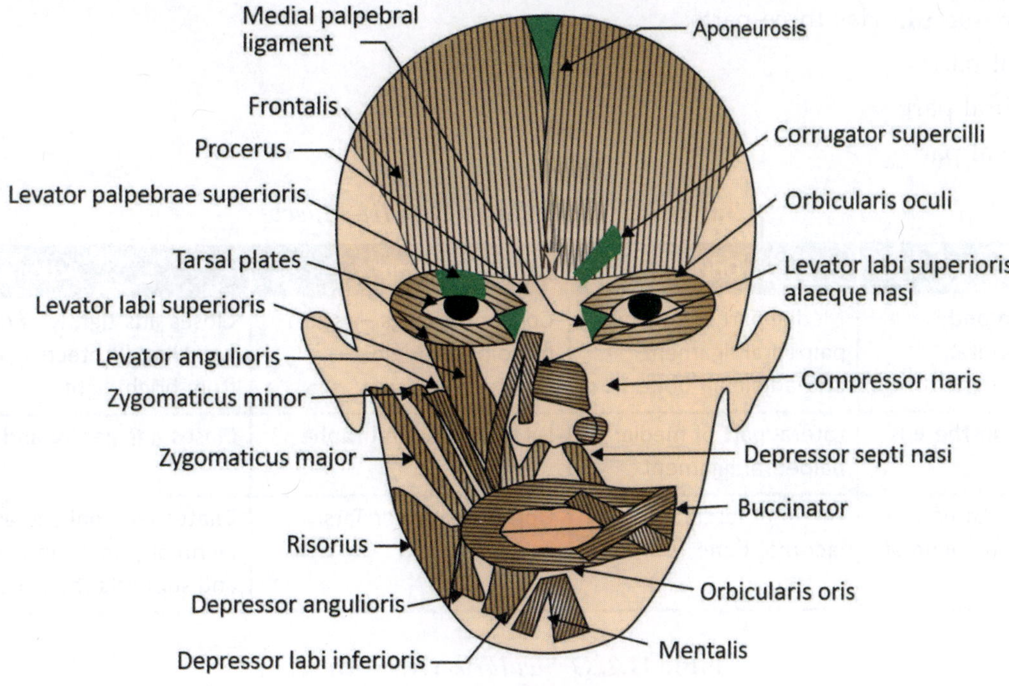

Fig. 11.1: *Facial muscles*

(c) Dilator naris

(d) Dilate nasal aperture

(e) Depressor septias in anger

E. Muscles around the mouth:

(a) Sphincter is – orbicularis oris

(b) Dilators are:

(i) Levator labii superioris – alaequae nasi

(ii) Levator labii superioris

(iii) Levator anguli oris (sadness)

(iv) Zygomaticus minor (contempt)

(v) Zygomaticus major (smiling)

(vi) Depressor labii inferioris

(vii) Depressor anguli oris

(viii) Mentalis

(ix) Buccinator

MUSCLES OF ORBIT

1. Corrugator supercilli:

Origin: Medial end of supercillary arch.

Insertion: Skin of mid eyebrow. (Skin and fascia above the supra orbital margin.)

Function: Draws the eyebrow medially. It forms vertical furrows on the eyebrow and causes the expression of frowning.

2. Levator palpebrae superioris: It is an eye opener.

Origin:

(a) Inferior surface of the lesser wing of the sphenoid bone.

(b) Orbital surface of the body of sphenoid bone anterior to the optic foramen.

Insertion: It expands towards the upper eyelid and divides into superficial and deep layers – are inserted into:

(a) Orbital septum

(b) Palpebral ligaments – medial and lateral

(c) Superior tarsal plate

(d) Skin of the upper eyelid.

- The smooth muscle fibres of this muscle are called as Muller's muscle.
- The aponeurosis of this muscle divides the lacrimal gland into palpebral and orbital parts.

Nerve Supply:

(i) Upper division of oculomotor nerve.

(ii) Sympathetic fibres from T_1 segment of spinal cord supplies smooth muscle fibres.

Action:

- It opposes the action of orbicularis oculi. So it elevates the upper eyelid.
- Paralysis of this muscle causes ptosis.

3. **Orbicularis-occuli:** Has three parts:
   (a) Orbital part
   (b) Palpebral part
   (c) Lacrimal part.

Table 11.1: ***Orbicularis-Occuli – Muscle***

Parts	Origin	Insertion	Action
(a) Orbital on and around orbital margin	Medial part of medial palpebral ligament and adjoining bone	Concentric rings – return to point of origin	Closes lids tightly and wrinkling (Protects eyes from bright light)
(b) Palpebral in the lids	Lateral part of medial palpebral ligament	Lateral palpebral raphe	Closes lids gently and blinking
(c) Lacrimal – Lateral and deep to lacrimal sac	Lacrimal fascia and lacrimal bone	Upper and lower Tarsi	Dilates lacrimal sac and directs lacrimal puncta into lacus lacrimalis and supports the lower lid.

Table 11.2: ***Orbicularis-Oris – Muscle***

Parts	Origin	Insertion	Action
(a) Intrinsic (deepest and thin layer)	Superior – Incisivus from maxilla and inferior incisivus from mandible	Angle of mouth	Closes and purses mouth
(b) Extrinsic two layers	Thickest middle (Buccinator) – Thick superficial – Elevators and Depressors	Lips and angle of mouth	Various types of Grimaces

MUSCLES OF MOUTH

1. **Orbicularis oris:** Has two parts – extrinsic and intrinsic.
2. **Buccinator (Muscle of cheek):** Trumphet muscle. It is pierced by parotid duct.

   Origin: Upper fibres – from maxilla – opposite upper molar teeth. Lower fibres from mandible – opposite lower molar teeth.

   Middle fibres from pterygo mandibular raphe (extending from pterygoid hamulus to mandible).

   Insertion: Upper fibres goes to upper lip, lower fibres goes to lower lip and middle fibres. Decussate before passing to lips (upper and lower lips).

   Action: It compresses the cheek against the teeth and prevents the accumulation of food in the vestibule and help in chewing. It also helps in sucking and blowing the cheek.
3. **The levator labii superiosis alaeque nasi:**

   Origin: Frontal process of maxilla.

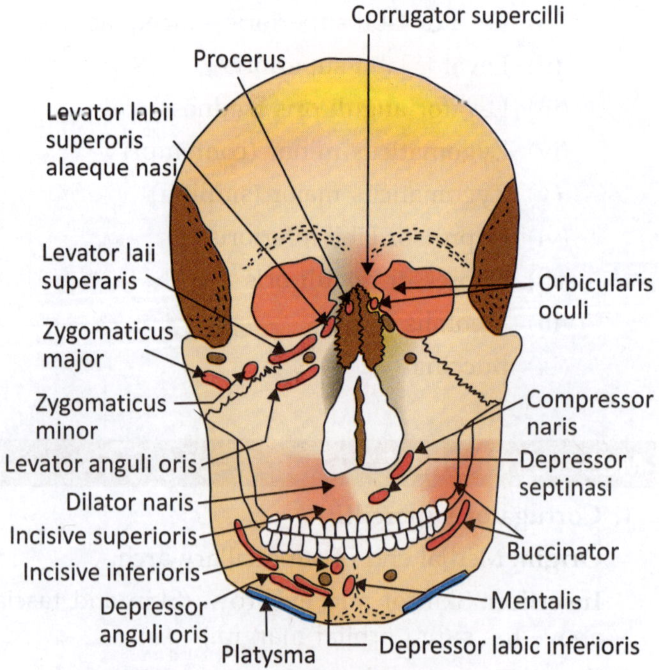

Fig. 11.2: ***Front view of skull showing attachments of facial muscles***

Insertion: It divides into nasal and labial parts:

- Nasal part is medially situated and inserted to the skin and cartilage of the ala of the nose.
- Labial part is laterally situated and is inserted into the orbicularis oris.

Nerve supply: Buccal branch of the facial nerve.

Action: The medial part dilates the nose by lifting the ala of the nose. The lateral part elevates the upper lip.

4. **The levator labii superioris:**

Origin:

(a) Infra orbital margin of the maxilla, above the infra orbital foramen.

(b) Zygomatic bone.

Insertion: Orbicularis oris (upper lip skin)

Nerve supply: Buccal branch of facial nerve.

Action: It elevates and everts the upper lip. Its action is required for the formation of naso labial furrow.

5. **Zygomaticus minor**

Origin: Outer surface of zygomatic bone, behind the zygomatico maxillary suture.

Insertion: Orbicularis oris (skin of upper lip).

Nerve supply: Buccal branch of facial nerve.

Action: It pulls the upper lip upwards and helps in formation of naso labial furrow.

6. **Zygomaticus major (Smiling muscle)**

Origin: Zygomatic bone infront of the zygomatico temporal suture.

Insertion: Orbicularis oris.

Nerve supply: Buccal branch of facial nerve.

Action: Elevation of the angle of the mouth and helps in forming naso labial furrow.

7. **Depressor anguli oris:**

Origin: Oblique line of mandible below buccinator.

Insertion: Blends with the orbicularis oris near the angle of mouth.

Nerve supply: Marginal mandibular branch of facial nerve.

Action: Draws the angle of mouth downwards and laterally.

8. **Depressor labii inferioris:**

Action: Oblique line of mandible near sympysis menti.

Insertions:

(i) Orbicularis oris.

(ii) Skin of the lower lip.

Nerve supply: Marginal mandibular nerve.

Action: Depressor of the lower lip.

9. **Mentalis:**

Origin: Incissive fossa of the mandible.

Insertion: Skin and fascia over the chin.

Action: It draws the lower lip downwards.

Nerve supply: Marginal mandibular nerve.

10. **Risorius (Grining muscle):**

Origin: Fascia covering the parotid gland.

Insertion: Angle of the mouth.

Nerve supply: Buccal branch of facial nerve.

Action: It retracts the angle of the mouth and expresses grining.

MUSCLES OF NOSE – NASALIS

1. **Compressor naris:**

Origin: Anterior surface of the maxilla, lateral to the nasal notch.

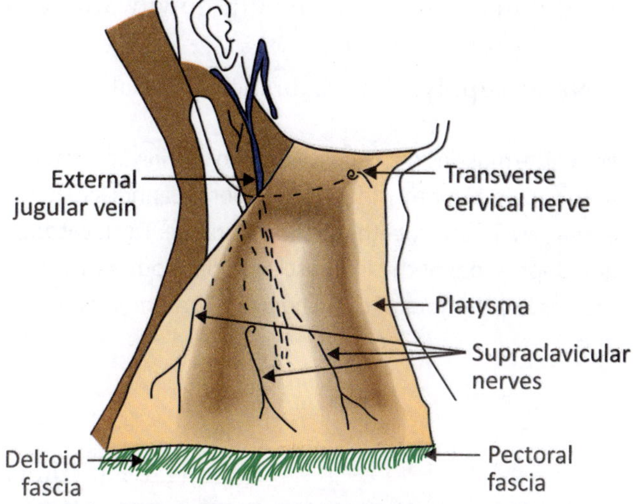

Fig. 11.3: *Platysma – neck muscle (subcutaneous plane)*

Insertion: Muscles of both sides meet along the bridge of the nose.

Action: It compresses the nose and reduces the size of the anterior nasal opening.

2. **Dilator naris:**

Origin: Anterior surface of maxilla inferior to origin of compressor naris.

Insertion: Ala of the nose.

Action: Dilates the nasal apperture.

3. **Depressor septi nasi**

Origin: Anterior surface of maxilla below the nasal notch near the midline.

Insertion: Septum of nose.

Nerve supply: Buccal branch of facial nerve.

Action: Helps in widening the nasal opening, i.e., dilates.

MUSCLE OF NECK

Platysma:

Origin: Upper part of pectoral and deltoid fascia below clavicle, fibres run upwards and medially for insertion.

Insertion: Anterior fibres – base of mandible, posterior fibres – skin of lower face and lip continuous with risorius.

Actions:

- Releases pressure of skin on veins
- Depresses mandible
- Pulls angle of the mouth downwards as in horror or surprise.

Nerve supply: Cervical branch of facial nerve.

Note: The muscle knot known as modiolus lying 1 cm lateral to the angle of mouth. Intersecting fibres cannot slip here as they are bound together by fibrous tissue. The levatores and depressors of the lip muscles radiate outward from the lips like the spokes of a wheel and form modiolus.

FACIAL NERVE TESTING

1. **Frontalis:** Look upwards without moving head, presence of normal horizontal wrinkles on forehead.
2. **Corrugator supercilli:** Frowning and making vertical wrinkles on forehead.
3. **Orbicularis oculi:** Tight closure of eyes.
4. **Orbicularis oris:** Whistling and pursing the mouth.
5. **Dilators of mouth:** Showing teeth.
6. **Buccinator:** Puffing the mouth and then blowing forcibly.

Platysma: Forcible pulling the angle of mouth – downwards and backwards. Prominent vertical fold on side of neck skin.

SENSORY OR CUTANEOUS NERVES OF FACE

Supplied by branches of trigeminal nerve and C_2 and C_3 of cervical plexus.

A. Ophthalmic Division (V_1): Branches are:

(a) Frontal branch:

(i) Supratrochlear nerve: Supply medial part of upper eyelid, forehead and skin of scalp medially.

(ii) Supra orbital nerve: Supply upper eyelid medially, forehead and skin of scalp upto vertex and conjunctiva.

(b) Lacrimal branch:

Lacrimal nerve: Supply upper eyelid laterally and conjunctiva.

(c) Nasociliary branch

(i) Infra trochlear nerve: Supply upper eyelid medially and skin of root of nose.

Table 11.3: Functional Groups of Facial Muscles

S.No.	Opening	Sphincter	Dilators
A.	Palpebral fissure	Orbicularis oculi	1. Levator palpebrae supererioris 2. Occipito frontalis (frontal belly)
B.	Oral fissure	Orbicularis oris	All muscles arround the mouth except orbicularis oris and mentalis (muscles of upper and lower lips)
C.	Nostrils	Compressor naris	1. Dilator naris 2. Depressor septi 3. Medial slip of levator labii superioris alaeque nasi.

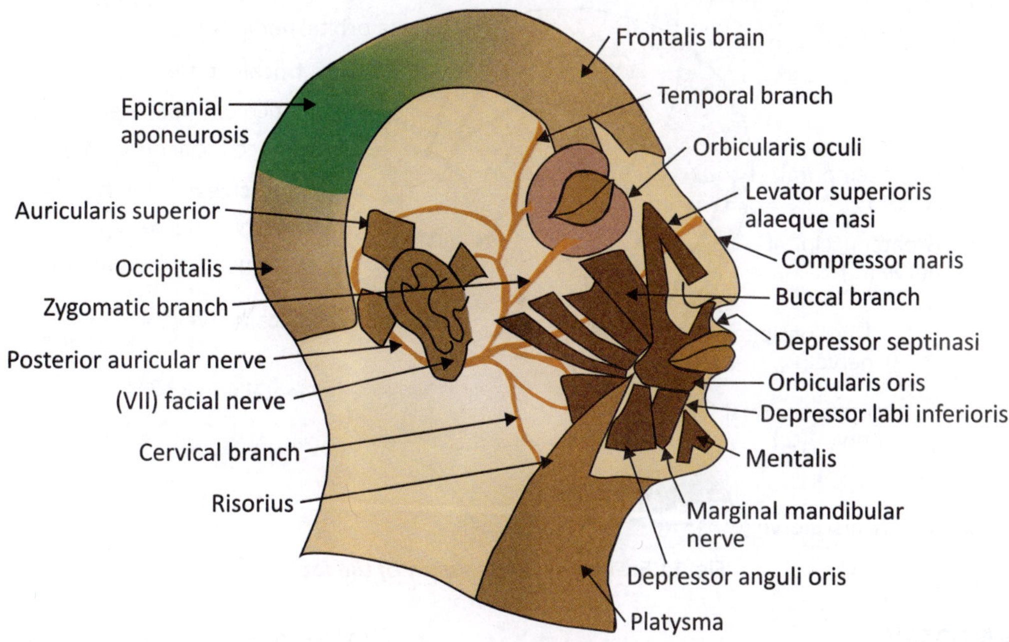

Fig. 11.4: ***Facial muscles and its nerve supply***

(ii) **Extrernal nasal nerve:** Supplies skin of dorsum of nose upto ala and tip of nose.

Area of Distribution:

- Scalp upto vertex
- Forehead
- Upper eyelid
- Conjunctiva of eyeball (Bulbar conjunctiva)
- Root, dorsum and tip of nose.

B. Maxillary Division (V_2): Branches are:

1. **Infra orbital nerve:** Nasal cavity, lower eyelid, maxillary air sinus, upper lip
2. **Zygomatico facial nerve:** Supply – skin of cheek
3. **Zygomatico temporal nerve:** Supplies skin of anterior temporal region.

Area of Distribution:

- Upper lip – mucous membrane and gums
- Palate – upper gums and teeth
- Side and ala of nose
- Lower eyelid
- Upper part of cheek – mucous membrane, gums and teeth of upper jaw
- Anterior part of temple.

C. Mandibular Division (V_3): Branches are:

1. Auriculo temporal nerve
2. Buccal nerve
3. Mental nerve.

Area of Distribution:

- Lower lip mucous membrane and gingiva near lower lip
- Chin
- Lower part of cheek – mucous membrane and gums
- Lower jaw except over angle and lower margin
- Upper 2/3 of lateral surface of auricle
- Side of head (temporal region).

D. Cervical Plexus: Branches are:

1. Anterior division of great auricular nerve (C_2, C_3)
2. Upper division of transverse (anterior) cutaneous nerve of neck (C_2 and C_3).

Area of Distribution:

- Skin over the angle of jaw.
- Skin over the parotid gland.
- Skin of lower margin of lower jaw.

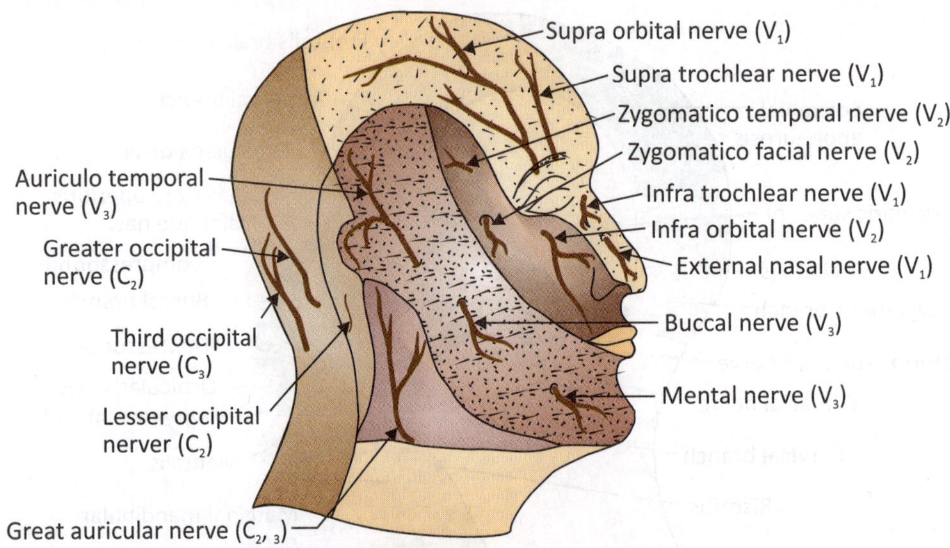

Fig. 11.5: *Sensory nerve supply of the face*

APPLIED ANATOMY

1. **Headache is common symptom in**
   - Common cold, boils on nose
   - Para nasal air sinuses (sinusitis)
   - Infection of teeth and gums
   - Eyes – refractive error, glaucoma
   - Meningitis etc. (supra tentorial part of duramater including lining of anterior and middle cranial fossa).

Clinically: Facial nerve is examined by testing facial muscles action.

Motor nerve supply of face is by facial nerve (VIIth nerve).

Branches of facial nerve in parotid gland:
- Temporal branch
- Zygomatic branch
- Buccal branch – upper and lower
- Mandibular branch
- Cervical branch.

In infra-nuclear lesion of VIIth nerve (Bell's palsy) whole of the face is paralyzed.
- Face becomes asymmetrical and drawn upto normal side.
- Affected side is motion less.
- Wrinkles disappear from forehead.
- Eye cannot be closed.
- Attempt to smile – draws the mouth to normal side.
- During mastication food accumulates between teeth and cheek.
- Articulation of labials is impaired.

In supra-nuclear lesion of VIIth nerve: Hemiplegia.
- Only lower part of face is paralyzed.
- Upper part escapes – due to its bilateral representation in the cerebral cortex (frontails and part of orbicularisoculi).

2. **Trigeminal neuralgia:** Involvement of one or more divisions of trigeminal nerve.

Causes: Attacks of very severe burning and scalding pain along the distribution of affected branch.

Relieved by: Injection of 90% of alcohol into affected division or by sectioning the affected nerve.

ARTERIAL SUPPLY OF FACE

Facial artery branch of external carotid artery in carotid triangle enters on the face at antero inferior angle of masseter muscle after crossing the lower border of mandible crosses the buccinator and reaches the angle of mouth, then runs along the lateral side of nose to reach the medial angle of eye. It is very tortuous, lies in front of facial vein.

Terminates – by anastomosing with the dorsal nasal branch of the ophthalmic artery. Its terminal part is known as angular artery.

Branches of facial artery on face are:

1. Inferior labial – supply lower lip
2. Superior labial – supply upper lip

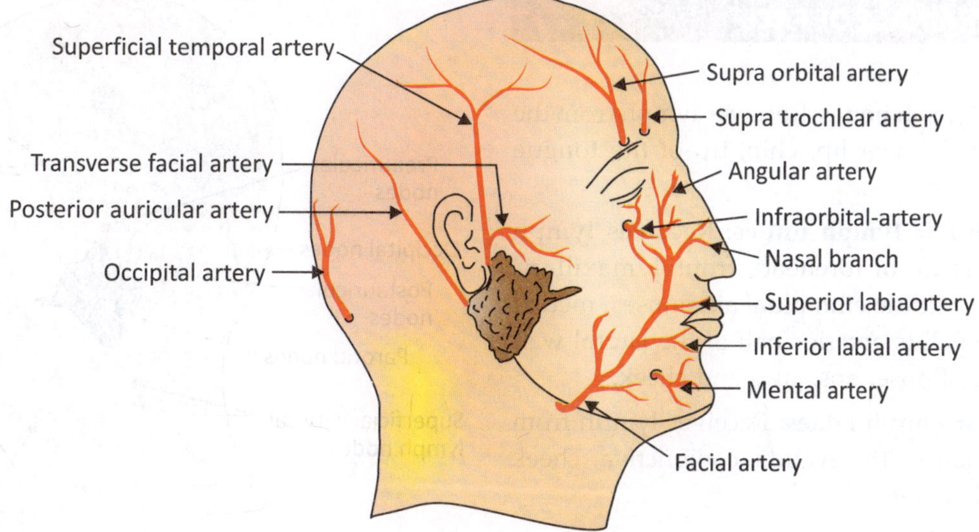

Fig. 11.6: ***Blood supply of face (arterial supply)***

3. Lateral nasal – supply skin of nose
4. Angular artery – skin of medial angle of eye
5. Muscular branches – to muscles of face.

Face develops: From sensory nerve supply of area.

1. **Fronto nasal process:** Ophthalmic branch of trigeminal nerve.
2. **Maxillary process:** Maxillary branch of trigeminal nerve.
3. **Mandibular process:** Mandibular branch of trigeminal nerve.

Muscles of face develops from mesoderm of second pharyngeal arch nerve of this arch is VIIth cranial nerve (facial nerve). So all the facial muscles are supplied by branches of facial nerve.

Venous drainage of face is by facial vein.

Commencement: Supratrochlear and supra orbital veins unite near the medial angle of the eye to form angular vein.

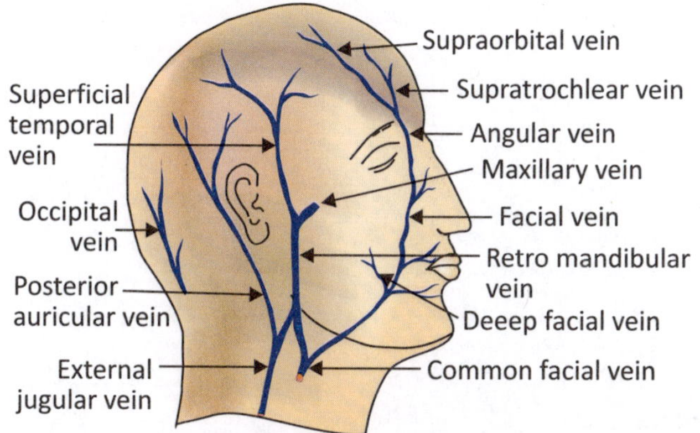

Fig. 11.7: ***Venous drainage of face***

Course: It passes downwards and backwards behind the facial artery. It crosses the antero-inferior angle of the masseter muscle and pierces the deep fascia of neck. It runs superficial to the submandibular gland.

Termination: It terminates by joining the anterior branch of retromandibular vein to form common facial vein, which terminates into internal jugular vein. It doesn't have valves.

DEEP CONNECTIONS

(a) Supra orbital vein communicate with superior ophthalmic vein via a communicating branch.

(b) With pterygoid plexus – via → deep facial vein passes over → Buccinator to → Cavernous Sinus by an emissary vein.

Infection from face → retro grade → thrombosis of cavernous sinus.

DANGEROUS AREA OF FACE

Danger areas of face is upper lip and lower part of nose – tip and philtrum of the nose and ala of nose.

The facial vein communicates with pterygoid venous plexus via deep facial vein. The pterygoid venous plexus communicates with the cavernous sinus via the emissary veins. Hence, infection from the face especially from the dangerous area of face spreads intra cranially and causes meningitis.

LYMPHATIC DRAINAGE OF FACE

Goes to:

1. **Submental lymph nodes:** Receives lymph from the midline of the lower lip, chin, tip of the tongue and related area.
2. **Submandibular lymph nodes:** Receives lymph from the middle of forehead, frontal, maxillary, anterior and middle ethmoidal air sinuses, medial part of the eyelids anterior half of the lateral wall and septum of nose, tips, jaws and cheek.
3. **Pre-auricular lymph nodes:** Receives lymph from the lateral half of the eyelids, conjunctiva, cheek and parotid region.

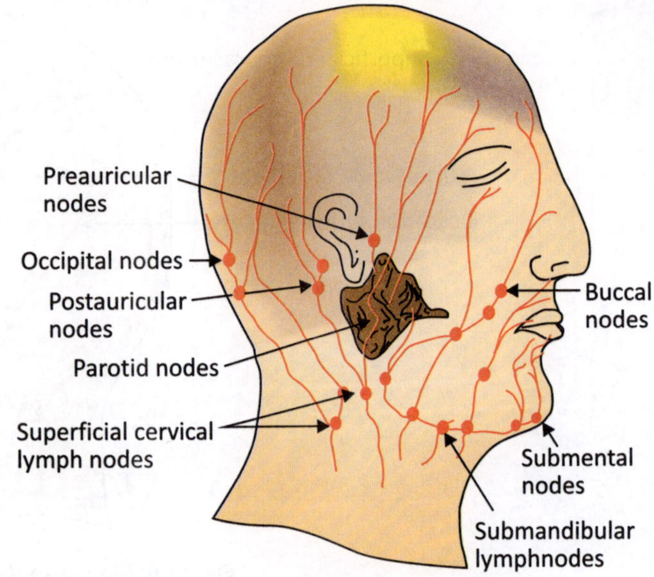

Fig. 11.8: *Lymphatic drainage of face*

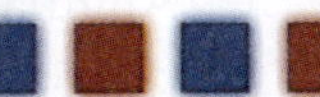

CHAPTER 12

Bony Landmarks of the Back

1. **External occipital protuberance (Inion) –** It is a palpable prominance in the midline.
2. **Superior nuchal line** – extends laterally from the prominance.
3. **External occipital crest** – extends downwards from the prominence in the midline.
4. **Inferior nuchal line** – starts from the mid-point of external occipital crest and runs parallel to superior nuchal line.
5. **Seventh cervical spine (C_7)** – is the first to be felt by the finger running downwards in the midline of the back of neck.
6. **Ligamentum nuchae** – It is a fibrous partition between the muscles of the two sides of the back of neck.
7. **Medial border of scapula** – is one or two inches lateral from the median line, when the arm hangs by the side.
8. **Superior angle of scapula** – overlies the second rib.
9. **Inferior angle of scapula** – overlies the seventh rib.
10. **Iliac crest** – is the bony ridge felt below the waist.
11. **Sacrum** – lies between the posterior ends of the iliac crest.
12. **Highest point of the iliac crest** – lies in the interval between the spines of third and fourth lumbar vertebrae.

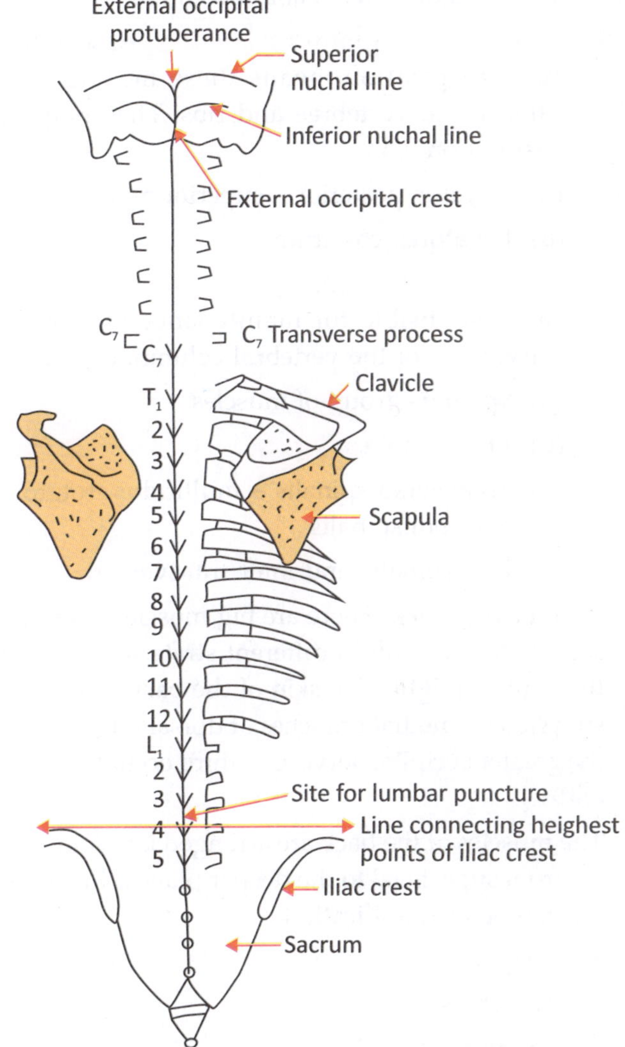

Fig. 12.1: *Bony landmarks of the back*

CLASSIFICATION OF MUSCLES OF BACK

These are classified as:

A. According to their functions are classified into three groups:

(i) **Superficial muscles:** Belong to upper limb, means these muscles are on one side attached to skull or vertebral column and on other side attached to pectoral girdle, i.e., bones of upper limb, e.g.,

(a) Trapezius
(b) Latissimus dorsi
(c) Levator scapulae
(d) Rhomboideus major and minor.

(ii) **Intermediate group of muscles:** Associated with respiration means these muscles are attached to vertebrae and ribs. They help in respiration, e.g.,

(a) Serratus posterior – superior and inferior.
(b) Levatores costarum.

(iii) **Deep or postvertebral group of muscles:** They are responsible for maintenance of normal curvatures of the vertebral column, e.g.,

(a) Splenius group of muscles
(b) Erector spinae
(c) Transverso spinalis – multifidus, rotators and semispinalis
(d) Interspinalis and inter transversari.

Back of the Neck: There are big muscles from the sacrum to the skull in different strata which keep the spine straight. The skin of the back of neck is supplied by medial branches of dorsal rami of C_2 – the greater occipital nerve, C_3 – third occipital nerve and C_4.

B. The muscles of the back are arranged into four layers from superficial to the deeper plane. This is another type of classification.

First layer:

1. Trapezius
2. Latissimus dorsi

Second layer:

1. Splenius:
   (a) Splenius capitis
   (b) Splenius cervicis
2. Levator scapulae
3. Rhomboideus minor and major
4. Serratus posterior superior
5. Serratus posterior inferior.

Third layer:

1. Erector spinae
2. Semispinalis capitis
3. Semispinalis cervicis
4. Semispinalis thoracis.

Fourth layer:

1. Suboccipital muscles
2. Multifidus
3. Inter transversari
4. Interspinalis
5. Rotators.

MUSCLES OF BACK

1. Trapezius: It is a paired muscle, connect the upper limb with vertebral column. Two muscles together resemble a trapezium so it is called trapezius. It forms roof of suboccipital triangle and its lateral margin forms the posterior border of the posterior triangle of the neck. It is large, flat and triangular in shape.

Origins:

(a) Medial 1/3 of superior nuchal line of occipital bone.
(b) External occipital protuberance.
(c) Ligamentum nuchae.
(d) Spines of seventh cervical and all the thoracic vertebrae and corresponding supraspinous ligaments.

Insertions:

(a) **Upper fibres:** Descends downwards laterally and are inserted to posterior border of lateral 1/3 of clavicle.

(b) **Middle fibres:** Directed horizontally and inserted to medial margin of acromion and suprior lip of the crest of spine of scapula.

(c) **Inferior fibres:** Ascends upwards, laterally and inserted to tubercle at the apex of the triangular surface at the medial end of spine, i.e., root of the spine of scapula.

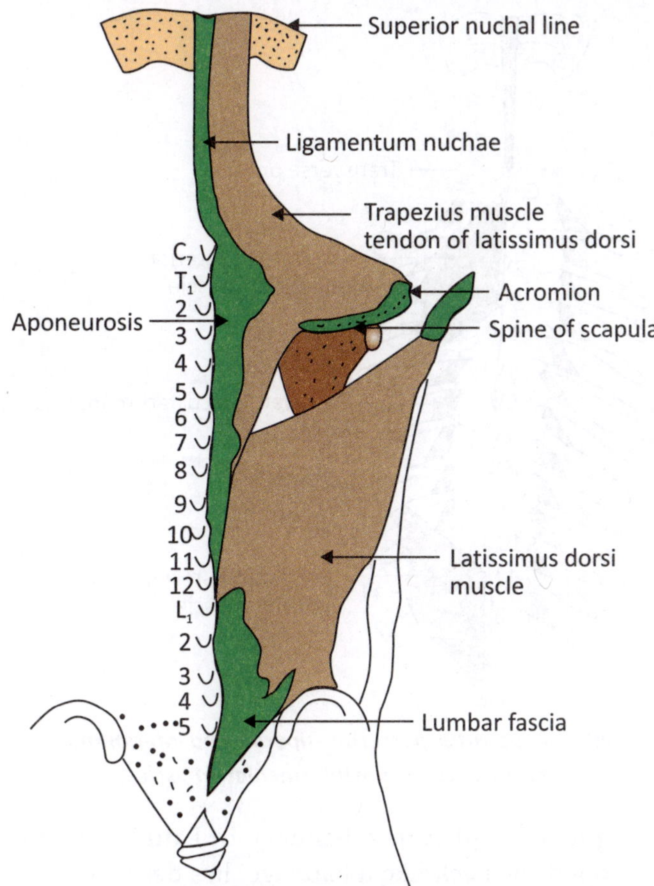

Fig. 12.2: *Superficial muscles of back (trapezius and latissimus dorsi)*

Nerve supply: Subtrapezoid plexus formed by spinal accessory and ventral rami of C_3 and C_4 nerves.

Actions:

1. Both the muscles fix the scapula and controls it during active movements of upper limb.
2. Maintains level and position of shoulder.
3. Elevates the shoulder alongwith levator scapulae.
4. Acting with serratus anterior raises the hand above the head.
5. Braces back the shoulder and retracts the scapula when acting with rhomboids.
6. It suspends the shoulder girdle from skull and vertebral column.

Upper fibres: Elevate the scapula.

Middle fibres: Pull the scapula medially.

Lower fibres: Pull the medial border of scapula downward.

2. **Latissimus Dorsi:** It is large wide flat and triangular thin muscle, extends over lumbar region and lower part of thorax.

Origin: From:

1. Posterior border of posterior part of iliac crest.
2. Lumbar fascia.
3. Spines of lower six thoracic vertebra deep to attachment of trapezius.
4. Lower three or four ribs – outer surface.
5. Few fibres also arise from inferior angle of scapula – posterior surface.

Insertion: Fibres ascends upwards laterally converge into a tendon which wraps round the lower border of teres major muscle and is inserted into the floor of bicipital groove of humerus.

Action: It extends, adducts and medially rotates the arm.

Nerve supply: Thoraco dorsal nerve C_6, C_7 and C_8 branch of posterior cord of brachial plexus.

3. **Levator Scapulae:** It is a thick elongated muscle.

Origin: From posterior tubercles of transverse processes of upper four cervical vertebrae.

Insertion: On medial border of scapula from the upper angle to the spine. The upper most fibres are inserted lowest down.

Nerve supply:

1. Ventral rami of C_3 and C_4.
2. Twigs from dorsal scapular nerve C_5.

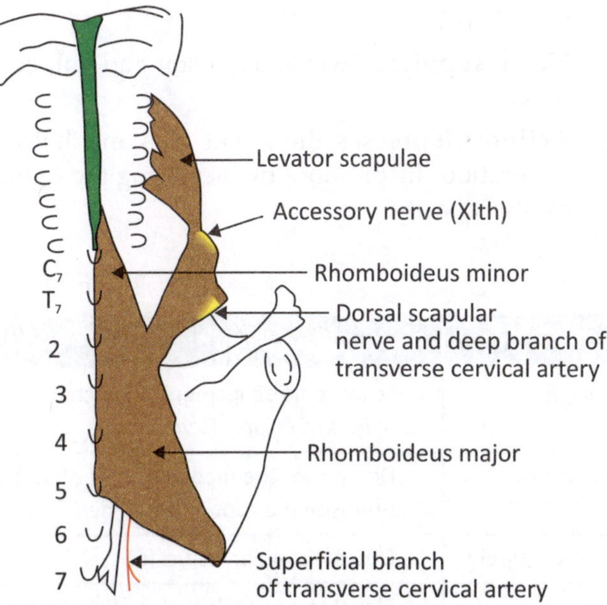

Fig. 12.3: *Levator scapulae and rhomboidei*

Action: Elevation and medial rotation of the scapula (Braces the shoulder backwards).

4. **Rhomboidei:** They expand as parallel bands obliquely downwards and laterally from the spines of the vertebrae to the scapula.
   - Spinal root of accessory nerve accompanied by the superficial branch of transverse cervical artery lies superficial to the levator scapulae and rhomboidei.
   - The dorsal scapular nerve accompanied by the deep branch of the transverse cervical artery lies deep to the levator scapulae and rhomboidei.
5. **Serratus Posterior Superior:** It runs infero laterally.

   Origin:

   (i) Lower part of ligamentum nuchae.

   (ii) Spines of C_7, T_1, T_2 and T_3 vertebrae.

   Insertion: On the outer surface of 2nd, 3rd, 4th and 5th ribs.

   Nerve supply: Second to fourth intercostal nerves.

   Action: Elevates the upper ribs and helps in respiration.
6. **Serratus Posterior Inferior:** It runs supero laterally.

   Origin:

   (i) From spines of T_{11}, T_{12}, L_1 and L_2 vertebrae.

   (ii) Lumbar fascia.

   Insertion: On the outer surface of lower four ribs, i.e., 9th to 12th rib.

   Nerve supply: Lower inter costal and sub costal nerves.

   Action: Depresses the lower ribs and helps in respiration (inspiration) by increasing the thoracic cavity capacity.

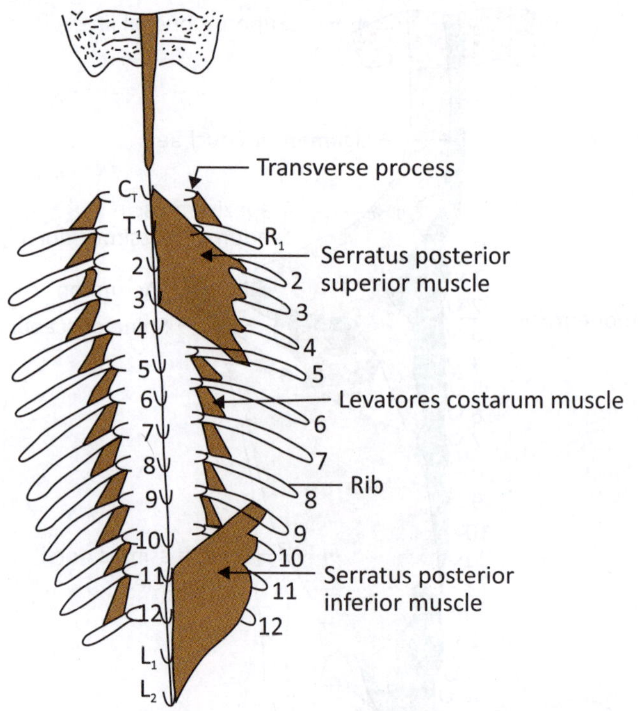

Fig. 12.4: *Serratus posterior superior and inferior and levatores costarum intermediate muscles*

7. **Splenius (splenius = bandage in Latin):** It wraps round the neck like a bandage, lies deep to trapezius and sternocleido mastoid muscle but superficial to semispinalis capitis and levator scapulae. It is divided into two parts, upper part reaching to skull is splenius capitis and lower part remains in the neck called splenius cervicis part.

   (a) Splenius Capitis

   Origin:

   (i) Lower part of ligamentum nuchae.

   (ii) Spines of C_7, T_1, T_2, T_3 and T_4 vertebra.

   Insertions:

   (i) Mastoid process – lateral part.

Table 12.1: *Rhomboidei Muscles*

	Rhomboideus Minor	Rhomboideus Major
Origin	– Lower part of ligamentum nuchae – Spines of C_7 and T_1 vertebra	– Spines of T_2, T_3, T_4 and T_5 vertebrae – Supraspinous ligaments
Insertion	– Dorsum of the medial border of scapula opposite the root of the spine	– Dorsum of the medial border of the scapula from the root of the spine to the inferior angle
Nerve supply	– Dorsal scapular nerve (C5)	– Dorsal scapular nerve (C_5)
Action	– Elevates and pulls the medial border of scapula medially and backwards	– Pulls the scapula upwards and backwards and help in its rotation

(ii) Occipital bone below the superior nuchal line (lateral part).

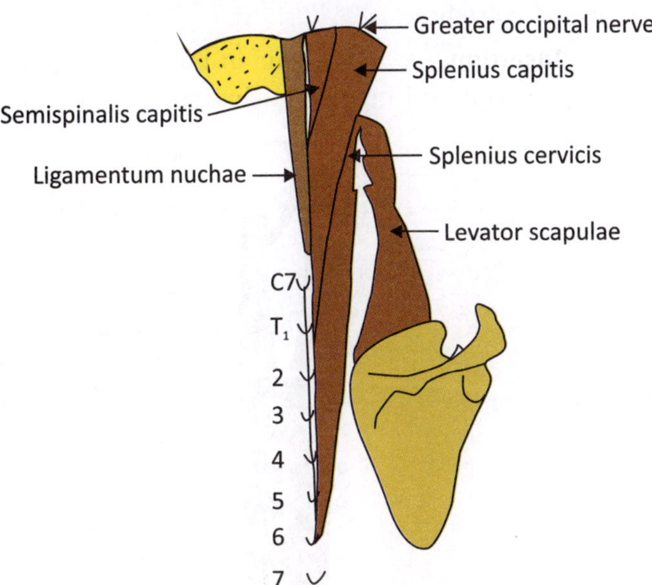

Fig. 12.5: *Deep muscles – splenius muscle*

Nerve supply: Dorsal rami of C_3, C_4 and C_5 nerves.

Action: Extension of head and rotates the face to the same side.

(b) Splenius Cervicis:

Origin: Spines of T_3, T_4, T_5 and T_6 vertebrae.

Insertion: On posterior tubercle of transverse process of upper three or four cervical vertebrae deep to levator scapulae.

Nerve supply: Dorsal rami of C_5, C_6 and C_7 nerves.

Action:

(i) Extensor of the head.

(ii) Turning of the face towards the same side.

- Both parts are acting together.

8. Levators Costarum: Series of 12 pair of muscles.

- Present in the deepest part of thoracic region.
- Helps in respiration.

Origin: From the tips of transverse processes of C_7 vertebra down to eleventh thoracic vertebra.

Insertion: On posterior part of the shaft of the rib below.

9. Erector Spinae (sacro-spinalis): It extends from the sacral region to the head. The breadth of the muscle is from the spines to the angles of the ribs (equal to the breadth of the palm).

Origin:

(i) Median sacral crest

(ii) Sacrotuberous ligament

(iii) Dorsal sacro iliac ligament

(iv) Lateral sacral crest

(v) Dorsal segment of iliac crest

(vi) Spines of all the lumbar vertebrae

(vii) Spines of T_{11} and T_{12} vertebrae

(viii) Ligaments connecting these spines.

Parts: It has three parts: lateral, intermediate and medial part:

(i) Lateral portion called ilio costalis: cervicalis. It divides into:

(a) Ilio costo lumborum

(b) Ilio costo thoracis

(c) Ilio costo cervicis.

(ii) Intermediate portion called longissimus. It is the thickest part and divided into:

(a) Longissimus thoracis

(b) Longissimus cervicis

(c) Longissimus capitis.

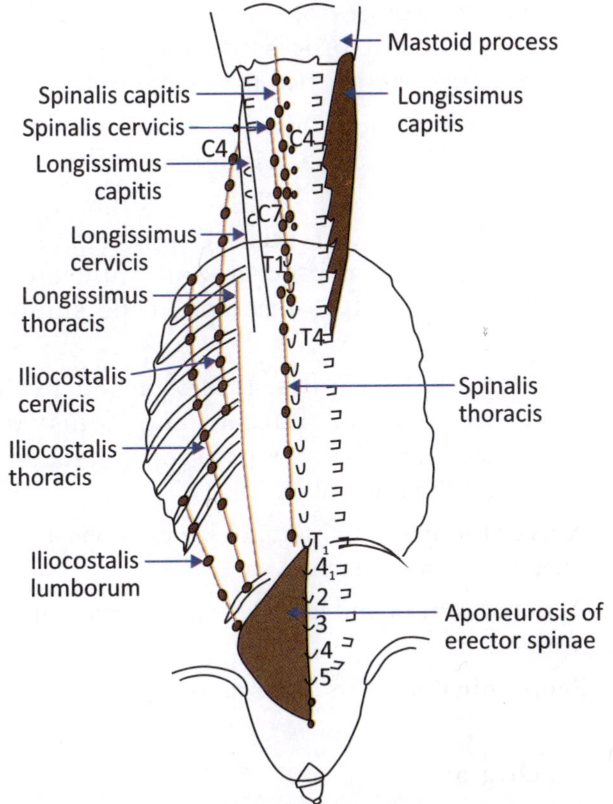

Fig. 12.6: *Deep muscles – erector spinae muscle*

(iii) Medial portion called spinalis and divided into:

(a) Spinalis thoracis

(b) Spinalis cervicis

(c) Spinalis capitis.

Insertions:

(i) Ilio costo lumborum is inserted to the lower six ribs near the angle.

- Ilio costo thoracis originates from the angle of lower six ribs and inserted to the upper six ribs near the angle.
- Ilio costo cervicis originates from the angle of 2-6 ribs. It is inserted to the transverse process of the C_4-C_6 vertebrae.

(ii) Longissimus thoracis: Originates from the accessory process and transverse process of all lumbar vertebrae and thoraco lumbar fascia. It is inserted to the transverse process of all the thoracic vertebrae and lower 9-10 ribs.

Longissimus cervicis: Originates from transverse process of the upper thoracic vertebrae and inserted to the posterior tubercle of transverse process of 2-6 cervical vertebrae.

Longissimus capitis: Originates from the transverse process of upper 4 thoracic vertebrae and articular process of lower 4 cervical vertebrae and inserted to the mastoid process.

(iii) Spinalis thoracis: Originates from spines of T_{11}, T_{12}, L_1, L_2 vertebrae. It is inserted into spinous process of T_1-T_8 vertebrae.

(a) Spinalis cervicis: Originates from ligamentum nuchae and spine of C_7 vertebra. It is inserted to the spinous process of axis.

(b) Spinalis capitis: It is attached to the ligamentum nuchae and joins the semispinalis capitis (area between superior and inferior nuchal lines).

Nerve supply: Dorsal rami of lower cervical, thoracic and lumbar nerves.

Action: Extensor and lateral flexor of vertebral column.

10. Semi Spinalis: It has three parts

(a) Semispinalis capitis:

Origin:

(i) Transverse process of upper 6 thoracic vertebrae.

(ii) Spine of C_7 vertebrae.

(iii) Articular process of 4th, 5th and 6th cervical vertebrae.

Insertion: Occipital bone in the area between superior and inferior nuchal lines.

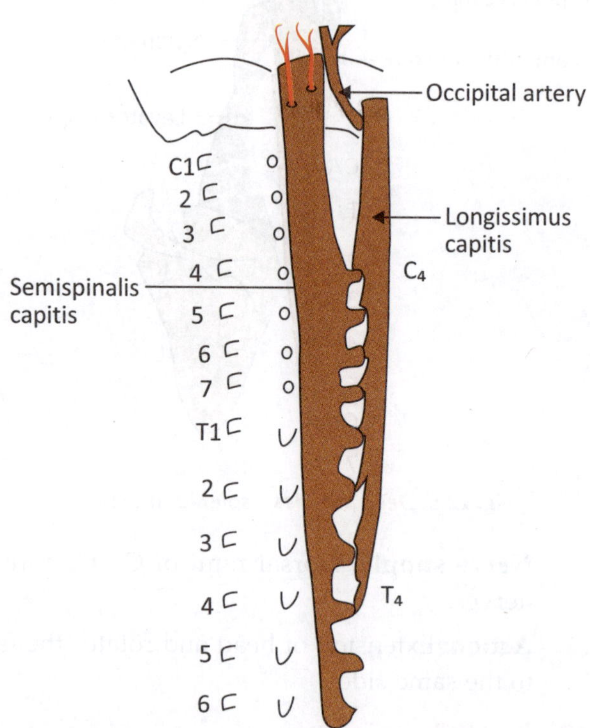

Fig. 12.7: *Semispinalis capitis and longissimus capitis*

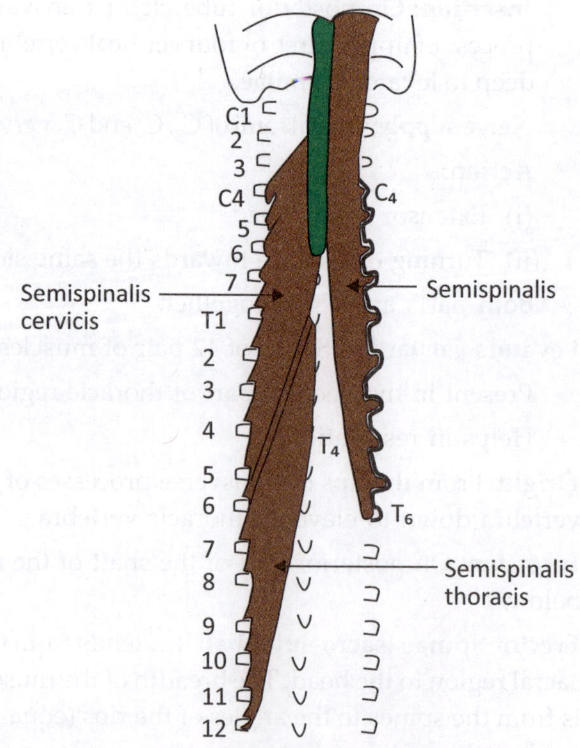

Fig. 12.8: *Deep muscles – semispinalis muscle*

Nerve supply:

(i) Dorsal rami of cervical and thoracic nerves.

(ii) Suboccipital nerve (C_1).

Actions:

(i) Extension of head.

(ii) Rotation of the face towards opposite side.

(b) **Semi spinalis cervicis:**

Origin: Transverse process of T_1-T_6 vertebrae.

Insertion: Spines of C_2-C_6 vertebrae.

Nerve supply: Dorsal rami of cervical and upper thoracic nerves.

Action: Extensor and lateral flexor of the vertebral column.

(c) **Semisphinalis thoracis:**

Origin: Transverse process of T_6-T_{10} vertebrae.

Insertion: Spines of upper 4 thoracic and lower 2 cervical vertebrae.

Action: Extensor of vertebral column and rotates the vertebral column to the opposite side.

11. **Transverso Spinalis:** As the name implies – run from transverse process to spines and are usually oblique and short, arranged in three layers of muscles – semispinalis, rotators and multifidus. Their breadth is equal to the breadth of the thumb.

    Rotators are present only in thoracic region and are eleven on each side, extends from base of transverse process to the root of the spine of the vertebra above. In occipital region they are modified into obliques and recti, forming sub- occipital triangle.

    Multifidus: Extends from upper part of sacrum to the upper part of neck. Fibres slope downwards and medially from the transverse processes to the spines.

12. **Interspinalis:** They are medial connecting spines of adjacent vertebrae. They are poorly developed in the thoracic region.

13. **Inter Transversari:** Join adjacent transverse processes. They are best developed in the cervical and lumbar regions.

14. **Sub-Occipital Muscles:** They are situated deeply, below the occipital bone, in the fourth layer.

(a) **Rectus capitis posterior major:**

Origin: Spine of axis (C_2) fibres are directed upwards and laterally.

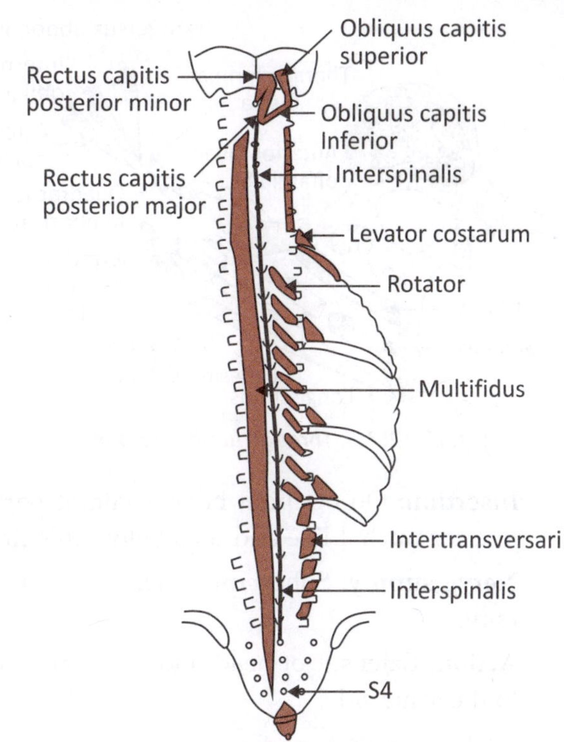

Fig. 12.9: *Deep muscles – multifidus and rotators, intertransversari and interspinalis*

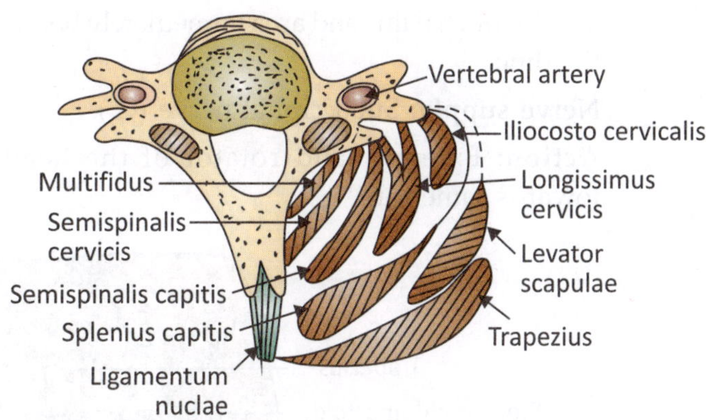

Fig. 12.10: *T.S. Through cervical region*

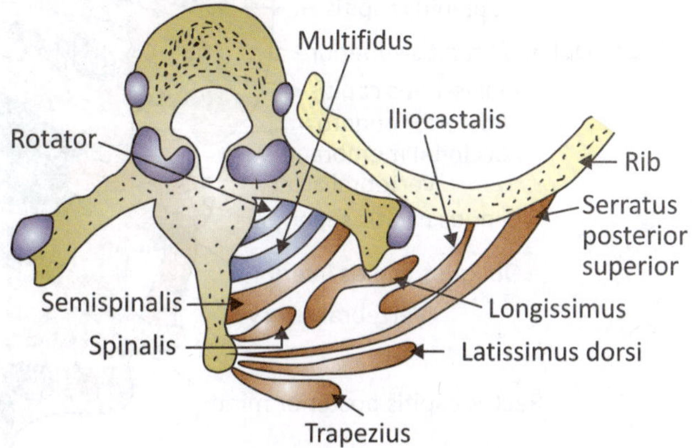

Fig. 12.11: *T.S. Through thoracic region*

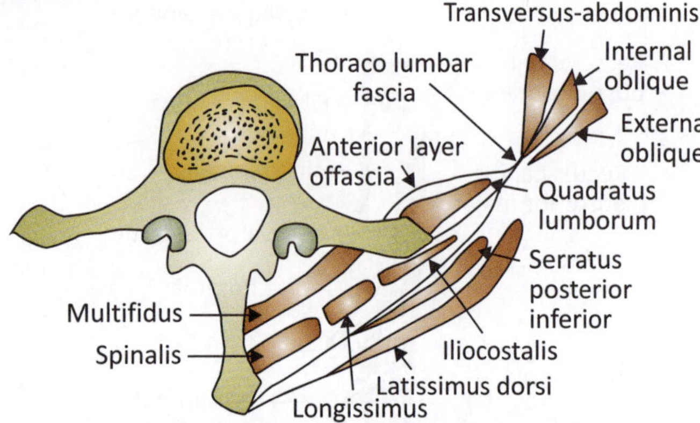

Fig. 12.12: *T.S. Through lumbar region*

Insertion: On occipital bone – lateral part of inferior nuchal line and area below this line.

Nerve supply: Suboccipital nerve (C_1) dorsal rami.

Action: Extensor of head and rotate the head to the same side.

(b) **Rectus capitis posterior minor:**

Origin: Tubercle of posterior arch of atlas (C_1).

Insertion: On occipital bone – medial part of inferior nuchal line and area immediately below this line.

Nerve supply: Suboccipital nerve (C_1).

Action: Extensor and rotator of the head towards same side.

(c) **Obliquus capitis superior:**

Origin: Transverse process of atlas.

Insertion: On occipital bone – area in between the superior and inferior nuchal lines.

Nerve supply: Suboccipital nerve (C_1).

Action: Extensor and rotator of head towards same side.

(d) **Obliquus capitis inferior**

Origin: Spine of axis.

Insertion: Transverse process of atlas.

Nerve supply: Suboccipital nerve (C_1).

Action: Turns the face towards same side.

Suboccipital-Triangle

Situation: It lies in the muscles of fourth layer of back, just below the occipital bone.

Boundaries

Medial – Rectus capitis posterior major

Above and lateral – Obliquus capitis superior.

Below and lateral – Obliquus capitis inferior.

Roof – Semi-spinalis capitis and longissimus capitis.

Floor is formed by posterior arch of atlas and posterior atlanto occipital membrane.

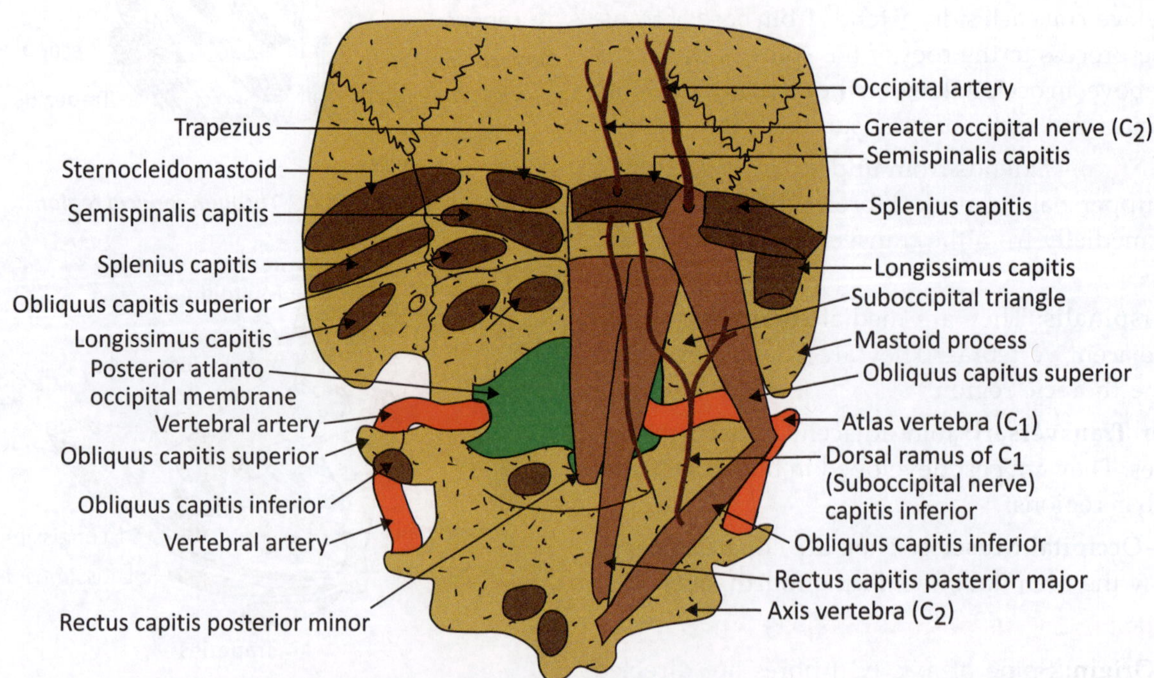

Fig. 12.13: *Boundaries and contents of suboccipital triangle Suboccipital triangle*

Contents are:

1. Suboccipital nerve (Dorsal rami of C_1)
2. Third part of vertebral artery
3. Suboccipital plexus of veins
4. Dense connective tissue.

The vertebral artery grooves the posterior arch of the atlas.

- The suboccipital nerve intervenes between them.
- Vertebral artery enters the cranial cavity either through the lateral border or it may pierce the posterior atlanto occipital membrane.
- The suboccipital nerve communicates with the greater occipital nerve (C_2, C_3) and supplies muscles of suboccipital triangle.
- The occipital artery crosses lateral boundary of the triangle.
- The greater occipital nerve (C_2, C_3) winds round the obliquus capitis inferior and crosses along the roof of the triangle.

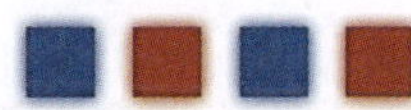

CHAPTER 13

Orbit and Eyeball

BONY ORBIT

Orbit are paired pyramidal cavities situated one on each side of the root of nose. Each orbit lodges one eyeball and it's associated structures.

Parts: It has

- Apex
- Base
- Medial walls are parallel to each other.
- Lateral walls are at right angle to each other.
- Roof
- Floor.

Base is formed by orbital margin.

- **Superiorly:** Frontal bone has a notch or foramen supra orbital notch or foramen.
- **Laterally:** Zygomatic bone and frontal bone.
- **Medially:** Maxilla and frontal bone.
- **Inferiorly:** Zygomatic and maxilla bone.

Apex: It is formed by superior orbital fissure.

Medial wall: Formed by

1. Formed by frontal process of maxilla.
2. Lacrimal bone.
3. Ethmoid bone (labyrinth).
4. Body of sphenoid.

- Lacrimal fossa present in it and lodges lacrimal sac.

Lateral wall: Formed by:

1. Zygomatic bone.
2. Greater wing of sphenoid
   - Whitnall's tubercle present along it's anterior part it gives attachment to lateral check ligament.

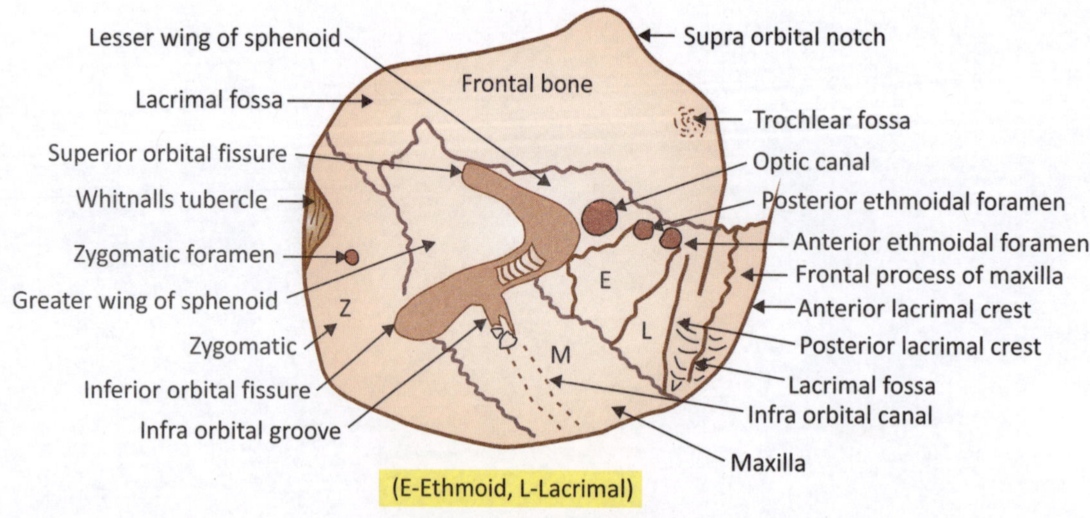

Fig. 13.1: *Orbit-bony features*

- Suspensary ligament of lock wood – Lateral palpebral raphe.
- Levator palpebrae superioris.
- Inferior orbital fissure present between floor and lateral wall.
- Superior orbital fissure present between roof and lateral wall.

Roof:

- Orbital surface of frontal bone.
- Lesser wing of sphenoid.
- Laterally lacrimal fossa is present which lodges lacrimal gland.

Floor: Orbital surface of maxilla, zygomatic bone, greater wing of sphenoid and orbital process of palatine bone.

RELATIONS OF ORBIT

- **Superiorly:** Anterior cranial fossa
- **Inferiorly:** Maxillary air sinus
- **Medially:**
  - Ethmoidal air sinuses
  - Sphenoid air sinus
- **Laterally:**
  - Temporal fossa
  - Middle cranial fossa

Openings in the Orbit

1. **Anteriorly it opens on the face.**
2. **Posteriorly, through infra orbital groove:** Via inferior orbital fissure opens into pterygo palatine fossa. Infra orbital nerve and vessels along with an emissary vein pass through it.
3. **Superior orbital fissure:** This opens into middle cranial fossa. It is divided into three parts by a common tendinous ring:
   (a) **Supero lateral compartment:** This is lateral to ring and transmits – lacrimal nerve, trochlear nerve, frontal nerve, superior ophthalmic vein and recurrent meningeal artery.
   (b) **Intermediate compartment:** (within the ring) it transmits upper and lower divisions of oculomotor nerve (IIIrd nerve), nasociliary nerve (V_1) and abducent nerve.
   (c) **Infero medial compartment:** This lies medial to ring and transmits inferior ophthalmic vein.
4. **Optic foramen:** This opens into cranial cavity, transmits optic nerve (IInd) and ophthalmic artery.
5. **Zygomatico temporal and facial foramina:** This transmits zygomatico temporal and facial nerve and vessels.
6. **Anterior and posterior ethmoidal foramina:** This transmits anterior and posterior ethmoidal nerve and vessels.
7. Medial wall has fossa for lacrimal sac via naso lacrimal duct it opens into nasal cavity.

ORBITAL FASCIA (TENON'S CAPSULE)

- Thick fascia derived from periosteum of orbital bones. This extends from sclero corneal junction to the entery of the optic nerve on the back.
- Orbital fascia is loosely attached to sclera. It forms the socket for eyeball in which eyeball moves. Inferiorly it becomes thick and forms the suspensary ligament of Lockwood.
- Tendons of ocular muscles pierce the capsule and are attached to sclera.
- A sleeve of fascia is continued over muscles as facial sheath.
- Where medial and lateral recti pierce the fascia it forms strong check ligaments which are attached to Whitnall's tubercle laterally and a posterior compartment lodges the retrobulbar strurctures.

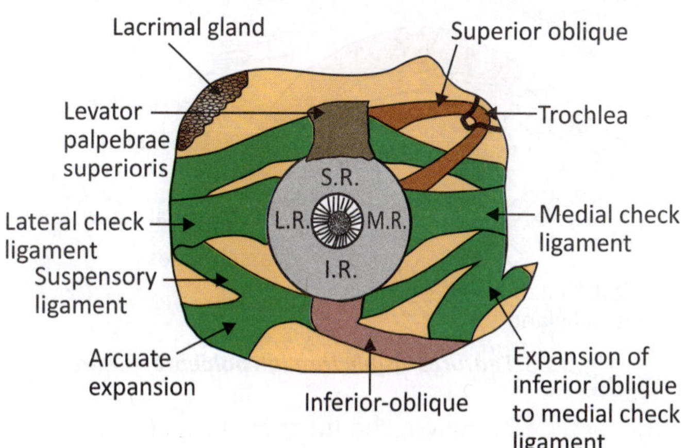

Fig. 13.2: *Fascia bulbi (Tenon's capsule)*

EYELIDS OR PALPEBRAE

Eyelids are movable curtains found in front of the eye. The upper eyelid is longer and more movable than the lower eyelid. The space between two eyelids is known as palpebral fissure. The eyelids meet along the lateral and medial angles of the eye. The lower border of the upper eyelid crosses the upper border of the cornea. The deep surface of the eyelids are lined by the conjunctiva. When the eyelids are separated the conjunctival sac is open. When the lids are closed the conjunctival sac is a closed sac or chamber.

FEATURES ON EYELIDS

When eyes are open few things are noted:

1. **Lacrimal caruncle:** A small triangular space in the medial part called Lacus Lacrimalis – with a reddish, fleshy elevation in the centre – called lacrimal caruncle.
2. **Plica semilunaris:** A small semilunar fold of conjunctiva present lateral to lacrimal caruncle.
3. **Margins of eyelids:** These are divided into two parts –
   (a) **Ciliary part:** This is lateral 5/6th part and is flat having eyelashes or cilia.
   (b) **Lacrimal part:** This is medial 1/6th part and is smooth devoid of eyelids.
4. **Lacrimal papilla:** At the junction of these two parts of eyelid margin, there is a small conical projection called lacrimal papilla. On the summit of papilla a small aperture is present known as Lacrimal Punctum.

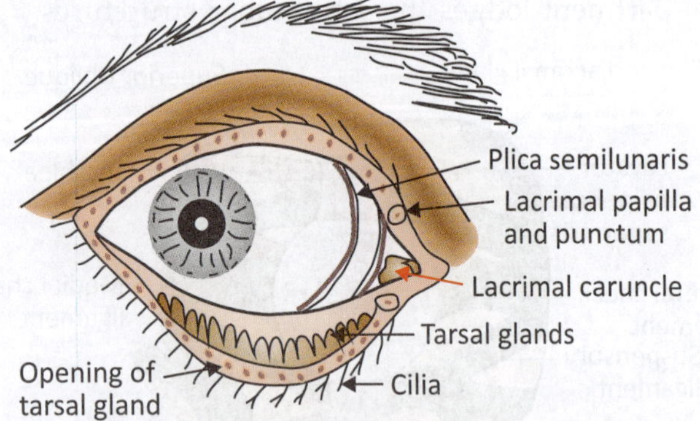

Fig. 13.3: *Features visible through palpebral fissure*

5. **Tarsal glands:** On the inner surface of eyelids – a number of yellowish parallel streaks of tarsal glands are seen whose ducts open on the posterior margin of the eyelids. The cilia project from the anterior edge.

LAYERS OF EYELIDS

1. **Skin** is the outer layer, thin and loosely attached to underlying tissue. At lower and outer border hairs are arranged in two or more rows. Along the roots of hair there are sebaceous glands called Zeis glands are present. The lid margin has well developed sweat glands called gland of Moll.
2. **Superficial fascia:** This is almost devoid of fat and contains loose areolar tissue.
3. **Muscular layer:** It is formed by orbicularis oculi (sphincter) and palpebral part of Muller muscle is found in both eyelids. But levator palpebrae superioris is found only in the upper eyelid, this is called opener of the eye.

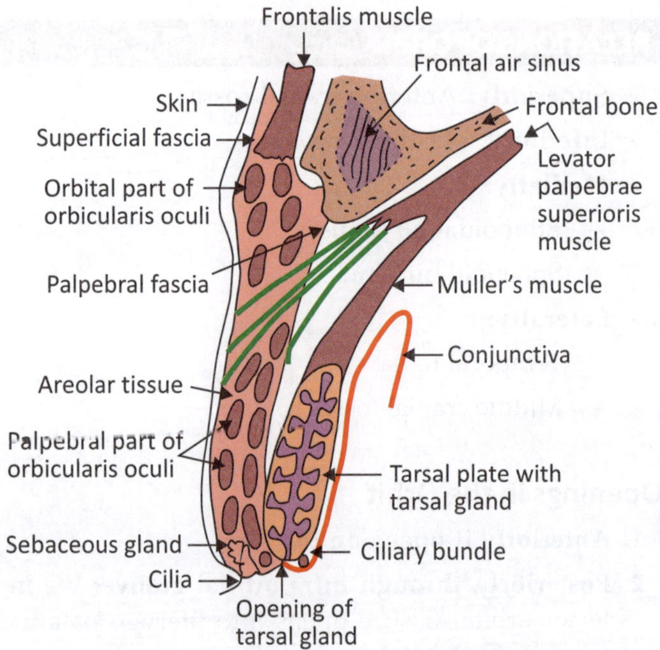

Fig. 13.4: *Structure of eyelid–seen in section*

4. **Orbital septum:** It is made up of fibrous membranous sheath attached to the upper and lower borders of the orbital margin. It is thickened anteriorly and forms tarsal plate.

   Laterally it is connected by the lateral palpebral ligament and medially by medial palpebral ligament. Borders of the tarsal plate contain 30 to 40 sebaceous glands known as Meibomian glands which lie in grooves on the deep surface of the tarsal plates parallel to each other in a single row.

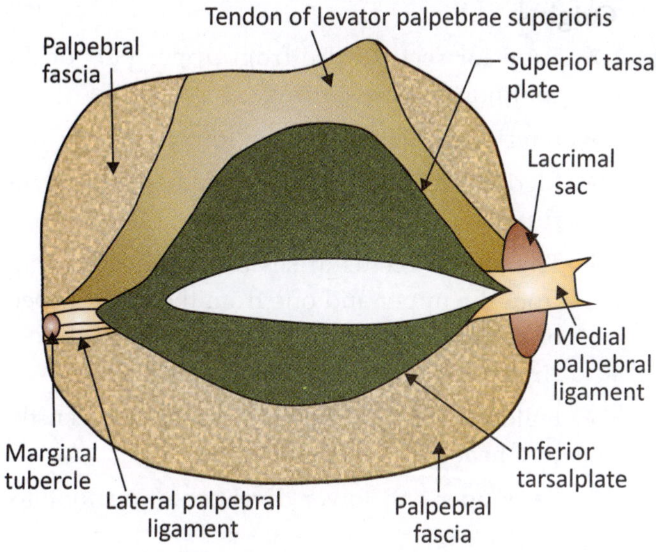

Fig. 13.5: ***Orbital septum***

Palpebral fascia is a layer of connective tissue attached to the orbital margins and extending into the eyelids to become continuous with the tarsus.

5. **Conjunctiva:** It is made up of non-keratinized stratified squamous epithelium and is transparent vascular mucous membrane. It lines the upper surface of the lower eyelid and lower surface of the upper eyelid. At the fornices conjunctiva is reflected over the front of eye (sclera) and extends upto the corneal margin.

NERVE SUPPLY

1. **Upper eyelid** is supplied by branches of lacrimal, supra orbital, supratrochlear and infra trochlear nerves.
2. **Lower eyelid** is supplied by palpebral branch of infra orbital nerve.
3. Same nerves supply the conjuctiva that lines each eyelid.

BLOOD VESSELS

Both eyelids are supplied by palpebral branches of the ophthalmic artery. Lower eyelid has an additional supply by palpebral branch of infra orbital artery.

VEINS

Follow the course of arteries and drains into superior and inferior ophthalmic veins and infra orbital vein.

LYMPHATIC DRAINAGE

Lateral part of eyelids drain into preauricular lymphnodes and medial part of lids drain into buccal and submandibular group of lymph nodes.

Applied Anatomy

1. **Blepharitis:** Chronic inflammation of the eyelid margins.
2. **Stye (Hardeolum externum):** Acute inflammation of the lid margin and glands of hair follicles, i.e., Zeis glands.
3. **Chalazion:** It is a chronic granulomatous inflammation of the Meibomian gland (Tarsal glands).
4. **Entropeon:** Inward tilting of the eyelid margins along with eye lashes (inversion).
5. **Ectropion:** It is the eversion of the lid margin.
6. **Ptosis:** This may be congenital or acquired drooping of the upper eyelid due to paralysis of the levator palpebrae superioris.

CONTENTS OF ORBIT

1. Eyeball
2. Extra ocular muscles of eyeball
3. Lacrimal apparatus
4. Orbital fascia
5. Ophthalmic artery and its branches
6. Superior and inferior ophthalmic veins
7. Central vein of retina
8. Ciliary ganglion
9. Optic, oculomotor, trochlear, ophthalmic and maxillary division of trigeminal and abducent nerves.
10. Sympathetic plexus around the arteries.
11. Orbital pad of fat and lymphatics.

1. EYEBALL

Anterior $1/6^{th}$ is cornea which is transparent, posterior $5/6^{th}$ is sclera – which is opaque made-up white fibrous sheath.

- Antero posterior diameter is 24 mm.
- Optic nerve enters through optic disc – which lies 3 mm medial to posterior pole.
- Macula lies on posterior pole and has maximum visual acuity due to collection of cones in the retina.

2. EXTRA OCULAR MUSCLES OR MUSCLES OF THE ORBIT

Within the orbit there are four recti, two oblique and one levator palpebrae superioris are situated.

Recti muscles are:

(a) Superior rectus
(b) Inferior rectus
(c) Medial rectus and
(d) Lateral rectus.

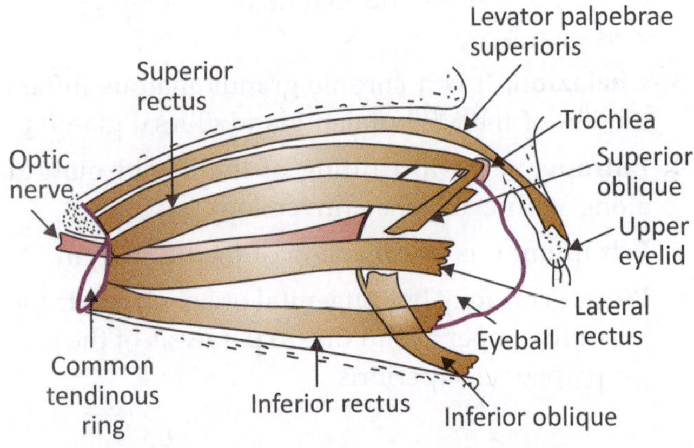

Fig. 13.6: *Extrinsic muscles of the eyeball*

All rectus muscles: Originate from the common tendinous ring, which is situated around the superior, medial and inferior borders of the optic foramen.

Origins:

- Superior rectus arise from upper part of the common tendinous ring.
- Inferior rectus arises from lower part of ring.
- Medial rectus arises from medial part of the ring.
- The lateral rectus arises by two heads – one from the upper and one from the lower aspect of the lateral part of the common tendinous ring.
- Following structures are passing between the two heads of the lateral rectus
  - Upper and lower divisions of oculomotor nerve.
  - Nasociliary nerve.
  - Abducent nerve.
- From the origin recti muscles widen forwards and form the cone of muscles.

Insertion: They are inserted to the corresponding surface of the sclera, behind the corneal margin at the various distances, ranging from 6.5 mm to 8 mm away.

Nerve supply:

- Superior rectus is supplied by upper division of oculomotor nerve.

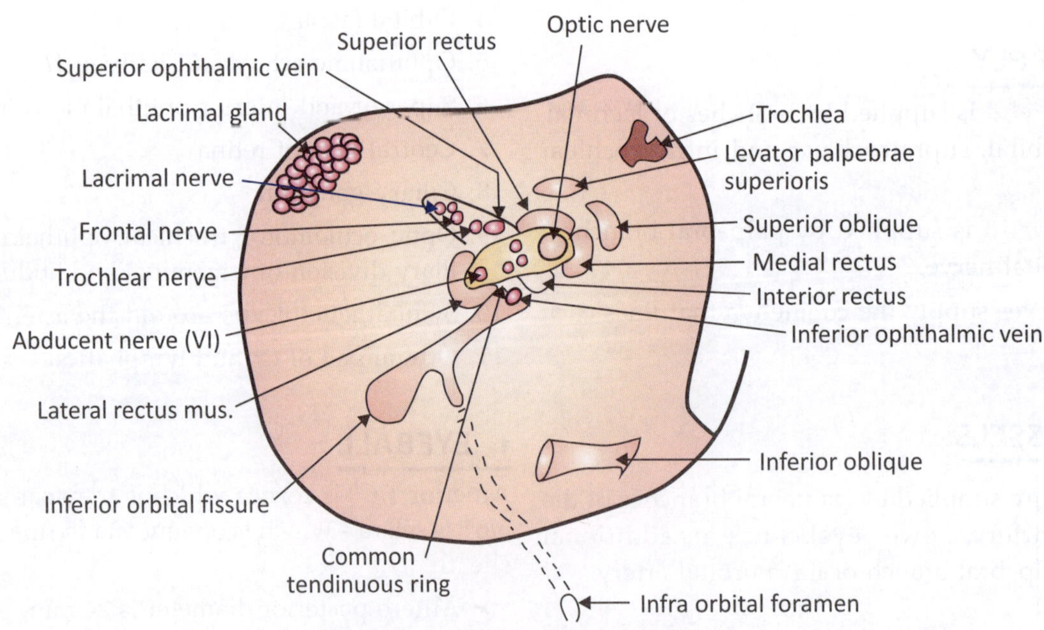

Fig. 13.7: *Origin of orbital muscles*

- Medial rectus and inferior rectus are supplied by inferior division of oculomotor nerve.
- The lateral rectus is supplied by the abducent nerve.

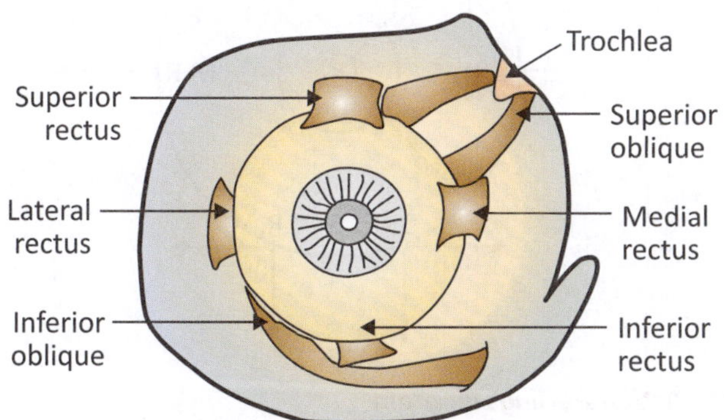

Fig. 13.8: *Insertion of orbital muscles*

Actions:

- **Lateral rectus:** Moves the cornea horizontally and laterally.
- **Medial rectus:** Moves the cornea horizontally and medially.
- **Superior rectus:** Moves the cornea upwards and slightly medially.
- **Inferior rectus:** Moves the cornea downwards and slightly medially.

Superior Oblique Muscle

Origin: It arises from orbital surface of the body of sphenoid bone above and medial to optic foramen and inferior surface of lesser wing of sphenoid bone.

Course and insertion: Superior oblique muscle forms a tendon, which winds round the fibro cartilagenous pulley like trochlea and expands for insertion on the upper surface of the sclera, which lies below the insertion of superior rectus muscle, and behind the equator.

Nerve supply is by trochlear nerve, i.e., 4th cranial nerve.

Action: It rotates the eyeball downwards and laterally.

Inferior Oblique Muscle

Origin: It arises from upper surface of floor of the orbit, lateral to the lacrimal groove.

Insertion: On lateral surface of the sclera behind the equator.

Action: It rotates the eyeball – upwards and laterally.

Movements of the Eyeball

Occurs on three axis:

I. Vertical axis of movement:

(a) Adduction:

- Main adductor is medial rectus.
- Accessory adductors are superior rectus and inferior rectus.

(b) Abduction:

- Main abductor is lateral rectus.

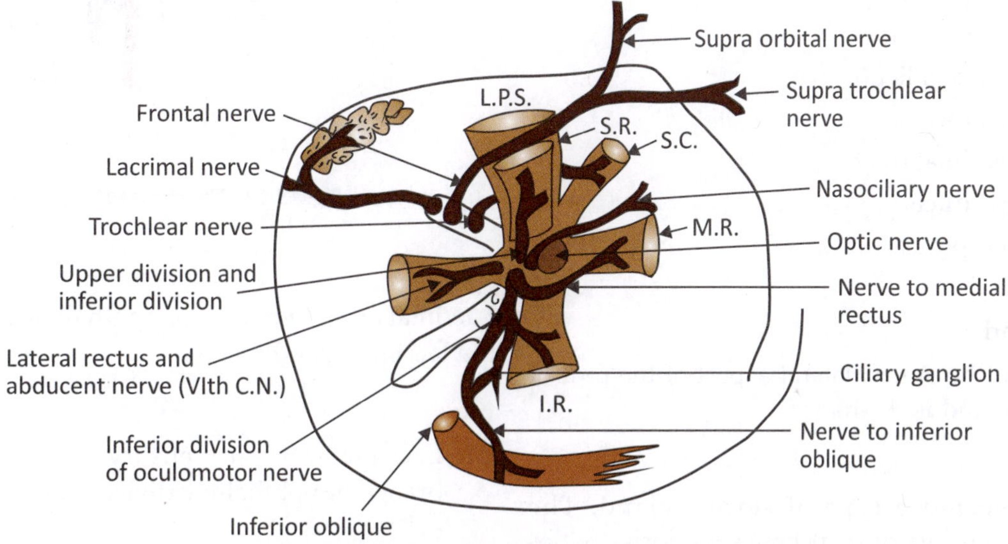

Fig. 13.9: *Nerve supply of the orbital muscles*

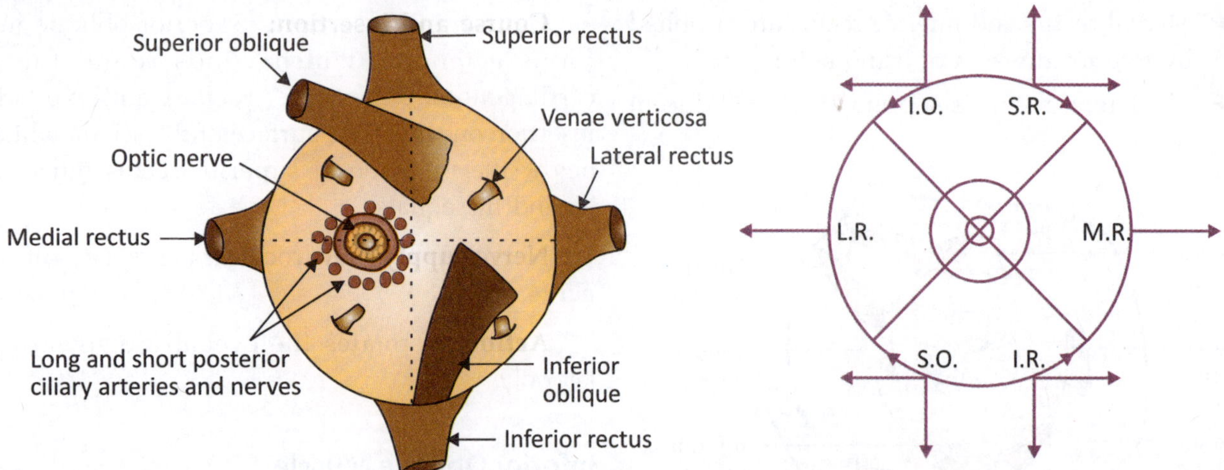

Fig. 13.10: *Insertion of ocular muscles – Action starlings diagram*

- Accessory abductors are superior oblique and inferior oblique.

II. Transverse axis movements

(a) **Elevation:** Superior rectus and inferior oblique.

(b) **Depression:** Inferior rectus and superior oblique.

III. Antero posterior axis movements

(a) **Intorsion:** Superior rectus and superior oblique muscle.

(b) **Extorsion:** Inferior rectus and inferior oblique muscle.

3. LACRIMAL APPARATUS

It is formed by lacrimal gland and its drainage system. For example:

(i) Lacrimal gland
(ii) Conjunctival sac
(iii) Lacrimal canaliculi
(iv) Lacrimal sac
(v) Naso lacrimal duct
(vi) Lacrimal ducts
(vii) Lacrimal puncta

Lacrimal Gland

It is situated on the antero lateral aspect of the roof of the orbit. The gland is 'J' shaped.

Type

Compound recemose type of serous gland. The aponeurosis of the levator palpebrae superioris divides the gland into:

(a) A large deeper orbital part and

(b) A small palpebral part is superficial, lying within the eyelid.

The two parts are continuous with each other around the lateral aspect of the aponeurosis. The ducts of the orbital part pass through the palpebral part and opens into the lateral part of superior conjunctival fornix. There are about 8-10 ducts.

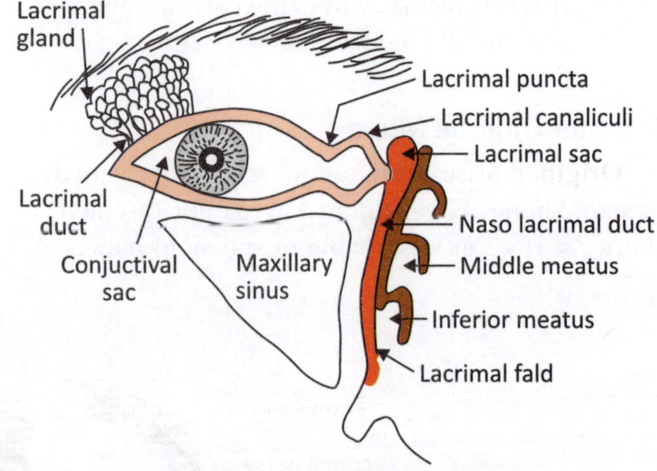

Fig. 13.11: *The lacrimal apparatus*

Blood Supply:

Lacrimal artery a branch of ophthalmic artery supplies the lacrimal gland.

Nerve Supply:

1. Lacrimal nerve is sensory for the gland and is branch of ophthalmic division of trigeminal nerve (V^{th}).

2. Parasympathetic supply comes from – Lacrimatory nucleus situated in the pons. Pre-ganglionic fibres pass through geniculate ganglion of facial nerve → greater superficial petrosal nerve → joins deep petrosal nerve (sympathetic) → to form the nerve of pterygoid canal → relayed into pterygo palatine ganglion → post ganglionic fibres join maxillary nerve → zygomatic nerve → zygomatico temporal nerve → parasympathetic fibres leave and joins lacrimal nerve → reaches to lacrimal gland and are secretomotor for the gland.

Functions of the Tears

1. Keeps the cornea and front of the eyeball moist.
2. Removes the foreign bodies from the surface of the eye.
3. Lacrimal fluid contains enzymes called lysozymes.
4. It has bacterio static function.

Accessory Lacrimal Glands

(Glands of Krause) are situated along the fornices of the conjunctival sac.

Conjunctival Sac

This is the space between the inner surface of the eyelids and anterior surface of eyeball. When lids are closed the sac is a closed space.

Lacrimal Canaliculi

It commences from the lacrimal punctum.

- Each duct is 10 mm long.
- The upper canaliculus is directed upwards and medially, it then dilates, form an ampulla and then directed downwards and medially to open into the lacrimal sac.
- The inferior canaliculus passes downwards and then horizontally and medially to open into the lacrimal sac behind the medial palpebral ligament.
- Some times superior and inferior canaliculi may unite to form the sinus of Meir which opens into the lacrimal sac.

Lacrimal Sac

- It is a membranous sac, about 12 mm long and 5 mm wide, situated in the lacrimal fossa or groove behind the medial palpebral ligament. It's upper end is blind and lower end is continuous with the nasolacrimal duct.
- The sac is covered by the lacrimal fascia derived from the orbital perioteum. Between the fascia and sac a venous plexus is present.

Relations:

Anterior:

1. Medial palpebral ligament.
2. Anterior lacrimal crest giving origin to orbicularis oculi.

Posterior: Lacrimal part of the orbicularis oculi is attached.

Laterally: Lacrimal fascia and lacrimal part of orbicularis oculi.

Medially: Lacrimal groove separates it from the nose.

Applied: Inflammation of the lacrimal sac is called dacrocystitis.

Naso Lacrimal Duct

- It is a membranous passage about 18 mm long. It extends from lacrimal sac to the inferior meatus of the nose, runs downwards, backwards and laterally.
- The terminal part of the duct is oblique. The opening is guarded by a mucous valve called Hasner's valve. It prevents entry of air into the sac.

Lacrimal Circulation

The watery lacrimal fluid secreted by the gland flows into the conjuctival sac where it lubricates the front of the eye and deep surface of the lids. Periodic blinking helps to spread the fluid over the eye. Most of the fluid evaporates, rest is drained by the lacrimal canaliculi. When excessive it overflows as tears. Through the canaliculi it reaches the sac. From the lacrimal sac via naso lacrimal duct the tears drip into the inferior meatus of the nose.

Applied Anatomy

1. **Epiphora:** Over flow of tears on the cheek due to excessive secretion or obstruction of lacrimal passage.
2. **Acute Dacryo Adenitis:** Acute inflammation of the lacrimal gland.
3. **Dacryo Cystitis:** Inflammation of lacrimal sac due to obstruction of the naso lacrimal duct.

4. ORBITAL FASCIA

(Described on page 94).

5. OPHTHALMIC ARTERY

It is a branch of internal carotid artery arises within the middle cranial fossa.

Course

It runs forwards and enters the optic canal. It lies infero lateral to the optic nerve and enters the orbit. It crosses superior to the optic nerve from lateral to medial side, accompanied by the nasociliary nerve and superior ophthalmic vein. It reaches the medial side of the orbit and terminates by dividing into supratrochlear and dorsal nasal branches.

Branches

1. **Muscular branches:** To supply extrinsic muscles of the eyeball.
2. **Central artery of retina:** It is an end artery, arises from the ophthalmic artery when it comes medial to optic nerve. It pierces the postero-medial aspect of the optic nerve about 1 cm behind the eyeball and runs forwards enters the retina and divides into temporal and nasal branches. It supplies the optic nerve and retina.
3. **Two long posterior ciliary arteries:** To supply eyeball.
4. **About seven short posterior ciliary arteries:** To supply the choroids and outer layers of the retina.
5. **Lacrimal artery supplies lacrimal gland and eyelids.**
   - It gives a pair of lateral palpebral arteries to supply each eyelid. They anastomose with medial palpebral arteries.
   - It also gives a recurrent meningeal branch – passes through superior orbital fissure and anastomose with anterior branch of middle meningeal artery and supply meningies of middle cranial fossa.
6. **Posterior ethmoidal artery:** Supplies posterior ethmoidal and sphenoidal air sinus and nose.

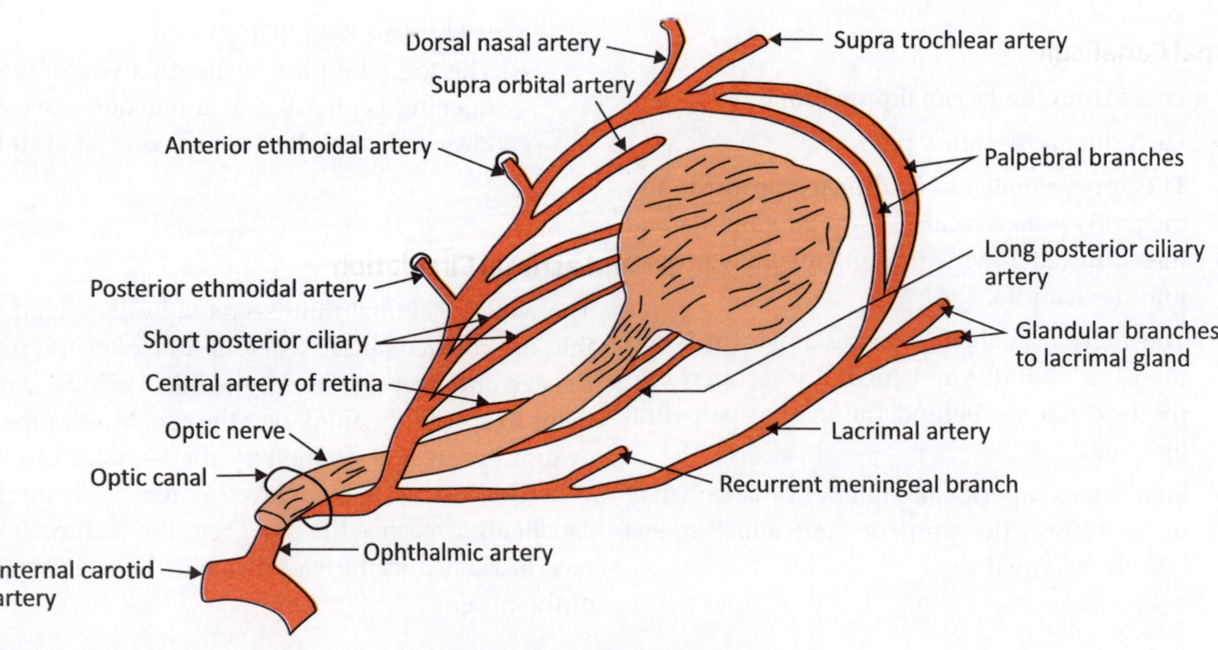

Fig. 13.12: *Ophthalmic artery*

7. **Anterior ethmoidal artery:** Supplies nose, anterior and middle ethmoidal air sinuses.
8. **Medial palpebral arteries:** These anastomoses with lateral palpebral branches.
9. **Supra orbital and supra trochlear arteries:** Supplies forehead and scalp.
10. **Dorsal nasal artery:** Supplies dorsum of the nose and ends by anastomosing with the branches of facial artery.

6. OPHTHALMIC VEINS

There are two ophthalmic veins:

(a) **Superior ophthalmic vein:** It begins along the medial aspect of upper eyelid, crosses superior to optic nerve from medial to lateral side, accompanied by ophthalmic artery and naso ciliary nerve. It passes through superior orbital fissure and terminates into cavernous sinus.

Tributaries: These are small veins accompanying the branches of the ophthalmic artery joins and form superior ophthalmic vein.

(b) **Inferior ophthalmic vein:** It is situated along the floor of the orbit. It drains orbital muscles, lacrimal sac and eyelids ect. It terminates by draining into cavernous sinus, passing through medial part of superior orbital fissure.

Applied Anatomy

Facial vein is communicated with the superior ophthalmic vein. So infections from face spreads via superior ophthalmic vein to cavernous sinus causing thrombosis of the sinus.

7. CENTRAL VEIN OF RETINA

It joins the superior ophthalmic vein or separately drains into cavernous sinus.

8. LYMPHATICS OF THE ORBIT

Drains into preauricular parotid lymph nodes.

9. NERVES OF THE ORBIT

These are optic nerve, oculomotor nerve, trochlear nerve, branches of ophthalmic and maxillary divisions of the trigeminal, abducent nerve and sympathetic nerves.

(a) **Optic nerve** is the nerve of sight and 2nd cranial nerve, made up of axons, i.e., central processes of the ganglionated cell layer of the retina. It pierces the choroids and sclera at lamina cribrosa, situated 3 or 4 mm medial to the posterior pole of the eyeball.

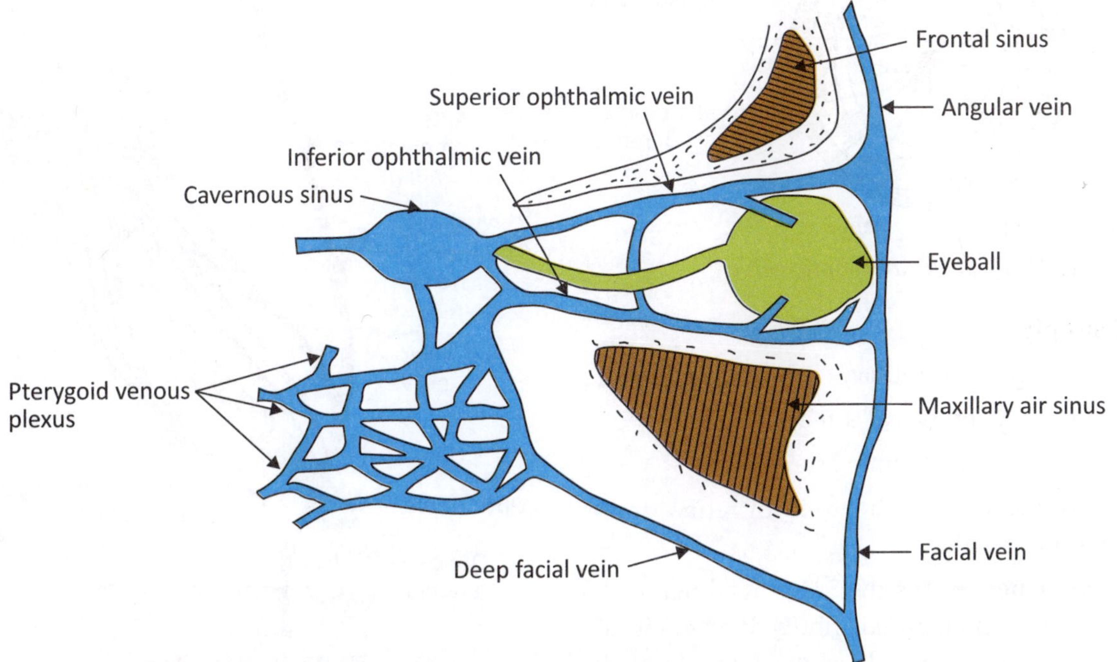

Fig. 13.13: *Ophthalmic veins and its connections*

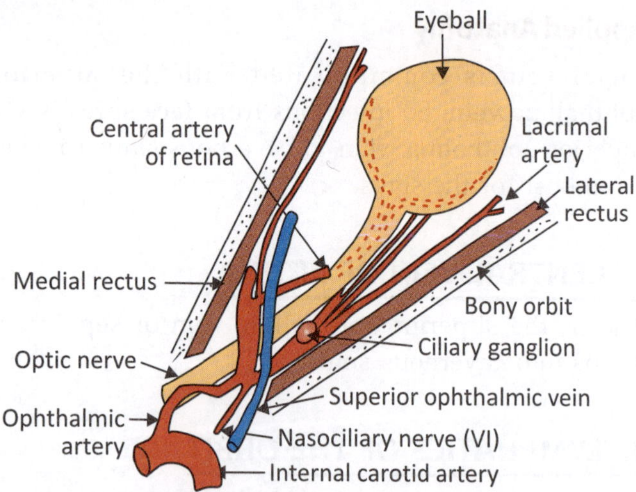

Fig. 13.14: ***Relations of optic-nerve***

The nerve passes through the retrobulbar compartment of the orbit, enters the optic canal through the optic foramen and reaches the anterior cranial fossa. It terminates by joining the nerve of the opposite side and form the optic chiasma.

Length is about 40 mm.

Parts:

1. Intra orbital part – 25 mm long
2. Part within the optic canal – 5 mm long
3. Intra cranial part – 10 mm long.

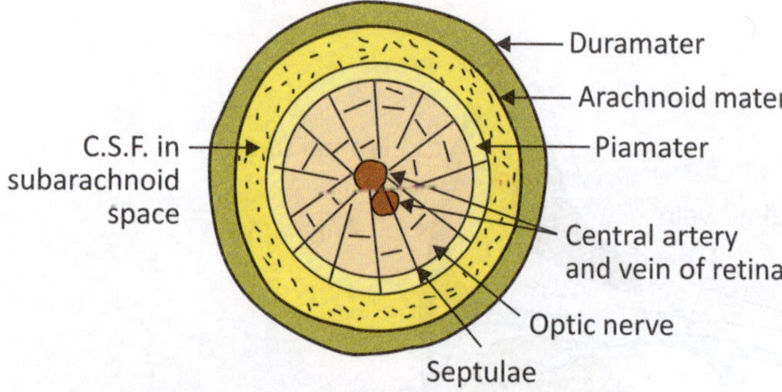

Fig. 13.15: ***Structure of optic-nerve***

Blood supply:

1. Central artery of retina
2. Superior hypophyseal artery
3. Branches of ophthalmic artery.

Venous drainage by central vein of retina drains into cavernous sinus.

(b) Oculomotor nerve: It is the 3rd cranial nerve has motor and parasympathetic fibres. It enters in the orbit as upper and lower divisions within the common tendinous ring. It supplies extra ocular muscles except superior oblique and lateral rectus muscle. Para-sympathetic fibres supply ciliaris muscle and sphincter puplae muscles which helps in accommodation. These fibres are relayed into ciliary ganglion.

(c) Trochlear nerve: It is the fourth cranial nerve, motor in nature, supply only superior oblique muscle, enters the orbit through lateral compartment of superior orbital fissure passes upwards medially.

(d) Abducent nerve: Is the sixth cranial nerve, motor in function, supply only lateral rectus muscle, enters the orbit within the common tendinous ring, i.e., intermediate compartment of superior orbital fissure.

(e) Ophthalmic division of trigeminal nerve: It is one of the branch of 5th cranial nerve. Pure sensory, divides into frontal, lacrimal and nasociliary nerves, enters into the orbit through superior orbital fissure to supply – scalp, lacrimal gland, eyelids, eyeball conjunctina, ethmoidal and sphenoidal air sinues and nose.

10. CILIARY GANGLION

It is situated near the apex of the orbit on the lateral side of optic nerve, medial to lateral rectus. It is a peripheral parasympathetic ganglion.

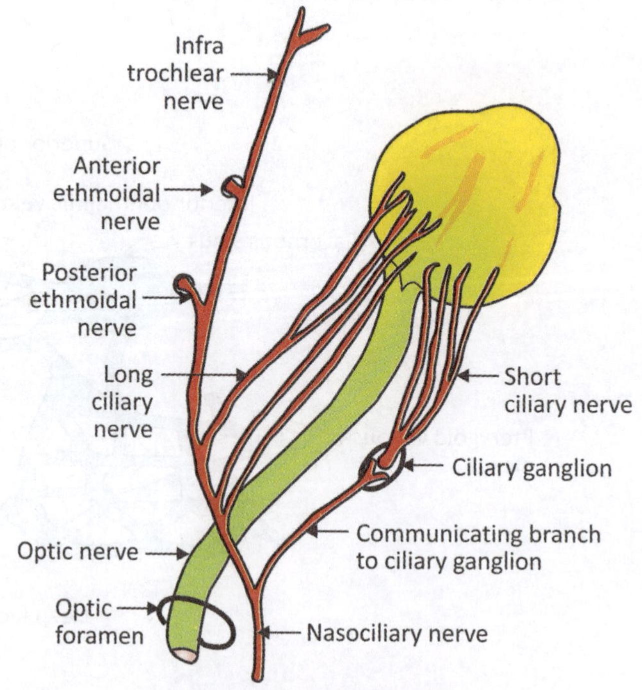

Fig. 13.16: ***Nasociliary nerve***

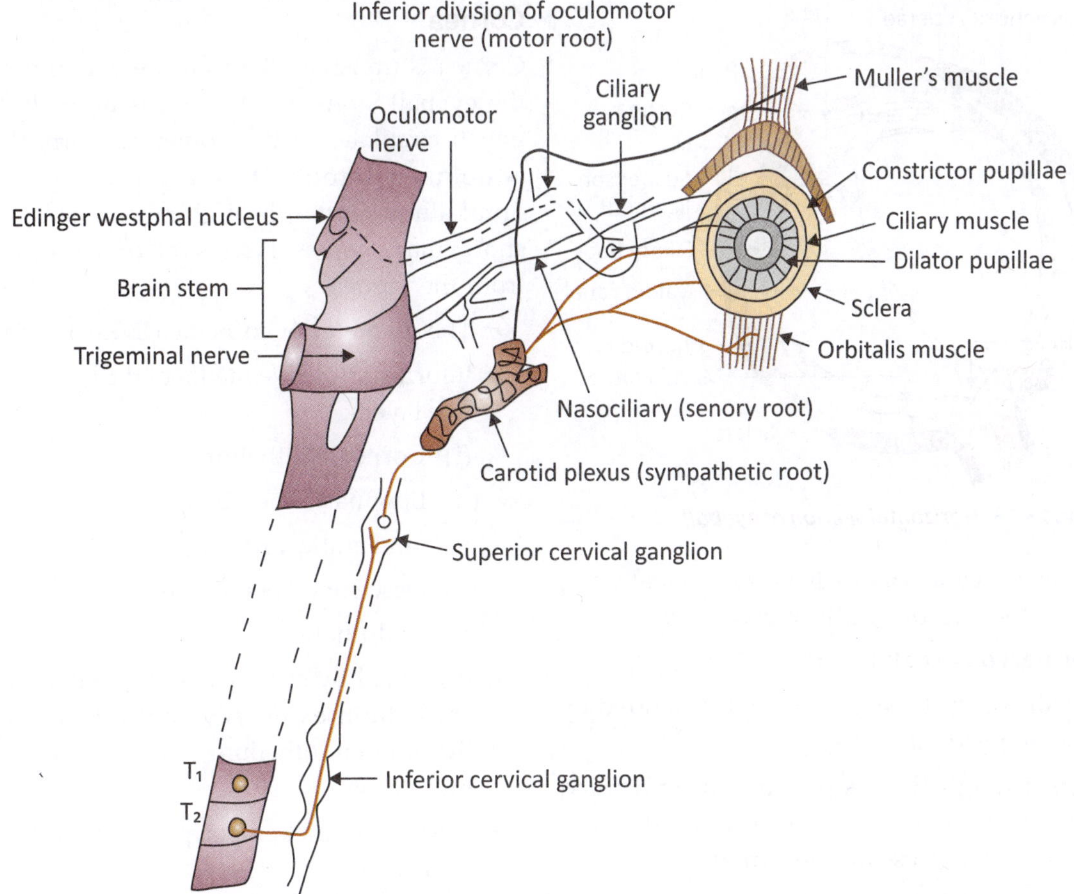

Fig. 13.17: ***Ciliary ganglion and its roots***

Size:

Pin head – 2 mm

- Topographically it is connected to naso ciliary nerve.
- Functionally connected to oculomotor nerve.

Structure:

Multipolar neurons present in it.

Roots:

1. **Motor root:** Comes from nerve to inferior oblique. This is a parasympathetic root – to supply sphincter pupillae and ciliaris muscle. Preganglionic fibres come from Edinger Westphal nucleus and relayed in the ganglion. Post ganglionic fibres arise and pass through short ciliary nerves.
2. **Sensory root:** Comes from naso ciliary nerve. It contains sensory fibres from eyeball.
3. **Sympathetic root:** Comes from internal carotid plexus to supply – dialator pupillae. These are post ganglionic fibres coming from superior cervical sympathetic ganglion.

Branches:

15 to 20 short ciliary nerves arise from the ganglion to supply ciliary body muscles and muscles of the iris, i.e., sphincter and dilator pupillae. These nerves pierce the sclera around the enterance of the optic nerve, containing fibres from all the three roots of the ganglion.

THE EYEBALL

It is a highly differentiated end organ, is the organ of sight and one of the five special senses. It is almost spherical in shape and its diameter is about 2.5 cm. There are two eyeballs, situated within the bony orbital cavity.

Eyeball is made up of three concentric coats:

1. **Outer or fibrous coat:** Comprises sclera and cornea.

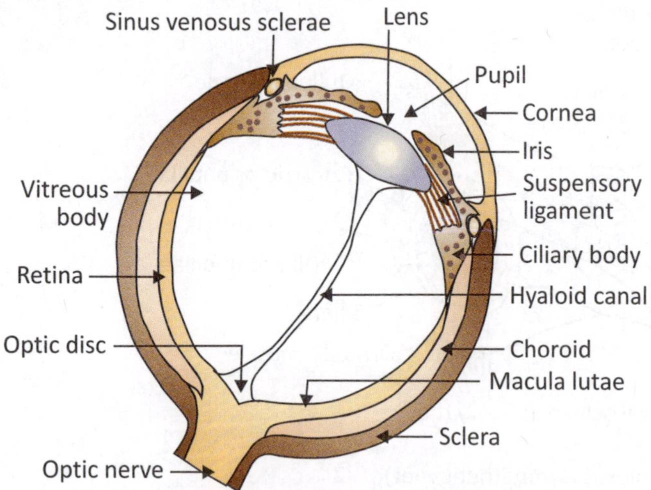

Fig. 13.18: ***Horizontal section of eyeball***

2. **Middle or vascular coat:** Also called uveal tract, consists of the choroids, ciliary body and iris.
3. **Inner or nervous coat:** It is the retina.
   - Eyeball is a cystic structure kept distended by pressure inside it.
   - It has a tough fibrous coat and a fluid filled cavity that maintains the shape and distributes the hydraulic pressure uniformly.
   - It lies embedded in a orbital pad of fat inside the orbital cavity, covered by "Tenon's capsule".
   - It is made up of two segments:
     (a) Anterior $1/6^{th}$ is segment of a small sphere, i.e., Cornea.
     (b) Posterior $5/6^{th}$ is segment of a large sphere, i.e., Sclera.
   - Antero posterior diameter is about 24 mm (vertical).
   - Transverse diameter is about 23 mm or equal.
   - Light entering the eyeball passes through several refracting media. From before backwards these are:
     - Cornea, aqueous humour, the lens, the vitreous body and retina.

1. THE OUTER FIBROUS COAT

Consisting of a cup- like expansion of dural sheath of optic nerve. It is tough fibrous tunic formed by sclera and cornea. Sclera is opaque and forms posterior 5/6th part.

Cornea

Cornea is transparent and forms anterior 1/6th part of the eyeball, non-vascular and is nourished by lymph which circulates in the numerous corneal spaces, i.e., aqueous humour. It is supplied by branches of ophthalmic nerve (through ciliary ganglion) and the short ciliary nerves. Pain is the only sensation aroused from the cornea.

- The diameter of cornea is about 11 mm.
- It forms refractive media of the eye and made up of five layers:
  (i) Corneal epithelium
  (ii) Bowman's membrane
  (iii) Substantia propria
  (iv) Descemet's membrane
  (v) Endothelium.
- It is lined by stratified squamous non-keratizined epithelium externally continuous with conjunctiva and endothelium lining the anterior chamber internally.
- Cornea is thicker peripherally and thinner centrally.
- At the periphery, the cornea meets the sclera at sclerocorneal junction called limbus – on the inner aspect lies a circular canal known as sinus venosus sclerae or canal of schlemn, which drains excessive amount of aqueous humour.

Applied Anatomy

1. **Keratitis:** Inflammation of cornea.
2. **Leucoma:** A white scar on cornea.
3. **Exposure keratitis:** Epithelium of the cornea becomes dry and hazy due to exposure.
4. **Arcus senilis:** It is a lipoid degeneration of the corneal border in elderly individuals.
5. Corneal transplantation

Sclera (Skleros = hard)

Sclera is opaque and forms posterior 5/6th of the eyeball. It is made up of dense fibrous tissue which is firm white and maintains the shape of the eyeball.

- Its average thickness is about 1 mm and covered by membrane called Tenon's capsule.

- The anterior part is covered by conjunctiva and is white.
- The sclera is almost avascular. However, the loose connective tissue between conjunctiva and sclera called as episclera is vascular.
- The recti and oblique muscles of the eyeball are inserted over the sclera.
- Lamina cribrosa is situated on the posterior surface of the sclera and is pierced by optic nerve fibres.
- Posteriorly sclera is continuous with the dural sheath of the optic nerve.
- Anteriorly it is continuous with the cornea at the sclero corneal junction.
- Sclera is pierced by the following vessels and nerves:
  1. A pair of long posterior ciliary arteries.
  2. Short posterior ciliary arteries about 6 to 9 in number.
  3. Long and short ciliary nerves.
  4. Long ciliary arteries.
  5. Venae verticosae – about 4 in number.
  6. Anterior ciliary arteries about 7 in number.
  7. Optic nerve.

Applied Anatomy

1. **Staphyloma:** Localised bulging of sclera.
2. **Blue sclera:** Congenital condition – bluish discolouration of the sclera due to thining of sclera.
3. **Cupped disc:** Due to increased intra cranial tension lamina cribrosa will buldge outwards – Papillaedema.
4. **Scleritis:** Inflammation of sclera.

2. VASCULAR PIGMENTED COAT (UVEAL TRACT)

It has three parts – choroid, ciliary body and iris diaphragm. Iris has an aperture in its centre called pupil. It is formed by expansion of archnoid mater and piamater. It is vascular and pigmented layer.

Choroid

It is a soft thin pigmented membrane. Anteriorly it ends at the ora serrata by merging with the ciliary body; posteriorly it is perforated by optic nerve.

- It is 0.2 mm thick.
- The choroid supplies nutrition to the retina.
- It shows blood vessels arranged in three layers. All layers are held, together by connective tissue stroma which contains pigmented chromatophores.
- It has rich sensory nerve supply from naso ciliary nerve.

Ciliary Body

It is the anterior continuation of the choroid upto limbus which lies between choroid and iris. It is triangular shaped in cross-section. It has a base and an

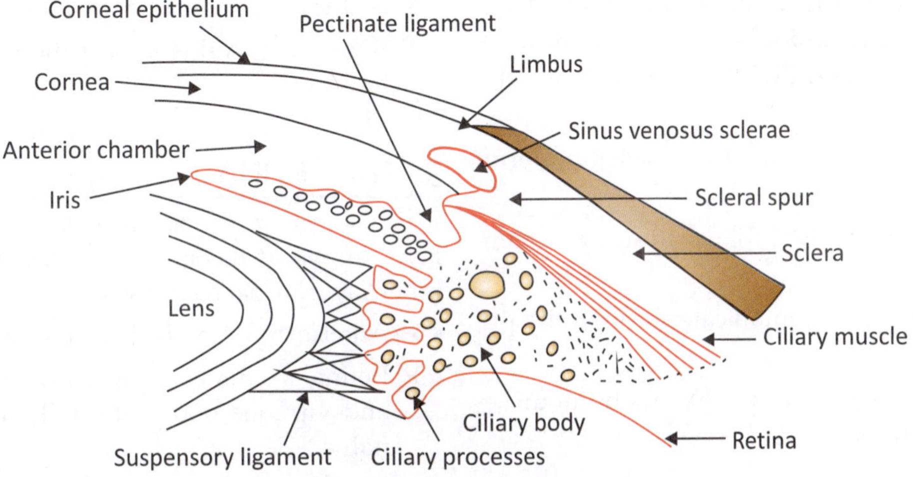

Fig. 13.19: *Sclero corneal junction*

apex. To the middle of the base iris is attached. The apex is continous with the choroid.

It consists of three parts:

(i) **Ciliary ring:** Flattened circular band.

(ii) **Ciliary processes:** 60 to 80 in number, formed by inward folding of layer of choroids – connected with suspensory ligament of lens.

It secretes aqueous humour.

(iii) **Ciliary muscles** are plain muscles on outer side of choroid run from base to limbus.

- Outer fibres called Brucke's muscle, run antero posterior.
- Inner fibres are called Muller's muscle run, circularly.

Action:

The contraction of the muscle relaxes the suspensory ligament so that lens becomes more convex and helps in accommodation and are also responsible for opening the canal of schlemn and helps in the drainage of the aqueous humour.

Nerve Supply of Muscle:

Parasympathetic fibres coming from Edinger-Westphal nucleus, pass through oculomotor nerve are relayed in the ciliary ganglion to supply ciliary muscles.

Iris

It is pigmented diaphragm:

- Iris is the anterior part of the uveal tract. It forms a circular curtain with an opening in the centre called pupil.
- It is hanging down from the ciliary body. It lies between the cornea and lens, i.e., with in the anterior compartment and divides it into anterior and posterior chambers.
- The space between lens and iris is called posterior chamber.
- The space anterior to the iris is called anterior chamber.
- The two chambers communicate through the pupil.
- Both chambers containing aqueous humour secreted by ciliary processes.
- Pupil controls the amount of light entering the eye. It is made up of four layers:

1. **Endothelial layer.**
2. **Stroma** is formed by connective tissue, containing pigment loaded chromato phores, vessels and nerves. Vessels are arranged in a radiating fashion, near the pupil they anastomose.
3. **Muscles of the iris:** Circular muscles forming sphincter pupillae and radial muscles forming dilator pupillae.
4. **Epithelial layer:** Covers the back of the iris are pigmented epithelial cells.

Blood Supply to Iris:

Greater arterial circle of iris is situated in the ciliary body, formed by pair of long posterior ciliary arteries.

Nerve Supply:

Sphincter pupillae is supplied by parasymphathetic fibres from oculomotor nerve (Edinger-Westphal nucleus).

Dilator Pupillae:

Supplied by sympathetic fibres from T_1 ganglion.

Actions:

- Sphincter pupillae – constricts the pupil during bright light.
- Dilator pupillae dilates the pupil during dim light.

Applied Anatomy

1. **Iritis:** Inflammation of the iris.
2. **Cyclitis:** Inflammation of ciliary body.
3. **Iridodialysis:** Tear of iris at its ciliary attachment.
4. **Synechiae:** Adherence of the iris to the cornea or lens.

3. THE RETINA

It is also called as nervous coat and is photosensitive layer of eye. It has an outer pigmented layer and an inner layer of nervous tissue.

- Anteriorly retina ends at the ora serrata.
- Retina is situated between the hyaloid membrane and vitreous body internally and choroid externally.

- Macula lutea is a yellow spot situated at the posterior pole of the eye. It is about 1 to 2 mm in diameter. It is the site of maximum acuity due to collection of cones.
- The optic disc is situated 3 mm medial to the maculalutea. Disc is slightly depressed and is pierced by the central artery of the retina. Rods and cones are absent in the optic disc. It is insensitive to light and is known as blind spot.
- Microscopically retina has ten layers from without inwards:
  - (i) Layer of pigmented epithelim
  - (ii) Layer of rods and cones
  - (iii) External limiting membrane
  - (iv) Outer nuclear layer
  - (v) Outer plexiform layer
  - (vi) Inner nuclear layer
  - (vii) Inner plexiform layer
  - (viii) Ganglion cell layer
  - (ix) Layer of nerve fibres
  - (x) Internal limiting membrane.

Colour Vision:

Cones of the retina are responsible for colour vision. Rods may perceive blue colour.

Blood Supply:

1. Chorio capillaries supply outer layers of retina.
2. Central artery of retina supplies inner layers.

Venous Drainage:

Blood from retina is drained into choroidal veins and central vein of retina. Which drains into Caverneous Sinus.

SEGMENTS AND CHAMBERS OF EYEBALL

Eyeball can be divided into two segments anterior and posterior.

1. Anterior Segment

It lies anterior to lens which is suspended from the ciliary body by zonules, i.e., suspensory ligament. Structures anterior to lens – are iris cornea and two aqueous filled spaces, i.e., anterior and posterior chambers.

(a) **Anterior chamber:** It is bounded anteriorly by cornea and posteriorly by the iris and part of ciliary body. It communicates with posterior chamber through pupil its peripheral recess is called the angle of the anterior chamber irido – corneal angle formed by trabecular meshwork. Next to it canal of schlemn is present in the substance of sclera. Aqueous humour produced by ciliary processes is drained from the anterior chamber through this meshwork and canal.

(b) **Posterior chamber:** It is present behind the iris and in front of lens. It is a triangular space containing aqueous humour.

2. Posterior Segment

It is present behind the lens and infront of retina and optic disc, filled with vitreous humour. It is transparent, colourless and jelly like, consisting of 99% of water with small amount of mucoprotein.

Blood Supply:

The short posterior ciliary arteries divide into 10 to 20 branches, pierce the sclera and supply the choroid and sclera. Two long posterior ciliary arteries supply the ciliary body and iris. They reach the ciliary muscle and divide into two branches which enter the substance of muscle at its anterior end and anastomose with anterior ciliary arteries – form circulus iridis major and supply ciliary body and iris.

Applied Anatomy

1. Retinitis – inflammation of retina.
2. Sudden occlusion of the central artery of retina causes blindness.
3. Thrombosis of retinal vein – occur in elderly.
4. Pigmentosa – Degenerative disease. Night blindness and deposition of melanin in the retina.
5. Retinal detachment – separation of retina from choroid.

CONTENTS OF THE EYEBALL

1. Aqueous Humour

It is a clear fluid secreted by ciliary process of the ciliary body in the posterior chamber, passes through pupil and enters the anterior chamber. From here, it is drained away through the spaces at the irodo corneal angle into the canal of schlemn, passes away through venae verticosae.

When there is obstruction in the circulation – intra ocular pressure is raised – causes glaucoma – it is a severely painful condition.

2. The Lens

It is a transparent biconvex structure, forms one of the constituents of the refractive media of the eye. Its main function is to converge light rays and form images on the retina.

Diameter is about 9 mm.

Thickness is about 4 mm.

- It is suspended by the suspensory ligament.
- The posterior surface is more convex than anterior surface.
- It is covered by an elastic capsule.

Nutrition of the lens is provided by:

1. Aqueous humour present in the anterior chamber.
2. Auto oxidation system within the lens.

3. Accommodation

Ability of the eye to adjust for both distant and near vision. It is done by the following mechanisms –

1. Contraction of ciliary muscle.
2. Choroid is pulled forwards and inwards.
3. Relaxation of the suspensory ligament caused by ciliary process.

Accommodation Reflex

It is constriction of pupil while looking at a near object.

Pathway for Accommodation Reflex

Visual receptors (rods and cones) → bipolar cells of retina → ganglion cells → optic nerve → optic chiasma → optic tract → lateral geniculate body → optic radiation → visual area of occipital lobe (area 17) → frontal lobe through the association fibres → third nerve nucleus → oculomotor nerve → ciliary ganglion → short ciliary nerves → ciliary muscles.

Applied Anatomy

(i) Cataract – lens become opaque.

(ii) Congenital cataract – since after birth.

(iii) Senile cataract – due to old age.

(iv) Extraction of lens – may be extra ocular or intra ocular.

4. The Vitreous Body

This is a jelly-like body with in the posterior compartment of the eye – lies behind the lens. It is transparent and enclosed by the hyaloid membrane. Hyaloid canal is a passage in the central part of the vitreous, extends from the posterior surface of the lens to the optic disc. In the fetus hyaloid artery passes through it, later on it oblitrates.

It forms one of the refractive media of the eye.

- **Development:** Optic vesicle forms optic cup. It is an out growth from the forebrain vesicle.
- **Lens:** Develops from lens placode (Ectodermal in origin).
- **Retina:** Pigment layer from the outer layer of optic cup and nervous layers from the inner layer of optic cup.
- **Choroid and sclera:** Develops from mesoderm.
- **Cornea:** This develops from surface ectoderm.

Visual Pathway

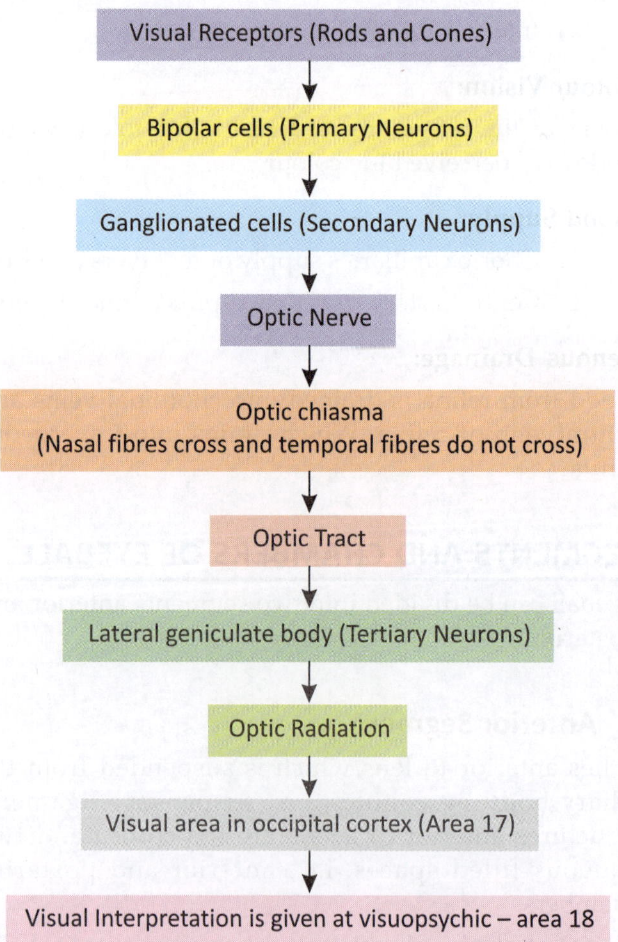

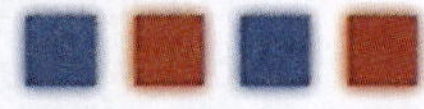

CHAPTER 14

Neck

INTRODUCTION

- Neck is that part of body which connects the head to the upper part of trunk.
- It is cylindrical in shape and is like a tube.

BOUNDARIES

Superior:

- Lower border of the body of mandible, i.e., the line joining angle of mandible to mastoid process.
- Superior nuchal line.
- External occipital protuberance.

Inferior:

From anterior to posterior neck is bounded by:

- Supra sternal notch of manubrium sterni.
- Upper surface of clavicle.
- Acromion process of scapula and spine of C_7.
- Line extending from the acromion process to spine of C_7 vertebra.

ANATOMICAL FEATURES OF NECK

Consists of following layers:

1. **Skin** is thin.
2. **Superficial Fascia**
   - Containing loose connective tissue.
   - A thin sheet of muscle – Platysma.
   - Cutaneous nerves, blood vessels and lymphatics.

   Cutaneous nerves: These are branches of cervical plexus formed by upper four cervical nerves:

   (a) Lesser occipital nerve (C_2).

   (b) Great auricular nerve (C_2 and C_3).

   (c) Transverse cervical nerve (C_2 and C_3).

   (d) Supra clavicular nerves (C_3 and C_4). It divides into three branches – medial, intermediate and lateral supra clavicular nerves. They supply skin of upper part of thorax and shoulder down to 2nd intercostal space.

3. **Deep Cervical Fascia (Fascia colli):**
   - Deep fascia of the neck is a fibrous sheet that encircles the neck from all sides just like a collar.
   - It is divided into following layers:

     (a) Investing layer of fascia

     (b) Pre-tracheal fascia

     (c) Pre-vertebral fascia

     (d) Carotid sheath

     (e) Bucco-phyaryngeal fascia.

(a) Investing Layer of Deep Fascia of Neck

- It invests the neck from all sides.
- It covers all cervical structures except—platysma, superficial vessels and nerves.
- Forms roof of the posterior triangle of the neck.
- It splits and encloses.
  - **Two muscles:** Trapezius and sternocleido-mastoid.
  - **Two glands:** Parotid and submandibular gland.

- **Two spaces:** Supra sternal and supra clavicular space.
- It forms two pulleys to bind the respective tendons of the digastric and omohyoid muscles.

Attachments

Superiorly:

- External occipital protuberance
- Superior nuchal line
- Mastoid process
- Lower border of zygomatic arch.

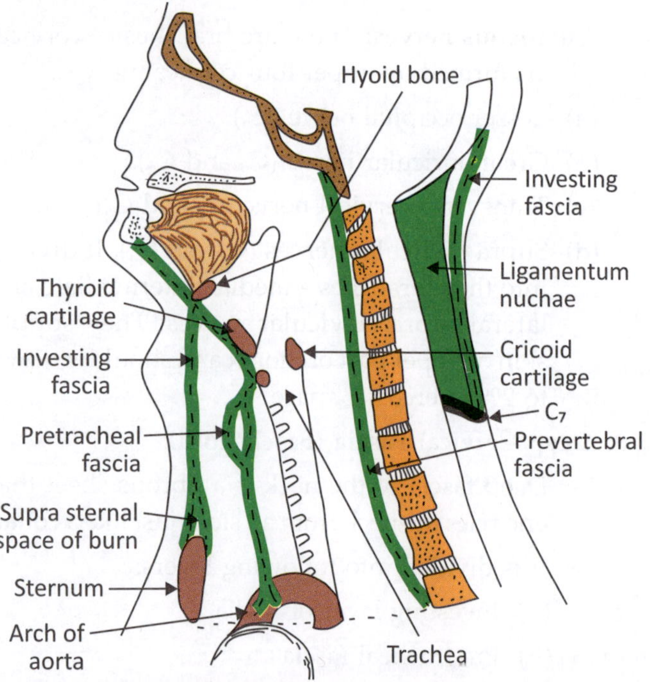

Fig. 14.1: *Vertical extent of deep fascia of neck*

Posteriorly:

- Ligamentum nuchae
- Spine of C_7 vertebra.

Postero inferiorly:

- Spine of scapula
- Acromion process of scapula.

Antero-inferiorly:

- Clavicle
- Manubrium sterni.

Antero-superiorly:

- Symphysis menti.
- Lower border of mandible.
- An imaginary line joining the angle of mandible and mastoid process.
- Fascia forming the roof of posterior triangle pierced by
  - External jugular vein and
  - Supra clavicular nerves (medial, intermediate and lateral branches)
- Between the angle of mandible and styloid process of temporal bone this fascia is thickened to form stylomandibular ligament, which separates parotid gland from sub-mandibular gland, this ligament is pierced by facial artery.

Supra sternal space of burn's: Near the lower part of midline of neck fascia splits and encloses this space. Structures present in this space are:

1. Jugular venous arch – connecting two anterior jugular veins.
2. Lymph glands – 1 or 2.
3. Sternal head of sternocleidomastoid muscle.
4. Inter clavicular ligament.

Supra clavicular space – Contains:

1. Lower portion of external jugular vein and
2. Supra clavicular nerves.

(b) Pre-tracheal Fascia

Enclosing visceral compartment of neck.

Attachments

- **Superiorly:** Hyoid bone.
- **Inferiorly:** Extends into thorax and joins fibrous pericardium.
- **Laterally:** It fuses with carotid sheath. Through this sheath it is continous with the investing layer of deep fascia.
- **Medially:** It splits and encloses the thyroid gland.
- The pre-tracheal fascia invests the infra-hyoid muscles.
- It is attached to thyroid and cricoid cartilages as suspensory ligament of Berry. It binds the thyroid gland to the larynx.

(c) Pre-vertebral Gascia

Attachments

- **Superiorly:** It extends to the base of skull.
- **Inferiorly:** Extends into posterior mediastinum and attached to T_4 vertebral body and even extends into abdomen.
- **Laterally:** It extends to the carotid sheath and via this sheath, it is connected to investing layer of deep fascia on the medial surface of sternocleido mastoid muscle.

Visceral Compartment of Neck

- Space between pretracheal and prevertebral fascia is occupied by viscera of neck, e.g., pharynx, larynx, oesophagus, trachea and thyroid gland.
- Prevertebral fascia covers the scalene muscles and forms fascial floor of posterior triangle and continued downwards as axillary sheath, which contains axillary vessels and brachial plexus. It extends upto elbow.

(d) Carotid Sheath

Carotid sheath is formed by:

Anteriorly: Pre-tracheal fascia.

Posteriorly: Pre-vertebral fascia.

Extends from base of skull to the root of neck.

- Above to arch of aorta below.
- Ansa cervicalis is situated on the surface of carotid sheath.

Carotid sheath encloses:

- Internal carotid artery
- Common carotid artery
- Internal jugular vein
- Vagus nerve.

(e) Bucco-pharyngeal Fascia

Extends from base of skull downwards.

- It covers posterior and lateral surfaces of pharynx.
- Retropharyngeal space is found between this fascia and pre-vertebral fascia – containing lymph nodes.
- A fascial septum connects this fascia to pre vertebral fascia and divides into right and left retro pharyngeal space.

Applied Anatomy

1. Cold abscess from cervical vertebra may pass behind prevertebral fascia – it may push forward to the middle of posterior wall of pharynx. It may

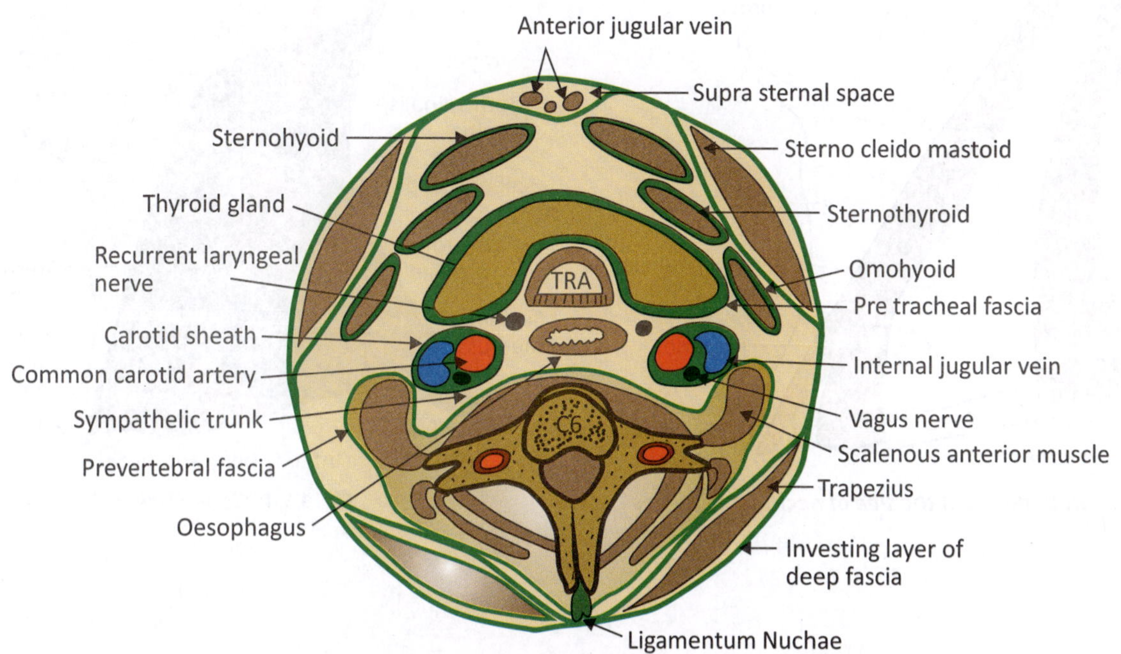

Fig. 14.2: *Deep cervical fascia in T.S. of neck (attachments)*

track down along the floor of posterior triangle of neck to the axilla via axillary sheath.

2. Abscess – formed from retro pharyngeal lymph nodes may be unilateral and pressing one side of pharynx forwards.
3. Fasciaitis: This is inflammation of fascial sheath due to infection.
4. Pre-vertebral and pre-tracheal fascia are slippery in nature allows free movement of trachea, oesophagus and pharynx during swallowing and neck movements.
5. Thyroid gland moves on swallowing because of attachment of pre-tracheal fascia to hyoid bone and thyroid cartilage.

SIDE OF THE NECK (QUADRILATERAL SPACE)

- It is rectangular space.
- Divided into following two triangles by sternocleidomastoid muscle:
  1. Anterior triangle neck.
  2. Posterior triangle neck.

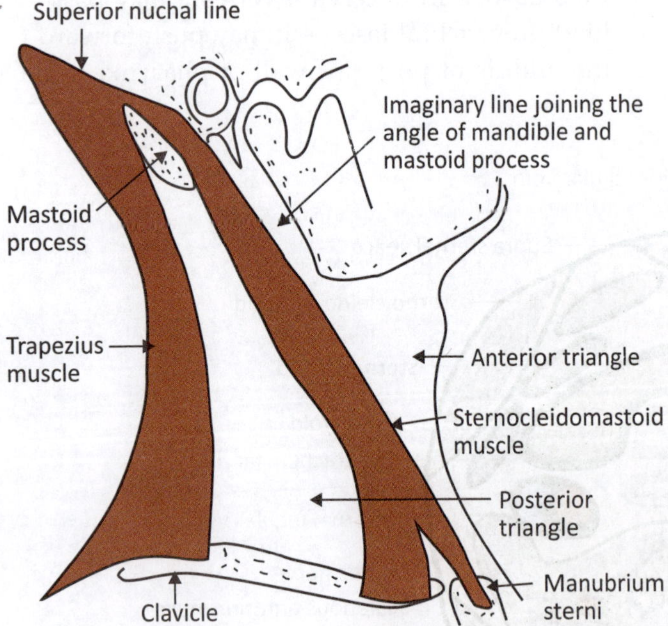

Fig. 14.3: *Boundaries of the side of neck and triangles*

1. Anterior Triangle Neck

Boundaries:

Anterior: Anterior midline of neck extending from symphysis menti above to middle of sternal notch below.

Posterior: Anterior border of sternocleido mastoid muscle.

Base: Lower border of mandible and line joining the angle of mandible with mastoid process.

Apex: Suprasternal notch.

2. Posterior Triangle Neck

Situation: Postero lateral aspect of neck.

Boundaries:

Anteriorly: Posterior border of sternomastoid muscle.

Posteriorly: Anterior border of trapezius muscle.

Base: Middle 1/3 of clavicle.

Apex: At superior nuchal line on overlapping of sternomastoid on trapezius muscle.

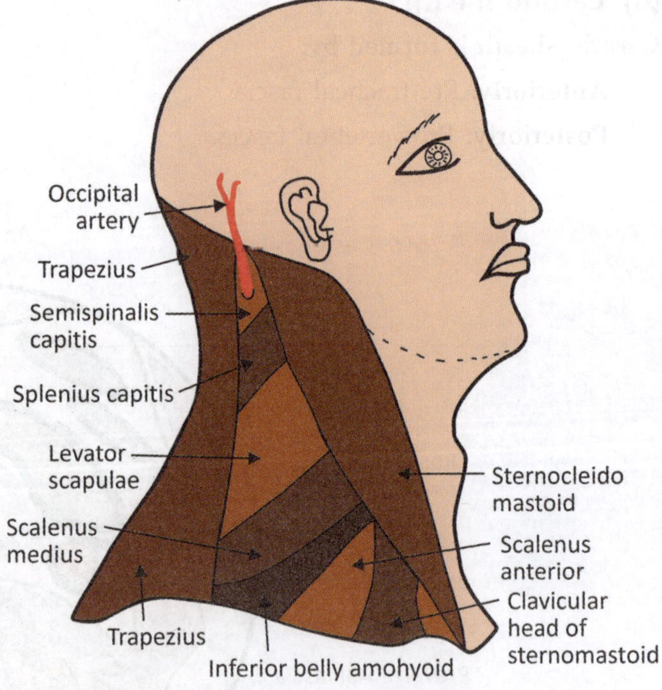

Fig. 14.4: *Floor of triangle*

Floor:

Musculo fascial: Prevertebral fascia carpets the muscles forming the floor.

- Semispinalis capitis
- Splenius capitis
- Levator scapulae
- Scalenus medius
- Scalenus anterior.

Roofs:

- Skin
- Superficial fascia: containing platysma and cutaneous nerves and vessels.
- Investing layer of deep cervical fascia it is pierced by:
  - Supra clavicular nerves.
  - External jugular vein – injury may lead to air embolism.

Parts:

Inferior belly of omohyoid divides the triangle into two parts:

(a) Occipital triangle above

(b) Subclavian triangle below.

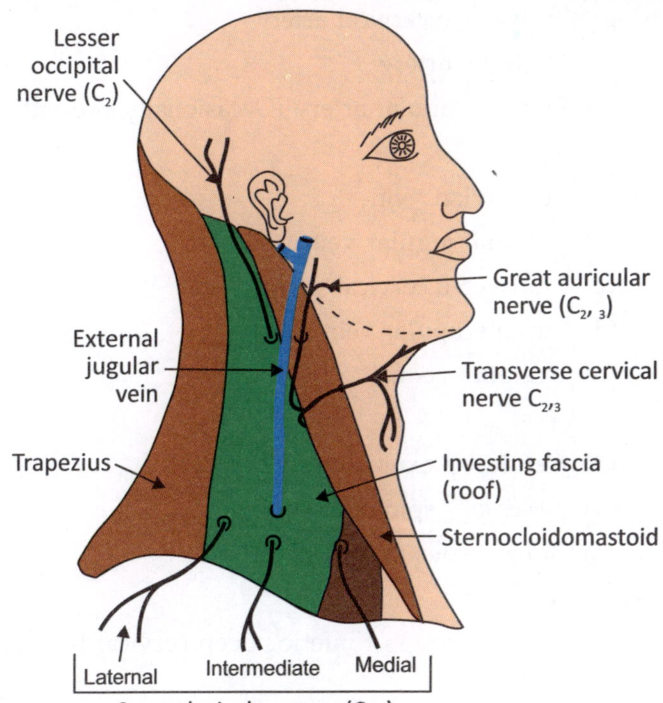

Fig. 14.5: *Roof of triangle*

Contents of Posterior Triangle

1. Arteries:

(a) IIIrd part of subclavian artery

(b) Supra scapular artery

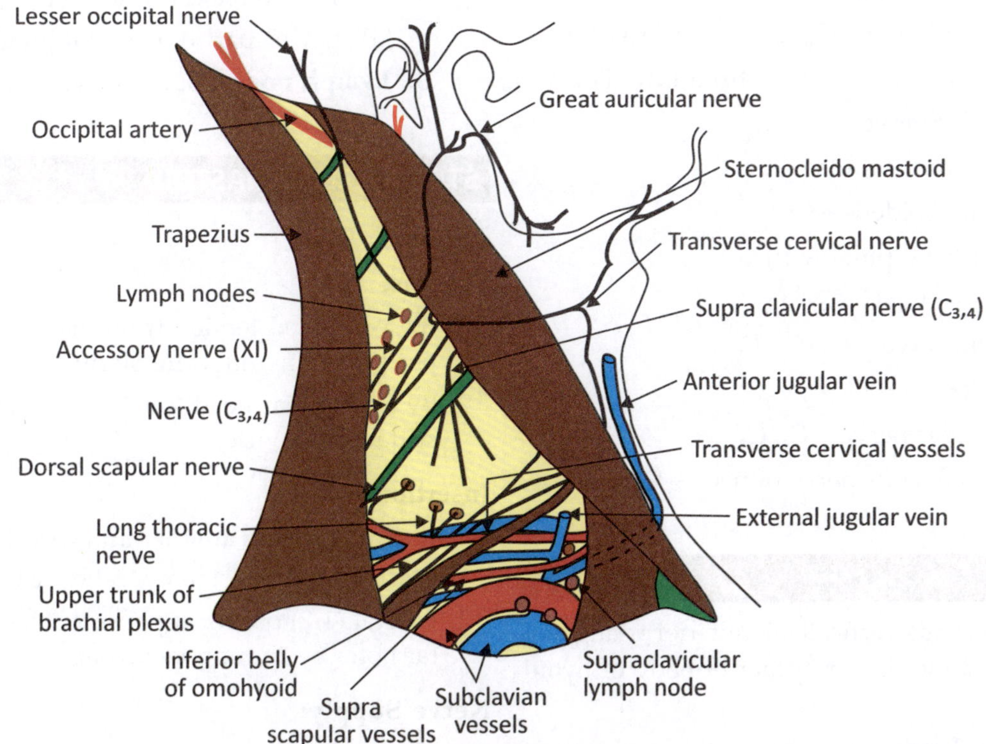

Fig. 14.6: *Contents of posterior triangle*

(c) Transverse cervical artery
(d) Occipital artery
(e) Dorsal scapular artery (Occasionally present).

2. **Veins:**
(a) Subclavian vein
(b) External jugular vein
(c) Transverse cervical vein
(d) Supra scapular vein
(e) Occipital vein.

3. **Nerves:**
(a) Cervical plexus with its branches
(b) Accessory spinal nerve root
(c) Brachial plexus and its branches.

4. **Lymph Nodes**
(a) Lateral group of inferior deep cervical lymph nodes.
(b) Supra clavicular group of lymph nodes.

5. **Fat and connective tissue.**

6. **Muscle –** inferior belly of omohyoid.

Nerves in Posterior Trianagle

1. Trunks of brachial plexus between scalenus anterior and scalenus medius.
2. Supra scapular nerve – C_5, C_6 – from Erb's Point
3. Nerve to subclavius – C_5, C_6 – from Erb's Point
4. Supraclavicular nerves – C_3, C_4
5. Nerve to Levator Scapulae – C_3, C_4
6. Nerve to Rhomboideus – C_5
7. Accessory nerve (Spinal root)
8. Phrenic nerve – C_3, C_4, C_5
9. Long thoracic nerve – C_5, C_6, C_7
10. Lesser occipital nerve – C_2, C_3
11. Greater auricular nerve – C_2, C_3
12. Transverse cutaneous nerve of neck – C_2, C_3.

OMOHYOID

Superior belly ascends vertically in anterior triangle of neck and inserted into lower border of body of hyoid bone.

Intermediate Tendon is held in position by loop of deep fascia that slings the tendon to clavicle and Ist rib.

Inferior belly: Arises from supra scapular ligament and the bone of superior border of scapula near the ligament and crosses the posterior triangle in its lower part and it divides into two triangles – occipital and subclavian triangle.

Action: Depresses the hyoid bone.

Nerve supply: C_1, C_2 and C_3 via – Ansa cervicalis loop.

A. **Contents of occipital triangle:**
(a) Occipital artery and vein.
(b) Spinal root of accessory nerve.
(c) Lymph nodes – along accessory nerve and occipital lymph nodes.
(d) Branches of cervical plexus of nerves – cutaneous and muscular branches.

B. **Contents in subclavian triangle:**

1. **Nerves:**
(a) Three trunks of brachial plexus.
(b) Nerve to serratus anterior (Long thoracic C_5, C_6, C_7).
(c) Nerve to subclavius (C_5, C_6).
(d) Supra scapular nerve C_5, C_6.

2. **Vessels:**
(a) Third part of subclavian artery and vein.
(b) Supra scapular artery and vein.
(c) Transverse cervical artery and vein.
(d) Lower part of external jugular vein.

3. **Lymph nodes:** Supra clavicular chain.

STERNOCLEIDOMASTOID

Strap like muscle.

Origins:

1. By a rounded tendon from the – Front of the upper part of manubrium sterni.
2. By a muscular head from the medial 1/3 of upper surface of clavicle.

Insertion:

Two heads join one another and inserted on:

1. Mastoid process of temporal bone by thick tendon.
2. Lateral (1/2) part of superior nuchal line of occipital bone by thin aponeurosis.

Nerve Supply:

Spinal part of accessory nerve and anterior rami of C_2 and C_3 proprioceptive in nature.

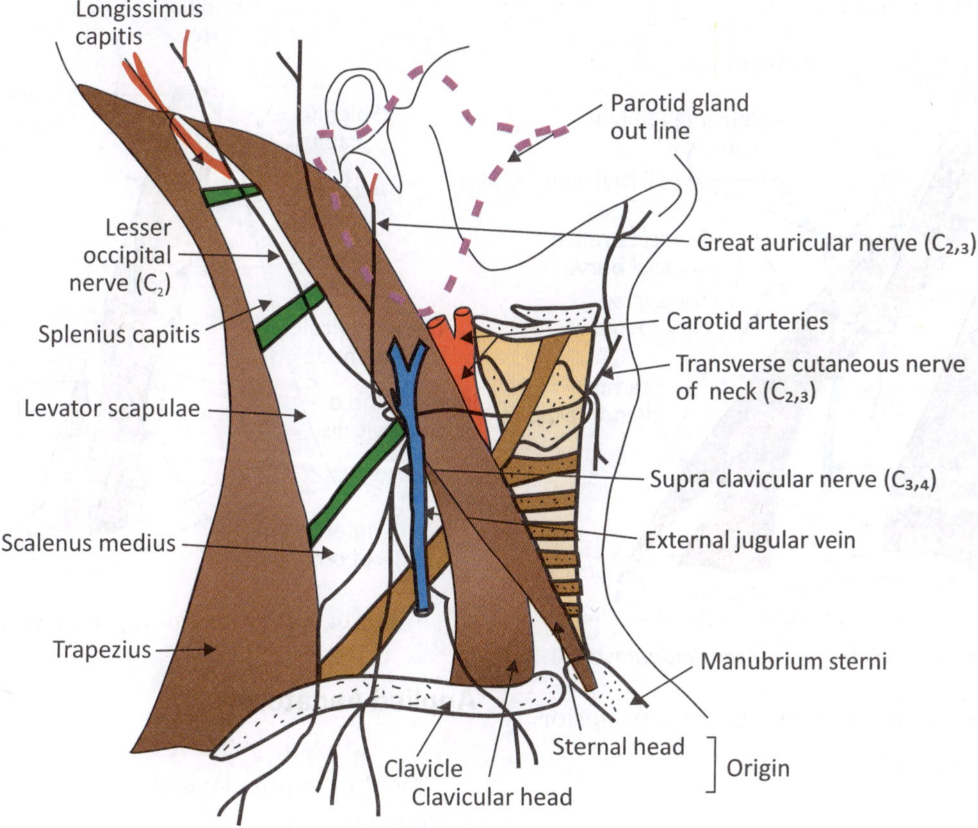

Fig. 14.7: ***Sternocleido mastoid and its relations***

Actions:

- **Both muscle acting together:** Extend the head at the atlanto occipital joint and flex the head during eating and lifting from pillow – flex cervical part of the vertebral coloumn.
- **Contraction of the muscle:** Pulls the ear down to the tip of the shoulder on the same side and rotates the head, so that the face looks upward to the opposite side.

Also acts as accessory muscles of inspiration – when origin is moving and insertion end is fixed.

When head is fixed by pre and post-vertebral muscles.

Enclosed in two layers of investing layer of deep fascia.

Pierced by

- Accessory nerve.
- 4 sternomastoid arteries and 2 branches from occipital artery.
  - 1 branch from superior thyroid artery.
  - 1 branch from supra scapular artery.

Arterial supply by sternomastoid arteries – 4 branches.

RELATIONS OF STERNO MASTOID

- **Anteriorly:** Aneterior triangle.
- **Posteriorly:** Posterior triangle.

Superficial:

1. Skin.
2. Superficial fascia with platysma.
3. Deep fascia – superficial lamina.
4. External jugular vein and superficial cervical lymph nodes.
5. Great auricular, transverse cervical and medial supraclavicular nerves.
6. Parotid gland overlaps the muscle.

Deep:

1. **Bones** – Mastoid process above.
2. **Joints** – Sternoclavicular joint below.
3. **Carotid sheath** with its contents.
4. **Muscles:**
   (a) Sternohyoid
   (b) Sternothyroid
   (c) Omohyoid

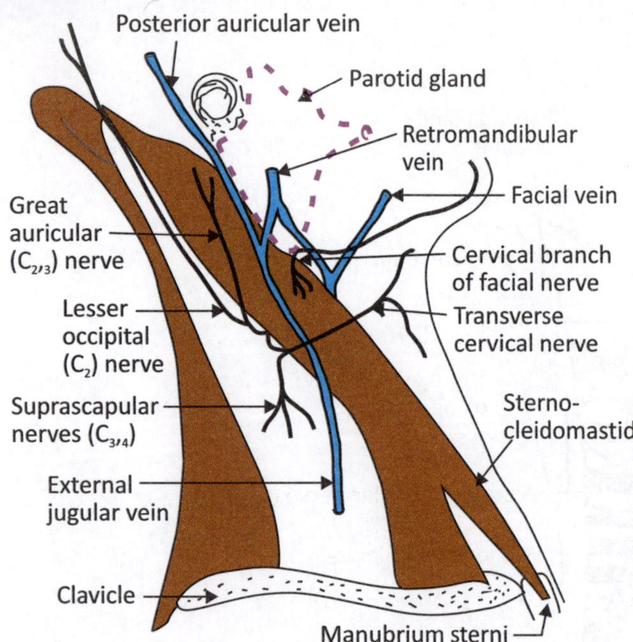

Fig. 14.8: *Superficial relations of sternocleidomastoid*

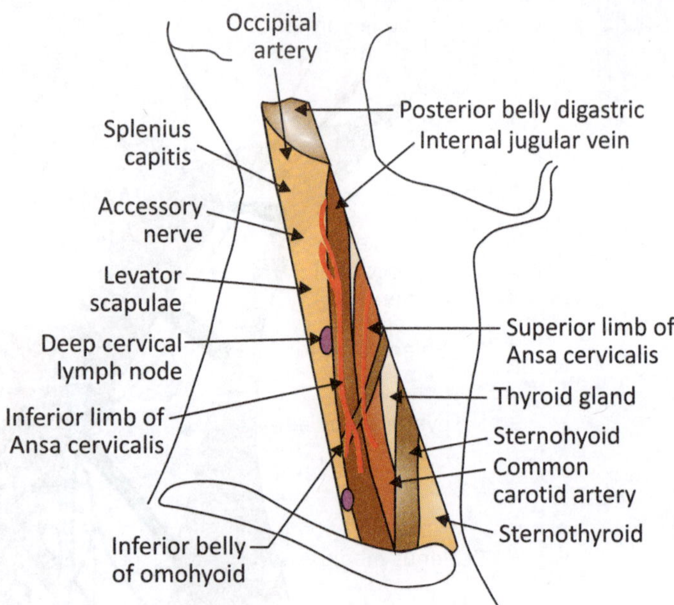

Fig. 14.9: *Deep relations of sternocleidomastoid*

(d) 3 Scalenus – anterior, medius and posterior
(e) Levator scapulae
(f) Splenius capitis
(g) Semi spinalis capitis
(h) Posterior belly of digastric

5. **Arteries:**
   (a) Common carotid
   (b) Internal carotid artery
   (c) External carotid artery.
   (d) Occipital artery
   (e) Subclavian artery
   (f) Supra scapular artery
   (g) Transverse cervical artery.
6. **Veins:**
   (a) Internal jugular vein
   (b) Anterior jugular vein
   (c) Facial and lingual veins.
7. **Nerves:**
   (a) Vagus nerve
   (b) Accessory nerve
   (c) Cervical plexus
   (d) Upper part of brachial plexus
   (e) Phrenic and ansa-cervicalis.
8. **Lymph nodes:** deep cervical group.

Applied Aanatomy

1. **Swelling in posterior triangle** is due to enlargement of supra clavicular lymph nodes
   (a) Lipoma
   (b) Cystic hygroma
   (c) Lymphangioma
   (d) Cervical rib
   (e) Pharyngeal pouch
   (f) Hodgkin's disease
   (g) Tuberculosis – cold abscess
   (h) Secondaries – from CA breast, CA stomach (G.I.T.) or chest.

   Left supraclavicular lymph nodes or Virchow's or Scalene nodes also known as signal nodes enlarged in cases of CA stomach, testis and other abdominal organs – due to vast territory drained by thoracic duct.
2. **Torticollis or Wry Neck** is deformity caused by spasm or contracture of muscles supplied by spinal accessory nerve. Rheumatic Torticollis due to exposure to cold or draught.
   (a) Reflex torticollis due to inflammed lymph nodes which irritate the spinal accessory nerve.
   (b) Congenital torticollis – due to contracture of muscle since birth or due to injury at birth.

3. **Cervical rib:** May compress subclavian artery and brachial plexus – radial pulse decreases, tingling, numbness etc.
4. **Block dissection of neck** is done in malignancies.

DIGASTRIC MUSCLE

Digastric muscle has three parts:

- Posterior belly – muscular
- Intermediate tendon – fibrous
- Anterior belly – muscular.

POSTERIOR BELLY

Arises from medial surface of mastoid process of temporal bone (mastoid notch).

This passes – downwards and forwards across carotid sheath and ends in intermediate tendon. It pierces the stylohyoid insertion and held in position by a loop of deep fascia – bounds the tendon to the junction of body and greater cornu of hyoid bone.

Anterior Belly:

Attached to the lower border of the body of mandible near median plane (Digastric notch of mandible).

Nerve Supply:

Facial nerve supplies posterior belly. Anterior belly by nerve to mylohyoid (V_3).

Action:

Depresses the mandible or elevates the hyoid bone.

Relations of Posterior Belly of Digastric

I. Superficial relations

1. Mastoid process.
2. Muscles attached to mastoid process – sternocleido mastoid, splenius capitis and longissimus capitis.
3. Lower part of parotid gland.
4. Retro mandibular vein.
5. Stylohyoid muscle.
6. Submandibular gland.
7. Submandibular lymph nodes.
8. Angle of mandible with insertion of medial pterygoid.

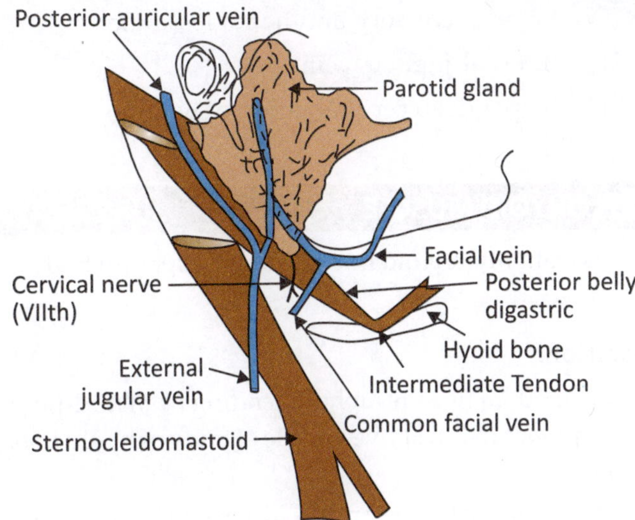

Fig. 14.10: *Superficial relations of posterior belly digastric*

Upper border is related to:

- Posterior auricular artery
- Stylohyoid muscle.

Lower border is related to: Occipital artery.

II. Deep relations

1. Transverse process of atlas.
2. Rectus capitis lateralis.
3. Obliquus capitis superior.
4. External carotid artery.
5. Lingual artery.
6. Facial artery.
7. Occipital artery.
8. Internal carotid artery.

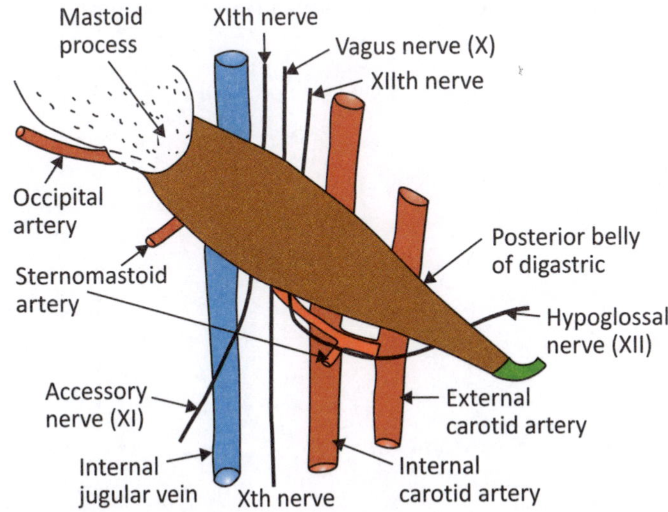

Fig. 14.11: *Deep relations of posterior belly of digastric*

9. Vagus, accessory and hypoglossal nerve.
10. Internal jugular vein.
11. Upper deep cervical group of lymph nodes.

MYLOHYOID MUSCLE

Arises from mylohyoid line on medial aspect of body of mandible.

Insertion:

On median fibrous raphe extending from mid-point of symphysis menti above middle of body of hyoid bone below.

It forms a diaphragm for floor of mouth and is continuous with the mylohyoid muscle of opposite side through mid-line raphe that extends from the mandible to the hyoid. Superficial to mylohyoid is anterior belly of digastric muscle both derived from mandibular arch in embryo and are innervated by V_3 (mylohyoid nerve).

HYOGLOSSUS

Arises from greater cornu and body of hyoid bone and inserts into tongue.

Important relation with XIIth nerve (hypoglossal) on its external surface and lingual artery on its internal surface in digastric triangle.

MIDDLE CONSTRICTOR OF PHYARNX

Arises from V shaped union of greater and lesser omohyoid bone and from stylohyoid ligament that attaches to lesser cornu. Its fibres pass posteriorly to lateral wall of pharynx.

STYLOHYOID MUSCLE

Origin:

From styloid process of temporal bone.

Insertion:

Into junction of the body with greater cornu of hyoid bone. Tendon is pierced by intermediate tendon of digastric near its insertion.

Action:

- Pulls the hyoid bone upward and backward
- Keep the hyoid in its position.

Nerve supply:

Branch from facial nerve.

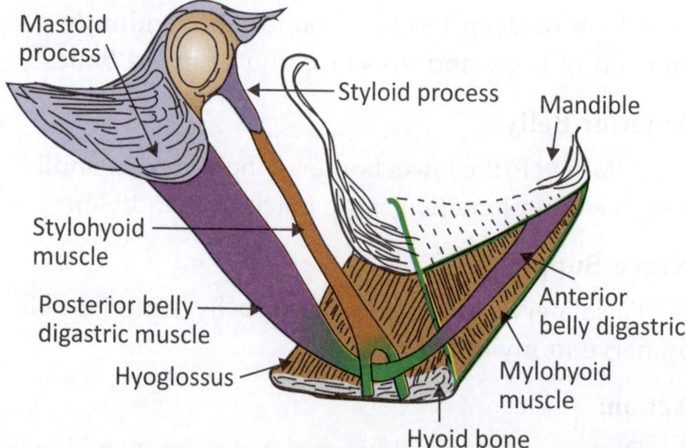

Fig. 14.12: *Digastric, mylohyoid and stylohyoid muscles*

CHAPTER 15

Subdivisions of Anterior Triangle of Neck

It is divided by digastric muscle and superior belly of omohyoid into four parts:

1. Submental triangle
2. Digastric triangle
3. Carotid triangle
4. Muscular triangle.

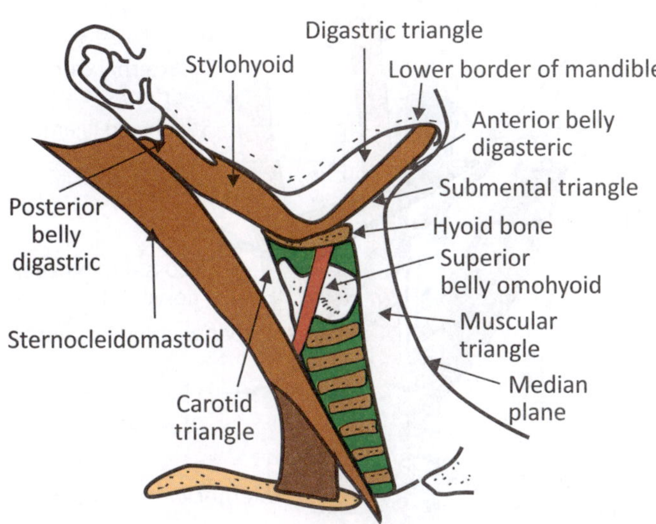

Fig. 15.1: *Subdivisions of anterior triangle of neck*

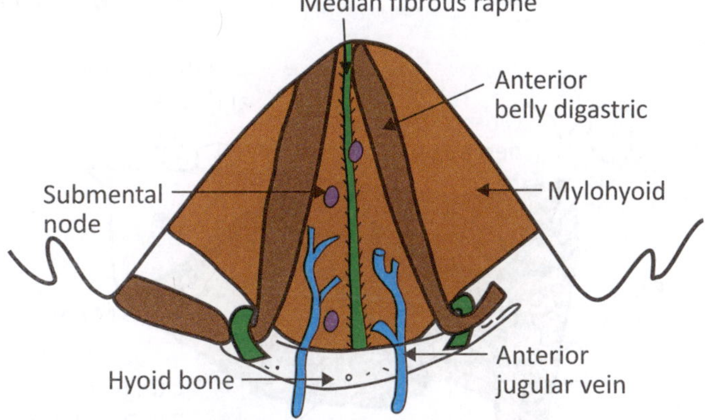

Fig. 15.2: *Submental triangle*

SUBMENTAL TRIANGLE

Boundaries

- On each side – Anteior belly of digastric.
- Base – Body of hyoid bone.
- Apex – Chin or symphysis menti.
- Floor – Mylohyoid muscles both side.
- Roof – Skin, superficial fascia, platysma and fascia colli (investing layer).

Contents

1. Submental lymph nodes (2-3).
2. Submental veins and commencement of anterior jugular vein.

DIGASTRIC TRIANGLE

Boundaries

- Antero-inferior – Anterior belly of digastric
- Postero-inferior – Posterior belly of digastric
- Base – Lower border of mandible and an imaginary line-joining angle of mandible to mastoid process.
- Apex – Intermediate tendon of digastric muscle bound down to hyoid bone by a facial sling.
- Floor – Mylohyoid muscle anteriorly.

  Hyoglossus muscle and a small portion of middle constrictor posteriorly.
- Roof – Skin, superficial fascia, platysma, investing layer of deep cervical fascia.

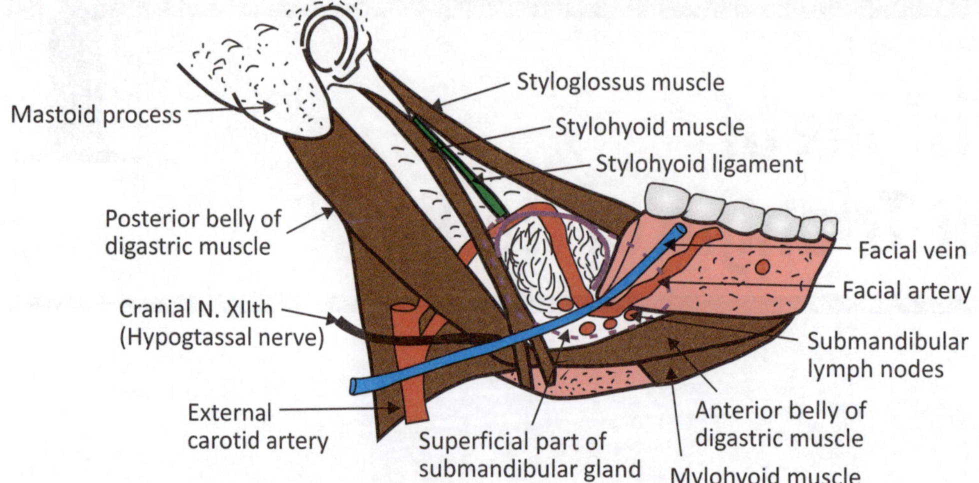

Fig. 15.3: *Digastric triangle boundaries and contents*

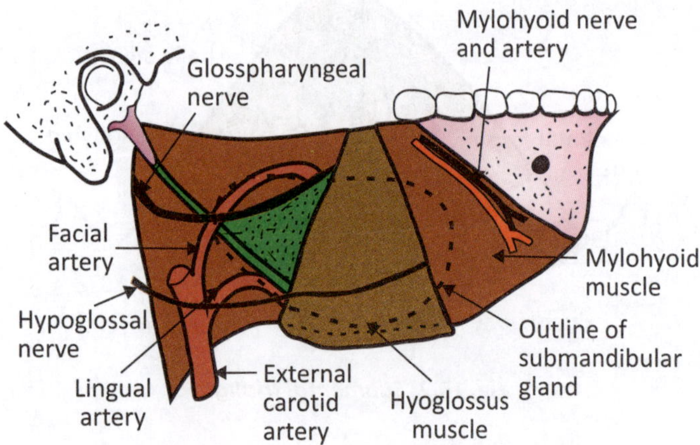

Fig. 15.4: *Floor of digastric triangle mylohyoid muscle*

MAIN CONTENTS OF DIGASTRIC TRIANGLE

1. Submandibular gland.
2. Submandibular lymph nodes.
3. Hypoglossal nerve (XIIth C.N.).
4. Submental artery and vein, branches of facial artery.
5. Mylohyoid nerve and vessels.
6. Carotid sheath with its contents poheteriorly and external carotid artery with its brances anteriorly.
7. External carotid artery with its branches – lingual artery, facial artery and posterior auricular artery.
8. Structures passing between external and internal carotid artery are:
   - Styloid process
   - Styloglossus musle
   - Stylopharyngeus muscle
   - Glassopharyngeal nerve
   - Lower end of parotid gland
   - Pharyngeal branch of vagus nerve (X).

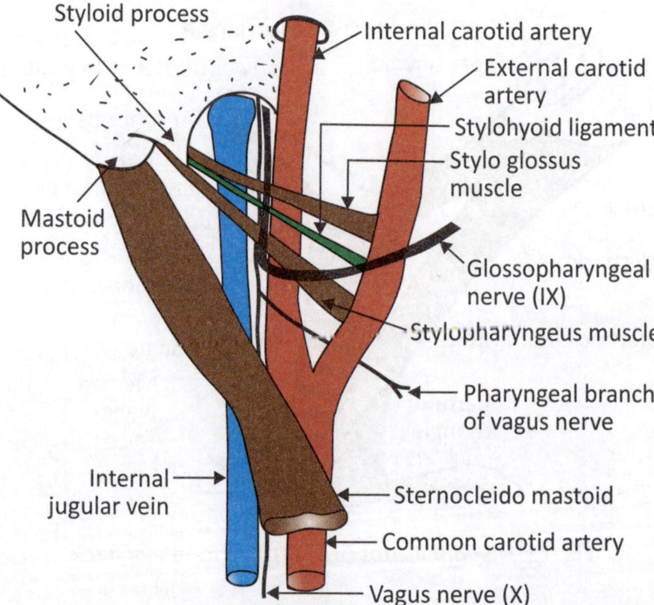

Fig. 15.5: *Structures intervening between internal and external-carotid arteries*

CAROTID TRIANGLE

Boundaries

- Antero-superiorly – Posterior belly of digastric and stylohyoid muscle
- Antero-inferiorly – Superior belly of omohyoid muscle

- Posteriorly – Anterior border of sterno-cleidomastoid muscle
- Roof – Skin, superficial fascia, platysma, cervical branch of facial nerve, transverse cutaneous nerve of neck. Investing layer of deep cervical fascia.
- Floor – Thyrohyoid and hyoglossus muscle – anteriorly, middle and inferior constrictor of pharynx posteriorly.

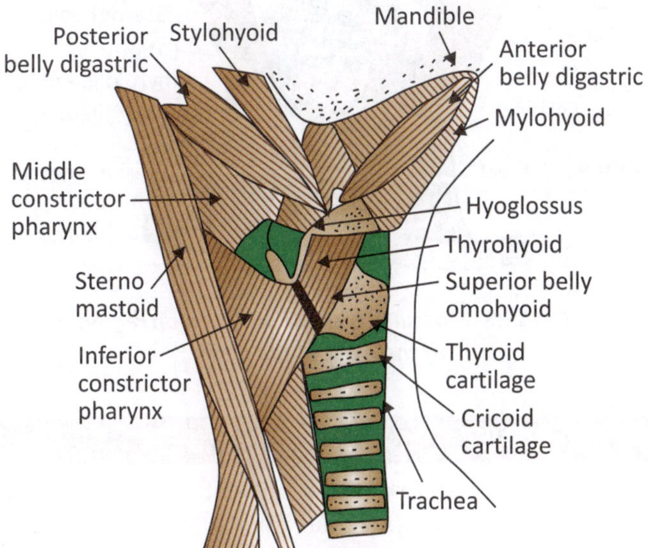

Fig. 15.6: ***Boundaries of carotid triangle and its floor***

CONTENTS OF CAROTID TRIANGLE

A. Arteries:

1. Common carotid artery with carotid sinus and carotid body at its termination.
2. Internal carotid artery.
3. External carotid artery with its superior thyroid, lingual, facial, ascending pharyngeal and occipital branches.

B. Veins:

1. Internal juglar vein.
2. Common facial vein – draining into internal jugular vein.
3. Pharyngeal vein – open into internal jugular vein or common facial vein.
4. Lingual vein – open into internal jugular vein

C. Nerves:

1. Vagus nerve – running – vertically downwards postero medial to internal jugular vein.
2. Superior laryngeal branch of vagus nerve dividing into external and internal laryngeal nerve.
3. Spinal accessory nerve – running downwards on internal jugular vein.

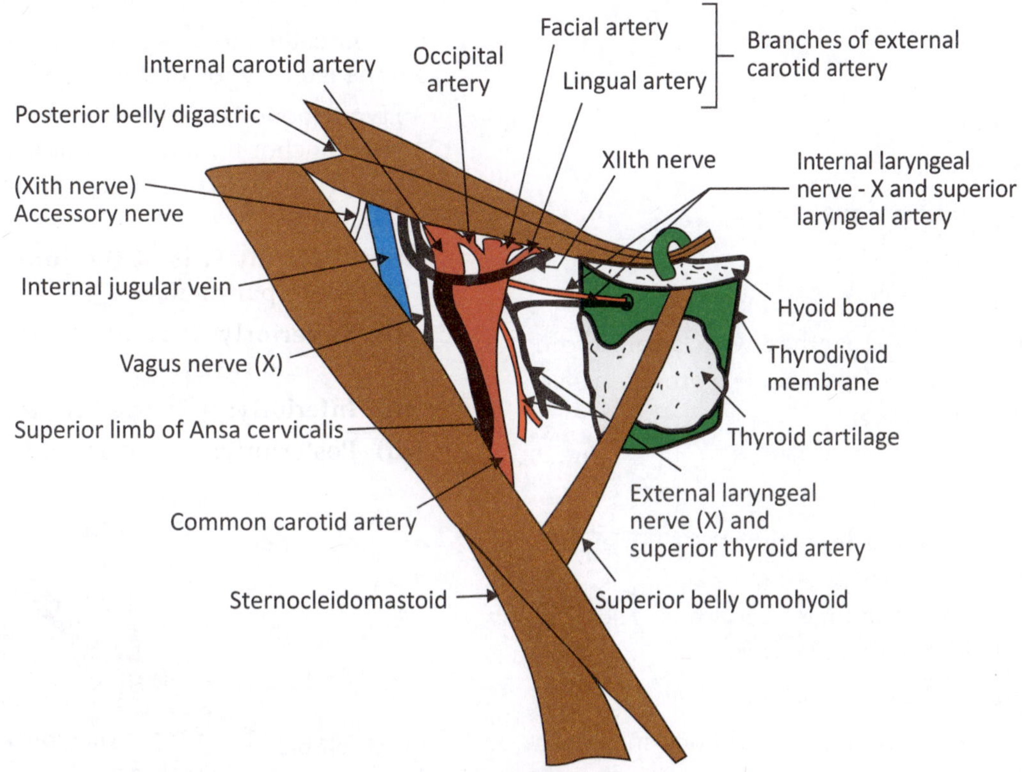

Fig. 15.7: ***Contents of carotid triangle***

4. Hypoglossal nerve – running forwards over external and internal carotid artery. Hypoglossal nerve gives off upper root of ansa cervicalis C_1 fibres (Descendens Hypoglossi) and another branch to thyrohyoid.
5. Sympathetic chain–runs vertically downwards posterior to carotid sheath.

D. Carotid sheath and its contents.

E. Lymph nodes:

Deep cervical lymph nodes along internal jugular vein (jugulo digastric and jugulo omohyoid).

MUSCULAR TRIANGLE

Lies below the hyoid bone.

Boundaries

- Anteriorly – Mid-line of the neck.
- Supero-Laterally – Superior belly of omohyoid.
- Infero-Laterally – Anterior border of sterno cleidomastoid muscle.
- Floor – Sternohyoid and sternothyroid muscle.
- Roof – Skin, superficial fascia, investing layer of deep fascia with platysma and cutaneous nerves and vessels.

Deep to it lies:

- Thyroid gland
- Larynx and trachea
- Pharynx and oesophagus.

Actions

- Infrahyoid muscles together with suprahyoid muscles – stabilize the hyoid bone to provide a base for movements of tongue.
- Participate in movements of larynx in swallowing.
- Thyrohyoid is supplied by C_1 branch of XIIth nerve; other infrahyoid muscles are supplied by C_1, C_2 and C_3 via branch from ansa cervicalis. They depress the hyoid bone and larynx.
- Thyrohyoid – elevates the larynx.
- They move the larynx and hyoid bone in speech and swallowing.

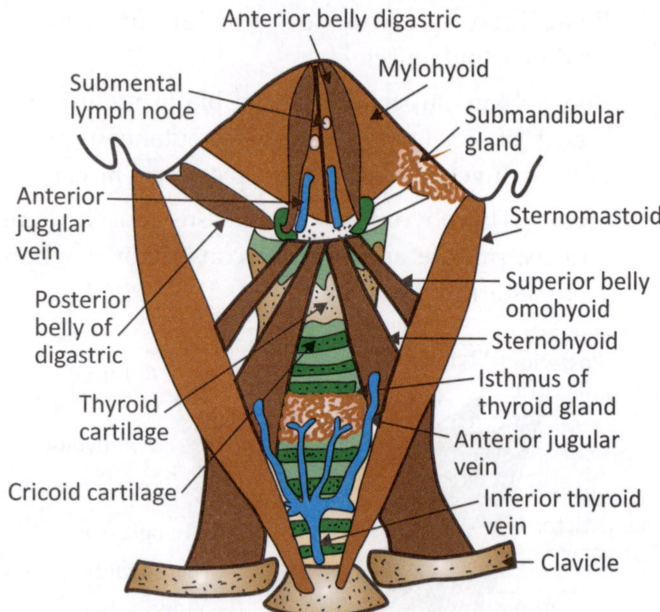

Fig. 15.8: ***Muscular triangle and median region of the front of the neck***

HYOID BONE

It is a small 'U' shaped bone present in the horizontal plane just superior to the larynx.

Parts

1. **Body:** It is anterior and forms the base of the 'U'.
2. **Horns:** Greater and lesser horn, project posteriorly from the lateral ends of the body.
   - Hyoid bone is a highly movable and strong bony anchor for a number of muscles and soft tissue structures, e.g., membranes and ligaments.
   - **Significantly it is at the junction between three compartments:**
     (i) **Superiorly:** It is attached to the floor of the oral cavity.
     (ii) **Inferiorly:** It is attached to the larynx.
     (iii) **Posteriorly:** It is attached to the pharynx.

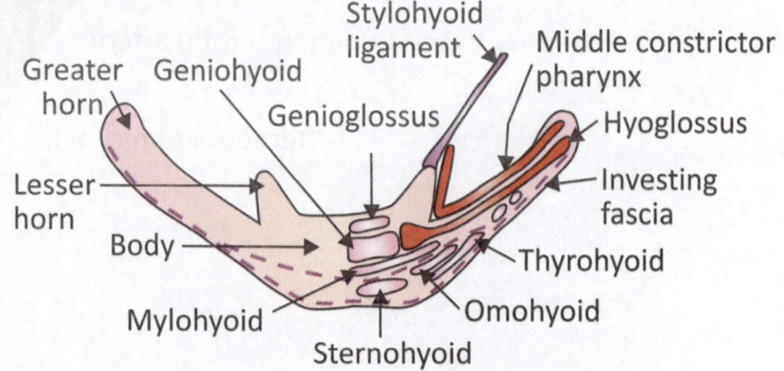

Fig. 15.9: ***Hyoid bone-front viens***

MUSCLE IN THE ANTERIOR TRIANGLE OF NECK

I. Suprahyoid Muscles:

Muscle	Origin	Insertion	Nerve supply	Function
Stylohyoid	Base of styloid process	Lateral surface of body of hyoid bone at the junction of greater and lesser horn	Branch of facial nerve (VII)	Pulls hyoid bone postero superiorly
Digastric Anterior belly	Digastric fossa of mandible below genial tubercles	Intermediate tendon at body of hyoid bone	Mylohyoid nerve (V_3)	Assist in opening mouth and raises hyoid bone
Posterior belly	Digastric notch present on medial side of mastoid process	Intermediate tendon at body of hyoid bone	Branch of facial nerve (VII)	Assist in opening mouth and raises hyoid bone
Mylohyoid	Mylohyoid line on inner surface of body of mandible	Median fibrous raphe and mid of body of hyoid bone	Mylohyoid nerve (V_3)	Elevation of floor of mouth and hyoid bone during swallowing
Geniohyoid	Inferior mental spine	Anterior surface of body of hyoid bone	C_1 fibres (via-XIIth nerve)	Hyoid bone is fixed depresses mandible, when mandible is fixed elevates hyoid bone.

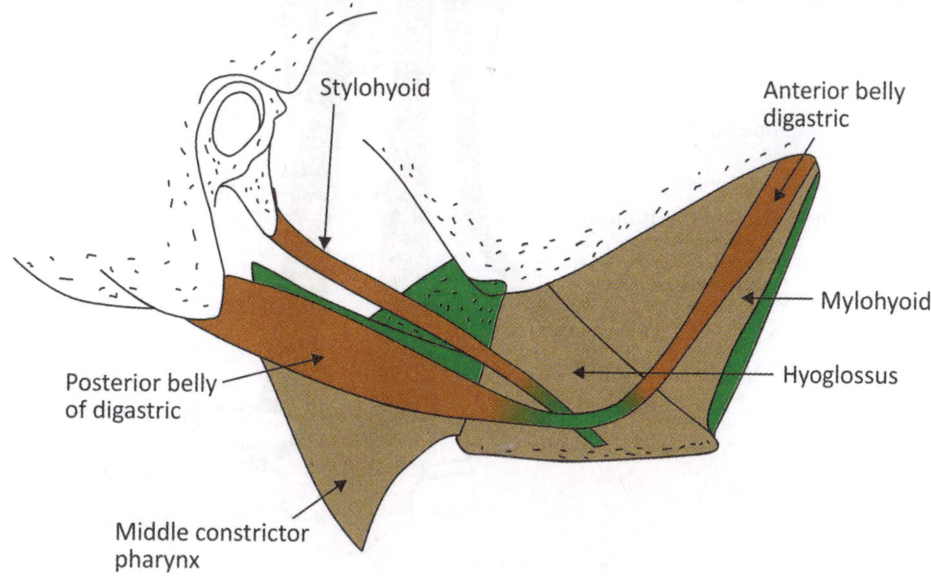

Fig. 15.10: *Suprahyoid muscles of neck*

II. Infrahyoid Muscles:

Muscle	Origin	Insertion	Nerve supply	Function
Sternohyoid	Posterior aspect of sterno clavicular joint and manubrium sterni	Body of hyoid bone medial to omohyoid	C_1, C_2 and C_3 via ansa cervicalis	Depresses hyoid bone after swallowing
Omohyoid	Superior border of scapula medial to suprascapular notch and suprascapular ligament	Lower border of body of hyoid bone lateral to sternohyoid	Anterior rami of C_1, C_2 and C_3 (via ansa cervicalis)	Depresses and fixes hyoid bone
Thyrohyoid	Oblique – line of lamina of thyroid cartilage	Greater horn and body of hyoid bone	Anterior Rami of C_1 (via XIIth nerve)	Depresses hyoid bone, when hyoid is fixed it raises larynx
Sterno Thyroid	Posterior surface of manubrium sterni	Oblique line on lamina of thyroid cartilage	Anterior Rami of C_1, C_2 and C_3 (Ansacervicalis)	Draws larynx downward

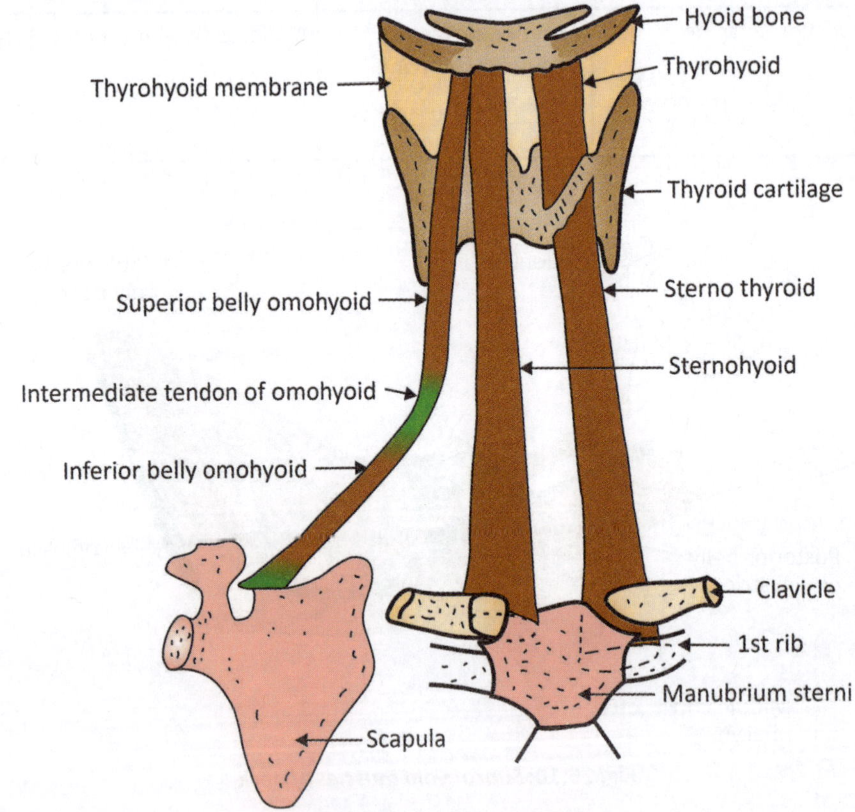

Fig. 15.11: *Infrahyoid muscles*

CHAPTER 16

Parotid Gland

This is a Greek word comprising *para* means near or around and *otos* – Ear.

This is the largest salivary gland and is a compound tubulo-acinar-serous type of gland. It secrets water saliva.

- **Weight:** About 15 to 30 gms
- **Shape:** Irregular-wedge shaped
- **Development:** Buccal ectoderm
- **Situation:** Parotid bed in parotid region is bony, muscular and fascia lined space.

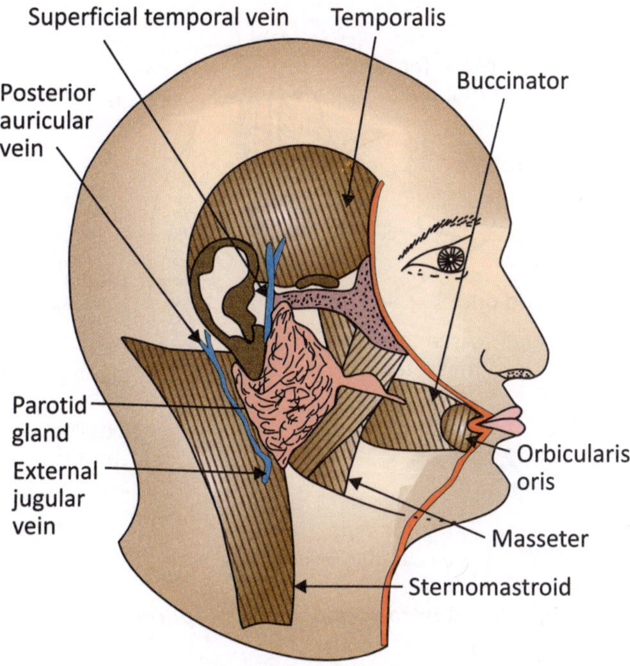

Fig. 16.1: *Situation of parotid gland*

BOUNDARIES OF PAROTID BED

- **Anterior:**
  - Posterior border of ramus of mandible
  - Medial pterygoid muscle
  - Masseter muscle.
- **Posterior:**
  - Mastoid process
  - Anterior border of sternocleido mastoid muscle.
- **Superiorly:**
  - Capsule of temporo-mandibular joint
  - External auditory meatus.

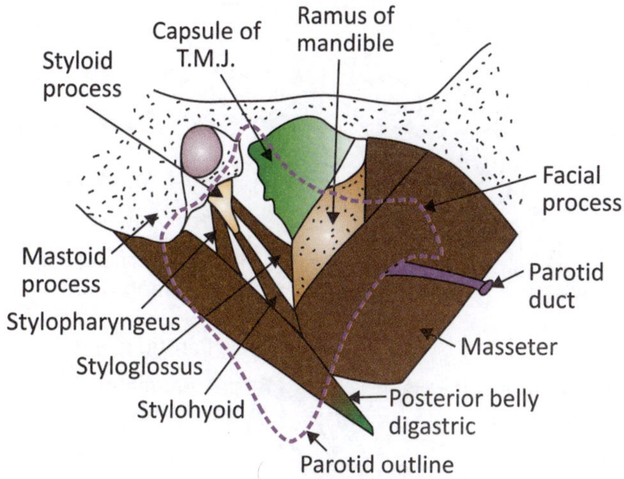

Fig. 16.2: *Parotid bed*

- **Inferiorly:**
  - Posterior belly of digastric
  - Stylohyoid.

➢ Floor
- Styloid process
- Styloglossus, stylopharyngeus and stylohyoid muscle
- Gland overflows out of structures of parotid bed.

EXTERNAL FEATURES

Surfaces: There are four surfaces of this gland:

1. Superficial surface – lower end is called apex
2. Superior surface or base
3. Antero medial surface
4. Postero medial surface.

RELATIONS OF PAROTID GLAND

1. **Superficial Surface:** It is related to:
   - Skin
   - Superficial fascia
   - Great auricular nerve (C_2 and C_3)
   - Pre-auricular lymph nodes
   - Parotid masseteric fascia.

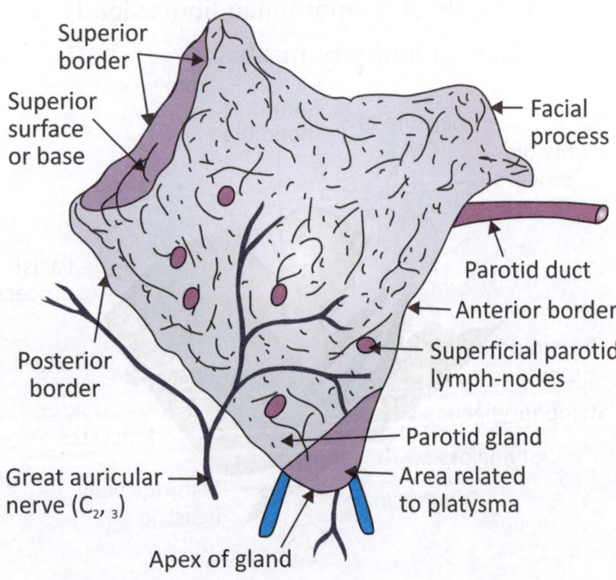

Fig. 16.3: *Superficial surface of parotid gland*

Apex: Lower end of superficial surface is called apex. It crosses the posterior belly of digastric muscle and enters the carotid triangle. It is pierced by cervical branch of facial nerve, anterior and posterior divisions of retro-mandibular vein.

2. **Superior Surface (base of the gland):**

➢ It is concave upper aspect of the gland and is related to:

(a) Temporo mandibular joint
(b) External auditory meatus.

➢ **This surface is pierced by:**

(a) Superficial temporal vessels
(b) Auriculo temporal nerve
(c) Temporal branch of facial nerve.

➢ An abscess formed in this surface may burst and open into the external auditory meatus.

➢ It is not covered by parotid fascia.

3. **Antero-medial Surface:**

➢ Posterior border of ramus of mandible grooves this surface.

➢ **Surface is related to:**

(a) Masseter muscle
(b) Posterior border of ramus of mandible
(c) Capsule of temporo mandibular joint
(d) Medial pterygoid muscle.
(e) Branches of facial nerve leaves the gland through this surface.

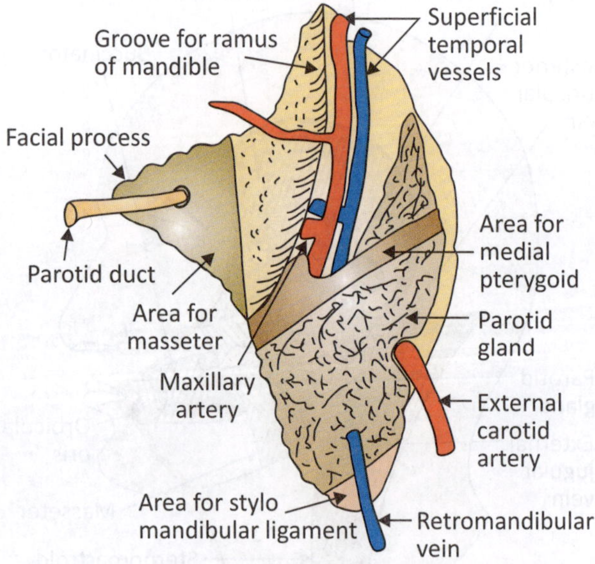

Fig. 16.4: *Antero-medial surface of parotid gland*

4. **Postero-medial Surface:** It is a large surface and related to:

(a) Mastoid process of temporal bone
(b) Sternocleido mastoid muscle

(c) Posterior belly of digastric muscle
(d) Styloid apparatus
(e) External carotid artery enters the gland.

Styloid process separates the gland from the following structures:

(i) Internal jugular vein
(ii) Internal carotid artery
(iii) Glossopharyngeal, vagus and accessory nerves.

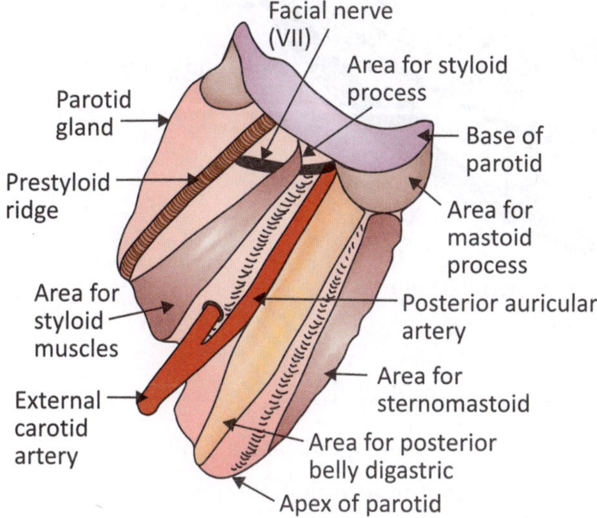

Fig. 16.5: *Postero-medial surface of parotid gland*

Anterior Border

Separates the superficial surface from the antero medial surface. From this border following structures are emerging:

(i) Zygomatic branch of facial nerve
(ii) Transverse facial vessels
(iii) Upper buccal branch of facial nerve
(iv) Parotid duct
(v) Lower buccal branch of facial nerve
(vi) Marginal mandibular branch of facial nerve.

- Accessory parotid gland (Sociaparotid) when present it may be situated above the parotid duct.

CAPSULE OF THE GLAND

Investing layer of deep cervical fascia splits at the lower pole of the gland divides into superficial and deep layers. Deep layer passes deep to gland and attached to the base of the skull. Superficial layer is called parotido-masseteric fascia, it is attached to the lower border of zygomatic arch. This fascia is not elastic and hence inflammations of the gland are highly painful.

Superior aspect of the gland has no proper capsule, posteriorly the capsule is defective. Here, parotid space communicates with pharyngeal space.

STRUCTURES PRESENT WITHIN THE GLAND

(i) Facial nerve with its branches
(ii) Retro mandibular vein
(iii) External carotid artery.

- Facial nerve is sandwiched between superficial and deep lobes of the parotid gland. An isthmus connects the two lobes:
- Facial nerve crosses superficial to the retro-mandibular vein and external carotid artery.

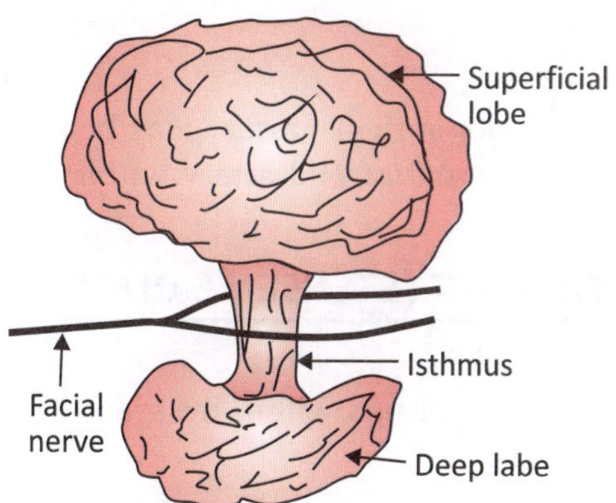

Fig. 16.6: *Lobes of parotid gland*

(i) Facial nerve: Divides into following branches:

A. Temporo facial branch divides into:

(a) Temporal branch
(b) Zygomatic branch.

B. Cervico facial branch divides into:

(a) Upper and lower buccal branch
(b) Marginal mandibular branch
(c) Cervical branch.

(ii) Retro mandibular vein: This is formed by union of superficial temporal vein and maxillary vein within the lower part of the gland and it divides into anterior and posterior divisions.

(iii) External carotid artery: This is deeply situated within the gland. It terminates by dividing into superficial temporal and maxillary arteries.

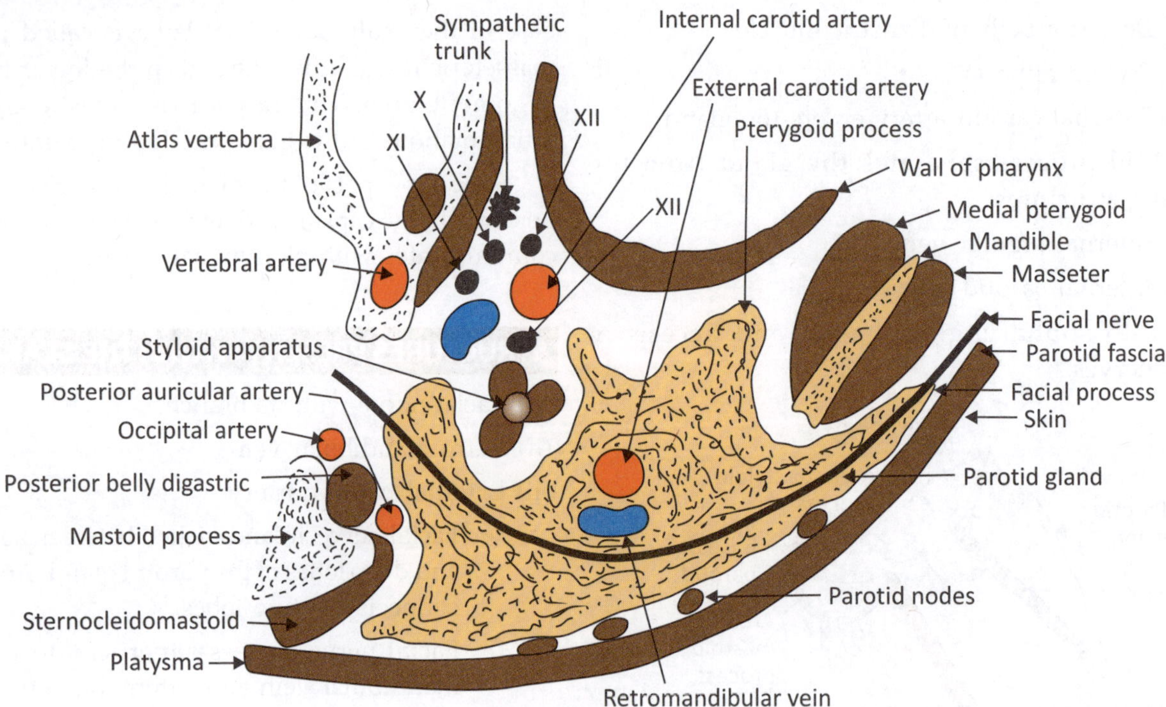

Fig. 16.7: ***T.S. through parotid gland***

- Posterior auricular artery may be formed from the external carotid artery within the gland.

PAROTID DUCT (STENSEN'S DUCT)

- **Length:** 5 cm
- **Formation:** Formed within the gland by fusion of two ducts.
- **Emergence:** It emerges through the anterior border of the parotid gland.
- **Course:** It runs forwards on the lateral surface of the masseter muscle.

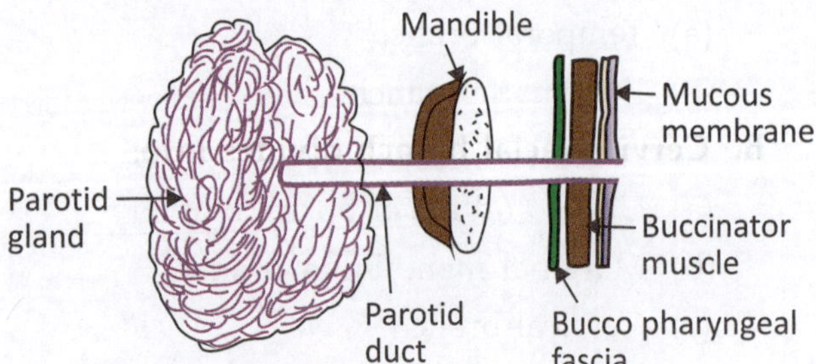

Fig. 16.8: ***Structures pierced by parotid duct***

- It is situated in between the upper and lower buccal nerves. At the anterior border of the masseter muscle it turns medially and pierces the following structures:
  - Buccal pad of fat
  - Bucco pharyngeal fascia
  - Buccinator muscle
  - Mucous membrane of the mouth.
- **Termination:** It terminates in the vestibule of the mouth at the level of upper second molar tooth. The terminal part of the duct is oblique. This oblique direction is acting like a valve.
- **Blood supply:** From branches of external carotid artery.
- **Venous drainage:** External jugular vein.
- **Lymphatic drainage:** Parotid lymph nodes.

NERVE SUPPLY OF PAROTID GLAND

A. **Sympathetic supply**: Plexus around external carotid artery. These fibres are vasomotor in function and derived from the superior cervical sympathetic ganglion.

B. **Parasympathetic supply (Secretomotor supply):** Inferior salivatory nucleus → glossopharyngeal nerve → tympanic branch of glossopharyngeal → tympanic plexus → lesser superficial petrosal nerve → otic ganglion → postganglionic fibres join auriculo temporal nerve → parotid gland.

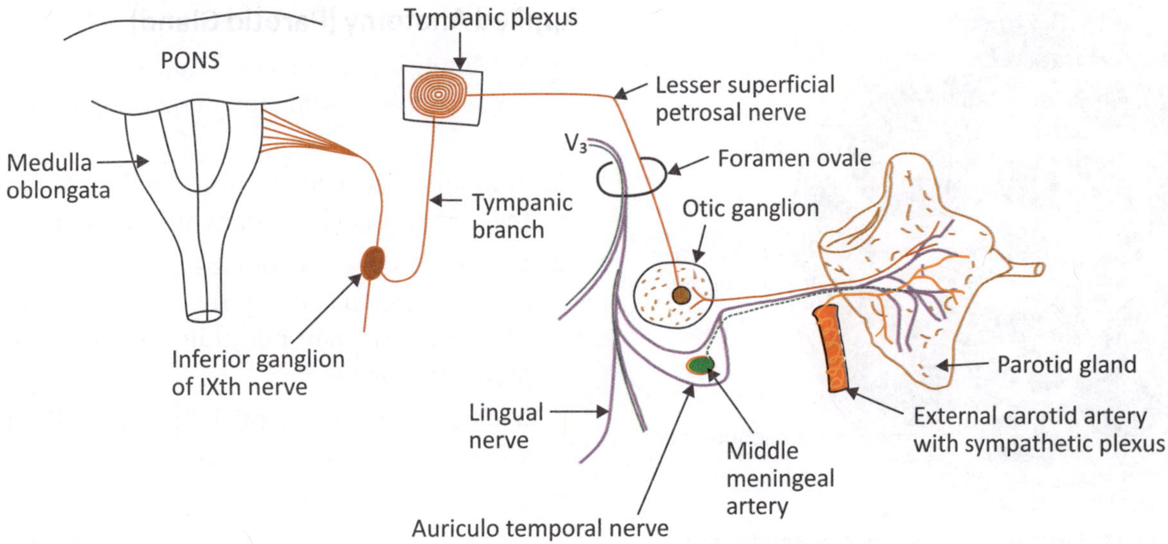

Fig. 16.9: *Nerve supply of parotid gland*

C. **Sensory supply:**
- Auriculo temporal nerve
- Great auricular nerve.

Important structures that radiate from the periphery of the parotid gland:

1. **Superiorly:**
   - Superficial temporal vessels
   - Auriculo temporal nerve
   - Temporal branch of facial nerve.

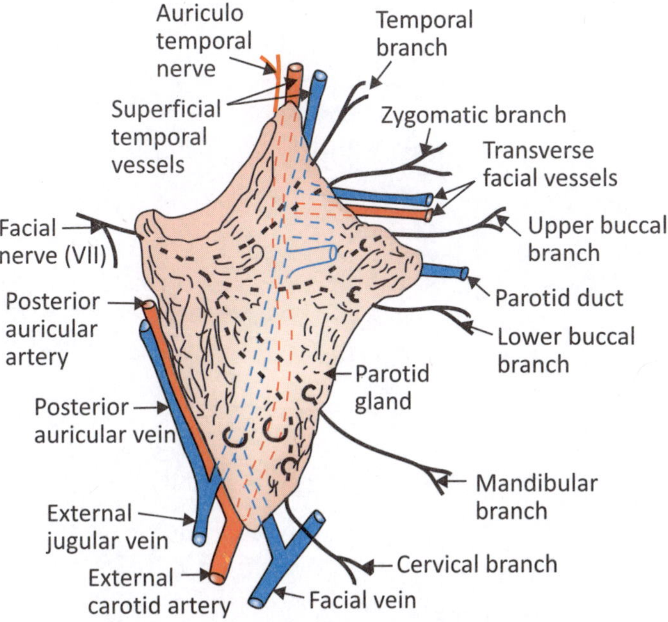

Fig. 16.10: *Structures radiating from parotid gland*

2. **Anteriorly:**
   - Transverse facial vessels
   - Zygomatic branch of facial nerve
   - Upper buccal branch of facial nerve
   - Parotid duct
   - Lower buccal branch of facial nerve
   - Marginal mandibular nerve (VII).
3. **Inferiorly:**
   - Cervical branch of facial nerve
   - External jugular vein
   - Great auricular nerve.
4. **Posteriorly:**
   - Occipital vessels
   - Posterior auricular vessels and nerve.

MICROSCOPIC STRUCTURE OF PAROTID GLAND

- Serous type of salivary gland.
- Glandular mass is covered by fibrous capsule.
- Capsule invades the gland as fibrous septae and divides the gland into lobes and lobules.
- Each lobule is formed by collection of alveoli.
- Each alveolus has pyramidal shaped cells containing zymogen granules.
- Nucleus is kept along the base of the cell.

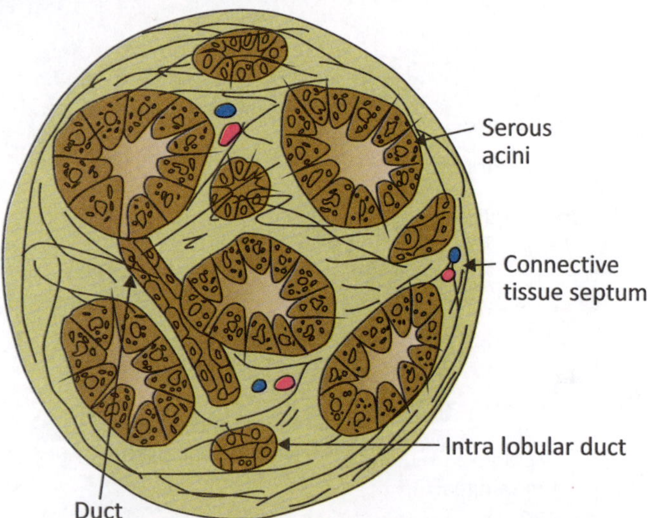

Fig. 16.11: ***Microscopic structure of parotid gland***

- Cells are anchored to the basement membrane.
- Zymogen granules are utilized in the synthesis of enzymes of the saliva.
- Basket cells support the serous cells of the alveolus. They help in squeezing the alveoli while releasing the saliva.
- Secretory canaliculi open into the lumen of follicle, and are lined by cuboidal epithelium.

Applied Anatomy (Parotid Gland)

1. Swelling of parotid gland causes severe pain because of non-yielding tough parotid masseteric fascia.
2. Tumours arise usually from the lateral portion of the gland. Mixed tumours are commonest.
3. Parotid abscess may burst superiorly into external auditory meatus or may run medially towards the pharynx or it may perforate the fascia inferiorly and enter the neck.
4. **Mumps:** This is a viral infection of the parotid gland and involves both sides.
5. Calculus formation.
6. Parotid sialography – radiopaque dye is injected into the duct – to study the anatomy of parotid duct and gland.
7. While draining parotid abscess horizontal incision should be given to save the branches of facial nerve – Hiltons Law.

Infection from mouth can spread by parotid duct and involve parotid gland.

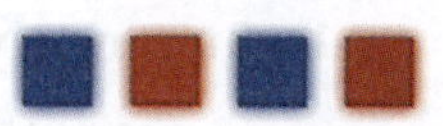

CHAPTER 17

Submandibular Gland

Situation: Digastric triangle and in the submandibular fossa of the mandible.

Type: Compound and tubulo acinar mixed type of gland (serous and mucous).

Development: This develops from buccal ectoderm.

Weight: About 15 gms.

Shape: 'J' shaped, size of a walnut. Indented by posterior border of mylohyoid.

Parts: Superficial and deep part.

Two parts are continuous around the posterior border of mylohyoid muscle.

Superficial part is larger than deep part.

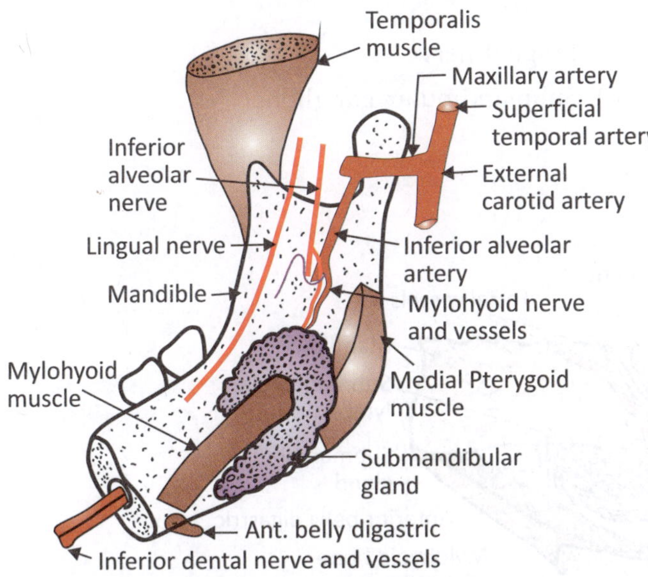

Fig. 17.1: *Submandibular gland*

SUPERFICIAL PART OF SUBMANDIBULAR GLAND

Is large and fills the digastric triangle.

Extends:

- Upwards deep to mandible upto mylohyoid line.
- Anteriorly – upto anterior belly of digastric muscle.
- Posteriorly – upto stylomandibular ligament.

Surface: It has three surfaces:

1. Inferior surface
2. Lateral surface
3. Medial surface

Relations:

1. **Inferior surface:** On this surface submandibular lymph glands are situated.

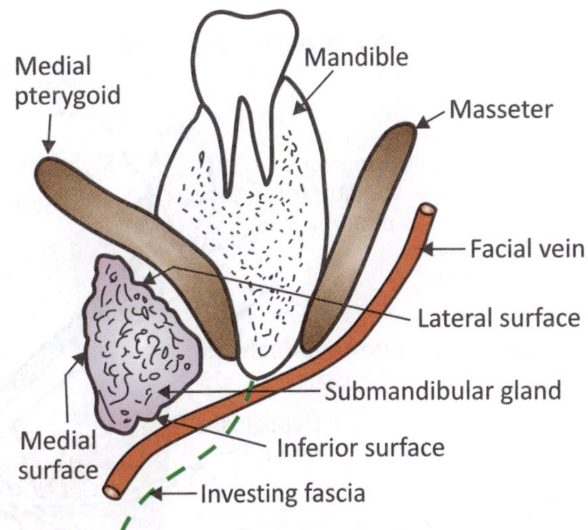

Fig. 17.2: *Inferior relations of submandibular gland*

It is related to:

(i) Skin
(ii) Superficial fascia containing
(iii) Platysma and cutaneous nerves and vessels
(iv) Investing layer of deep cervical – fascia
(v) Common facial vein
(vi) Cervical branch of facial nerve.

2. **Lateral surface:** It is related to:
   (i) Mandible – Submandibular fossa
   (ii) Medial pterygoid muscle
   (iii) Facial artery.
3. **Medial surface:** It is related to:
   (a) Anterior part: Mylohyoid muscle with its nerve and vessels.

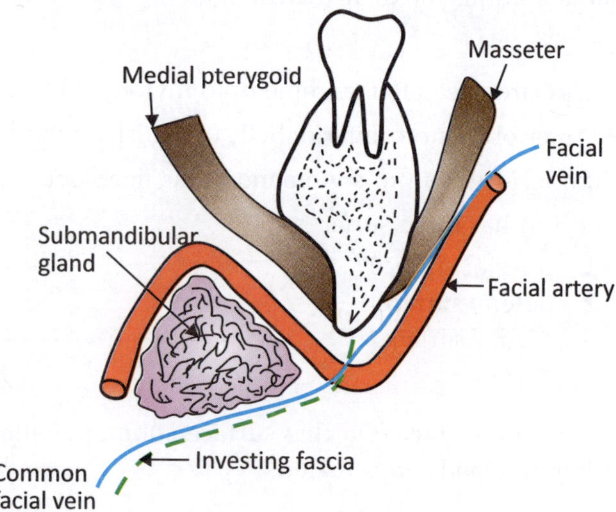

Fig. 17.3: ***Lateral relations of gland***

(b) Middle part:
(i) Hyoglossus muscle
(ii) Lingual nerve
(iii) Submandibular ganglion
(iv) Hypoglossal nerve (XII).

(c) Posterior part:
(i) Styloglossus muscle
(ii) Stylopharyngeal muscle
(iii) Glossopharyngeus nerve (IX)
(iv) Posterior belly of digastric muscle
(v) Wall of pharynx – middle constrictor muscle
(vi) Lingual artery
(vii) Hypoglossal nerve (XII)
(viii) Stylohyoid muscle and ligament.

DEEP PART

- Situated above the mylohyoid muscle.
- Contacts anteriorly – sublingual gland.
- Smaller than the superficial part.
- Wedged between hyoglossus and mylohyoid muscle.

Relations:

- **Superiorly:**
  (i) Lingual nerve
  (ii) Submandibular ganglion.

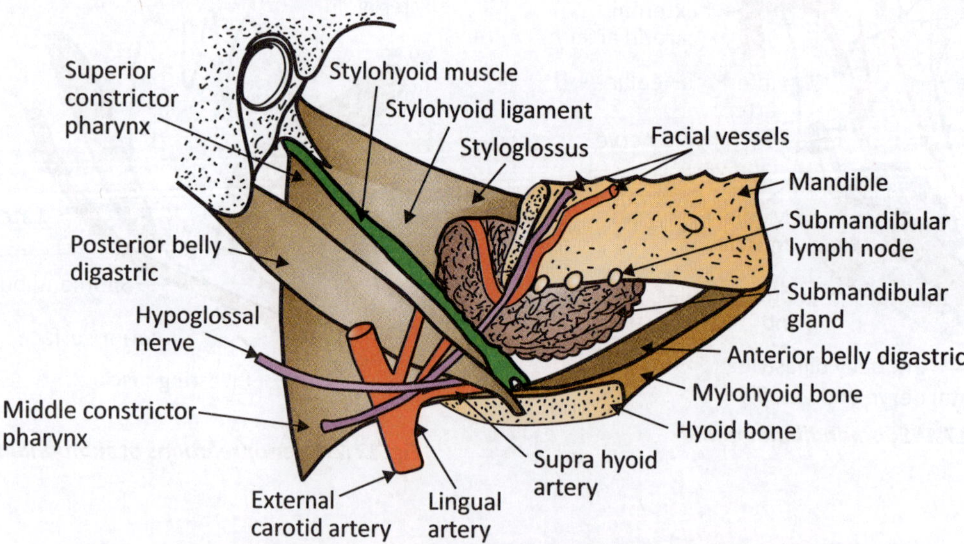

Fig. 17.4: ***Medial relations of superficial part of submandibular gland***

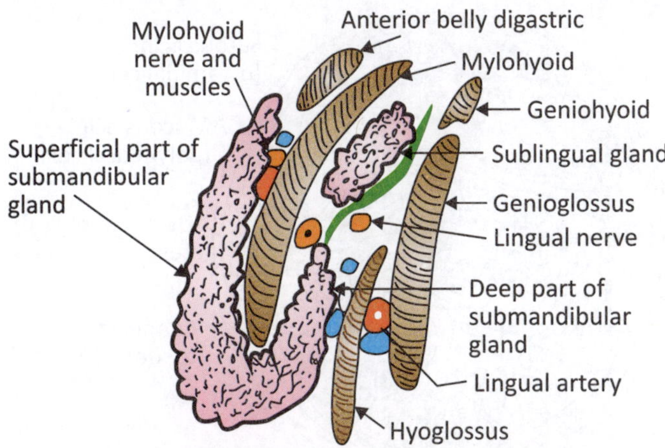

Fig. 17.5: *Horizontal section through submandibular region showing location of submandibular and sublingual glands*

- **Inferiorly:** Hypoglossal nerve
- **Medially:** Hyoglossus muscle

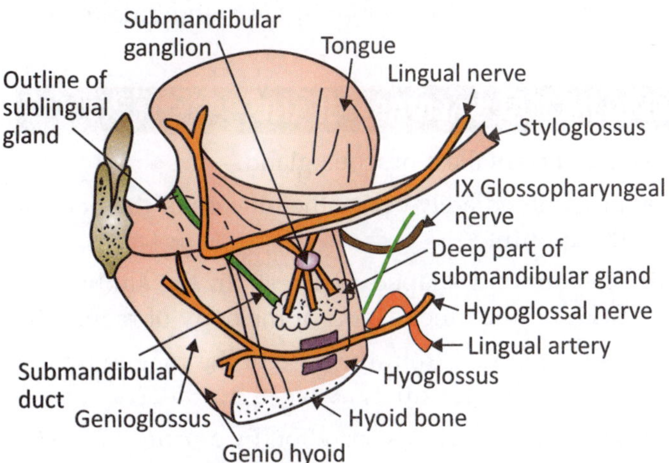

Fig. 17.6: *Relations of deep part of submandibular gland and its duct*

- **Laterally:** Mylohyoid muscle
- **Anteriorly:** Sublingual gland (Salivary).
- **Posteriorly:**
  - (i) Posterior belly of digastric muscle
  - (ii) Stylomandibular ligament
  - (iii) Parotid gland.

CAPSULE OF SUBMANDIBULAR GLAND

- Investing layer of deep cervical fascia splits into two layers – superficial layer is attached to lower border of mandible.
- Deep layer covers medial surface of gland and attached to mylohyoid line of the mandible.

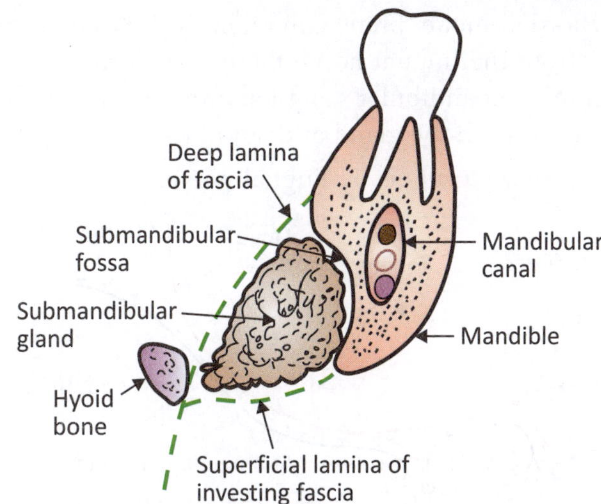

Fig. 17.7: *Fascial covering of gland (Capsule)*

Blood Supply:

- **Arterial supply** is by branches of facial and lingual arteries.
- **Venous drainage** by common facial and lingual veins.
- **Lymphatic drainage**: Submandibular lymph nodes.

SUBMANDIBULAR DUCT (WHARTON'S DUCT)

- Thin walled, about 5 cm long.
- Emerges out of anterior end of deep part of gland.

Course: Runs forwards on hyoglossus muscle, after it lies between genioglossus and sublingual gland.

Termination: On surface of sublingual papilla at the root of frenulum linguae.

- Duct can be felt below the mucous membrane of the mouth along the sides of the tongue.
- Lingual nerve hooks round the lower border of duct and reaches medial to the duct.

NERVE SUPPLY OF SUBMANDIBULAR GLAND

1. **Sympathetic supply** by plexus around facial artery. These fibres are the post ganglionic fibres from the superior cervical sympathetic ganglion. These fibres are vasomotor in function.
2. **Parasymphathetic supply (Secreto motor):** Preganglionic fibres are coming from superior salivatory nucleus with the sensory part of the facial nerve, they leave the facial nerve in its

chordatympani branch and join the lingual nerve – from the lingual nerve these fibres are relayed into submandibular ganglion and postganglionic fibres reach the gland and supplies.

3. **Sensory supply** is by lingual nerve.

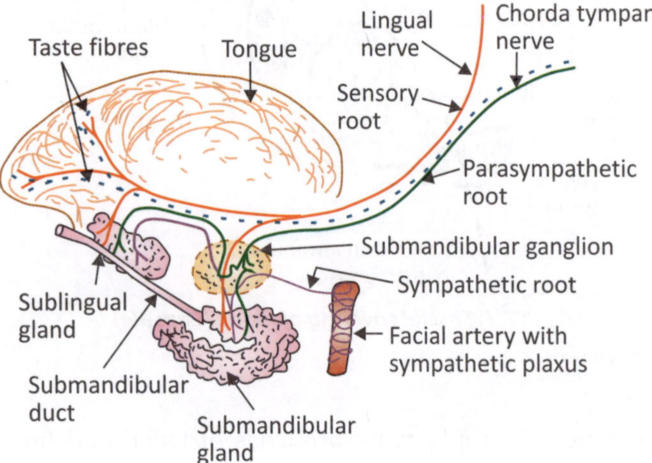

Fig. 17.8: *Submandibular ganglion*

Submandibular Duct and Lingual Nerve – Relation

- Nerve is situated above the duct.
- It then crosses lateral to the duct.
- It is then situated below the duct.
- It hooks round the lower border of the duct and reaches the medial surface of the duct.

STRUCTURE OF SUBMANDIBULAR GLAND

- Mixed type of gland.
- Gland shows large number of serous alveoli lined by pyramidal shaped cells with zymogen granules.
- Mucous alveoli have large irregular shaped (polyhedral) cells; contain mucous granules in the cytoplasm.
- Basket cells are absent.
- Usually, along the terminal part of the mucous alveolus, the serous cell clusters to form the demilunes of Giannuzi.
- Duct is lined by cuboidal epithelium and similar to parotid gland.

Applied Anatomy

1. Calculus formation.
2. Infection from oral cavity can reach to gland and causes inflammation to gland.

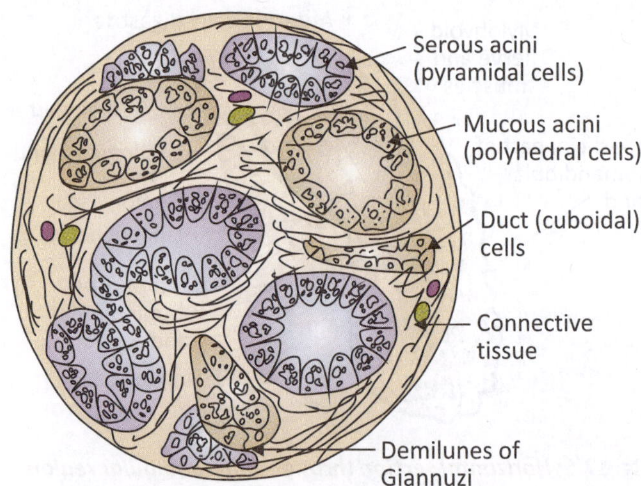

Fig. 17.9: *Microscopic structure of submandibular gland*

3. Secondaries deposited in the gland from oral cancer.
4. Carcinoma or tumour of the submandibular gland.

SUBLINGUAL SALIVARY GLAND

- It is the smallest mucous gland.
- Lies immediately below the mucosa of the floor of the mouth.
- It is almond shaped and rests in the sublingual fossa on the inner aspect of the body of mandible.
- It is separated from the base of the tongue by the submandibular duct.
- The gland pours its secretion by a series of ducts, about 10 to 15 in numbers into the oral cavity on the sublingual fold.

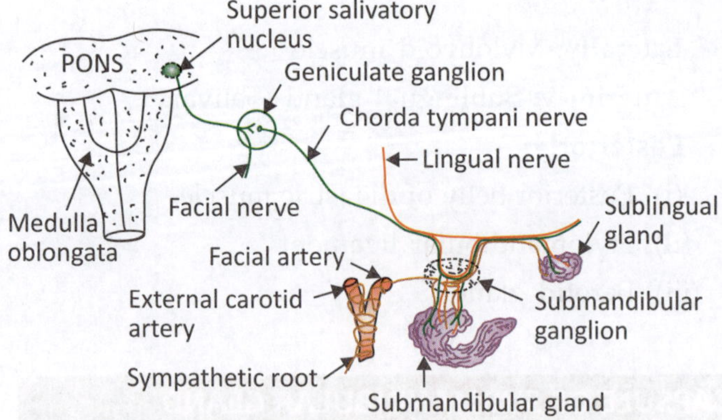

Fig. 17.10: *Nerve supply of submandibular and sublingual gland*

Blood supply: By sublingual branches of lingual artery.

Venous drainage: Lingual vein drains into internal jugular vein.

Nerve supply:

- **Sympathetic:** Via plexus around lingual artery.
- **Parasympathetic:** From submandibular ganglion (superior salivatory nucleus and chorda tympani).

Sensory: Lingual nerve.

Nature of secretion: Predominently mucous.

Styloid apparatus: Styloid process is the part of temporal bone. Structures which are attached to this process form styloid apparatus.

STRUCTURES ARE MUSCLES AND LIGAMENTS

Muscles are:

- Stylohyoid
- Styloglossus
- Stylopharyngeus.

Ligaments are:

- Stylomandibular ligament and
- Stylohyoid ligament.

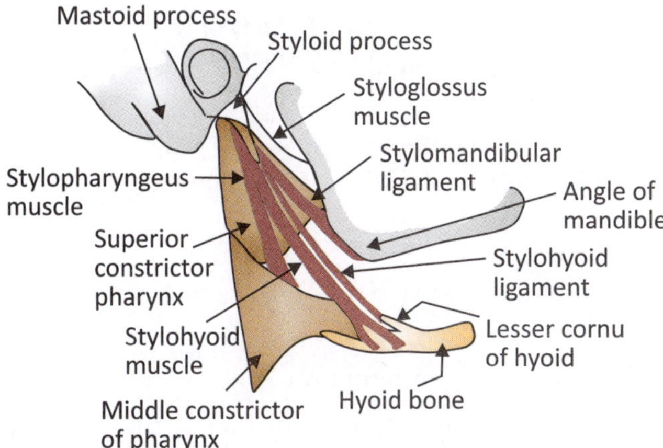

Fig. 17.11: *Styloid apparatus*

1. **Styloid process:** It is long slender and pointed bony process projecting – downwards, forwards and medially.
   - It lies between external and internal carotid arteries to reach the side of pharynx.
   - Laterally it is related to parotid gland and medially related to internal jugular vein.
2. **Styloglossus:** It arises from tip and anterior surface of styloid process and upper end of stylohyoid ligament. Passes downwards and forwards inserted into the side of the tongue, intermingling with the fibres of hyoglossus. It is supplied by hypoglossal nerve and pulls the tongue upwards and backwards.
3. **Stylopharyngeus:** It arises from the medial surface of the styloid process, passes between external and internal carotid arteries, enters the pharynx through the gap between superior and middle constrictors and is inserted to posterior border of lamina of thyroid cartilage.
   - It is supplied by glossopharyngeal nerve (IX) and pulls the larynx upwards during swallowing and phonation.

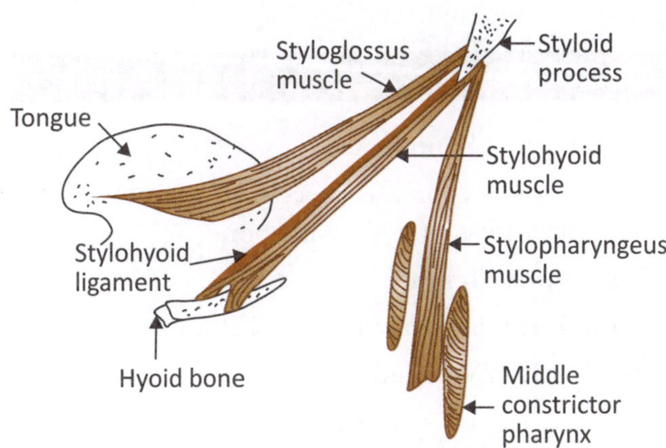

Fig. 17.12: *Styloid apparatus*

4. **Stylohyoid muscle:** It arises from tip and posterior surface of styloid process, runs downwards to get inserted at the junction of greater cornu and body of hyoid bone, before insertion it bifurcates and embrace the digastric tendon.
   - It is supplied by branch of facial nerve (VII) and pulls the hyoid bone upwards and backwards (keep it in position or helps in stabilizing the hyoid bone when other muscles act on hyoid).
5. **Stylomandibular ligament:** It is formed by thickening in the investing layer of deep fascia neck, stretches from tip of styloid process to the angle of mandible. It separates the parotid gland from submandibular gland. It is an accessory ligament of temporo-mandibular joint.
6. **Stylohyoid ligament:** Extends from the tip of styloid process to the lesser cornu of hyoid bone keep it in position.

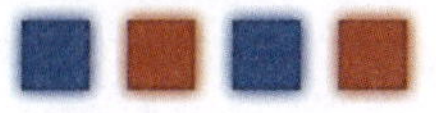

CHAPTER 18

Temporal and Infra Temporal Fossa

TEMPORAL FOSSA

Boundaries: It is bounded:

- **Anteriorly:** Zygomatic process of frontal bone and frontal process of zygomatic bone.
- **Posteriorly:** Temporal line.
- **Superiorly:** Superior temporal line.
- **Inferiorly:** Zygomatic arch.
- **Floor:** Parts of – frontal, parietal, temporal and greater wing of sphenoid bone.

Contents:

1. Temporalis muscle and fascia.
2. Deep temporal nerves – two
3. Deep temporal vessels – two
4. Auriculo – temporal nerve
5. Superficial temporal vessels.

INFRA TEMPORAL FOSSA

Situation: It is situated below the zygomatic arch and temporal fossa, in the deeper aspect of the lateral surface of the face.

Boundaries of Infra Temporal Fossa

Anterior: Posterior surface of maxilla

Posterior:

1. Styloid process
2. Tympanic plate of temporal bone
3. Carotid sheath

Medial: Lateral pterygoid plate.

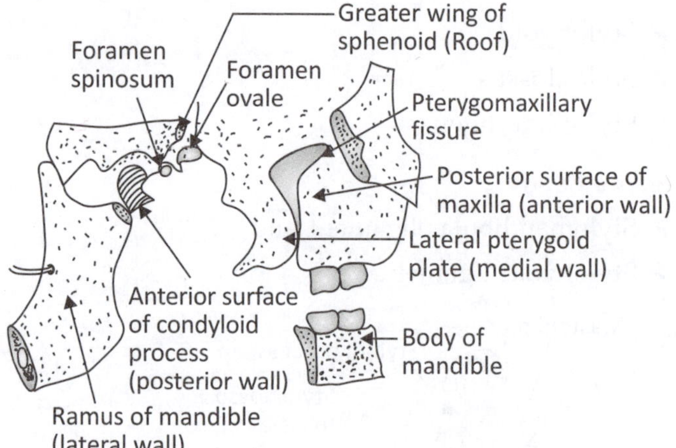

Fig. 18.1: *Bony walls of infratemporal fossa*

Superiorly:

1. Infra temporal surface of greater wing of sphenoid bone.
2. Squamous part of temporal bone.

Inferiorly: This fossa is continuous with parapharyngeal spaces.

Lateraly: Inner surface of ramus of mandible.

Communications

Anteriorly: With orbit through inferior orbital fissure.

Medially: With pterygo palatine fossa through pterygo maxillary fissure.

Superiorly: With temporal fossa deep to zygomatic arch, and middle cranial fossa via foramen ovale, foramen spinosum and foramen lacerum.

Inferiorly: With para pharyngeal spaces.

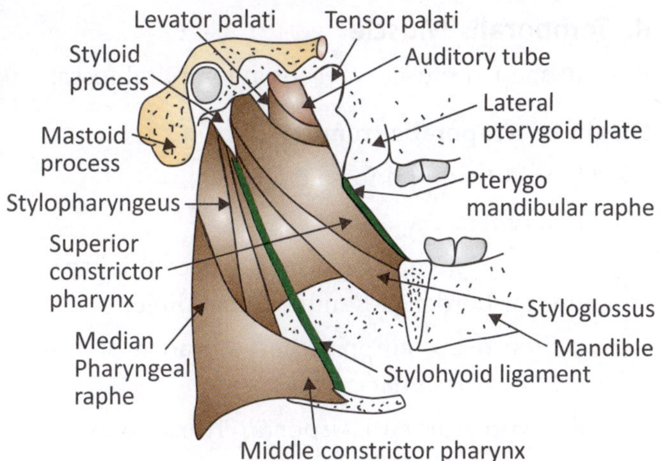

Fig. 18.2: *Medial limit of infra temporal fossa*

Contents

1. Mandibular nerve and its branches.
2. Maxillary artery and its branches.
3. Chorda tympani nerve.
4. Otic ganglion.
5. Pterygoid plexus of veins.
6. Lower part of temporalis muscle, medial and lateral pterygoid muscles.
7. Spheno mandibular ligament.
8. Fat and connective tissue.

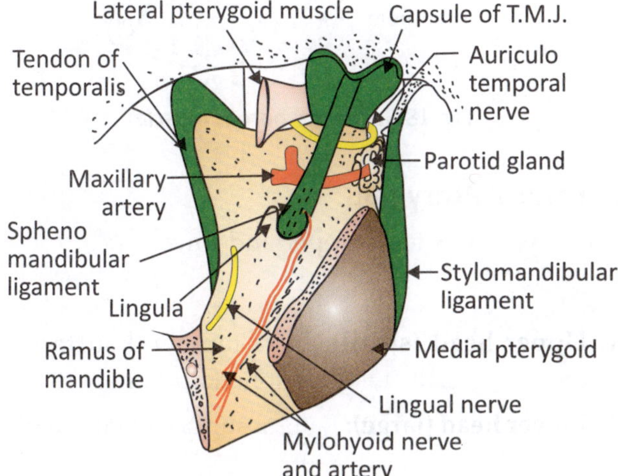

Fig. 18.3: *Lateral wall of infratemporal fossa and related structures*

Applied Anatomy of Infra Temporal Fossa

1. Head of mandible may dislocate forwards into the infra temporal fossa and compresses the structures present in it, e.g., mandibular nerve, maxillary artery etc.
2. Any growth from maxillary air sinus may grow posteriorly and involve the contents of infra temporal fossa.
3. Infection from dangerous area of face spread to cavernous sinus through pterygoid venous plexus communicates through emissary veins.
4. Collection of pus or blood in the infratemporal fossa may pass downwards to para pharyngeal spaces.

MUSCLES OF MASTICATION

Mastication is a process by which food is made into small particles. This function is done by muscles of mastication and temporo mandibular joint.

Muscles involved are:

- Masseter
- Temporalis
- Medial pterygoid and
- Lateral pterygoid.

Development: The muscles of mastication are developed from mesoderm of first pharyngeal arch. The nerve of this arch is mandibular nerve – supplies all the muscles of mastication (V_3).

I. Masseter Muscle

Gr = Masseter = a Chewer

Origin:

- Anterior 2/3 of zygomatic arch by tendinous fibres.
- Entire medial surface of arch by fleshy fibres.

Insertions:

- Outer surface of ramus and
- Angle of mandible

Relations:

Deep:

- Buccal pad of fat
- Masseteric nerve and vessels
- Buccal branch of anterior division of mandibular nerve.

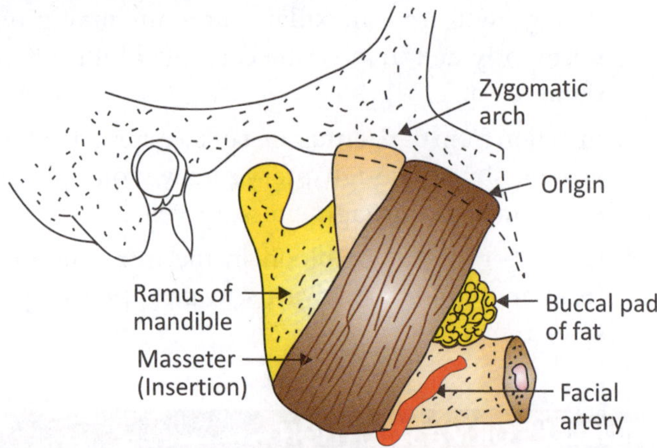

Fig. 18.4: *The masseter muscle*

Superficial:

- Transverse facial artery and vein
- Parotid duct and gland
- Branches of facial nerve.

Nerve Supply:

Masseteric nerve branch of mandibular nerve.

Action:

Elevation of mandible. It locks the jaw and clinches the teeth.

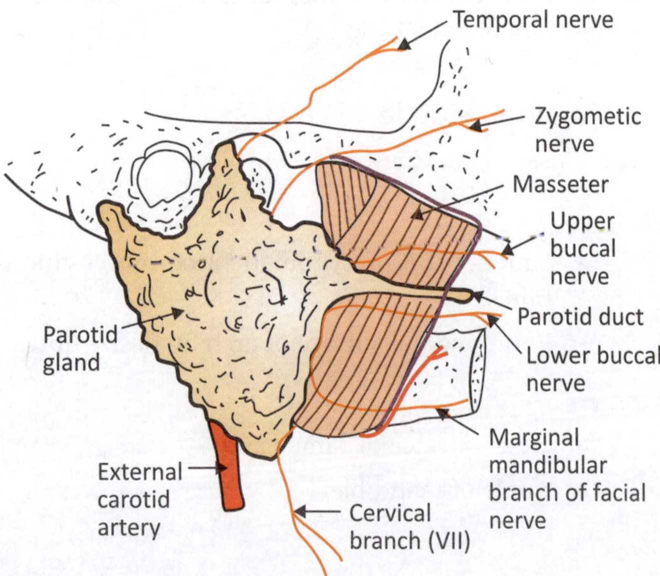

Fig. 18.5: *Superficial relations of masseter muscle*

Applied Anatomy

1. In Tetanus – Spasm of this muscle causes lock jaw or trismus.
2. Facial artery crosses lower border of mandible at antero inferior angle of masseter muscle. Pulsations of artery can be felt here.

II. Temporalis Muscle

It is fan shaped muscle present in temporal fossa.

Origin of temporalis from:

- Floor of temporal fossa and
- Temporal fascia.

Insertion: Margins and deep surface of coronoid process and anterior border of Ramus of mandible.

Nerve: Two deep temporal nerve branch of anterior division of mandibular nerve.

Action: Anterior and superior fibres elevate the mandible.

Posterior Fibres: Retract the protruded mandible.

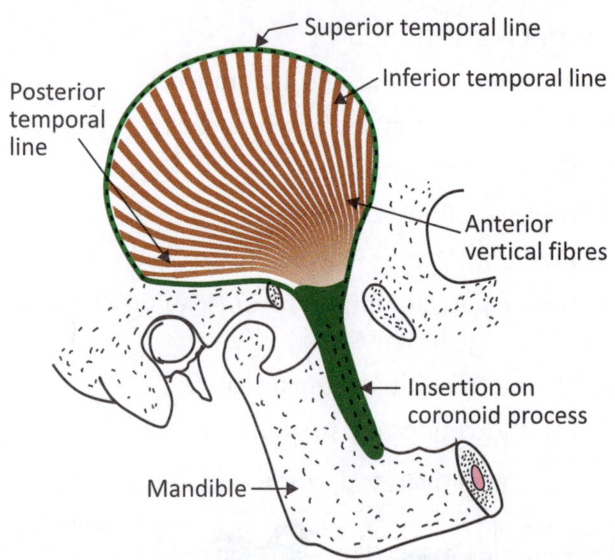

Fig. 18.6: *The temporalis muscle*

III. Lateral Pterygoid

Arises by two heads – upper and lower.

Origin:

A. **Upper head (small):** Infra temporal surface and crest of greater wing of sphenoid bone.

B. **Lower head (large):** Lateral surface of lateral pterygoid plate.

Insertion: Fibres run backwards laterally converge and inserted on pterygoid fovea present on anterior surface of neck of mandible.

- Anterior margin of articular disc and capsule of temporo mandibular joint.

Nerve supply: Pterygoid branch of anterior division of mandibular nerve.

Action: It depresses the mandible to open mouth.

- Lateral pterygoid of one side and medial pterygoid of other side – protrudes the mandible and causes side to side movement as in chewing, when act alternatively.

Relations:

A. Superficial:
- Masseter
- Ramus of mandible
- Tendon of temporalis
- Maxillary artery.

B. Deep:
- Mandibular nerve
- Middle meningeal artery
- Sphenomandibular ligament
- Deep head of medial pterygoid muscle.

C. Structures emerging at upper border of lateral – pterygoid – deep temporal nerves and masseteric nerve.

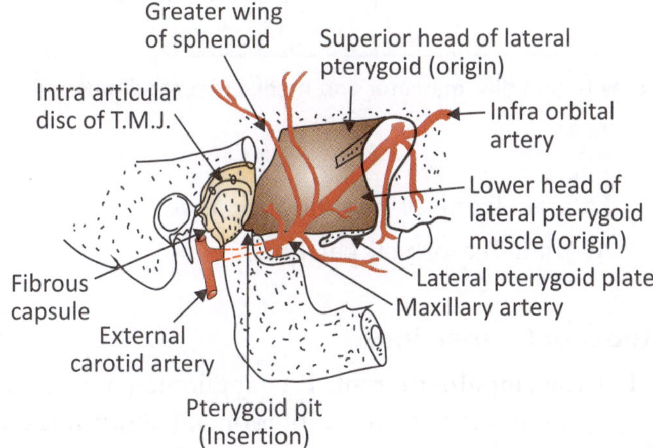

Fig. 18.7: *Lateral pterygoid muscle and its superficial relations*

D. Structures emerging at lower border of lateral – pterygoid:
- Lingual nerve.
- Inferior alveolar nerve.
- Middle meningeal artery passes upwards deep to it.

E. Structures passing through gap between two heads of lateral pterygoid:
- Maxillary artery enters the gap.
- Buccal branch of mandibular nerve comes out through gap.

F. Pterygoid venous plexus – surrounds lateral – pterygoid muscle.

IV. Medial Pterygoid

Origin by two heads:

A. **Superficial head (small slip):** Tuberosity of maxilla and adjoining bone.

B. **Deep head:** Medial surface of lateral pterygoid plate and adjoining part of palatine bone (Pyramidal process).

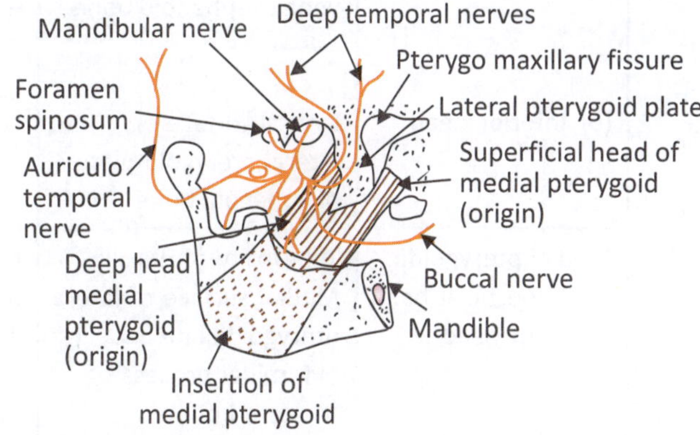

Fig. 18.8: *Medial pterygoid muscle and its superficial relations*

Insertion: Fibres run downwards, backwards and laterally to insert on medial surface of angle and ramus of mandible.

Nerve supply: To medial pterygoid from main trunk of mandibular nerve a branch arises and supplies it.

Applied Anatomy of Infra Temporal Fossa

1. Head of mandible may dislocate forwards into infra temporal fossa and compresses the structures like mandibular nerve and maxillary artery.
2. Any growth from maxillary air sinus may grow posteriorly and invade the contents of infra temporal fossa.
3. Infection from dangerous area of face spread into facial vein → deep facial vein → pterygoid venous plexus → emissary vein → cavernous sinus → may lead to meningitis or encephalitis.
4. Collection of fluid – pus or blood in infra temporal fossa may pass downwards to para pharyngeal space.

Table 18.1: *Muscles of Mastication*
(Nerve of 1st pharyngeal arch is mandibular nerve)
Develops from first pharyngeal arch

S.No.	Muscle	Origin	Insertion	Nerve	Action
1.	Temporalis fascia	Temporal fossa and Ramus of mandible	Coronoid process and	V_3	Elevate and retracts mandible
2.	Masseter	Lower border and medial surface of zygomatic arch	Lateral surface of Ramus and angle of mandible	V_3	Elevates mandible clinches teeth
3.	Lateral pterygoid: (a) Superior head (b) Inferior head	Infra temporal surface and crest of greater wing of sphenoid bone Lateral surface of lateral pterygoid plate of sphenoid bone	– Neck of mandible – Articular disc – Capsule of T.M.J.	V_3	Protrudes and depresses mandible with medial pterygoid of other side acting alternatively produces side to side movement as in chewing
4.	Medial pterygoid: (a) Superficial head (b) Deep head	Tuberosity of maxilla Medial surface of lateral pterygoid plate and pyramidal process of palatine bone	Medial surface of mandible on ramus and angle	V_3	Protrudes and elevates the mandible, with lateral pterygoid of other side acting alternatively produces side to side movement

Note: Jaws are opened by latral pterygoid muscle and are closed by temporalis, masseter and medial pterygoid muscles.

OTIC GANGLION

It is a peripheral parasympathetic ganglion.

Topographically:

Connected to the mandibular nerve, provides a relay station to secretomotor fibres for the parotid gland.

Functionally:

It is associated with glossopharyngeal nerve.

Size – Pin head – 2-3 mm.

Shape – Oval.

Location or situation:

Infratemporal fossa just below foramen ovale, medial to mandibular nerve and lateral to tensor palati surrounds origin of medial pterygoid nerve.

Relations:

Anterior: Medial pterygoid muscle

Posterior: Middle meningeal artery

Lateral: Trunk of mandibular nerve

Medial: Tensor veli palatini.

Roots or Connections

1. **Parasympathetic root:** Preganglionic parasympathetic fibres arise from inferior salivatory nucleus and pass via tympanic branch of glossopharyngeal nerve (IXth C.N.) and joins tympanic plexus of nerves in the middle ear. From plexus – lesser superficial petrosal nerve arises and passes through foramen ovale and these fibres are relayed into otic ganglion.
2. **Sympathetic root:** Derived from the sympathetic plexus around middle meningeal artery and conveys postganglionic fibres from superior cervical – sympathetic ganglion. These fibres do not relay in the otic ganglion.
3. **Motor root:** Nerve to medial pterygoid pass through the ganglion without relay.

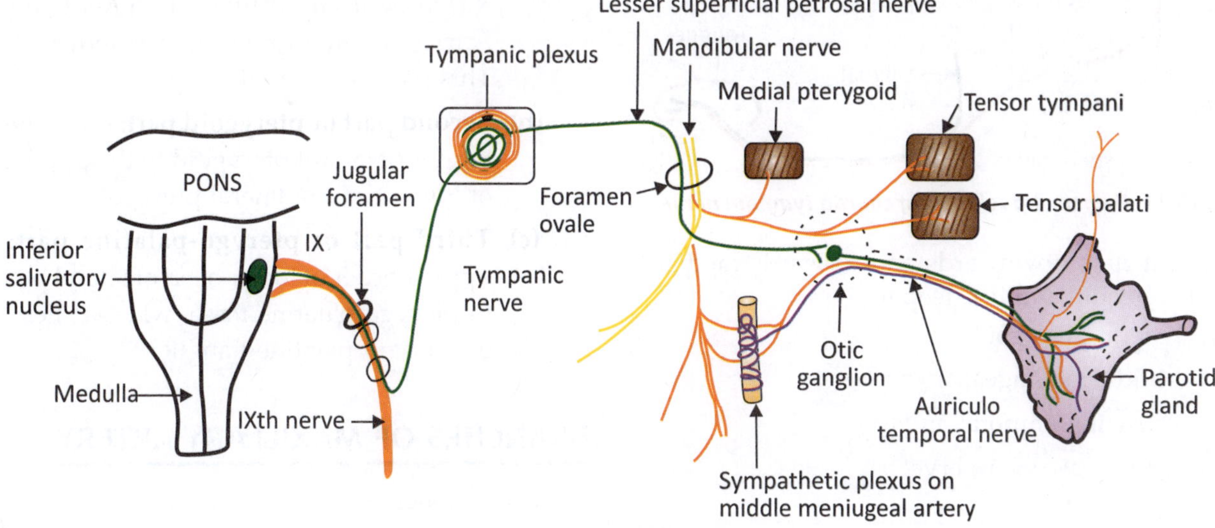

Fig. 18.9: *Otic ganglion*

4. **Sensory root:** Auriculo temporal nerve passes without relay.

Branches and Distributon

1. Nerve to tensor tympani.
2. Nerve to tensor palati.
3. Communicating branches to auriculotemporal nerve, these convey post ganglionic parasympathetic fibres which are secretomotor to parotid gland and sympathetic fibres are vasomotor for parotid, fibres of auriculo temporal are sensory for the gland.
4. Communicating branches to chorda tympani.
5. Communicate with nerve to pterygoid canal.

CHORDA TYMPANI NERVE

It is pre trematic branch of facial nerve.

Carries taste fibres from anterior 2/3 of tongue and parasympathetic fibres to submandibular and sublingual salivary glands.

Commencement and Course:

It arises in the facial canal about 6 mm above the stylomastoid foramen from the facial nerve and enters the middle ear through posterior canaliculus. Passes forwards across the inner surface of tympanic membrane internal to the handle of malleus and then leaves the middle ear by passing through the petrotympanic fissure to appear at the base of skull.

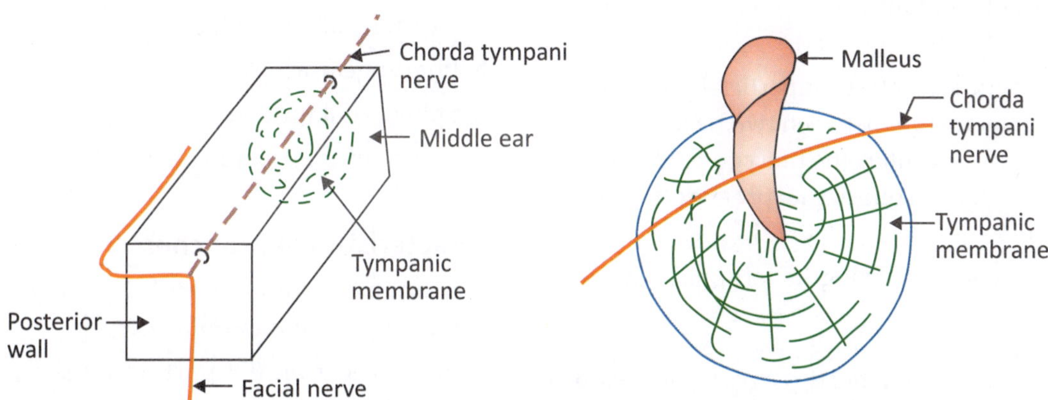

Fig. 18.10: *Course and relation of chorda tympani nerve*

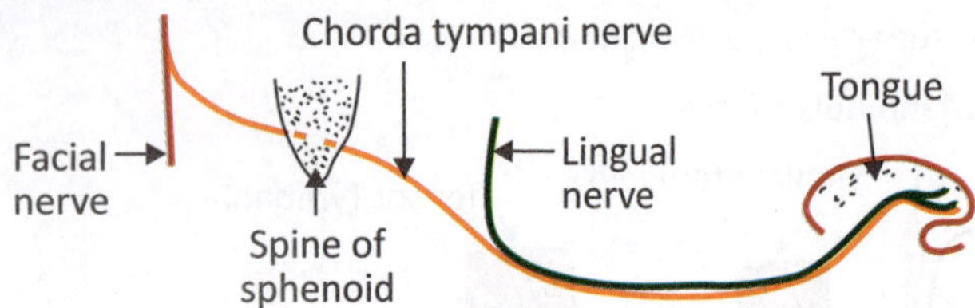

Fig. 18.11: ***Course and relation of chorda tympani nerve***

Here, it runs downwards and forwards medial to spine of sphenoid and lies deep to:

(i) Lateral pterygoid
(ii) Middle meningeal artery
(iii) Auriculo temporal and
(iv) Inferior alveolar nerve.

Terminates:

By joining the posterior aspect of lingual nerve at an acute angle and distributed with the branches of lingual nerve to anterior 2/3 of tongue, submandibular, sublingual and anterior lingual glands.

MAXILLARY ARTERY

(Syn. Internal Maxillary artery or mandibulo – maxillary artery)

- This artery supplies the structures present on a deeper plane and supplied by branches of mandibular and maxillary nerve.
- It is the larger terminal branch of external carotid artery.

Course:

It begins behind the neck of mandible and runs forwards, medially and upward upto the lower border of lower head of lateral pterygoid.

- Crosses the lower head superficially sometimes deep and emerges between two heads of lateral pterygoid and enters the pterygo palatine fossa by passing through the pterygomaxillary fissure.
- Here, it ends by giving its terminal branches.

Parts:

Maxillary artery is divided into three parts by the lower head of lateral pterygoid muscle.

(a) **First part or mandibular part:** From its origin to the lower border of lateral pterygoid. It lies between the neck of the mandible laterally and the sphenomandibular ligament medially. Auriculo temporal nerve lies above this part. This part is horizontally placed.

(b) **Second part or pterygoid part:** From the lower border of lateral pterygoid to the upper border of lower head of lateral pterygoid muscle.

(c) **Third part or pterygo-palatine part:** From upper border of lower head of lateral pterygoid to pterygo palatine fossa, where it lies infront of pterygo palatine ganglion.

BRANCHES OF MAXILLARY ARTERY

From first part:

1. Deep auricular artery
2. Anterior tympanic artery
3. Middle meningeal artery
4. Accessory middle meningeal artery
5. Inferior alveolar or dental artery.

From second part: Gives muscular branches and buccal branch.

1. Two deep temporal artery (anterior and posterior).
2. Pterygoid branches – for pterygoid muscles.
3. Masseteric artery – for masseter muscle and T.M.J.
4. Buccal artery – for skin and mucous membrane of cheek.

From third part:

1. Posterior superior alveolar artery
2. Infra orbital artery
3. Greater palatine artery
4. Pharyngeal artery
5. Spheno-palatine artery
6. Artery of pterygoid canal occasionally.

Characteristics of Branches

- Branches from 1st and 2nd parts accompany branches of mandibular nerve.
- Branches from 3rd part accompany branches of maxillary nerve and pterygo palatine ganglion.
- Branches of 1st and 3rd part of maxillary artery enters through a bony canal or foramen to supply their area of distribution.

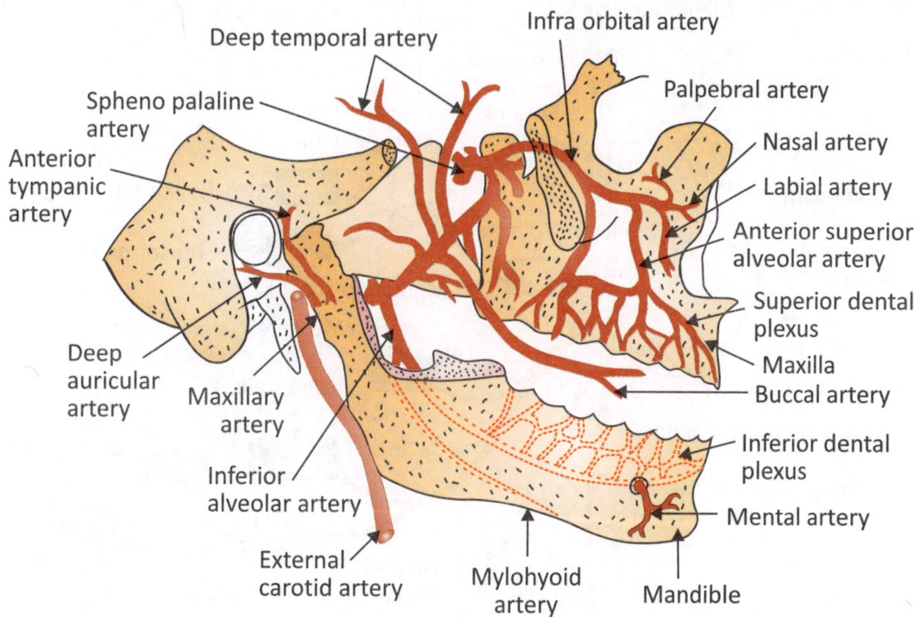

Fig. 18.12: *Maxillary artery and its branches*

Middle meiningeal artery: Largest branch from 1st part and most important passes through foramen spinosum and enters middle cranial fossa to supply periosteal dura of the cranial cavity. It ascends upwards deep to lateral pterygoid muscle and behind the mandibular nerve, passes between the two roots of auriculotemporal nerve and enters foramen spinosum along with nervous spinosus branch of mandibular nerve.

Inferior alveolar artery: Passes downwards and enters mandibular foramen to pass into mandibular canal to supply mandible, teeth of the lower jaw and passes through mental foramen to supply skin and mucous membrane of chin and lower lip. It also gives lingual branches to posterior part of the tongue.

Applied Anatomy

Angle of mandible has poor blood supply and is the site for alveolar osteitis after extraction of lower 3rd molar (wisdom tooth).

Deep auricular artery: Supply external auditory meatus. It passes through squamotympanic fissure.

Anterior tympanic artery: Accompanies chorda tympani nerve through petrotympanic fissure and reaches middle ear to supply.

Accessory meningeal artery: Passes through foramen – ovale to enter middle cranial fossa to supply trigeminal ganglion and surrounding dura.

MANDIBULAR NERVE

This is the largest of the three divisions of the trigeminal nerve.

- It is the nerve of the first branchial arch.
- It is a mixed nerve – consists of both sensory and motor fibres.

Origin: It is formed by two roots:

(a) **Larger sensory root:** Arises from the convex aspect of the trigeminal ganglion.

(b) **Small motor root:** Arises from ventral aspect of pons and passes below the trigeminal ganglion.

Course

Both roots pass through the foramen ovale and join to form the main trunk, which lies in the infratemporal fossa. After a short course the main trunk divides into a small anterior and a large posterior division.

Relations of the mandibular trunk:

Medial – Tensor veli palatini

Lateral – Lateral pterygoid muscle

Anterior – Otic ganglion and tensor palati

Posterior – Middle meningeal artery.

Branches:

I. Main Trunk:

(a) **Nervous spinosus or meningeal branch:** Enters through foramen spinosum and supplies duramater of middle cranial fossa.

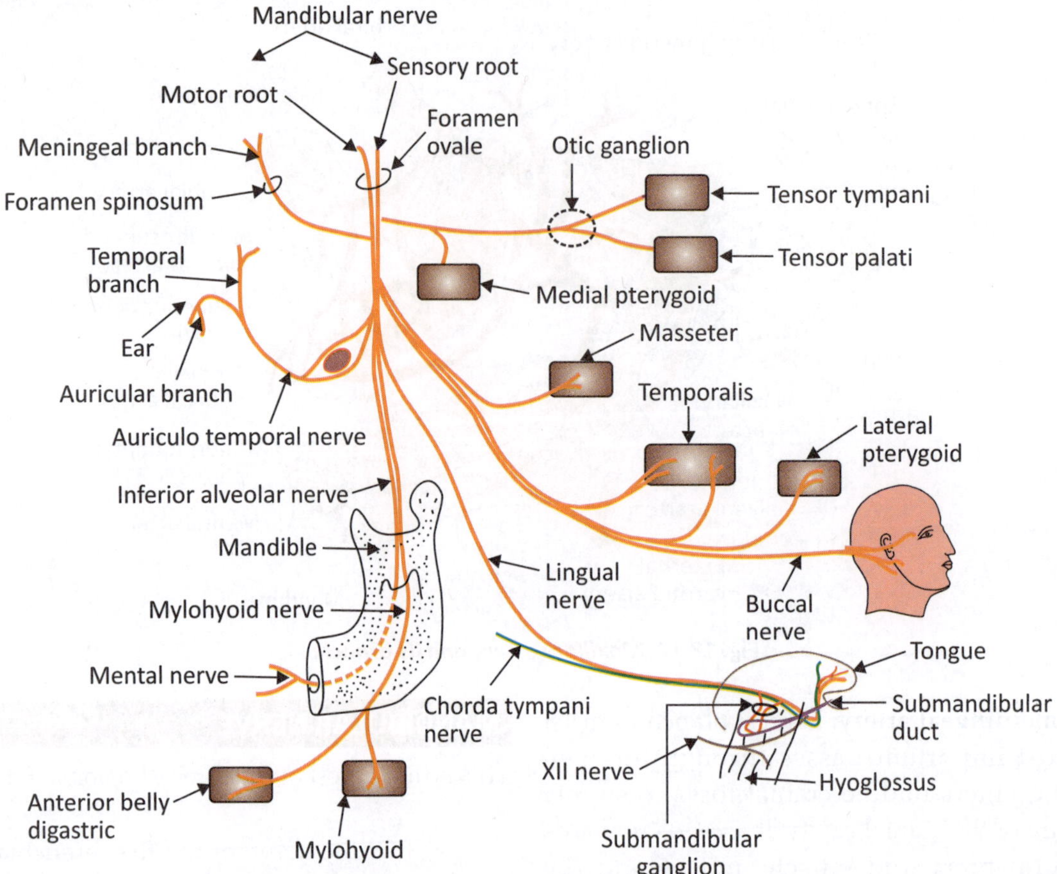

Fig. 18.13: ***Mandibular nerve and its branches***

(b) **Nerve to medial pterygoid:** It supplies medial pterygoid and then passes through otic ganglion and divides into two branches to supply tensor palati and tensor tympani. It forms the motor root of the otic ganglion.

II. Anterior Division: It consists major part of motor fibres and fewsensory fibres.

Motor branches:

1. Two deep temporal nerves to supply temporalis muscle from its deep surface.
2. **Nerve to lateral pterygoid:** Supplies lateral pterygoid muscle.
3. **Masseteric nerve:** Passes through mandibular notch and supplies masseteric muscle on its deep surface. It also gives a branch to temporo-mandibular joint to supply it.

Sensory Branch

Buccal nerve: Supplies skin and mucous membrane of cheek, passes between two heads of lateral pterygoid muscle – downwards and forwards pierces the buccinator muscle to reach its area of distribution, but it does not supply buccinator muscle.

III. Posterior Division: It consists of major sensory part with few motor fibres, gives rise three branches:

1. **Auriculo temporal nerve:** Arises by two roots and consists only sensory fibres. Two roots unite to form single trunk after encircling the middle meningeal artery.

   It runs backwards passing behind the insertion of lateral pterygoid muscle, around the neck of the mandible to reach the lateral side behind the temporo mandibular joint, superior to the parotid gland. It gives:

   (a) **Auricular branch:** To supply pinna, external acoustic meatus and adjoining part of tympanic membrane.

   (b) **Articular branch:** To temporo mandibular joint.

   (c) **Superficial temporal branches:** To supply area of skin over temple.

(d) Communicating branches: It receives postganglionic secretomotor fibres from otic ganglion to supply parotid gland. It also gives sensory fibres to parotid gland for its sensory supply.

2. **Inferior alveolar nerve:** It is the larger terminal branch of posterior division of mandibular nerve containing more sensory fibres and few motor fibres means – it is a mixed nerve.

   It emerges below the lateral pterygoid and runs over the ramus of mandible to enter the mandibular foramen alongwith inferior alveolar vessels.

   It traverses the mandibular canal and divides into terminal branches:

   (a) Nerve to mylohyoid: This branch is given before the inferior alveolar nerve enters the mandibular foramen; it consists all its motor fibres to supply mylohoid and anterior belly of digastric muscle and runs into mylohoid groove for its supply.

   (b) Dental branches: To supply teeth of lower jaw – these branches form inferior dental plexus before supplying the teeth – molar, premolar teeth and adjoining gum of lower jaw.

   (c) Mental nerve: Passes through mental foramen and supplies skin of chin and lower lip.

   (d) Incisive branch: Runs forwards into incisive canal of mandible and supplies canine and incisor teeth with the adjoining gum of lower jaw.

   (e) Communicating branch to lingual nerve.

3. **Lingual nerve:** It is the smaller terminal branch of posterior division of mandibular nerve. About 2 cm below the base of the skull chorda tympani nerve joins it posteriorly at an acute angle in the infra temporal fossa.

   Lingual nerve emerges below the lower border of lateral pterygoid muscle and runs downwards and forwards between the ramus of mandible and medial pterygoid.

   It comes in direct contact with mandible medial to the last molar teeth. Here, it is covered by mucous membrane of gum only.

   Then it crosses styloglossus and hyoglossus laterally.

   The submandibular ganglion is suspended from lingual nerve by two root on the surface of hyoglossus.

   Finally it curves under the submandibular duct at the level of genioglossus and turns up medially to the anterior part of tongue and floor of oral cavity.

Branches of Lingual Nerve:

(a) Sensory branches to mucous membrane of anterior 2/3 of tongue, floor of mouth and adjoining area of gum.

(b) Communicating branches with:

- **Chorda tympani:** The lingual nerve receives secretomotor fibres for submandibular and sublingual glands. It also conveys fibres for taste sensation from anterior 2/3 of tongue to the chorda tympani.
- **With hypoglossal nerve:** Lingual nerve transmits proprioceptive sensations from the lingual muscles via its communicating branches to the hypoglossal nerve.

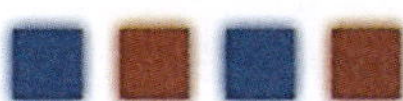

Chapter 19

Temporo Mandibular Joint

TYPES OF JOINT

Anatomically – Condyloid type of joint
Structurally – Synonial variety
Functionally – Biaxial joint (polyaxial).

Peculiarity of the Joint

- Only movable joint of head.
- Both sides of T.M.J. move together.

Bones taking part:

I. **Proximally:** Mandibular or condylar fossa of temporal bone and articular tubercle.

II. **Distally:** Head of mandible or condylar process.

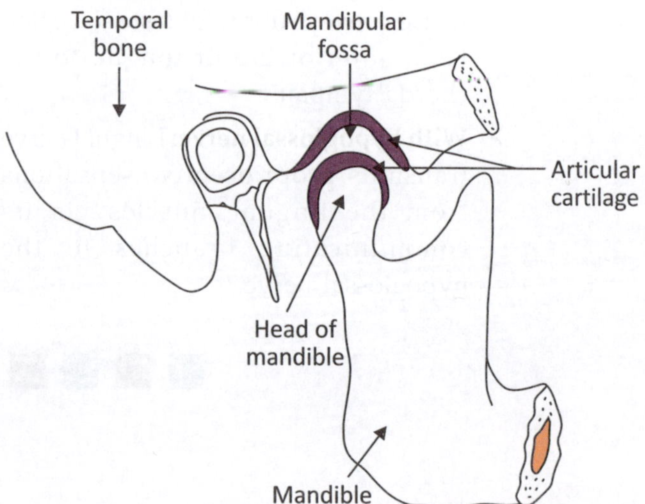

Fig. 19.1: *Proximal and distal articular surface of T.M.J.*

LIGAMENTS OF THE JOINT

1. Capsular ligament – is fibrous capsule
2. Lateral temporo – mandibular ligament
3. Spheno-mandibular ligament is pierced by mylohoid nerve and artery.
4. Stylo-mandibular ligament is pierced by facial artery.

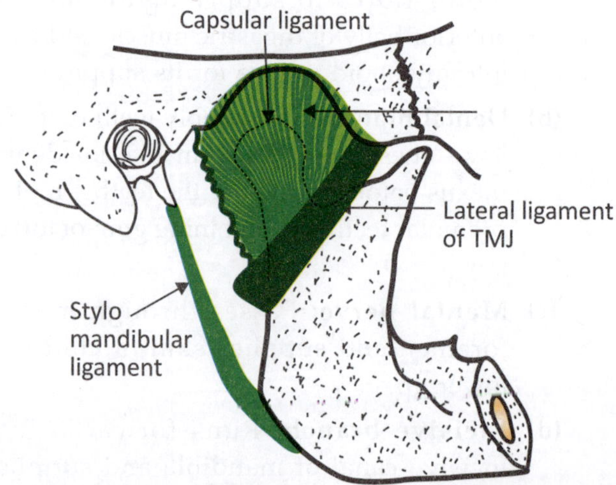

Fig. 19.2: *T.M.J. lateral surface and ligaments of the joint*

INTERIOR OF THE JOINT

Articular disc is fibro cartilaginous disc present with in the joint cavity and divides the cavity into superior and inferior compartments.

It is concavo-convex in shape. The center of disc is thin and avascular while its periphery is thick and rich in blood vessels and nerves.

- Disc is attached to inner aspect of the capsule of joint.

Morphology: From mesoderm of 1st arch articular disc is formed.

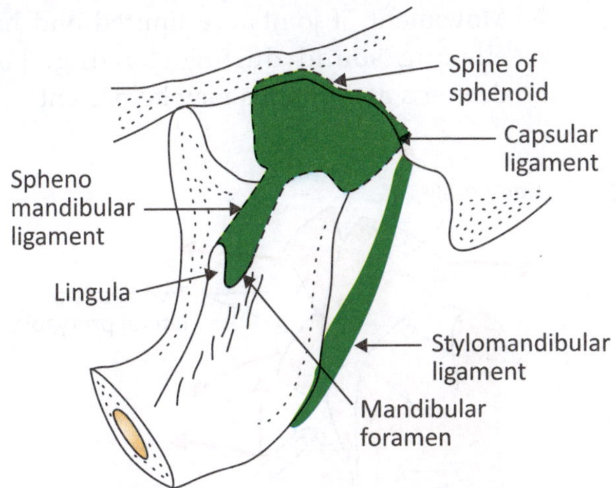

Fig. 19.3: *Accessory ligaments of T.M.J.*

- It represents degenerated tendon of lateral pterygoid muscle.

Parts of Disc:

- Anterior extension
- Anterior band
- Intermediate zone
- Posterior band
- Bilaminar zone – between two laminae venous plexus is present.

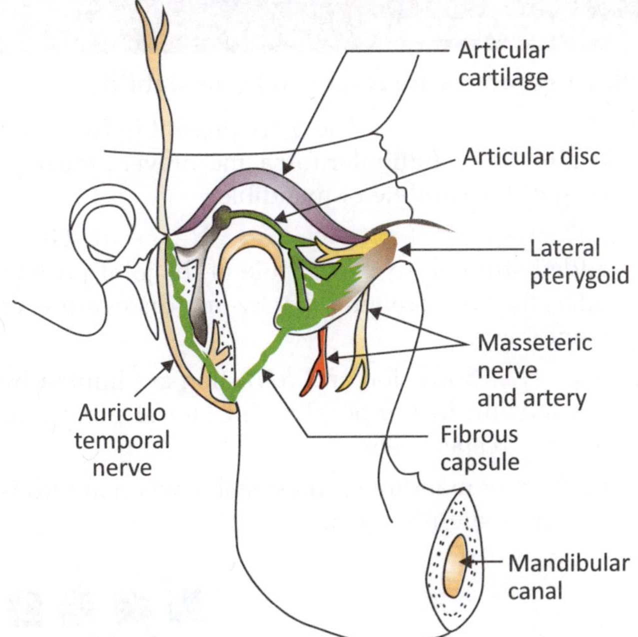

Fig. 19.4: *Sagittal section of T.M.J. interior of the joint*

Synovial membrane: Lines inner surface of capsule but does not line articulating surfaces.

- Both bony articular surfaces are covered by a layer of fibro cartilage identical with that of the disc and are not covered with hyaline cartilage so it is an atypical synovial joint.

RELATIONS OF TEMPORO MANDIBULAR JOINT

I. Lateral:

- Skin and fascia
- Parotid gland
- Temporal branches of VIIth Nerve.

II. Medial:

- Tympanic plate separates it from internal carotid artery.
- Spine of sphenoid with upper end of spheno mandibular ligament.
- Auriculo temporal and chorda tympani nerves.
- Middle meningeal artery.

III. Anterior: Lateral pterygoid muscle and masseteric nerve and vessels.

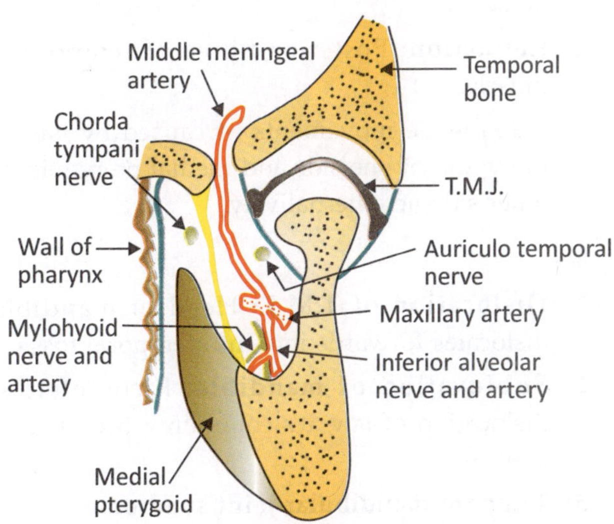

Fig. 19.5: *Oblique coronal section showing relations of joint*

IV. Posterior:

- Parotid gland separates it from external auditory meatus (Glenoid process).
- Superficial temporal vessels.
- Auriculo temporal nerve.

V. Superior:

- Middle cranial fossa.
- Middle meningeal vessels.

VI. Inferior: Maxillary artery and vein.

Nerve Supply:

1. Nerve to masseter – enters the joint anteriorly.
2. Auriculo temporal nerve (V_3) enters from the posterior aspect of joint.

Blood Supply:

Branches of:

1. Superficial temporal artery
2. Maxillary artery.

Lymphatic Drainage:

1. Pre-auricular lymph nodes.
2. Parotid lymph nodes.
3. Deep cervical lymph nodes.

Movements:

1. **Depression:** Lateral pterygoid, geniohyoid digastric and gravity.
2. **Elevation:** Masseter, temporalis and medial pterygoid muscle.
3. **Protraction:** Medial and lateral pterygoid muscles.
4. **Retraction:** Posterior fibres of temporalis muscle.
5. Side-to-side movements → caused by lateral pterygoid of one side and medial pterygoid of other side act alternatively.

Applied:

1. **Dislocation of T.M.J.:** Head of mandible dislocates forwards into infratemporal fossa.
2. **Subluxation of mandible:** Incomplete – dislocation of jaw, it's commonly occuring in females.
3. **Temporo mandibular joint syndrome:**
   - Severe pain around temporo mandibular joint.
   - Pain increases during chewing.
   - Movement of joints are limited and has clicking sound during chewing. H/o deafness and tinnitus may be present.

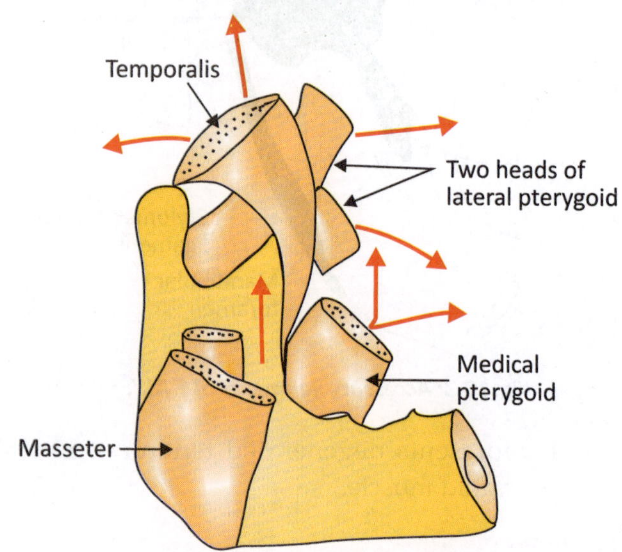

Fig. 19.6: ***Muscles acting on T.M.J. showing movements***

Development: The temporo mandibular joint develops very late. After all the other joints are fully formed, it is still incomplete. Only by the twelfth year of life it is fully developed in all respects.

STABILITY OF THE TEMPORO MANDIBULAR JOINT

Following factors are responsible for stability:

1. **Articular tubercles:** These are present in front and behind the mandibular fossa and prevent the slipping of the condyle of mandible.
2. **Lateral temporo mandibular ligament:** Gives added strength to the capsule of the joint postero laterally and prevents backward dislocation of mandible.
3. **Muscles:** Protrusion and retraction are limited by the tension in temporalis and lateral pterygoid muscles respectively.
4. Position of mandible is most stable when mouth is closed or slightly open.

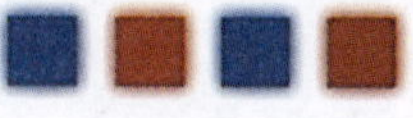

CHAPTER 20

The Pterygo Palatine Fossa

INTRODUCTION

It is a pyramidal shaped space situated deep to infratemporal fossa, below the apex of the orbit. This fossa is concerned with blood and nerve supply of upper jaw, nose, nasopharynx and lacrimal gland.

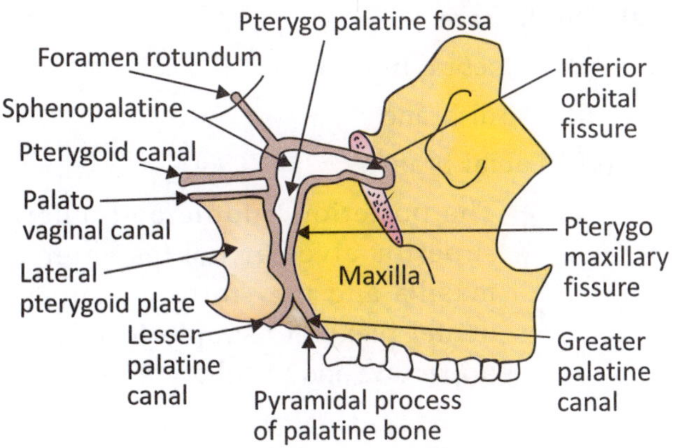

Fig. 20.1: *Pterygo palatine fossa*

Boundaries

Anterior: Medial part of the posterior surface of maxilla.

Posterior: Anterior surface of root of pterygoid process and adjoining part of sphenoid bone.

It presents with three openings in the posterior wall

1. **Foramen rotundum:** Connects it with middle cranial fossa.
2. **Anterior opening of pterygoid canal:** Connects it with foramen lacerum.
3. **Palato vaginal canal:** Connects it with nasopharynx.

Superior: Inferior surface of body of sphenoid bone.

Inferior orbital fissue – connects it with orbit.

Inferior: This is the apex of the fossa and is formed by meeting of the anterior and posterior boundaries, inferiorly in between them lies pyramidal process of palatine bone.

- Greater and lesser palatine canals are present inferiorly between the junction – connects it with oral cavity.

Medial: Perpendicular plate of palatine bone – posterosuperior part of lateral surface.

Lateral: Pterygomaxillary fissure connects it with infratemporal fossa.

Communications

1. Through foramen rotundum the maxillary nerve enters in this fossa and it communicates with middle cranial fossa.
2. Pterygoid canal – through this nerve and artery of pterygoid canal are passing and the fossa communicates with foramen lacercum.
3. Palatino vaginal canal – fossa communicates with roof of nasopharynx and pharyngeal nerves and a vessel passes through this canal to supply mucous membrane of nasopharynx.
4. Inferior orbital fissure – fossa communicates to orbital cavity anteriorly. Infra orbital nerve and vessels passes through this fissure.
5. Pterygo maxillary fissure – through this fossa communicates laterally to infratemporal fossa. IIIrd part of maxillary artery enters in the fossa through this fissure.

6. Via spheno palatine foramen situated in the medial wall, fossa communicates with nasal cavity. Spheno palatine artery and nasopalatine nerve passes through this foramen and enters the nose.
7. Through greater and lesser palatine canal situated inferiorly, fossa communicates with oral cavity. Greater and lesser palatine nerve and blood vessels passes through these canals.

CONTENTS OF PTERYGO PALATINE FOSSA

1. Maxillary nerve and its branches.
2. Pterygopalatine ganglion and its branches.
3. Third part of maxillary artery and its branches.

I. MAXILLARY NERVE (V_2)

This is a sensory nerve.

Commencement: From anterior border of trigeminal ganglion.

Courses:

- It passes forwards and laterally and enters the lateral wall of cavernous sinus.
- It leaves the cranial cavity through foramen rotundum and enters the pterygo palatine fossa.
- It then enters the orbit through inferior orbital fissure. The nerve is accompanied by the infra orbital artery. The part of this nerve in the floor of the orbit is called infra-orbital nerve. Here the nerve is passes within the infra orbital canal and leaves the orbit through the infra orbital foramen and enters the face.

Termination: It terminates by dividing into following branches:

(a) Palpebral branch
(b) Nasal branch
(c) Labial branch.

Branches

(a) Within the cranial cavity: Meningeal branch which supplies meninges of middle cranial fossa.

(b) Within the pterygo palatine fossa:

(i) 2 or 3 ganglionic branches to join pterygo palatine ganlion.
(ii) Zygomatic nerve divides into zygomatico-temporal and zygomaticofacial nerve.
(iii) Posterior superior alveolar nerve.

(c) Branches of V_2 nerve within the floor of the orbit:

(i) Middle superior alveolar nerve
(ii) Anterior superior alveolar nerve.

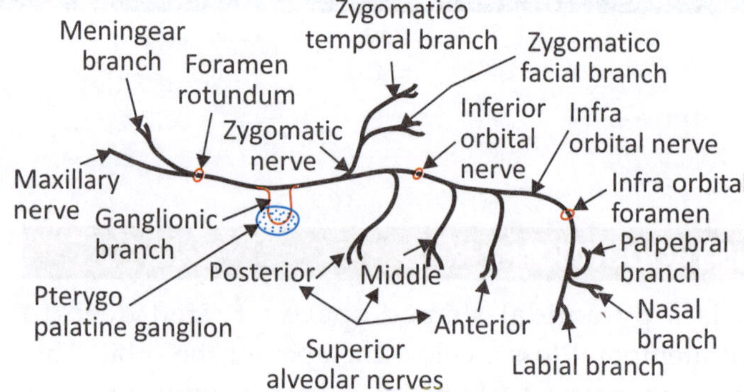

Fig. 20.2: *Maxillary nerve and its branches*

(d) On the face

(i) Palpebral branch
(ii) Nasal branch
(iii) Labial branch

- The posterior, middle and anterior superior alveolar nerves enter the maxilla and they form the superior dental plexus to supply teeth of the upper jaw and maxillary air sinus.

II. PTERYGO PALATINE GANGLION

Spheno-palatine ganglion or Meckel's ganglion or ganglion of Hey fever.

Situation: Pterygo palatine fossa.

Roots: Sympathetic and parasympathetic roots – Via nerve of pterygoid canal. It is formed by deep petrosal nerve from sympathetic plexus around internal carotid artery and greater superficial petrosal nerve from the geniculate ganglion of facial nerve unite to form the nerve of pterygoid canal also called as Vidian's nerve.

Sensory root: Maxillary nerve via its ganglionic branches.

Branches from the Ganglion

1. Orbital branches – supplies orbital periosteum and orbitalis muscle.

2. Greater and lesser palatine nerves – supplies mucous membrane of hard and soft palate.
3. Naso palatine nerve – to supply mucous membrane of medial and lateral wall of nose and anterior part of hard palate.
4. Nasal branches to nose – medial and lateral walls.
5. Pharyngeal branches to mucosa of nasopharynx.
6. Parasympathetic fibres to lacrimal gland – these fibres enters the maxillary nerve – pass through its zygomatico temporal branch – ultimately these fibres leave the zygomatico temporal nerve and join lacrimal nerve and finally reaches the lacrimal gland. These are secretomotor fibres for the gland.

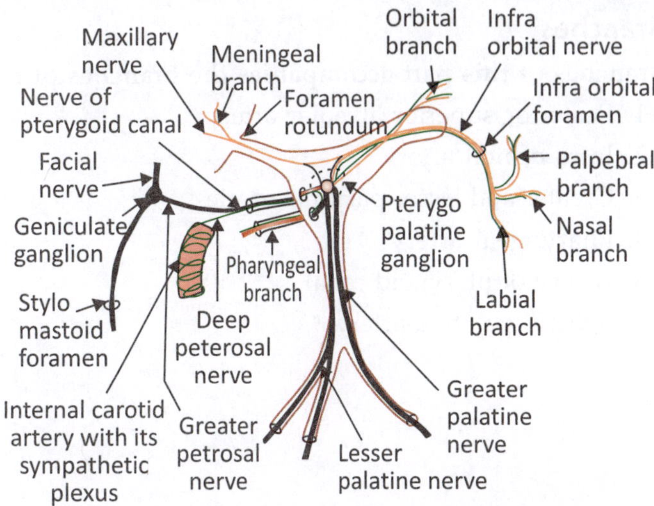

Fig. 20.3: *Schematic representation of pterygo palatine fossa and pterygo palatine ganglion, its branches and maxillary nerve*

Pathway

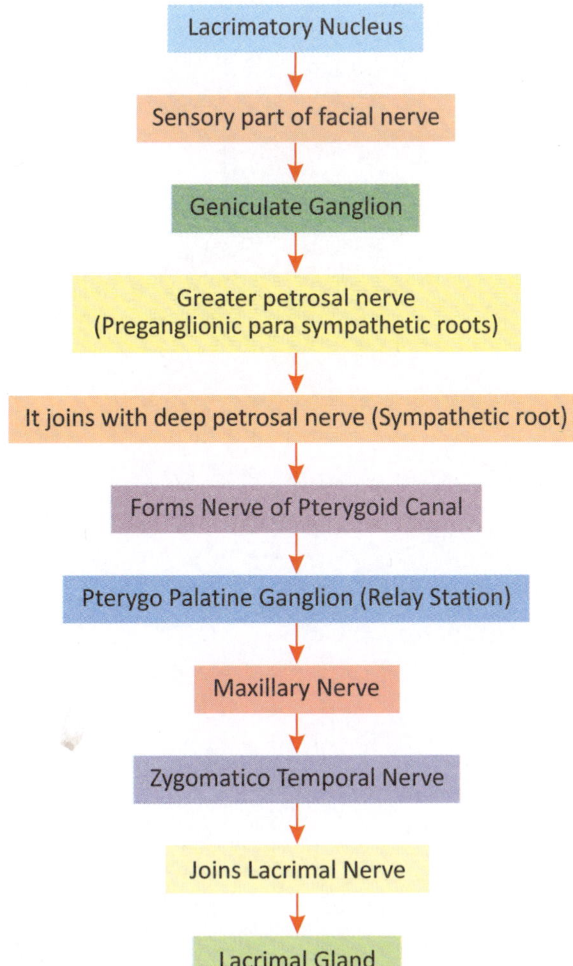

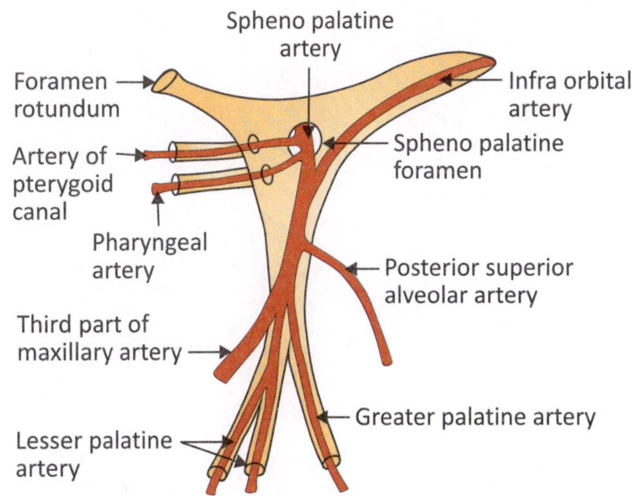

Fig. 20.4: *Maxillary artery in pterygo palatine fossa*

Applied: Stimulation of pterygo palatine ganglion causes nasal – Catarrh and lacrimation.

III. THIRD PART OF MAXILLARY ARTERY

- Enters the pterygo palatine fossa through lower part of pterygo maxillary fissure.
- It ascends upwards, medially and continued as sphenopalatine artery – which passes through sphenopalatine foramen and enters the nasal cavity to supply it.

Branches

Branches of this part accompanies the branches of maxillary nerve and pterygo palatine ganglion:

1. Posterior superior alveolar artery
2. Infra orbital artery
3. Greater and lesser palatine arteries
4. Pharyngeal artery
5. Artery of pterygoid canal
6. Spheno palatine artery.

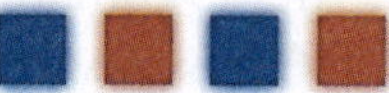

CHAPTER 21

Teeth

INTRODUCTION

Teeth are essential organs of mastication – arranged within sockets of maxilla and mandible. Human dentition is known as:

1. **Codont:** Arrangement – It is the situation of teeth in the sockets of upper and lower jaw.
2. **Heterodont:** Arrangement means – Various types of teeth e.g.,
   - Incisors
   - Canine
   - Premolars
   - Molars.
3. **Diphydont:** Means there are two types of dentition:
   A. **Primary dentition:** Milk or deciduous teeth are twenty in number and found in infants and children (I-2, C-1, M-2).
   B. **Secondary dentition:** Permanent teeth – 32 in number and found in adult (I-2, C-1, P-2, M-3). Milk teeth whither and permanent teeth appear.

ERUPTION OF TEETH

In primary dentition: First tooth appears in the child at the age of six to seventh month and eruption completed within 2 years.

In secondary dentition: Eruption begins at the age of 6 years and completed by 21-25 years. Teeth in the lower jaw erupt first than the upper jaw.

Incisors: They are situated on either side of the midline and are chisel shaped, necessary for cutting.

Canines: They are situated lateral to the incisors are conical shaped with blunt end. They project beyond other teeth and ment for tearing.

Premolars and molars are necessary for grinding having concavo convex flat surface.

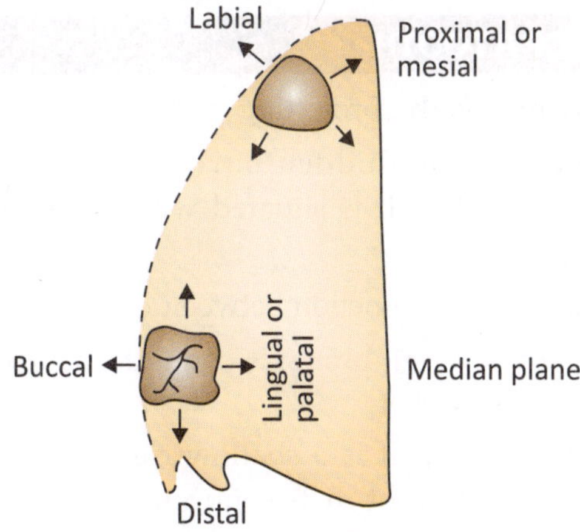

Fig. 21.1: *Dental terminology*

Time of Erruption

Deciduous teeth– Six to 24 months time.

E D C B A	A B C D E
E D C B A	A B C D E

B – Upper right lateral Incisor is caries

D – Right lower first Molar is caries

Permanent Teeth

Time of eruption in years – From six to 24 years.

8 7 6 5 4 3 2 1	1 2 3 4 5 6 7 8
8 7 6 5 4 3 2 1	1 2 3 4 5 6 7 8

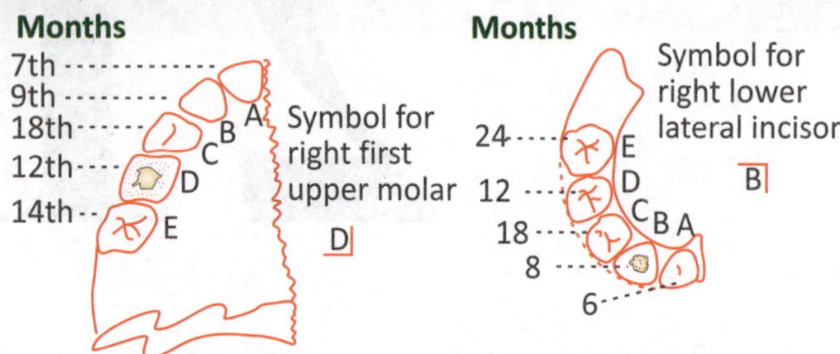

Fig. 21.2: *Deciduous or primary teeth (milk teeth)*

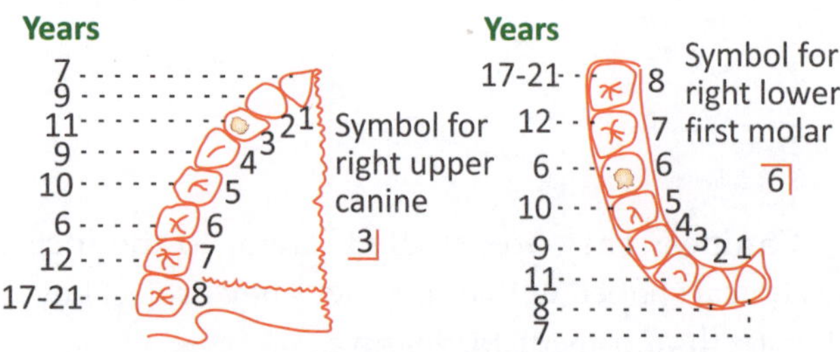

Fig. 21.3: *Permanent teeth*

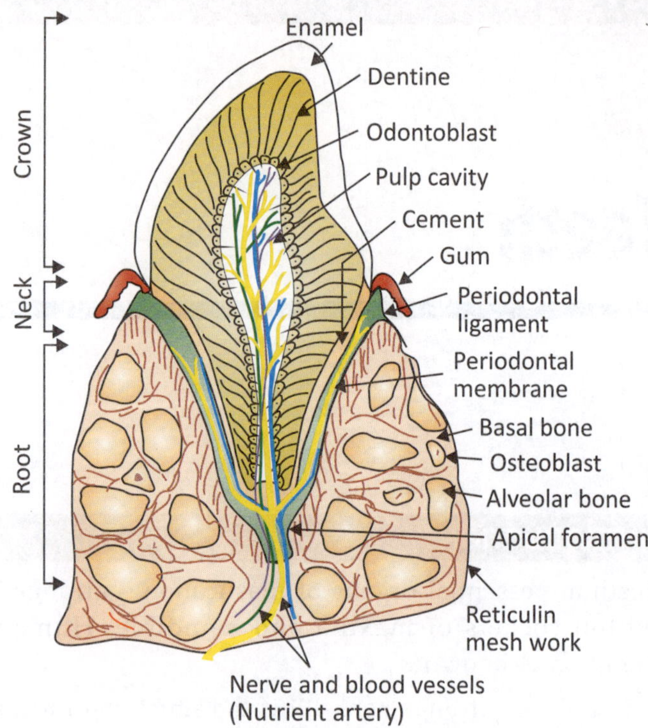

Fig. 21.4: *Structure of the tooth*

PARTS OF A TOOTH

1. **Crown:** It is the projecting part.
2. **Root:** It is the hidden buried part. It may be 1-3 in number. It is situated within the socket of the jaw.
3. **Neck:** It is the junction between crown and root.

Periodontal membrane: It connects the root with the wall of the socket.

Pulp chamber: It is a shallow cleft extends from the crown to the root. It is continuous with the root canal. The root canal has a terminal opening called apical foramen or apical pulp.

The wall of the tooth has three coverings:

1. **Enamel:** It is the hardest tissue of the body. It covers the crown, near the neck – it becomes thin and made mainly of inorganic salts – like calcium phosphate. It has enamel prisms.
2. **Dentine:** It is harder than bone, covers the entire tooth and chiefly formed by in organic salts. Dentin is produced by odontoblasts lining the pulp cavity.
3. **Cementum:** It covers the superficial surface of the dentin over the root. It is a binding material contains cementocytes and matrix.

Pulp cavity: It is the cavity of the tooth, opens at the floor of the socket through the apical foramen. It contains blood vessels, nerves and lymphatics. It is filled by a gelatinous substance. It is limited peripherally by the odontoblasts of the dentin.

NERVE SUPPLY OF TEETH

- Teeth of the upper jaw are supplied by superior alveolar nerves (posterior, middle and anterior) branches from the maxillary nerve.
- Teeth of the lower jaw are supplied by the branches of the inferior alveolar nerve (branch of mandibular – nerve – posterior division).
- Within the pulp cavity these nerves are unmyelinated, the nerves also passing between the odontoblasts.

BLOOD SUPPLY

- Teeth of upper jaw are supplied by superior alveolar arteries branches from the 3rd part of maxillary artery.

- Teeth of the lower jaw are supplied by inferior alveolar artery branch from 1st part of maxillary artery.

Lymphatics: Goes to submandibular, submental and finally – deep cervical group of lymph nodes. From both upper and lower jaw teeth.

Applied Anatomy

1. **Forensic dentistry:** Identification of unknown persons by the details of their dentition and tooth restorations.
2. **Polyphydent dentition:** Development of several successive sets of teeth during a lifetime.
3. **Praecoxdentia:** Premature eruption of teeth.
4. **Tardadentia:** Delayed eruption of teeth.
5. **Dental caries:** Decay of the teeth.
6. **Dental curve:** Curve of line along which the teeth of a jaw are situated.
7. **Hutchinson's tooth:** Lateral incisors of the upper jaw is pegged and a central incisor of the upper jaw has convex lateral borders and semilunar notches on their cutting edges found in congenital syphilis.
8. **Discolouration of tooth:** May occur as a side effect of certain drugs, e.g., Tetracycline.
9. **Twinning of tooth** is a dental abnormality in which two adjacent teeth are united together.
10. **Denticle:** A small tooth like projection within the pulp cavity of a tooth.
11. **Pyorrhoea alveolaris** (chronic periodontitis): Foul breath is present.
12. **Irregular dentition:** Found in rickets due to deficiency of Vitamin-D.
13. **Decalcification of enamel and dentin:** Softening and gradual destruction of tooth – forms caries in which tooth becomes tender and mastication is painful.
14. **Apical abscess** is formed when pulp is dead diagnosed by X-ray.

DEVELOPMENT OF TEETH

Starts from six week of intra uterine life up to early adulthood.

1. Oral epithelium thickens to form dental lamina at 6 weeks of intra uterine life.
2. Tooth bud stage begins and dental organ formed.
3. Dental organ becomes like a cap over dental papilla – begins to develop from underlying mesenchymal tissue, i.e., cap stage.
4. Bell stage: Cap like dental bud becomes like a bell over dental papilla, having outer and inner dental epithelium, containing ameloblasts surrounding dental papilla.
5. Dentin formation: Odontoblasts starts multiplying and forms dentinal tubules radiating at its periphery. Same time primordium of permanent tooth erupts from same epithelium. Tooth bud – enamel organ + dental papilla + dental sac.
6. Enamel formation – by deposition of inorganic salts over satellate reticulum.
7. Cementum and periodontal membrane formation. Tissue derived from two embryological sources, i.e.,
   A. Ectodermal epithelium – down growth of fetal oral mucosa forming enamel organ – ameloblasts – forms enamel.
   B. Dental papilla of mesenchymal – odontoblasts – form dentin.

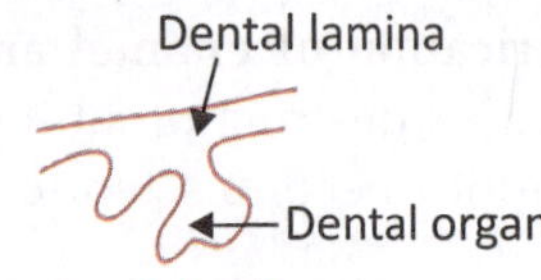

A. Tooth bud stage

Epithelial bud
Dental papilla (Mesenchyme)
B. Cap stage

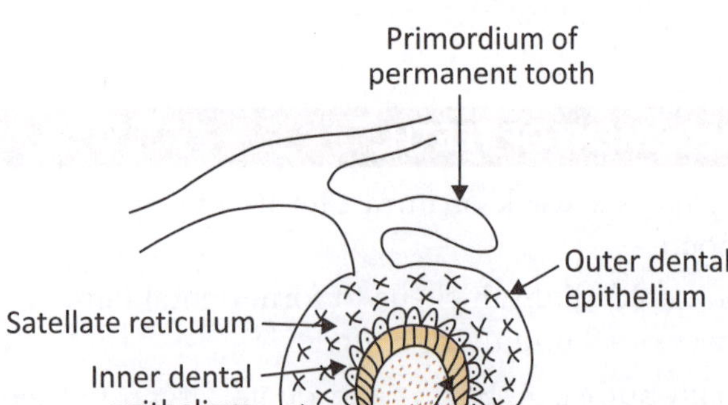

C. Bell stage

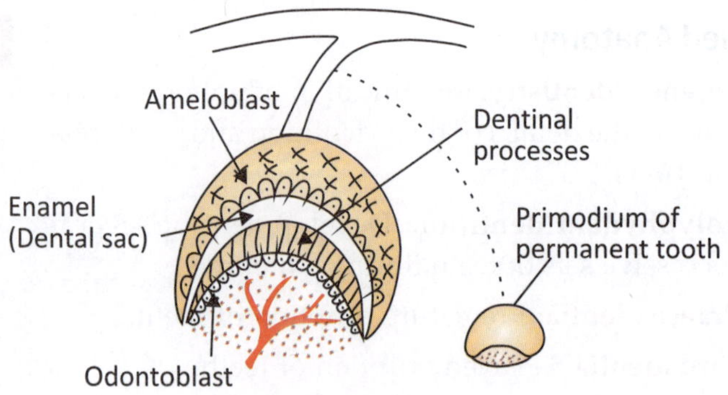

D. Dentine formation

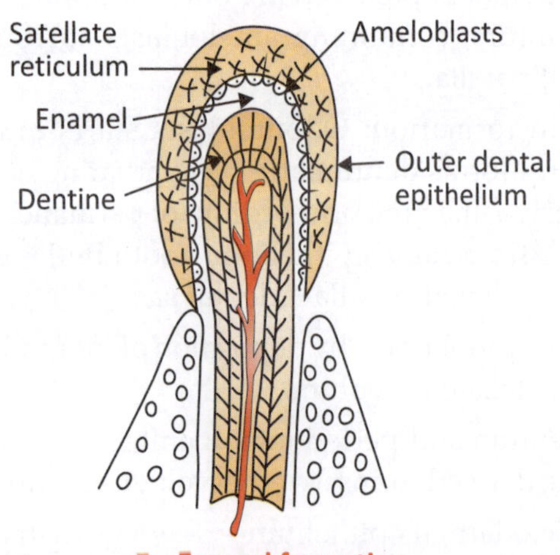

E. Enamel formation

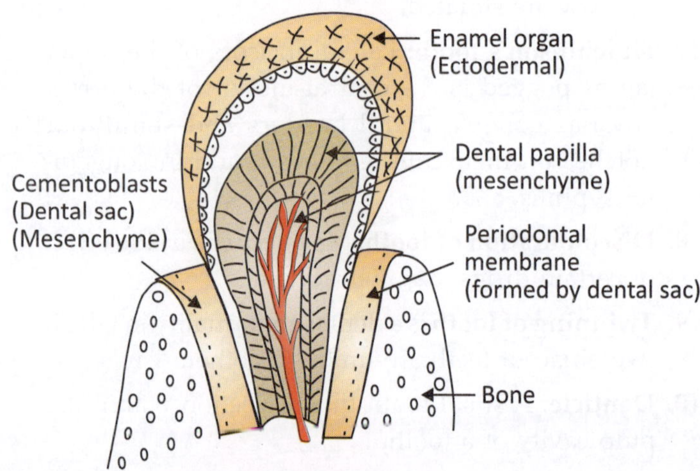

F. Cementum and periodental membrane formation

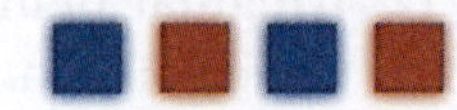

CHAPTER 22

The Palate

INTRODUCTION

- The palate forms concave roof of mouth and floor of nasal cavity.
- Upper surface is lined by respiratory epithelium which is ciliated columnar epithelium.
- Lower surface is lined by oral epithelium which is stratified squamous epithelium.

Parts

Divided into two parts:

I. Hard Palate and

II. Soft Palate.

I. Hard Palate

The bones taking part are:

1. Palatine process of maxillae.
2. Horizontal plates of palatine bone
   - Peripherally palate is bounded by alveolar arches.
   - Posteriorly midline of hard palate forms the posterior nasal spine.

Suture of Palate:

- Intermaxillary suture
- Inter palatine suture
- Palato-maxillary suture.

Blood Supply:

- **Arteries:** Greater palatine artery.
- **Veins:** Pterygoid venous plexus.

Nerves:

Greater palatine nerve and naso palatine nerve.

Lymphatic:

Upper deep cervical and retropharyngeal group of lymph nodes.

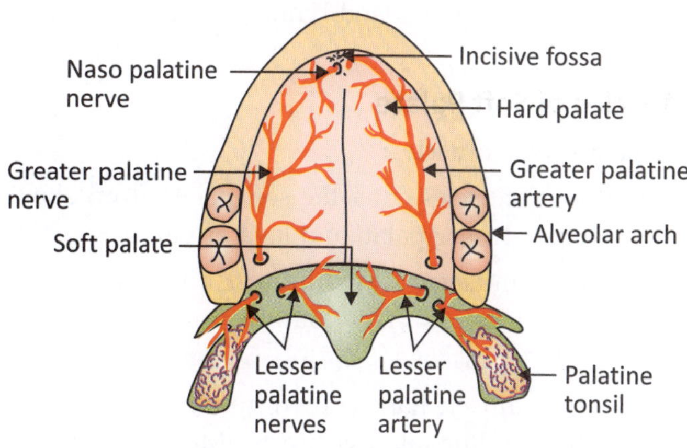

Fig. 22.1: *Blood and nerve supply of palate*

II. Soft Palate

It is a movable curtain and contains:

1. Aponeurotic palate
2. Muscles
3. Lymphatic tissue
4. Glands – mucous and serous salivary glands
5. Nerves
6. Vessels – artery, veins and lymphatics upper and lower surfaces are covered by mucous membrane.

Boundaries of Soft Palate

Anteriorly: It is attached to posterior border of hard palate.

Posteriorly: It has a free border from where a conical mass hangs down in middle part which is called as uvula.

Laterally: Two folds of mucous membrane – anterior – palatoglossal and posterior – palato-pharyngeus fold. Between these folds lies – palatine tonsil.

Structure: Composed of layers from above downwards.

- Mucous membrane of nasopharynx.
- Posterior-superior layer of palatopharyngeus muscle.
- Musculus uvulae.
- Levator palati muscle.
- Anterior inferior layer of palatopharyngeus.
- Tendon of tensor palati.
- Palato glossus muscle.
- Buccal mucous membrane with mucous salivary glands and lymph tissue.

Muscles of Soft Palate

These are five muscles:

- Two muscles enter the soft palate from above *viz.* – tensor palati and levator palati.
- Two muscles leave the soft palate and pass downwards *viz.* – palato pharyngeus and palatoglossus.
- One muscle hangs down from soft palate near the midline into uvula *viz.* – Musculus uvulae.

1. Tensor Palati

Origin from:

- Scaphoid fossa of pterygoid process of sphenoid bone.
- Lateral surface of auditory tube.
- Spine of sphenoid.

Insertion: Into crest of palatine bone on inferior surface near its posterior border by a tendinous sheath, i.e., palatine aponeurosis.

- Tendon hooks round the pterygoid hamulus.

Action: Tightens the soft palate.

Nerve supply: Mandibular nerve.

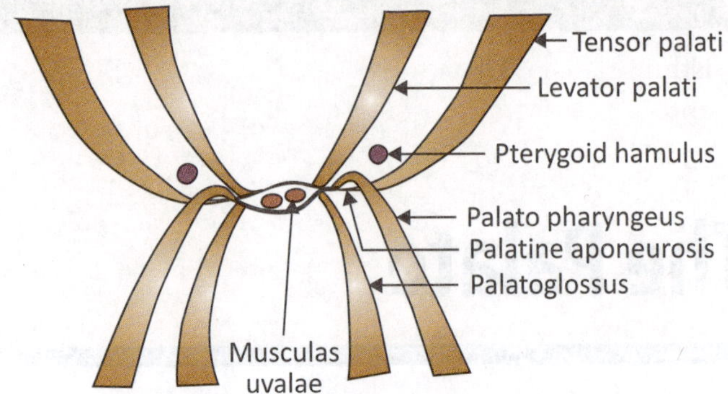

Fig. 22.2: *Coronal section of soft palate*

2. Levator Palati

Origin: Inferior surface of petrous part of temporal bone near its apex – antero medial to carotid canal.

- Medial surface of cartilaginous part of auditory tube.

Insertion: Upper surface of palatine aponeurosis. Between the two layers of palatopharyngeus.

Action: Elevation of soft palate.

Nerve supply: Pharyngeal plexus (X + cranial root of XIth C.N.).

3. Palatopharyngeus:

Arises from two layers, one on either side of levator palati.

Origin: Superior surface of palatine aponeurosis and posterior border of hard palate.

Insertion: Posterior border of lamina of thyroid cartilage along with salpingo pharyngeus muscle.

Action: Pulls the pharyngeal wall upwards.

Nerve supply: Pharyngeal plexus of nerves.

4. Palatoglossus

Origin: Inferior surface of palatine aponeurosis.

Insertion: Side of the tongue.

Action: Elevates the tongue upwards.

Nerve supply: Pharyngeal plexus of nerves.

5. Musculus Uvulae

Origin: Posterior edge of hard palate near midline.

Insertion: Mucous membrane of soft palate.

Action: Straightens the soft palate.

Nerve supply: Pharyngeal plexus of nerves.

Movement of soft palate: Closes the pharyngeal isthmus is the communication between nasopharynx and oropharyx.

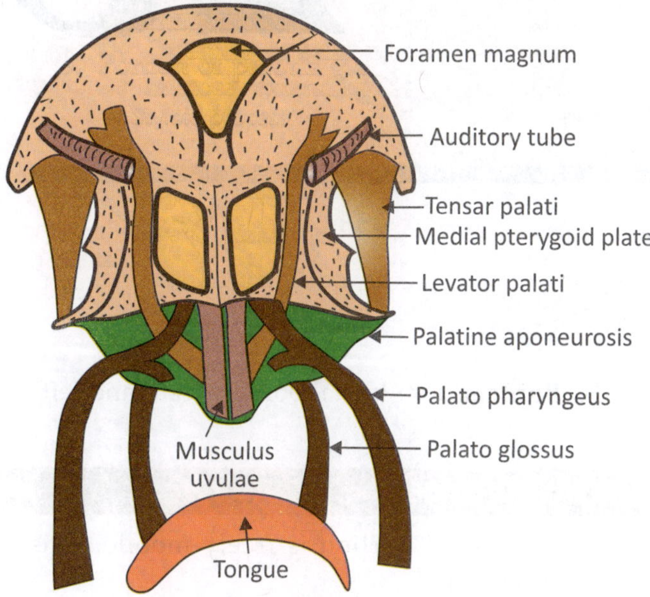

Fig. 22.3: *Muscles of soft palate*

Blood Supply of Palate

A. Arterial Supply

1. Greater palatine artery which is a branch of IIIrd part of maxillary artery.
2. Ascending palatine artery which is branch of facial artery.
3. Lesser palatine artery.
4. Tonsillar artery which is branch of facial artery.

B. Venous Drainage

1. Pterygoid venous plexus.
2. Pharyngeal venous plexus.
3. Para tonsillar vein.

Lymphatic Drainage

1. Submandibular group of lymph nodes.
2. Retro pharyngeal group of lymph nodes.

Nerve Supply:

A. Sensory supply:

1. Greater and lesser palatine nerves.
2. Glosso pharyngeal nerve (IXth).

B. Motor supply: Via pharyngeal plexus – Xth and cranial root of XIth cranial nerve.

C. Secretomotor: Lesser palatine nerve.

D. Gustatory (taste): From oral surface – lesser palatine and IXth Cranial Nerve.

Passavant's ridge: Upper fibres of palatopharyngeus pass circularly deep to mucosa of pharynx – act as sphincter internal to superior constrictor.

Applied Anatomy

1. **Torus palatinus:** Excessive bone growth at inter maxillary suture near palatine bone.
2. **Cleft palate:** It is a congenital defect due to:
   (a) Failure of fusion between medial nasal and maxillary processes.
   (b) Failure of fusion between two maxillary processes.
   - Cleft palate may be complete or incomplete.

   Complete Cleft Palate: In this type the cleft is present in entire part of palate there fore nose and mouth freely communicate with each other.

   Incomplete Cleft: Results in:
   (a) Bifid uvula.
   (b) Cleft in whole length of soft palate.
   (c) Cleft in whole length of soft palate and posterior part of hard palate.
3. **Sequestrum dermoid:** Cyst of epithelium formed within the cleft.
4. **Fibrochondroma of the palate:** Tumour formed of fibrous or cartilaginous tissue.
5. **Paralysis of soft palate** in lesions of Xth cranial nerve produces:
   - Nasal regurgitation of liquids
   - Nasal twang of voice
   - Flattening of palatal arches.

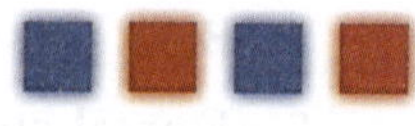

CHAPTER 23

Tongue

It is a muscular and mobile organ. It is concerned with swallowing, speech and taste.

Situation: Oral cavity and anterior wall of oropharynx.

Shape: Inverted shoe shaped.

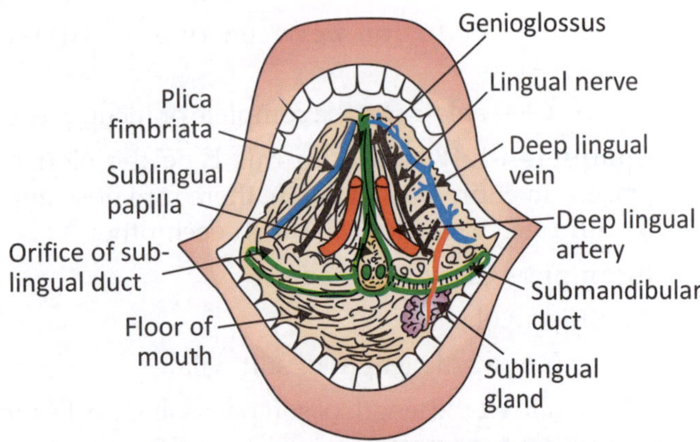

Fig. 23.1: *Ventral surface of the tongue*

Developments:

1. Muscles – occipital myotomes.
2. Mucous membrane of anterior 2/3 – Lingual swellings and tuberculum impar.
3. Mucous membrane of posterior 1/3 – Hypobronchial eminence.

Parts:

1. **Tip:** Contacts the incisor teeth.
2. **Base (root):** Directs towards oropharynx.
3. **Dorsal surface:** Convex in appearance.
4. **Ventral surface:** Directed towards floor of mouth.
5. **Borders:** Two lateral borders right and left.

DORSAL SURFACE

Anterior: Oral portion is freely mobile. This is horizontal at rest.

Posterior: Pharyngeal portion is more fixed and vertical. This has papillae and sensory nerve supply.

Sulcus terminalis: A 'V' shaped groove separates anterior 2/3 of dorsum from posterior 1/3.

Foramen caecum: Behind the apex of the sulcus there is a small depression called foramen caecum, this marks the site of origin of thyroid diverticulum.

Mucous membrane: This differs on the two regions of dorsum of the tongue – oral part and posterior 1/3. The oral part has small projections of lamina propria creating papillae which increase surface area of mucosa for taste receptors.

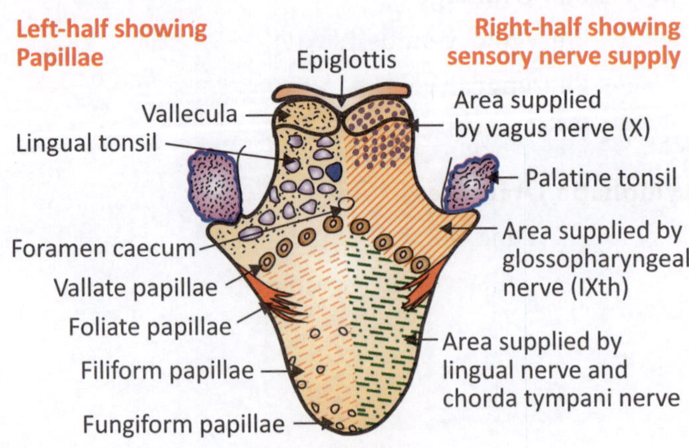

Fig. 23.2: *Dorsum of the tongue*

PAPILLAE ARE OF FOUR TYPES (MUCOUS MEMBRANE OF ANTERIOR 2/3 OF TONGUE)

1. **Vallate papillae:** These are 10 to 12 in number and present infront of sulcus terminalis in a single row, largest 2-4 mm in diameter. Papilla has a central circular elevation surrounded by a groove and a narrow wall. Taste buds are situated in the walls of groove.

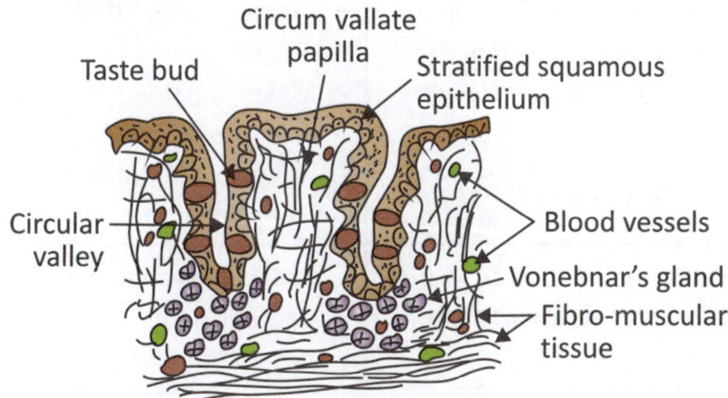

Fig. 23.3: *Structure of circum vallate papillae*

2. **Fungiform papillae:** Bright red, flat dots of about 1 mm in diameter, along the edges, dorsum and tip of tongue.
   - These contain taste buds.
3. **Filiform papillae:** They are conical projections on dorsal surface, arranged in 'V' shaped rows parallel to sulcus.
   - Apex of these papillae are keratinised.
   - No taste buds are found.
   - Giving velvety appearance of tongue.
4. **Foliate papillae:** They form transverse mucosal folds on the lateral aspect of the tongue.

Taste buds: They are found on and around the papilla in large numbers, present on mucous membrane of pharyngeal part of tongue, undersurface of soft palate and back of epiglottis.

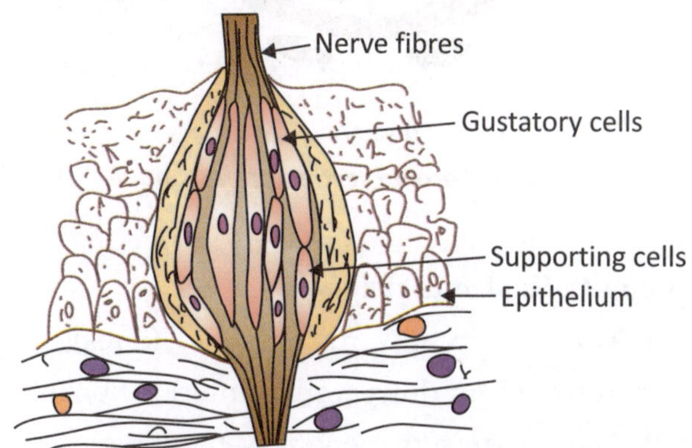

Fig. 23.4: *Structure of the taste bud*

FEATURES OF DORSAL SURFACE OF POSTERIOR 1/3 OF TONGUE

- Taste buds and papillae are absent.
- Collection of lymphoid tissue under mucous membrane called lingual tonsils – makes the surface humpy.
- Lingual tonsil with faucial tubal and pharyngeal tonsils make the lymphoid ring of Waldeyer.
- Mucous membrane reflected on epiglottis as median glosso epiglottic fold and lateral glosso-epiglottic folds between these folds on each side there is a depression called Vallecula.

MUSCLES OF TONGUE

Tongue is divided into two symmetrical halves by a median fibrous septum. Each half contains muscles arranged in two groups:

I. EXTRINSIC MUSCLES

These alters the position of tongue and are paired:

1. Hyoglossus (Chondro glossus)
2. Styloglossus
3. Genioglossus
4. Palatoglossus
   - All extrinsic muscles take origin from outside the tongue.

They change the position of the tongue and all are supplied by branches of hypoglossal nerve except palatoglossus – which is supplied by vago-accessory complex, i.e., through pharyngeal plexus of nerves.

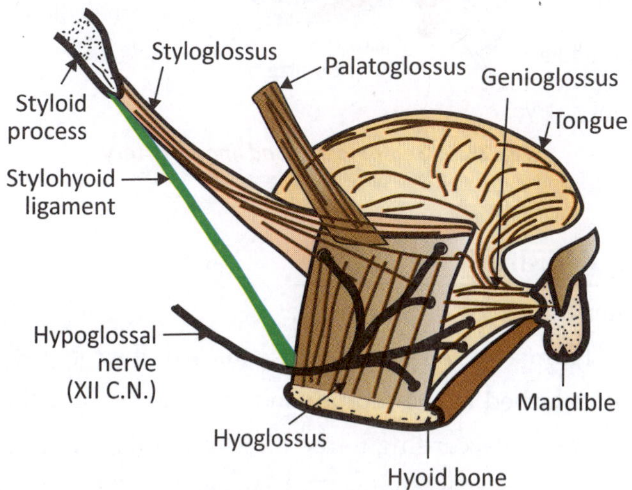

Fig. 23.5: *Extrinsic muscles of the tongue*

Table 23.1: ***Extrinsic Muscles of the Tongue***

Extrinsic muscle	Origin	Insertion	Action
1. Hyoglossus (Quadrilateral muscle)	Upper surface of greater cornu of hyoid bone and adjacent part of body of hyoid.	Fibres run upwards medially upto the side of the tongue and interdigitate with the fibres of styloglossus and inserted on the lateral border of tongue – posterior 2/3 part.	Depresses the sides of the tongue and makes the dorsal surface convex.
2. Genioglossus – Fan shaped – Forms the bulk of the tongue	From superior genial tubercles on the inner surface of symphysis menti to body of hyoid.	Fibres radiate and insert throughout the tongue from apex to root of the tongue lowest fibres are attached.	– Protrudes the tip of the tongue – Makes the dorsum concave – Prevents the tongue from falling back.
3. Styloglossus – Elongated slip like	Tip of styloid process and adjacent part of stylohyoid ligament.	Fibres run downwards and forwards for insertion along the entire length of side of the tongue.	– Draws the tongue upwards and backwards (Retract the tongue)
4. Palatoglossus – Slender slip	Oral or inferior surface of palatine aponeurosis.	Fibres lies in palato glossal arch and insert on the side of the tongue at the junction of anterior 2/3 with posterior 1/3.	– Pulls up the root of the tongue. Approximates the palatoglossal arches to close the oropharyngeal isthmus during swallowing.

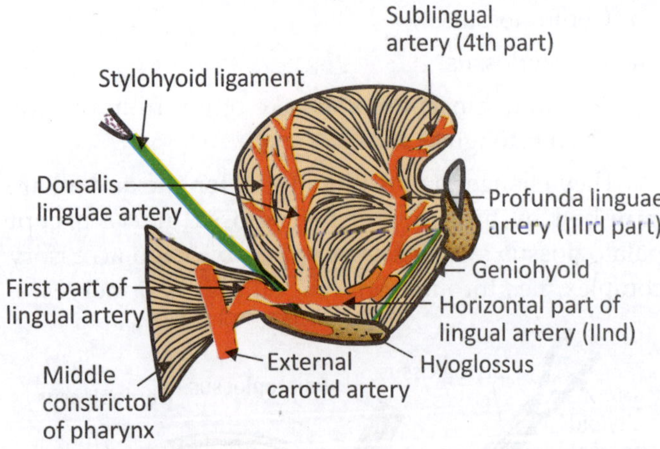

Fig. 23.6: ***Genioglossus and lingual artery***

II. INTRINSIC MUSCLES

Alter the shape of the tongue.

- Form a large part of muscle mass of the tongue.
- Attached to the septum and mucous membrane.
- Named according to the direction of their fibres:
  - Superior longitudinal muscle
  - Inferior longitudinal muscle
  - Transverse lingual muscle
  - Vertical muscle.

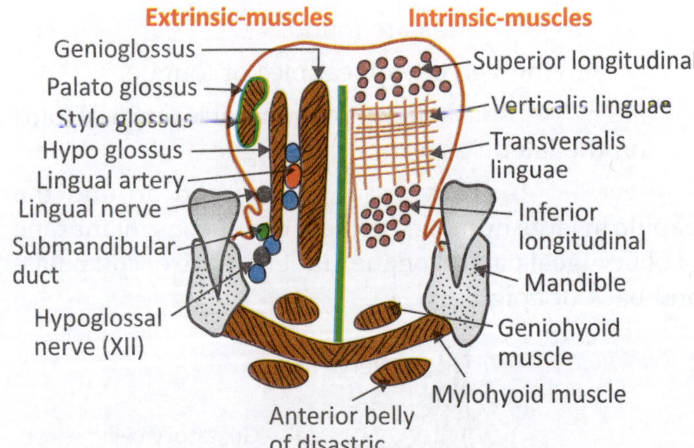

Fig. 23.7: ***Coronal section of the tongue***

Action:

- **Longitudinal muscle:**
  - Turn the tip upwards (superior fibres)
  - Turn the tip downwards (inferior fibres)
  - These reduce the length of the tongue during contraction.

Transversalis: This produces narrowing and lengthening of the tongue.

Verticalis: This flattens and broadens the tongue.

Nerve Supply:

1. **Motor supply:** All extrinsic and intrinsic muscles of the tongue are supplied by hypoglossal nerve (XII) except palatoglossus supplied via pharyngeal plexus of nerves.

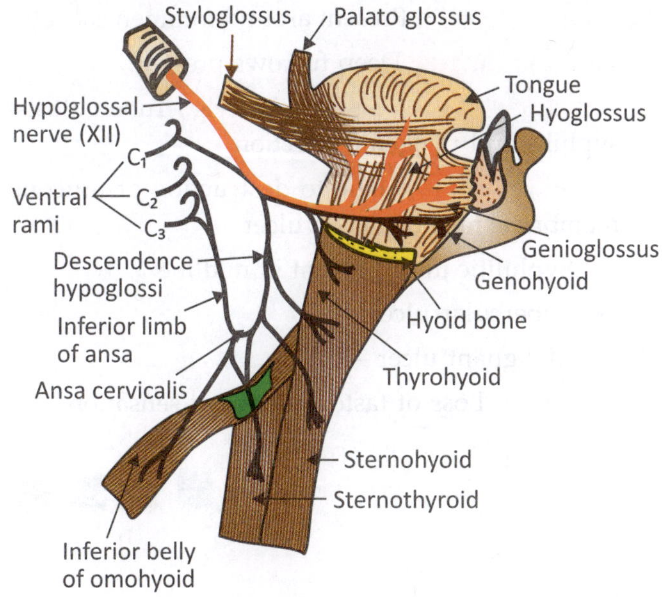

Fig. 23.8: *Hypoglossal nerve and ansa cervicalis*

2. **Sensory supply**
   (a) Anterior 2/3 – lingual nerve branch of mandibular division. This is sensory for general sensations (V_3).
   - Chordo tympani: This is a branch of VII and carries taste sensation from anterior 2/3 of tongue accompanies lingual nerve.

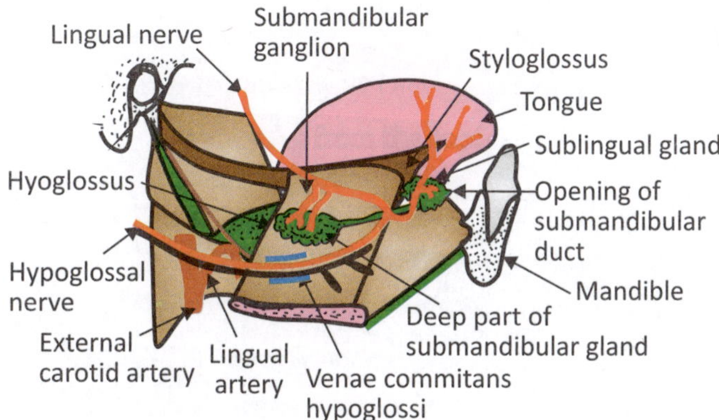

Fig. 23.9: *Muscles of tongue and its nerve supply*

   (b) Posterior 1/3 – glossopharyngeal – both sensory and carries taste sensation.
   - Also carries sensation and taste from circumvallate papillae.

Root of tongue near vallecula is supplied by internal laryngeal branch of Xth cranial nerve.

3. **Sympathetic:** Plexus around lingual artery.

BLOOD SUPPLY OF TONGUE

A. Arterial supply

1. Lingual artery and its branches.
2. Facial artery – Ascending palatine and tonsillar branches.
3. Ascending pharyngeal artery.

B. Venous drainage

1. **Superficial veins of tongue:** Drains inferior surface and tip – accompanies XIIth nerve joins with deep lingual and sublingual veins which ends in internal jugular vein.
2. **Deep veins:** Drains dorsum of tongue and follows lingual artery and ends in internal jugular vein.

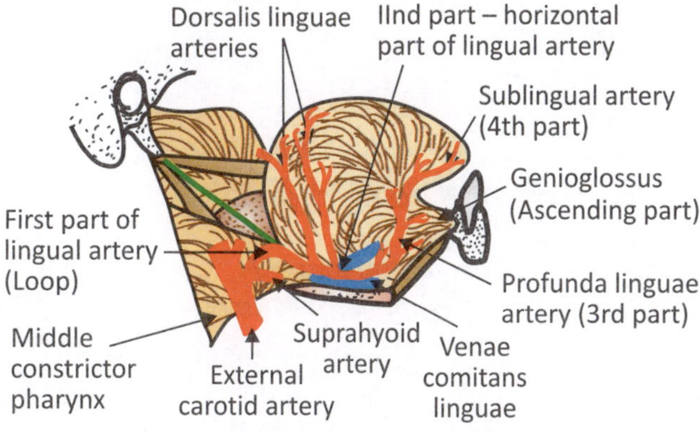

Fig. 23.10: *Blood supply of tongue*

LYMPHATIC DRAINAGE OF TONGUE

Divided into:

1. Apical vessels drain into submental lymph nodes → jugulo omohyoid lymph nodes.
2. Marginal vessels drain into submandibular, jugulo omohyoid and jugulo digastric group of lymph nodes.

3. Central vessels goes to jugulo omohyoid and jugulo digastric lymph nodes.
4. Basal or dorsal vessels go to retropharyngeal, jugulo digastric and jugulo omohyoid lymph nodes.

All lymph of tongue ultimately enters the *jugulo omohyoid nodes*, hence, known as lingual nodes.

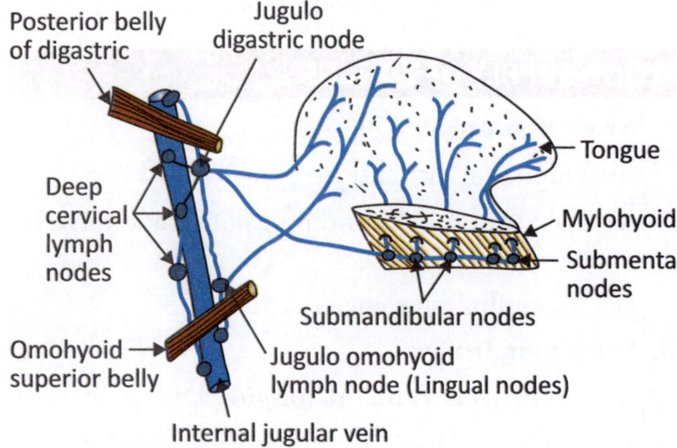

Fig. 23.11: *Lymphatic drainage of tongue*

Applied Anatomy

1. **Agenesis of tongue:** Aglossia.
2. **Bifid tongue:** Tip of tongue is divided.
3. **Microglossia:** Small tongue.
4. **Macroglossia:** Large tongue.
5. **Ankyloglossia or tongue tie:** Short frenulum linguae.
6. **Hemiglossia:** One-half of tongue is developed.
7. **Lingual thyroid:** Present around foramen caecum.
8. **Fissured tongue:** Deep furrows present.
9. **Infections of tongue:** Glossitis, e.g., Tuberculosis, syphilis and pyogenic infection.
10. **Ulcers of tongue:** Due to destruction of mucous membrane may be dental ulcer.
    - Syphilitic ulcer present in midline
    - Tubercular ulcer
    - Malignant ulcer – CA.
11. **Agueusia:** Loss of taste or reduced sensation.

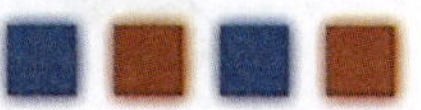

CHAPTER 24

Lymphatic Drainage of Head and Neck

INTRODUCTION

The lymph nodes draining the head and neck are classified into superficial and deep nodes.

Superficial lymphatics follow superficial veins while deep lymphatics follow arteries.

I. SUPERFICIAL NODES

Drain superficial tissues of head and neck.

A. **Circular group:** Arranged in the form of a circle round the neck called "Pericervical collar". It includes:

   (a) **Submental nodes:** Lie in submental triangle.

   (b) **Submandibular lymph nodes:** On the inferior surface of submandibular gland.

   (c) **Pre-auricular nodes:** Lie infront of auricle.

   (d) **Post auricular or mastoid nodes,** i.e., behind auricle on surface of mastoid process.

   (e) **Occipital nodes:** Lie in occipital region.

B. **Vertical group of superficial nodes:** These are:

   (a) Facial nodes – along facial vein.

   (b) Anterior cervical nodes – along anterior jugular vein.

   (c) Superficial cervical nodes – along external jugular vein.

   (d) Infrahyoid nodes – lie on thyrohyoid membrane, drains the larynx above the level of vocal cords.

   (e) Pre laryngeal nodes – lie on cricothyroid membrane drains larynx below the level of vocal cords.

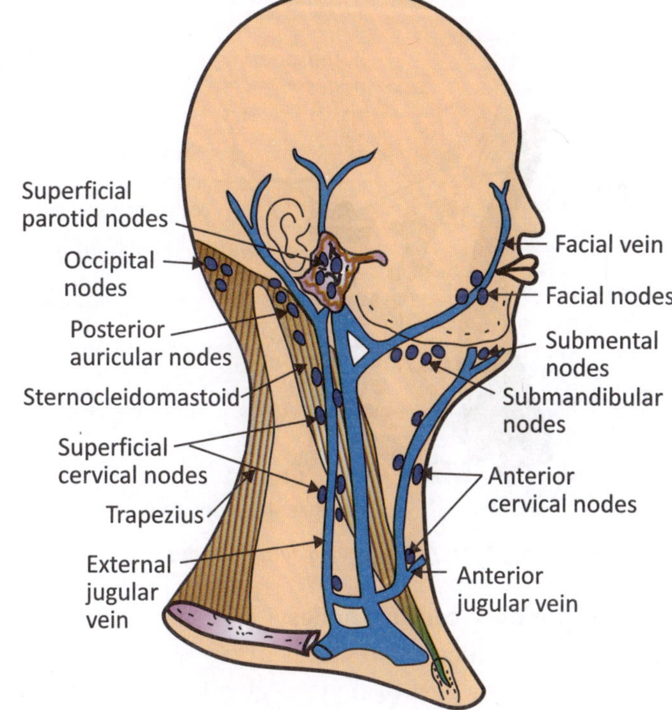

Fig. 24.1: ***Superficial cervical lymph nodes***

   (f) Pretracheal nodes – lie on trachea close to inferior thyroid vein.

Efferents: From all superficial nodes go to deep cervical nodes.

II. DEEP CERVICAL NODES

They drain deeper tissues of head and neck and are vertically disposed around the carotid sheath from the base of skull to the root of neck.

They are divided into superior and an inferior group by omohyoid muscle.

1. **Superior deep cervical nodes:** They drain cranial cavity, infratemporal fossa, parotid and submandibular nodes, root of the tongue, upper lateral part of thyroid gland, larynx and lower part of pharynx. Efferents pass to inferior deep cervical nodes.
   (a) **Jugulo digastric node:** Lies below the posterior belly of digastric muscle, where it crosses the internal jugular vein. It is the chief node draining the palatine tonsil, also called as tonsillar node.
   (b) **Inframastoid node:** Lies below the tip of mastoid process drains pharyngeal tonsil are known as adenoid nodes.

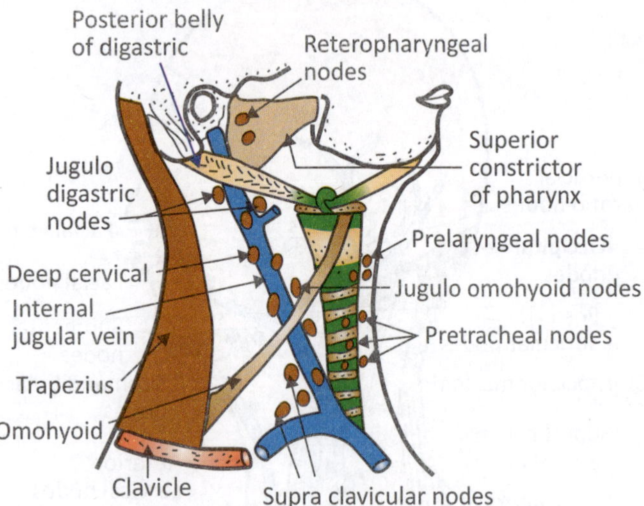

Fig. 24.2: *Deep cervical lymph nodes*

2. **Inferior deep cervical nodes:** Lie below the level of thyroid cartilage and drain upper deep cervical nodes, lower part of thyroid gland, lower part of larynx, trachea and cervical part of oesophagus.
   (a) **Jugulo omohyoid node:** Lies above the inferior belly of omohyoid where it crosses the internal jugular vein. It drains the tongue and so also called as lingual node.
   (b) **Supraclavicular nodes:** Lies in posterior triangle of neck above the clavicle. Accessory nerve is surrounded by these nodes.
   (c) **Para tracheal nodes:** Lie between trachea and oesophagus close to recurrent laryngeal nerve. They receive lymph from thyroid gland, oesophagus trachea and neighbouring areas.
   (d) **Retropharyngeal nodes:** Lie infront of lateral mass of atlas along lateral border of longus colli, situated between buccopharyngeal fascia and the prevertebral fascia.

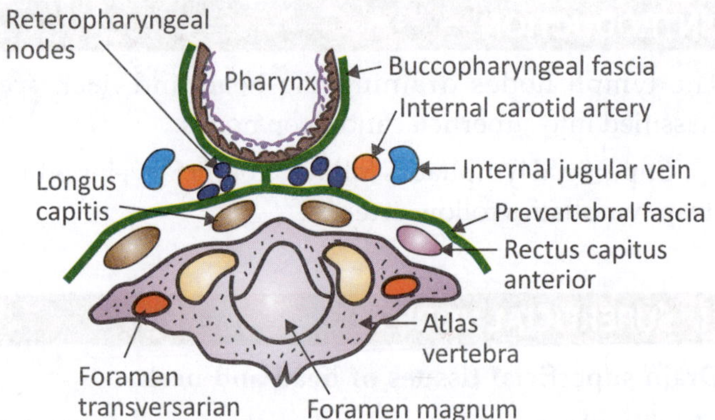

Fig. 24.3: *Relations of retropharyngeal lymph nodes*

They drain – nasopharynx, soft palate, posterior part of hard palate, nose and auditory tube. Efferents reach to upper deep cervical nodes and then lower deep cervical nodes draining entire head and neck either directly or indirectly. Efferents form jugular lymph trunk which on right side joins subclavian lymph trunk to form right lymph duct which joins the beginning of right brachiocephalic vein. On the left side jugular and subclavian lymph duct joins the thoracic duct which opens into the jugulo subclavian angle on left side.

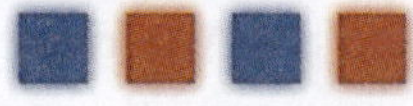

CHAPTER 25

Waldeyer's Ring

This is a collection of lymphoid tissue or follicles in the upper part of digestive system. This ring is formed by:

- **Superiorly:** Pharyngeal tonsils or Adenoids.
- **Inferiorly:** Lingual tonsil.
- **Laterally:** Palatine tonsils and tubal tonsils.

I. PALATINE TONSILS

Palatine tonsils are largest collection of lymphoid tissue present in the tonsillar fossa.

Development: From second pharyngeal pouch.

Boundaries of the tonsillar fossa:

- **Superiorly:** Soft palate
- **Inferiorly:** Dorsal surface of posterior 1/3 of tongue
- **Anteriorly:** Palato glossal arch
- **Posteriorly:** Palato pharyngeal arch
- **Laterally:** Superior constrictor muscle of the pharynx.

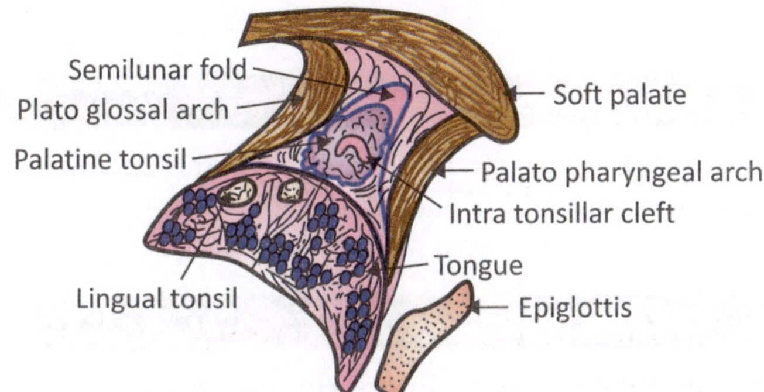

Fig. 25.1: ***Palatine tonsil in fauces (Oropharynx)***

- Lateral surface is covered with a fibrous – capsule. Between the fibrous capsule and superior constrictor of pharynx, the para tonsillar vein passes downwards. Plica triangularis, is a fold of mucous membrane connects the palato glossal and palatopharyngeal folds superiorly and inferiorly.
- **Tonsillar bed** or floor of the tonsillar fossa is formed by superior constrictor and palatopharyngeus muscles. It is separated from tonsil by a thick condensation of pharyngobasilar fascia forming capsule. Capsule is separated from superior constrictor muscle by a film of loose areolar tissue containing venous plexus of tonsil.

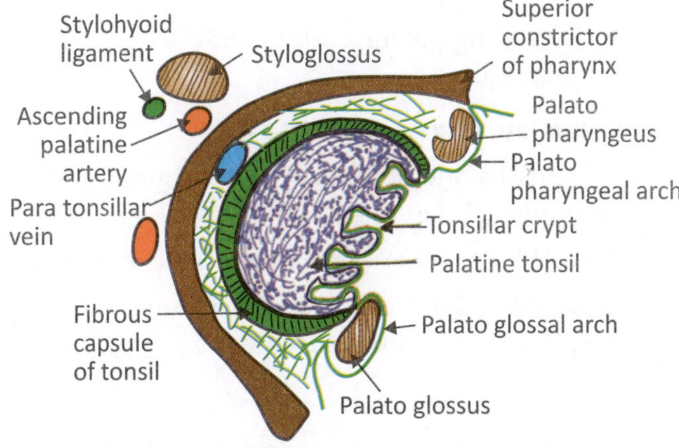

Fig. 25.2: ***Tonsillar bed – horizontal section through tonsil***

CHARACTERISTIC FEATURES OF TONSILS

- Tonsils are 1st line of defence of the body against bacterial invasion.

- Lymphoid tissue produces – antibodies which increases body resistance.
- They have no lymph sinus and so tissue fluid is filtered directly in them.
- Shape – ovoid – like a large almond (2 cm).

Parts:

- Two poles – upper and lower.
- Two borders – anterior and posterior.
- Two surfaces – medial surface is covered by buccal mucous membrane, i.e., stratified squamous epithelium.
- Lateral surface – covered by fibrous capsule – formed by pharyngo – basilar fascia.
- Number of septa extends from capsule into tonsil and conduct blood vessels and nerves into it.

Relations:

- **Medial surface:** It is covered by pharyngeal mucous membrane and has a superior intra tonsillar cleft (remains of 2nd pharyngeal cleft).
- And 12-15 tonsillar crypts that extend deeply into the lymphoid tissue.
- The crypts of the tonsil may lodge pus or food particles – causes infection of tonsil.
- **Lateral surface** related to
  - Superior constrictor of pharynx
  - Facial artery and its two branches
  - Ascending palatine artery and
  - Tonsillar artery.
- **Posterolaterally** are
- Styloglossus and stylopharyngeus muscles, glossopharyngeal nerve.

  Stylohoid ligament – Some times – styloid process.

  Upper pole: Related to – plica semilunaris **Lower pole:** Related to – plica triangularis.

Arterial Supply:

1. Tonsillar branch of facial artery (main).
2. Ascending palatine branch of facial artery.
3. Dorsal lingual branches of lingual artery.
4. Ascending pharyngeal branch of external carotid artery.
5. Descending palatine artery branch of IIIrd part of maxillary artery.

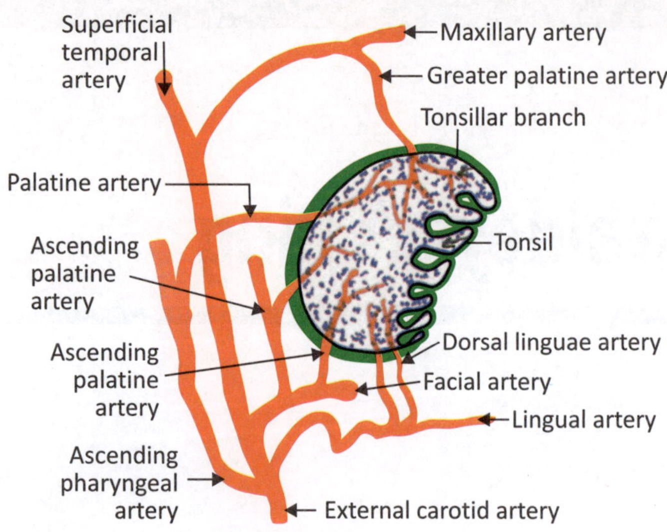

Fig. 25.3: ***Arterial supply of tonsil***

Venous drianage: Peri tonsillar venous plexus may be connected to pharyngeal venous plexus via para tonsillar vein – large vein.

- Main – tonsillar branch of lingual vein.
- Source of bleeding after tonsillectomy.

Nerve supply:

1. Tonsillar branches of glossopharyngeal nerve.
2. Lesser palatine nerves.

Lymphatic drianage: Mainly

1. Juglo digastric lymph node – called tonsillar lymph node because it is enlarged in tonsillitis.
2. Deep cervical group of lymph nodes.

II. PHARYNGEAL TONSIL

Lie postero superiorly under the mucous membrane of the roof and adjoining posterior wall of nasopharynx.

III. TUBAL TONSILS

These are present on each side around the opening of Eustachian tube into nasopharynx.

IV. LINGUAL TONSIL

This is present antero inferiorly and lies under the mucosa of posterior 1/3 of dorsum of tongue.

Collection of lymphoid tissue around the commencement of air and food passages arranged in a ring like patterns called *Waldeyer's lymphatic ring*. It prevents invasion of microorganisms into the air and food passages. The lymph from the ring drains into superficial and deep cervical group of lymph nodes, which form the external ring of Waldeyer.

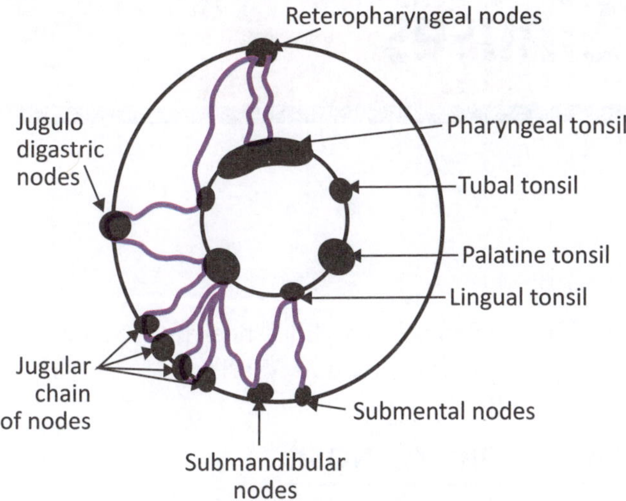

Fig. 25.4: *Waldeyer's lymphatic ring*

Applied Anatomy (Tonsil)

1. Tonsils are large in children and retrogress after puberty.
2. Tonsils are site of infection – causes tonsillitis.
3. Peritonsillar abscess – called Quincy – pus is collected in peritonsillar area due to recurrent infection.
4. Tonsilectomy is the surgical removal of large and infected tonsil.
5. Tonsillitis may cause pain in the ear – which is referred pain because both are supplied by glossopharyngeal nerve.
6. Septic focus can cause – pulmonary tuberculosis, meningitis, carditis and general ill health etc.
7. Tonsils produce antibodies and increases body resistance. They are more useful upto 5 years of age because of low immunity in children they act as safe guard and prevent infection.

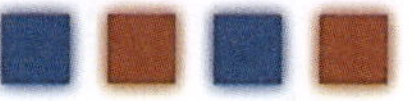

CHAPTER 26

Nose and Para Nasal Air Sinuses

Consists of external nose and nasal cavity.

I. EXTERNAL NOSE

It is a pyramidal projection on face which is covered with skin and subcutaneous tissue.

Parts:

1. A free tip.
2. A root at its junction with forehead.
3. Dorsum of nose is a rounded border between tip and root of nose.

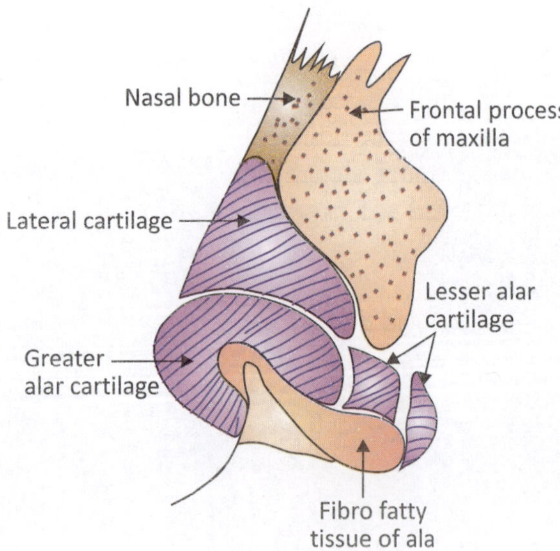

Fig. 26.1: *External nose*

NOSTRILS

Anterior nasal apertures – bounded medially by nasal septum and laterally by ala of nose.

- Skin of external nose lines nostrils – called vestibule has hairs known as Vibrissae.

FRAMEWORK OF NOSE

It is formed by bones, cartilage and fatty fibro areolar tissue.

1. **Bones:** At the root of nose – Paired nasal bones, nasal part of frontal bone and frontal process of maxilla.
2. **Nasal cartilages:** Septal cartilage, lateral cartilage and alar cartilage.
3. **Fibro areolar tissue:** Winged out from midline and forms postero lateral aspect of nares.

Nasal Muscles

Nasal muscles are dilator naris, compressor naris and procerus. All these muscles are supplied by branches of facial nerve.

Nerve Supply of External Nose

1. Nasal branch of infra orbital nerve – branch of (supplies lateral surface of nose) maxillary nerve.
2. Infratrochlear and external nasal branches of ophthalmic division of trigeminal nerve (supplies – root, dorsum and tip of nose).

Arterial Supply

1. Lateral nasal branch of facial artery.
2. Dorsal nasal branch of ophthalmic artery.
3. Nasal branch of infra orbital artery branch of maxillary artery.

Venous drainage: Same follows arteries.

Lymphatic Drainage:

- Submandibular nodes
- Superficial parotid nodes – drain skin of root of nose.

II. NASAL CAVITY

Extends from nostrils to choanae (posterior nasal aperture) through which it opens into nasopharynx. The median septum divides into two halves – right and left nasal cavity. It has – a roof, floor, medial wall and lateral wall.

A. ROOF

Anterior 1/3: This slopes downwards and forwards, formed by alar and lateral nasal cartilage, nasal bone and nasal part of frontal bone.

Middle 1/3: This is horizontal and formed by cribriform plate of ethmoid bone and transmits olfactory nerve filaments to anterior cranial fossa.

Posterior 1/3 of roof of nasal cavity: This slopes downwards and backwards and is formed by –

1. Body of sphenoid mainly.
2. Ala of vomer.
3. Vaginal process of medial pterygoid plate.

B. FLOOR

Formed by hard palate.

1. Palatine processes of maxilla – anterior 2/3.
2. Horizontal plate of palatine – posterior 1/3.

C. MEDIAL WALL (NASAL SEPTUM)

Partly bony and partly cartilaginous.

Bony Part:

1. Vomer – postero inferiorly.
2. Perpendicular plate of ethmoid postero superiorly.

Cartilagenous part is anterior and formed by septal cartilage.

Blood Supply of Medial Wall of Nose (Septum):

1. Long spheno palatine artery.
2. Greater palatine artery.

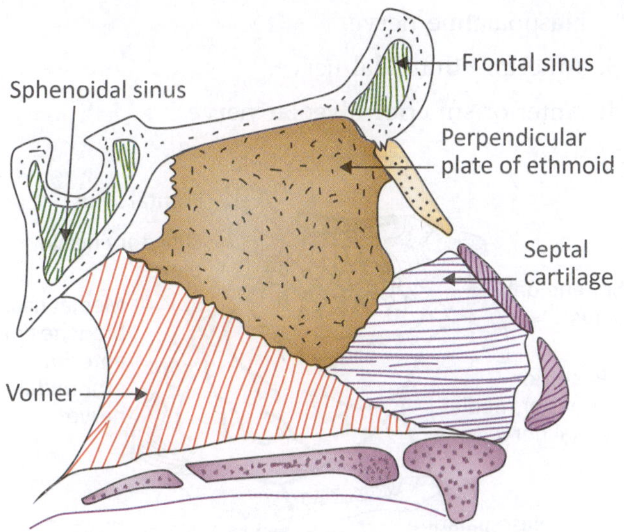

Fig. 26.2: *Nasal septum*

3. Superior labial branch of facial artery.
4. Anterior ethmoidal artery.
   - In the antero inferior quadrant of the nasal septum these arteries communicate freely to form the Kiesalbach's area (Little's area). Injury to this area causes bleeding, called Epistaxis.

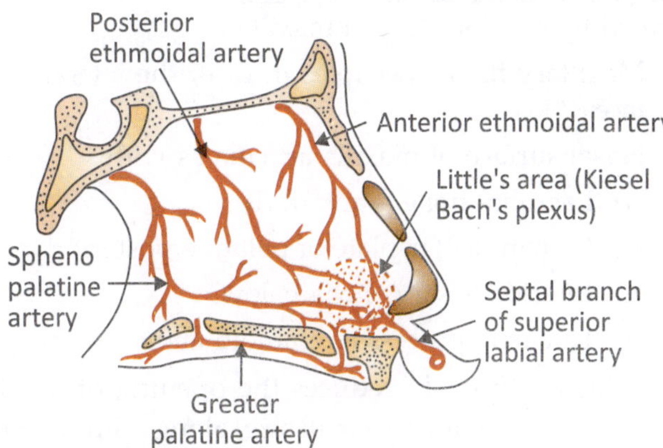

Fig. 26.3: *Arterial supply of nasal septum*

Venous Drainage:

1. Facial vein.
2. Pterygoid venous plexus.

Lymphatic Drainage:

1. Submandibular lymph nodes.
2. Reteropharyngeal lymph nodes.
3. Antero-superior group of deep cervical lymph nodes.

Nerve Supply:

1. Olfactory nerves carry the sense of smell from the upper part of septum.

2. Nasopalatine nerve.
3. Anterior ethmoidal nerve.
4. Anterior-superior alveolar nerve.

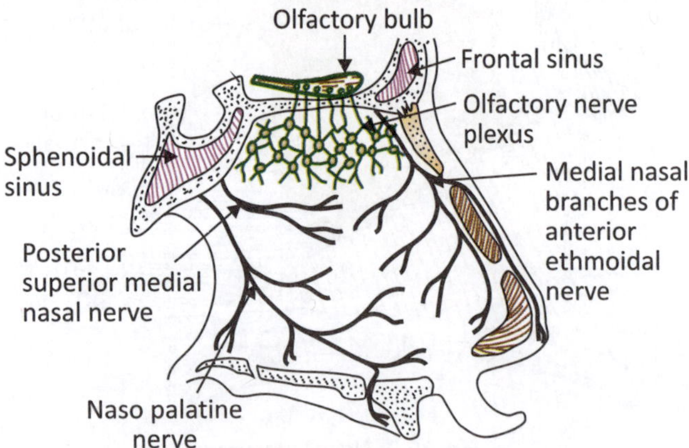

Fig. 26.4: *Nerve supply of nasal septum*

Autonomic Nerve Supply:

Vidians nerve through the spheno – palatine ganglion.

D. LATERAL WALL OF NOSE

Formed by nasal surface of maxilla.

- Maxillary hiatus occupies most of the lateral surface.
- Nasal surface of maxilla articulates with:
  - (i) Lacrimal bone – anteriorly.
  - (ii) Perpandicular plate of palatine posteriorly.
  - (iii) Inferior nasal concha below.
  - (iv) Uncinate process of ethmoid above.

  Which ultimately reduces the opening of maxillary– sinus to a very small size, along with it, thick nasal mucous membrane also helps in reducing the size of maxillary hiatus by 2-3 mm.

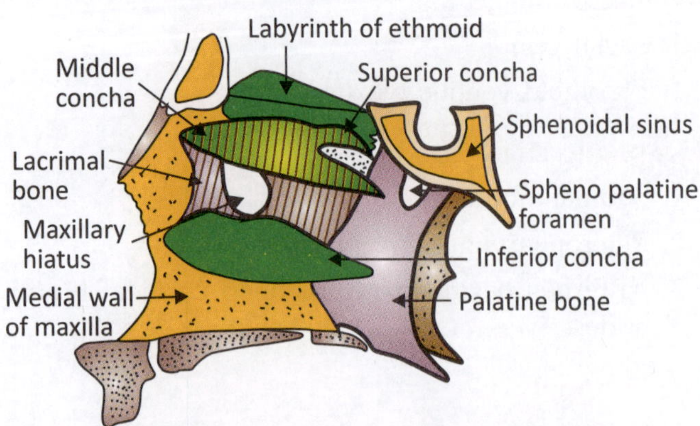

Fig. 26.5: *Bony framework of lateral wall of nose*

- Lateral wall is irregular becuase it has three bony elevations called conchae. The space between the adjacent conchae is known as the meatus.
- This wall is lined by mucous membrane called mucoperiosteum. The superior and middle conchae are formed by the labyrinthine part of the ethmoid bone.
- The inferior concha is formed by the conchal bone, it articulates anteriorly with the maxilla and posteriorly with the perpendicular plate of palatine bone.
- **Lateral wall is divided into three areas:**
  1. **Vestibule:** This area is lined by the skin having hairs called vibrissae. The vibrissae arising from the anterior wall of vestibule are directed backwards and from the posterior wall are directed forwards. They form a sieve at the nasal entry and filters the inspired air.
  2. **Atrium of the middle meatus:** A depressed area situated above the vestibule, but lies infront of the middle meatus. It is limited above by a ridge known as agger nasi.
  3. **Area of conchae and meatuses:** There are three conchae and four meatuses. Conchae are:
     - (a) Superior concha
     - (b) Middle concha and
     - (c) Inferior concha.

     Meatuses are: From above downwards –
     - (a) **Spheno ethmoidal recess:** Lies above the superior concha and below the body of sphenoid. It contains the opening of sphenoidal air sinus.
     - (b) **Superior meatus:** It is the narrowest space lies between the superior and middle concha. Posterior ethmoidal air cells opens into the space.
     - (c) **Middle meatus** is the space between middle and inferior nasal concha. Anteriorly it opens into the atrium of the middle meatus. The bulla ethmoidalis is an elevation caused by the middle air cells opens. Below the bulla ethmoidalis there lies a semilunar shaped gutter called hiatus semilunaris. It is bounded bleow by the uncinate process of ethmoid bone. Into the anterior part of the hiatus fronto nasal duct along with its

infundibulum opens which drains frontal sinus and anterior ethmoid air cells. The posterior part of the hiatus semilunaris receives the opening of maxillary air sinus one or two in number.

(d) *Inferior meatus* – It lies below the inferior nasal concha. In its anterior part naso lacrimal duct opens. Opening is guarded by the Hasner's valve. It does not permit entry of air into the naso lacrimal duct.

Blood Supply to the Lateral Wall of Nose:

Lateral wall is divided into four quadrants. Each quadrant has separate blood supply.

1. **Antero-superior quadrant:**
   (a) Anterior ethmoidal artery
   (b) Posterior ethmoidal artery
   (c) Facial artery.
2. **Postero-superior quadrant:** Sphenopalatine artery (maxillary artery) – Lateral nasal artery.
3. **Antero-inferior quadrant:**
   (a) Facial artery.
   (b) Perforating branches of greater palatine artery.
4. **Postero-inferior quadrant:** Greater palatine artery and its branches.

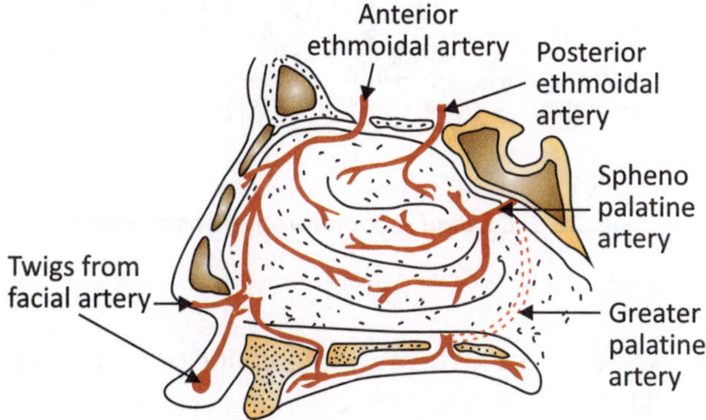

Fig. 26.6: *Blood supply of lateral wall of nose*

Venous Drainage:

(a) Anterior part drains into anterior facial vein.
(b) Middle part drains into pterygoid venous plexus.
(c) Posterior part drains into pharyngeal venous plexus

Lymphatic Drainage:

(a) Anterior part drains into submandibular lymph nodes.
(b) Posterior part drains into retropharyngeal lymph nodes.

Nerve Supply:

The sense of smell from the lateral wall is carried by the olfactory nerves above superior concha.

Parasymphathetic supply of lateral wall of nose is by vidians nerve (nerve of pterygoid canal).

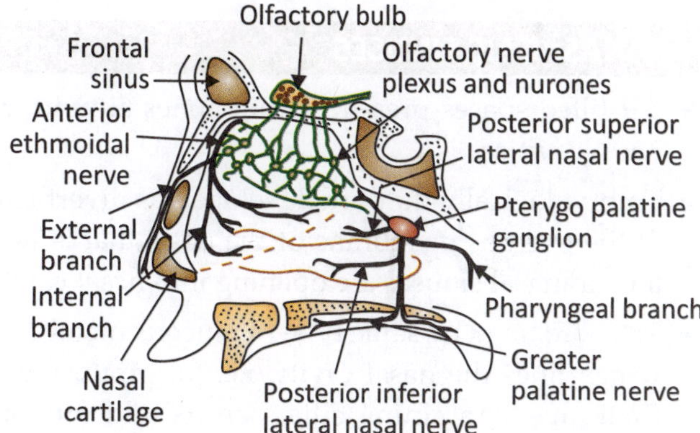

Fig. 26.7: *Nerve supply of lateral wall of nose*

Sensory Supply:

1. Antero superior quadrant – anterior ethmoidal nerve.
2. Postero superior quadrant – spheno palatine branches of spheno palatine ganglion.
3. Antero inferior quadrant – anterior superior alveolar nerve.
4. Postero inferior quadrant – greater palatine nerve.

Applied Anatomy

1. Dangerous area of the nose – olfactory area is considered as dangerous area of nose – because infection from this part may spread along the pia and arachnoid sheaths of the olfactory nerve to the interior of the cranial cavity.
2. Septal deviation to any side causes symptoms.
3. Septal haematoma – In this blood is collected in nasal septum.
4. Epistaxis – Bleeding from little's area of nose due to injury.
5. Vestibulitis – Inflammation of vestibule of nose.
6. Hypertrophy of conchae – This causes nasal obstruction.
7. Anosmia – Loss of sense of smell.

8. Parosmia – Perverted sense of smell.
9. Rhinorrhoea – C.S.F. leaking from number of anterior cranial fossa.
10. Caprosmia – Unpleasent odour due to decomposition of tissues of individual.
11. Rhinoscopy – The examination of nose by rhinoscope is called Rhinoscopy.

PARANASAL AIR SINUSES

- Air filled spaces present within bones around the nasal cavities.
- Embryologically they are developed as diverticula of the mucous membrane of the nose, that is why all paranasal sinuses are opening into nasal cavity.
- They are lined by same type of mucous membrane which lines the nasal cavity, i.e., respiratory epithelium – containing cilia, serous and mucous glands, i.e., ciliated columnar epithelium.

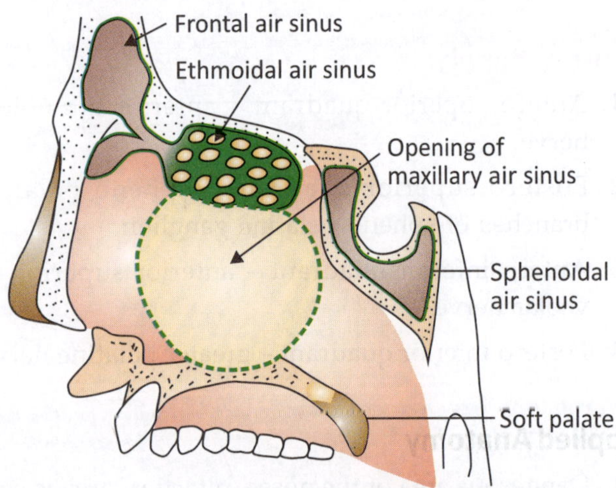

Fig. 26.8: ***Paranasal air sinuses***

CLASSIFICATION OF PARANASAL SINUSES

A. Anterior Group:

1. Maxillary air sinus
2. Frontal air sinus
3. Anterior ethmoidal sinuses.

B. Posterior Group:

1. Middle and posterior ethmoidal sinuses
2. Sphenoidal air sinuses.

FUNCTIONS OF PARANASAL AIR SINUSES

Exact function is not known.

1. Reduction of weight of skull.
2. Providing resonance for voice.
3. Protection of orbit by acting as a shock absorber.
4. Minimal respiratory function – by increasing surface area of mucous membrane and making the inspired air moist and warm (serving as air conditioning chamber).
5. Facial growth occurs rapidly after formation of sinuses.

I. Maxillary Air Sinus (Antrum of High More)

- Situated in the body of maxilla, largest among all sinuses, pyramidal in shape.
- Capacity – about 15 cc.
- Size – Height = 3.5 cm, Width = 2.5 cm Anterior depth = 3.5 cm.

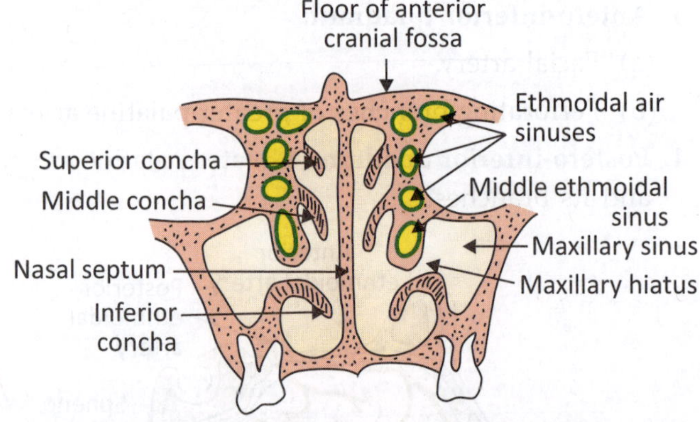

Fig. 26.9: ***Coronal section through nasal cavity***

Parts:

- **Apex:** Directed towards zygomatic process of maxilla.
- **Base:** Towards lateral wall of nose.
- **Roof** is formed by floor of orbit.
- **Floor** is formed by alveolar process of maxilla.

Roots of 1st and 2nd premolar and 3rd molar teeth projects into sinus – making conical projections in floor of sinus.

Drainage:

Into lower and posterior part of hiatus semilunaris in middle meatus of lateral wall of nose.

- Opening of the sinus is nearer to roof than the floor.
- Opening of maxillary sinus is a large aperture, made small by following bones –
  - Opening is still reduced by thick nasal mucosa, extending into sinus 2 to 3 mm.

Bones reducing opening of maxillary air sinus:

1. **Superiorly:** Uncinate process of ethmoid bone
2. **Inferiorly:** Conchal bone (inferior)
3. **Anteriorly:** Lacrimal bone
4. **Posteriorly:** Perpendicular plate of palatine bone.

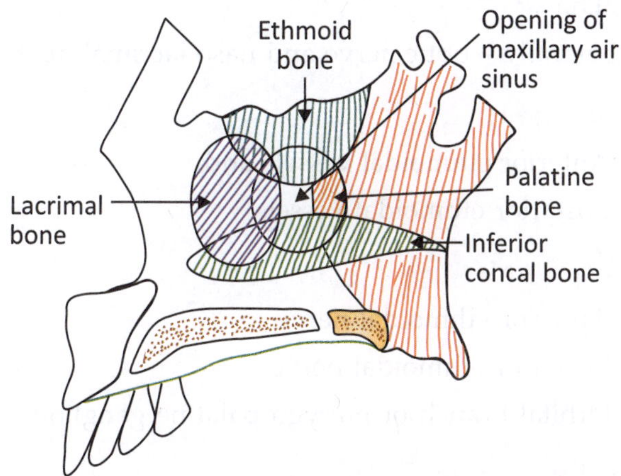

Fig. 26.10: *Bones reducing opening of maxillary air sinus*

Nerve Supply:

Anterior, middle and posterior superior alveolar nerves.

Blood Supply:

1. Facial artery
2. Greater palatine artery
3. **Infra orbital artery:** Anterior, middle and posterior superior alveolar arteries.

Lymphatic drainage: Submandibular lymph nodes.

Relations of Maxillary Sinus:

Superiorly: Orbit

Inferiorly: Oral cavity

Medially: Nasal cavity with

1. Naso lacimal duct
2. Lateral wall of nose

Posteriorly: Pterygo palatine – fossa and infra temporal fossa

Anteriorly: Face.

Applied Anatomy

1. During extraction of premolar teeth from upper jaw – a communication may be established accidentally between oral cavity and sinus – called antro-oral fistula.
2. Spheno palatine – fossa may be approached surgically through this air sinus.
3. **Tumour from maxillary sinus may grow:**
   (a) Superiorly and compress orbital structures.
   (b) Inferiorly – causing whithering (falling) of teeth of upper jaw and tumour may grow into mouth.
   (c) Medially it grows towards nose.
   (d) Posteriorly grows into pterygo palatine and infra temporal fossa.
4. Sinus may be tested clinically by torching a light within the mouth in a darkroom cheek will be glowing if it is normal.
5. Cald well – luck operation – sinus is opened through canine fossa and disease is treated via oral cavity.
6. Opening of maxillary sinus is situated superiorly, opening of other sinuses are directed inferiorly towards maxillary sinus spreading infections. Causing maxillary sinusitis – sinus is punctured called antral puncture – via canine fossa.

II. Frontal Air Sinus

Rudimentary at birth.

- Develop around 2nd year.
- Well developed at puberty.

Situation: Within frontal bone above supra orbital margin.

- Septum divides into right and left sinus. It may not be in centre.

Shape: Pyramidal shaped

Size-depth: 1.8 cm

Height: 3 cm

Breadth: 2.5 cm

Capacity: About 7 c.c.

Drainage: Into anterior part of hiatus semilunaris by fronto nasal duct.

Blood supply: Supra orbital artery

Nerve supply: Supra orbital nerve (V_1)

Venous drainage: Into anastomatic vein between supra orbital and superior ophthalmic vein.

Lymphatics: Submandibular lymph nodes.

Applied Anatomy

1. Frontal sinusitis.
2. Tenderness is elicited by pressing floor of frontal air sinus (orbital roof – medially).
3. In frontal sinusitis – fronto nasal duct is blocked.
   - Headache present on temporal and parietal area called vacauum frontal headache.
4. Fronto nasal duct is vertical – drainage is facilitated by vertical position.
5. Surgical drainage is called Howarth operation.
6. Sinus gallop – multiple sinus cavity formed.

III. Anterior Ethmoidal Sinuses

Present in ethmoid bone.

Number: Variable, about 20 in number.

Classified: According to location:

- Anterior – 11
- Middle – 1-5
- Posterior – 1-7
- Air cells present.

Drainage:

Anterior ethmoidal air cells joins ethmoidal infundibulum or fronto nasal duct and drains into anterior part of hiatus semilunaris.

Middle air cells: Open on bulla ethmoidalis.

Posterior air cells: Open into superior meatus.

Relations:

Superiorly – cranial cavity

Inferiorly – maxillary air sinus

Anteriorly – external nose

Medially – nasal cavity – superior and middle choncha

Laterally – optic nerve and naso lacrimal duct.

Blood Supply:

- Anterior ethmoidal vessels and
- Posterior ethmoidal vessels.

Nerve Supply:

- Anterior ethmoidal nerve
- Posterior ethmoidal nerve
- Orbital branch of pterygo palatine ganglion.

Lymphatic Drainage:

- Anterior and middle ethmoidal sinuses drains into submandibular lymph nodes.
- Posterior ethmoidal cells drain into retropharyngeal lymph nodes.

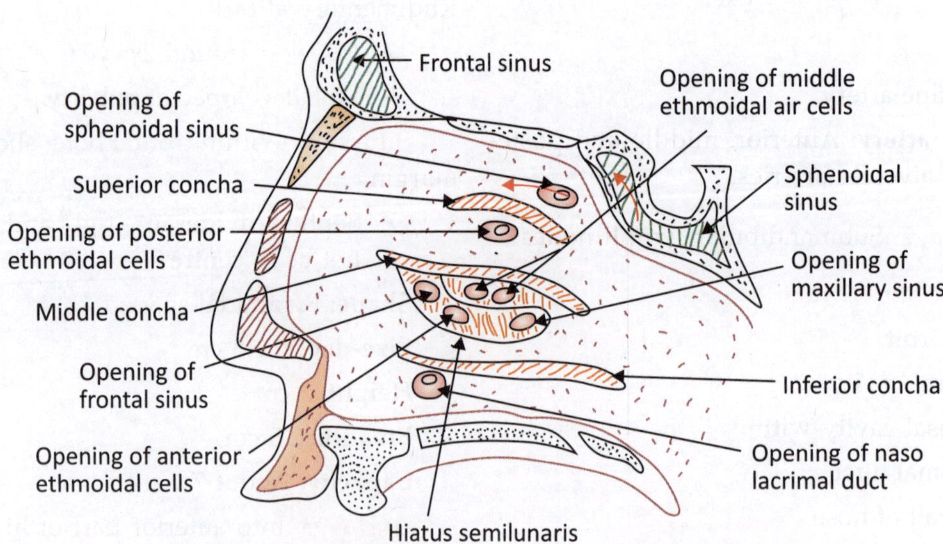

Fig. 26.11: *Lateral wall of nose showing openings of sinuses*

IV. Sphenoidal Air Sinus

- The right and left sphenoidal sinuses lie with in the body of sphenoid, above and behind the nasal cavity.
- They are separated by a septum.
- Two sinuses are usually asymmetrical.

Drainage:

Each sinus drains into spheno ethmoidal recess of nasal cavity present in the upper part of lateral wall of nose.

Measurements:

Vertical – 2 cm

Transverse – 1.8 cm

Antero – Posterior – 2 cm.

Relations:

(a) **Superiorly:** Pituitary gland and optic chiasma.

(b) **Inferiorly:** Roof of nasopharynx.

(c) **Laterally:** Cavernous sinus and internal carotid artery.

(d) **Posteriorly:** Pons and medulla oblongata.

(e) **Anteriorly:** Spheno ethmoidal recess.

Arterial supply: Posterior ethmoidal artery and branches of internal carotid artery.

Venous drainage: Cavernous sinus.

Nerve supply: Posterior ethmoidal nerve and orbital branch of pterygo palatine ganglion.

Lymphatic drainage: Into retro pharyngeal lymph nodes.

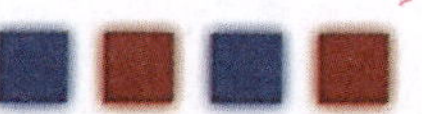

CHAPTER 27

Pre-Vertebral Region and Root of Neck

Bony framework: It is formed of seven cervical vertebrae.

- Superior surface of manubrium sterni.
- Ist rib – slopes downwards and forwards.
- Articulated cervical vertebrae when clothed with muscles attached to anterior tubercles of transverse processes, present a relatively flat pre-vertebral surface.

Deep cervical muscles are classified as:

A. **According to their position,** i.e.

I. **Pre-vertebral muscles:** Present infront of vertebral bodies, e.g.,

(i) Longus colli
(ii) Longus capitis
(iii) Rectus capitis anterior
(iv) Rectus capitis lateralis.

II. **Para-vertebral muscles:** Connect the cervical vertebral column with the thoracic cage, e.g.,

(i) Scalenus anterior
(ii) Scalenus medius
(iii) Scalenus posterior
(iv) Scalenus minimus
(v) Levator scapulae.

B. **Classification according to relation of muscles with cervical and brachial plexus:**

I. **Muscles medial to plexus:**

(i) Longus colli
(ii) Longus capitis
(iii) Rectus capitis anterior
(iv) Scalenus anterior.

II. **Muscles lateral to plexus:**

(i) Rectus capitis lateralis
(ii) Scalenus medius
(iii) Scalenus posterior
(iv) Levator scapulae.

Structure infront of neck of Ist rib: From medial to lateral side are:

1. Sympathetic trunk with T_1 ganglion or stellate ganglion.
2. First posterior intercostal vein.
3. Superior intercostal artery.
4. Ascending branch of ventral ramus of T_1 to join with C_8 ventral rami to from lower trunk of brachial plexus.
5. Apex of lung lies infront of all above structures.

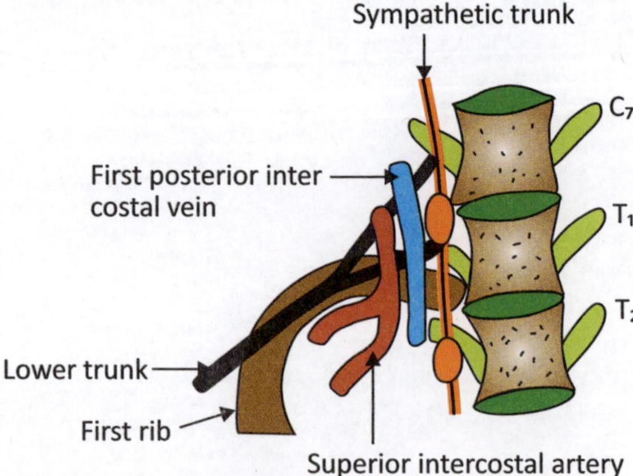

Fig. 27.1: *Structure present infront of neck of I[st] rib*

GENERAL FEATURES OF PRE-VERTEBRAL MUSCLES

1. Lie infront of vertebral column.
2. Are covered anteriorly by a thick pre-vertebral fascia.
3. Form the posterior boundary of retropharyngeal space.
4. Extend from base of skull to the superior mediastinum.
5. Are weak flexors of the head and neck. Rectus capitis lateralis causes lateral flexion.
6. Supplied by ventral rami of C_1 and C_2 cervical nerves except longus colli which is supplied by C_2 to C_6 nerves.

SCALENO VERTEBRAL TRIANGLE

This triangular space is present at the root of the neck on either side.

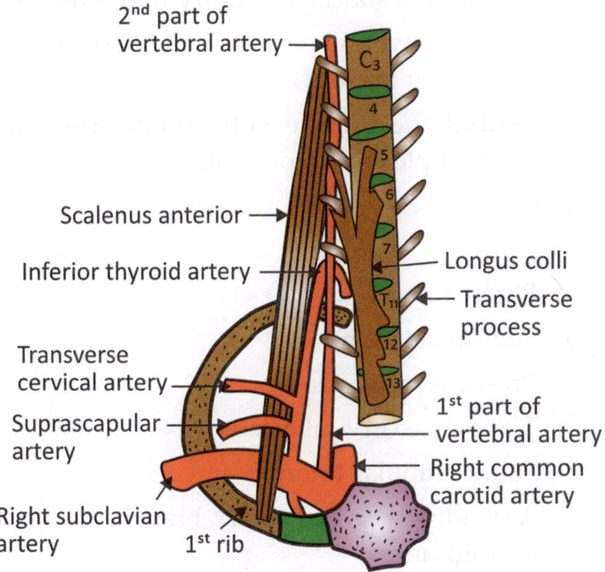

Fig. 27.2: *Vertebral triangle and first part of vertebral artery*

Boundaries:

- **Medial** – Lower oblique part of longus colli.
- **Lateral** – Scalenus anterior.
- **Apex** – At transverse process of C_6 vertebra.
- **Base** – First part of subclavian artery.
- **Floor** – Neck of 1st rib and cupola of the pleura.

Contents:

1. First part of vertebral artery and vertebral vein.
2. Cervical part of sympathetic trunk.

Paravertebral muscles:

1. Scalenus anterior
2. Scalenus medius
3. Scalenus posterior.

General Features

1. Scalenus medius is the largest and scalenus posterior is the smallest of the three scalene muscles.
2. Scalenus anterior is the 'Key' muscle of the paravertebral region.
3. Scalenus muscles extend from the transverse process of the cervical vertebrae to the first two ribs.
4. They can either elevate the ribs as in inspiration or bend the cervical part of the vertebral column laterally to ipsilateral side.

I. Muscles Medial to Plexus

1. **Longus colli** has three parts:

   (a) Upper oblique part:

   Origin: Anterior tubercle of transverse – process of C_3, C_4 and C_5 vertebrae.

   Insertion: Anterior arch of atlas.

   (b) Intermediate vertical part:

   Origin: Anterior surface of bodies of T_1, T_2 and T_3 vertebra.

   Insertion: Anterior surface of bodies of C_5, C_6, C_7 vertebra.

   (c) Lower oblique part:

   Origin: Anterior surface of bodies of T_1, T_2, T_3 vertebra.

   Insertion: Anterior tubercle of transverse process of C_5, C_6 vertebra.

   Nerve supply: Ventral rami of C_3, C_4, C_5 and 6 nerves.

   Action: Flexor of neck.

2. **Longus capitis:**

   Origin: Anterior tubercle of transverse process of C_3, C_4, C_5 and C_6 vertebra (typical cervical vertebra).

   Insertion: Basilar part of occipital bone.

Nerve supply: Ventral rami of C_2, C_3, C_4, C_5 and C_6 nerves.

Action: Flexor of neck.

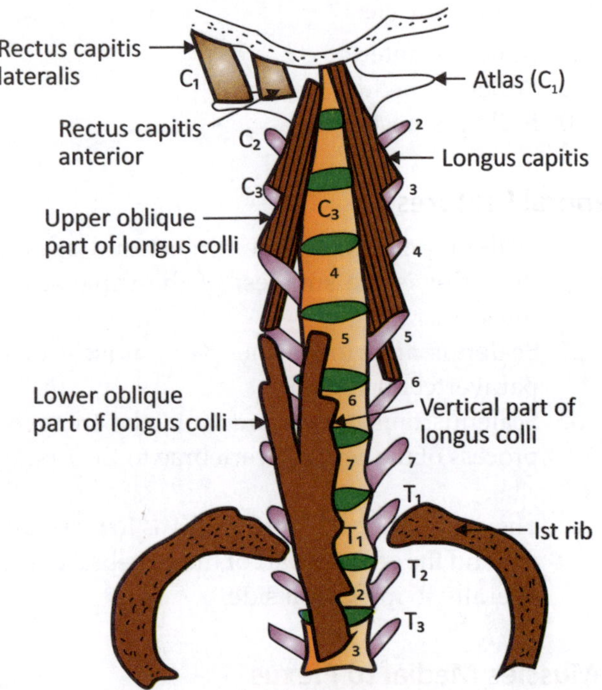

Fig. 27.3: *Pre vertebral muscles*

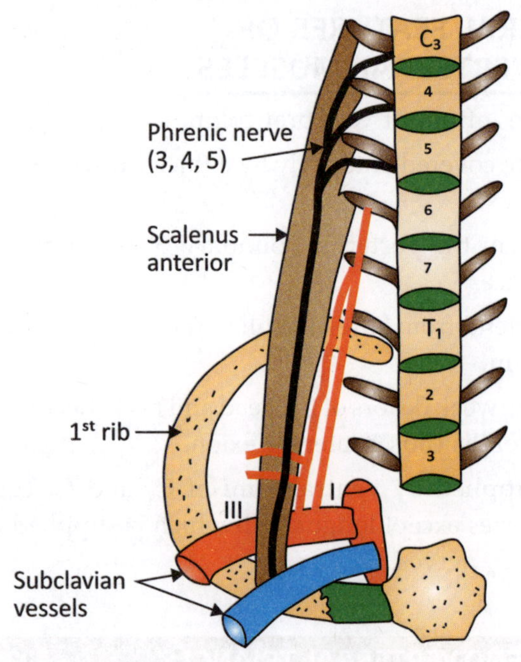

Fig. 27.4: *Scalenus anterior*

3. Rectus capitis anterior

Origin: Transverse process and lateral mass of atlas.

Insertion: Basilar part of occipital bone.

Nerve supply: Ventral rami of C_1, C_2 nerves.

Action: Flexor of neck.

4. Scalenus anterior: It is a flat and ribbon shaped 'Key' muscle of lower part of neck because of its relations to many important structures in this region, i.e., subclavian artery, vein and nerves (Phrenic and brachial plexus).

Origin: Anterior tubercle of transverse process of C_3, C_4, C_5 and C_6 vertebra (typical cervical vertebra).

Insertion: Scalene tubercle present on inner border of 1st rib.

Nerve supply: Ventral rami of C_4, C_5, C_6 nerves.

Actions:

1. It is an accessory respiratory muscle, i.e., lifts the first rib up and increases the vertical diameter of chest.
2. Flex the neck forwards.

Important Features:

1. Divides the subclavian artery into three parts.
2. Phrenic nerve and pre-vertebral fascia are found anterior to muscle.
3. Behind the muscle–subclavian artery and brachial plexus are present.

Relations of Scalenus Anterior

Anterior:

- Phrenic nerve
- Subclavian vein
- Pre-vertebral fascia
- Transverse cervical artery
- Supra scapular artery
- Ascending cervical artery branch of inferior thyroid artery
- Lateral part of carotid sheath containing internal jugular vein
- Descendens cervicalis – C_2 and C_3 nerve fibres
- Inferior belly of omohyoid
- Anterior jugular vein
- Sternomastoid branches of superior thyroid and supra scapular arteries
- Sternomastoid and clavicle.

Posterior:

- Brachial plexus – roots

- IInd part of subclavian artery
- Medial part of scalenus medius
- Cervical pleura covered by suprapleural membrane.

Medial:

- Carotid sheath
- Sympathetic chain
- Thyro cervical trunk
- Vertebral artery.

Lateral:

- Trunks of brachial plexus
- IIIrd part of subclavian artery
- Scalenus medius and posterior muscles.

II. Muscles Lateral to Plexus

1. **Rectus capitis lateralis**

   Origin: Transverse process and lateral mass of atlas.

   Insertion: Basilar part of occipital bone infront of jugular process.

   Nerve supply: Ventral rami of C_1 nerve.

   Action: Stabilizes atlanto occipital joints.

2. **Scalenus medius:** Forms part of floor of posterior triangle of neck.

   Origin: Posterior tubercle of transverse process of C_3, C_4, C_5 and C_6 vertebra (typical cervical vertebra).

   Insertion: Superior surface of 1st rib behind subclavian artery and brachial plexus.

   Nerve supply: Ventral rami of C_4, C_5, C_6 nerves.

   Action:

   - Elevation of 1st rib and
   - Forward flexion of cervical vertebral column.

   Structures Piercing the Muscle:

   1. Nerve to rhomboids (C_5)
   2. C_5, C_6 roots of long thoracic nerve.

   Relations of Scalenus Medius:

   Anterior:

   - Roots of brachial plexus
   - Second part of subclavian artery
   - Scalenus anterior muscle
   - Dorsal scapular nerve (C_5) and
   - Upper two roots of nerve to serratus anterior C_5 and C_6 – pierce it.

   Posterior:

   - Levator scapulae
   - Scalenus posterior.

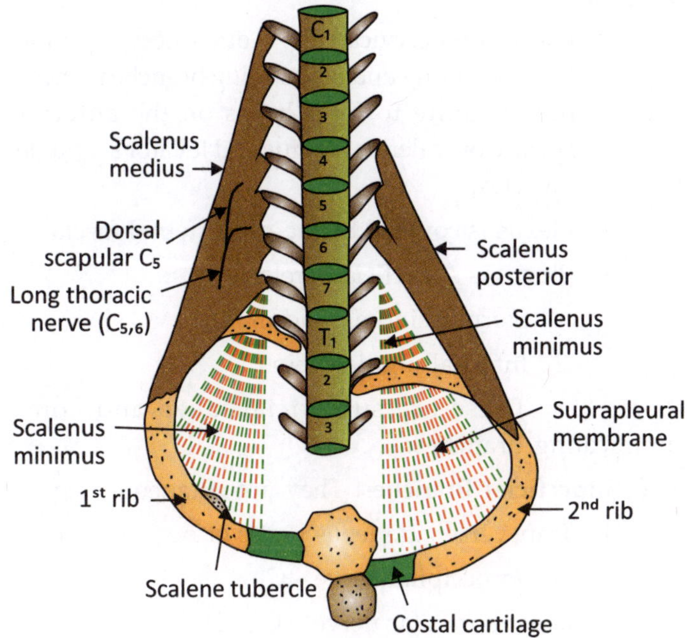

Fig. 27.5: *Scalenus medius and posterior*

3. **Scalenus posterior**

   Origin: Posterior tubercle of transverse process of C_4, C_5, C_6 vertebra.

   Insertion: 2nd rib.

   Nerve supply: Ventral rami of C_4, C_5, C_6 nerves.

   Action: Accessory respiratory muscle, lifts 2nd rib upwards → ↑ vertical diameter of chest and forward flexion of cervical vertebral column.

4. **Scalenus minimus:** Arises from transverse process of C_7.

   Inserted: On inner border of 1st rib and cervical pleura.

   Applied: Scalene anticus synodrome – cervical rib or spasm of scalene muscles or over crowding of scalene muscles may compress the subclavian artery and brachial plexus. The nerve usually involved is C_8 and T_1 (Lower Trunk).

   Fullness or swelling in posterior triangle.

Neurological Symptoms:

- Tingling, numbness, anaesthesia

- ➢ Hyperasthesia, parasthesia
- ➢ Wasting of hypothenar muscles.

Ischemia of upper limb: Cynosis of hand, necrosis of finger tips, digital gangrene etc.

Cervical plexus: It is a network of nerves formed in the upper part of neck by ventral rami of C_1 to C_4 nerves.

- ➢ Except first cervical nerve, other nerves divide into ascending and descending branches. These nerves unite to form loops on the anterior surface of scalenus medius and levator scapulae muscles.
- ➢ Plexus is covered by the prevertebral fascia.
- ➢ Plexus is superficially related to:
  1. Sternocleidomastoid muscle
  2. Internal jugular vein.

Branches: These are superficial, deep and communicating branches:

I. Superficial Branches: They are cutaneous, e.g.,

1. Transverse cutaneous nerve of neck – C_2, C_3.
2. Lesser occipital nerve – C_2.
3. Great auricular nerve – C_2, C_3.
4. Supra clavicular nerves – C_3, C_4.

II. Deep Branches:

A. Muscular

1. Phrenic nerve – C_3, C_4, C_5 – supplies diaphragm.
2. Rectus capitis lateralis – C_1.
3. Rectus capitis anterior – C_1.
4. Longus capitis – C_1 to C_4.
5. Longus colli – C_3 to C_8.
6. Inferior limb of ansa cervicalis – C_2, C_3.
7. Scalenus anterior – C_4, C_5, C_6.

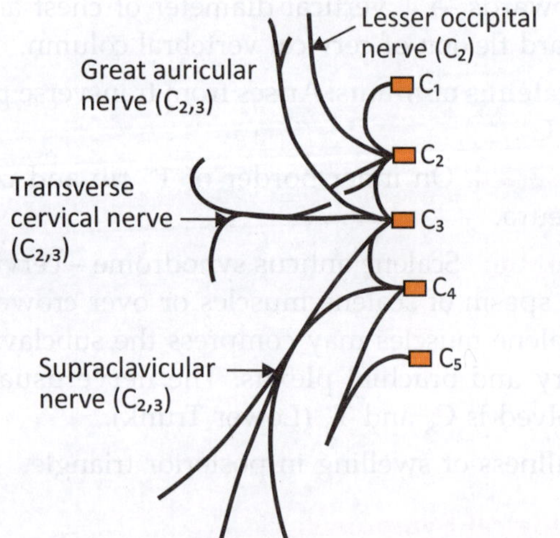

Fig. 27.6: *Cutaneous branches of cervical plexus*

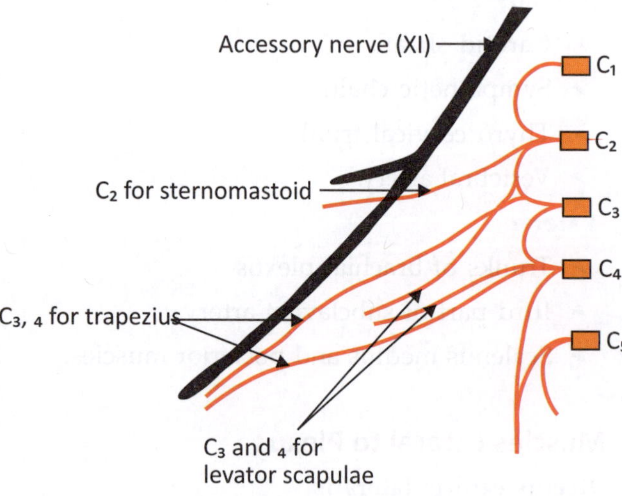

Fig. 27.7: *Deep and posterior muscular branches of cervical plexus*

B. Posterior branches to supply

1. Sternocleido mastoid – C_2, C_3.
2. Levator scapulae – C_3, C_4, C_5.
3. Trapezius – C_3, C_4.
4. Scalenus medius – C_3, C_4.

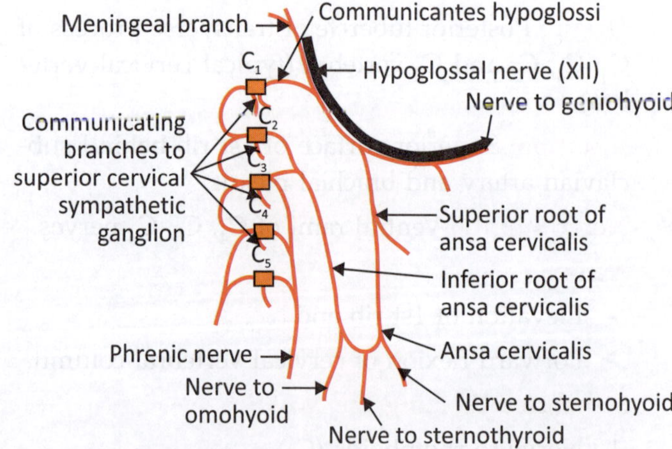

Fig. 27.8: *Deep inferior branches of cervical plexus*

III. Communicating Branches:

(a) Superior cervical sympathetic ganglion communicates with C_1 to C_4 nerves by grey rami communicants.

(b) A branch from C_1 joins hypoglossal nerve and forms superior limb of ansa cervicalis.

- Superior and inferior limb of ansa cervicalis joins and supplies infra hyoid muscles.

Some fibres of C_1 continue into hypoglossal nerve and supply thyrohyoid and geniohyoid.

Applied Anatomy

1. In case of meningitis – neck rigidity may occur due to involvement of cervical nerves.
2. Cervico occipital neuralgia.

BRACHIAL PLEXUS

It lies in the lower part of neck on the surface of scalenus medius deep to scalenus anterior and pre-vertebral fascia.

It is formed by ventral rami of lower four cervical nerves and T_1 with variable contribution from C_4 and T_2.

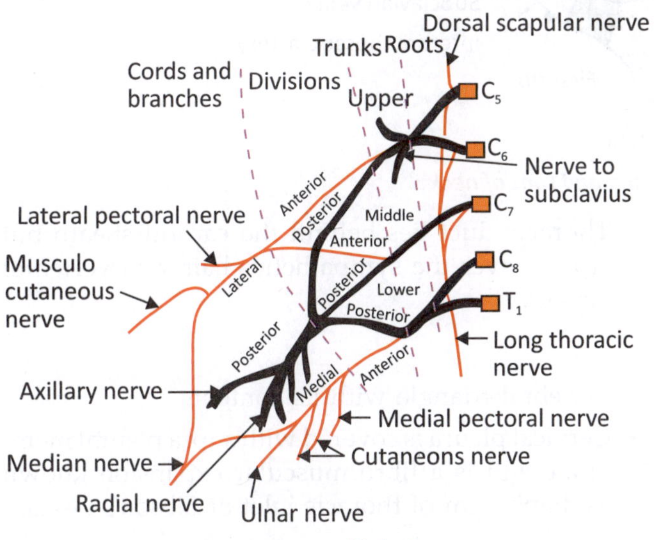

Fig. 27.9: ***Brachial plexus***

Parts of Brachial Plexus

1. **Roots**: C_5, C_6, C_7, C_8 and T_1 ventral rami.
2. **Trunks:**
   - C_5 and C_6 roots join and form upper trunk.
   - C_7 forms middle trunk.
   - C_8 and T_1 roots join and form lower trunk.
3. **Divisions:** Each trunk splits into an anterior and a posterior division behind the clavicle.
4. **Cords:** All three posterior divisions unite to form the posterior cord.
   - The upper two anterior divisions unite to form the lateral cord.
   - The lower anterior division forms the medial cord.
     - Cords are related to axillary artery – lateral, medial and posterior.
5. **Branches** are given off from roots, trunks and cord.

Branches from roots are:

- Dorsal scapular – C_5.
- Long thoracic – C_5, C_6 and C_7.

From trunks – Only upper trunk gives branches:

- Supra scapular–C_5, C_6
- Nerve to subclavius – C_5, C_6.

Location of Brachial Plexus

Roots and trunks: Lie in neck on scalenus medius muscle.

Divisions are behind the clavicle.

Cords and branches are in the axilla.

- The roots of the plexus lie behind scalenus anterior and the lower trunk is posterior to subclavian artery.

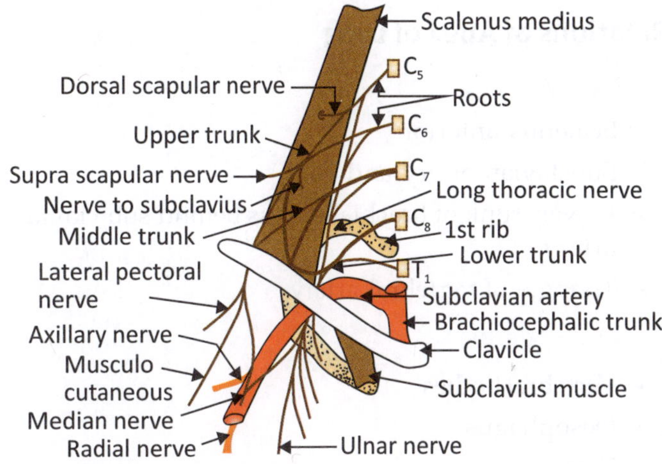

Fig. 27.10: ***In the neck only roots and trunks of brachial plexus lie and division is behind the clavicle***

Root of Neck:

- The cords are related to the axillary artery covered by pectoralis minor and major muscles in the axillary region.
- Lies above the apex of lung.
- Structures arching over the apex are costo-cervical trunk and its highest intercostal branch from anterior to posterior surface.

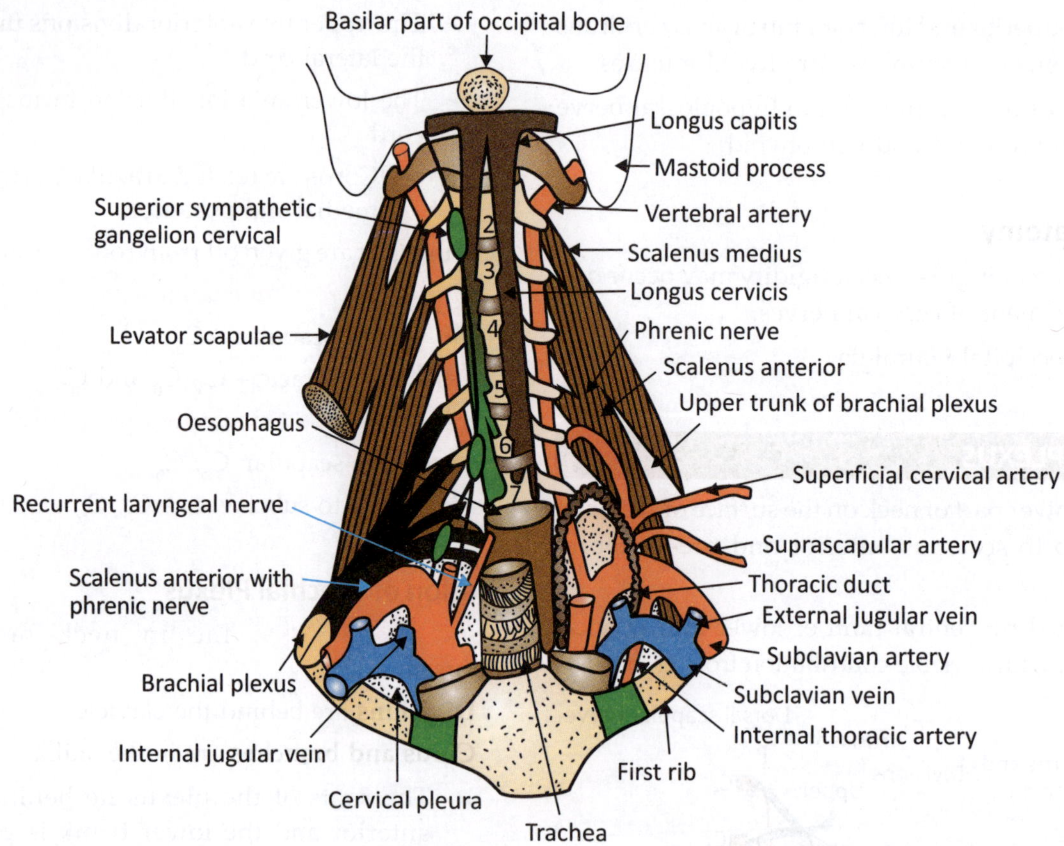

Fig. 27.11: ***Prevertebral region and root of neck***

Relations of Apex of Lung

Lateral:

- Scalenus anterior.
- Subclavian artery and vein.
- Lower trunk of brachial plexus behind sub-clavian artery.
- Triangle of vertebral artery.

Medial:

- Vertebral bodies
- Oesophagus
- Trachea
- Thoracic duct and recurrent laryngeal nerve on left side.

Anterior

- Great vessels of head, neck and upper limb, e.g., brachiocephalic trunk, common carotid and subclavian artery with its ascending and descending branches, e.g., vertebral, inferior thyroid and internal thoracic artery and vein.
- Phrenic nerve and vagus nerve (X).
- Thoracic duct and subclavian artery arches over the apex of left lung from medial to lateral side.
- Thoracic duct lies behind the carotid sheath but crosses over the sympathetic chain and vertebral vessels.

Superior:

- Vertebral triangle with its contents.
- Cervical pleura is covered with supra pleural membrane and is a fibro muscular expansion known as diaphragm of thoracic inlet or Sibson's fascia.

Sibson's Fascia

(Diaphragm of thoracic inlet)

It is a fibro muscular membrane.

- Contains muscle fibres of scalenus minimus.
- Dome of cervical pleura is attached to it's under aspect.

Attachments: From tip of transverse process of C_7 to inner border of I^{st} rib and its cartilage.

Function: Helps to limit recession of soft tissues of the root of neck during inspiration and ballooning during expiration.

Posterior: Apex of lung is related to neck of Ist rib and structures passing infront of neck are – from medial to lateral. Sympathetic trunk with its inferior cervical ganglion.

V – Superior inter costal vein

A – Superior inter costal artery

N – Ascending branch of T_1 spinal nerve joins with C_8 and forms lower trunk of branchial plexus.

SUBCLAVIAN ARTERY

Supplies: Upper limb, breast, anterior thoraco abdominal wall, considerable part of neck and brain.

Origin or Commencement:

- Right subclavian artery commences from brachio-cephalic artery behind right sternoclavicular joint.

Relations of Subclavian Artery

- Left subclavian artery commences from arch of aorta.

Termination: It terminates at the lateral border of first rib by becoming the axillary artery.

Parts: Divided by scalenus anterior muscle into three parts:

- Ist part medial to muscle
- IInd part behind the muscle
- IIIrd part lateral to muscle.

Cervical part of subclavian artery arches over the apex of lung, cervical pleura and supra pleural membrane – it will be posterior relation for all 3 parts of subclavian artery.

Table 27.1: *Anterior Relation*

Ist Part	IInd Part	IIIrd Part
– Skin – Superficial fascia – Platysma – Investing layer of deep fascia neck	– Skin – Superficial fascia – Platysma – Investing layer of deep fascia neck	– Skin – Superficial fascia – Platysma – Investing layer of deep fascia neck
Artery: – Common carotid artery – Sternomastoid artery branch of suprascapular artery	1. Transverse cervical artery 2. Suprascapular artery	Suprascapular artery
Veins: – Internal jugular vein – Anterior jugular vein – Vertebral vein	1. Subclavian vein 2. Anterior jugular vein	1. Subclavian vein 2. External jugular vein 3. Anterior jugular vein 4. Suprascapular vein 5. Transverse cervical vein
Muscles: – Sternomastoid – Sternohyoid – Sternothyroid	1. Scalenus anterior 2. Sternomastoid	1. Subclavius muscle 2. Posterior border of sternomastoid 3. Inferior belly of omohyoid
Nerves: – Vagus – Cardiac branches of X and sympathetic trunk – Ansa subclavia – Right recurrent laryngeal nerve		
On left side: – Phrenic nerve – Thoracic duct – Left brachiocephalic vein	1. Right phrenic nerve	1. Supra clavicular nerves 2. Nerve to subclavius
On right side: – Right lymphatic duct		
Bones		– Middle 1/3 of clavicle

Table 27.2: *Relations of subclavian artery*

Relation	Ist Part	IInd Part	IIIrd Part
Posterior – Relations	1. Supra pleural membrane 2. Cervical pleura 3. Apex of lung 4. Ansa subclavia 5. Right recurrent laryngeal nerve	1. Supra pleural membrane 2. Cervical pleura 3. Apex of lung	1. Scalenus medius 2. Lower trunk of brachial plexus 3. Supra pleural membrane 4. Cervical pleura 5. Apex of lung
Superior – Relations	–	1. Upper and middle trunks of brachial plexus 2. Inferior belly of omohyoid	Upper and middle trunks of brachial plexus
Inferior – Relations	–	–	First rib

Branches of Subclavian Artery

1. Vertebral artery
2. Internal thoracic artery
3. Thyrocervical trunk
   (a) Inferior thyroid artery
   (b) Suprascapular artery
   (c) Transverse cervical artery
4. Costo cervical trunk
   (a) Superior intercostal artery
   (b) Deep cervical artery
5. Dorsal scapular artery – occasionally present, goes posteriorly along the medial border of scapula and takes part in the anastmosis around the scapula with subscapular artery at the inferior angle of scapula.

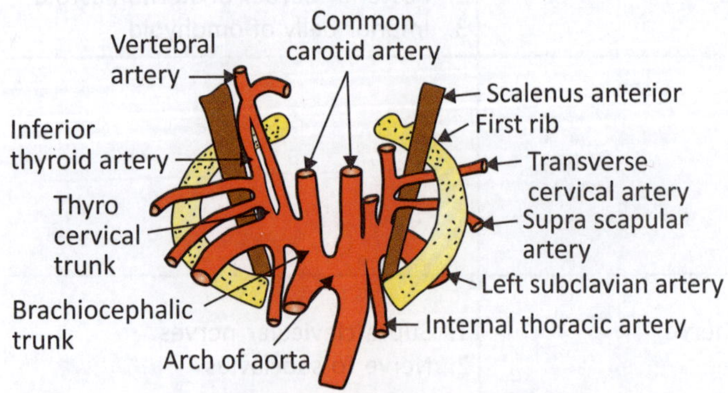

Fig. 27.12: ***Subclavian artery and its branches***

VERTEBRAL ARTERY

Branch of Ist part of subclavian artery with in the vertebral triangle.

It Supplies:

- Visual area of cerebrum
- Hind brain, cerebellum, pons and medulla
- Spinal cord
- Suboccipital muscles
- Bones and meninges.

Parts: It is divided into four parts according to its anatomical location.

Course: Passes upwards within the vertebral triangle (Ist part)

- Crosses transverse – process of C_7 vertebra.
- Enters the foramen – transversarium of C_6 vertebra.
- Passes upwards via foramen transversarium of all cervical vertebrae (IInd part).
- Passes behind the lateral mass of atlas and lies on the posterior arch of atlas (IIIrd part).
- Separated by posterior arch by dorsal rami of C_1 – suboccipital nerve.
- Passes upwards, medially and pierce the posterior atlanto-occipital membrane and enters the cranial cavity via foramen magnum.
- Within the cranial cavity artery lies anterior to the medulla oblongata, i.e., (IVth part).

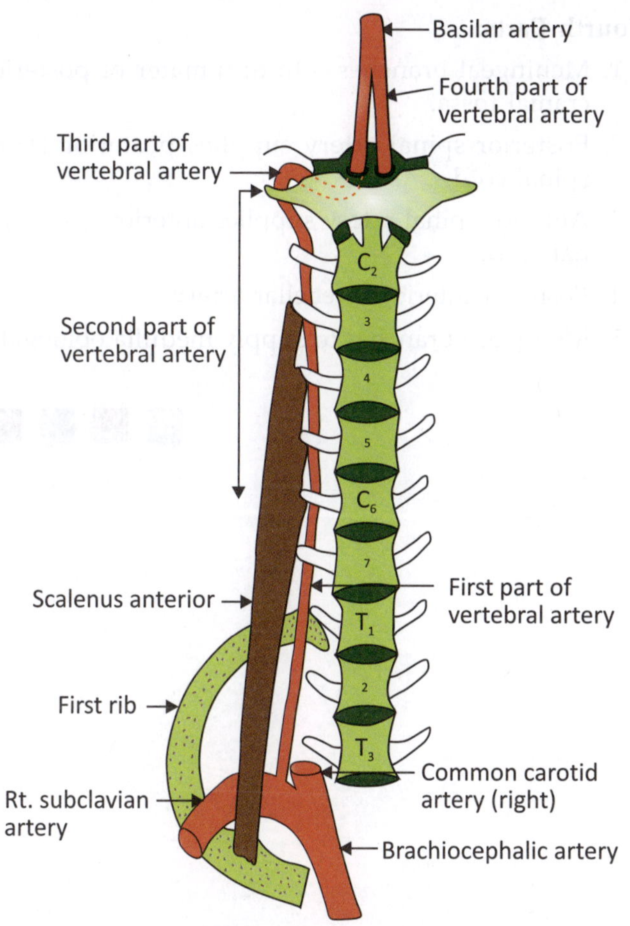

Fig. 27.13: *Vertebral artery*

Termination: At the lower border of pons vertebral artery of both sides unite to form basilar artery.

Part of Vertebral Artery

First part: Found within vertebral triangle.

Relations:

Anterior:

1. Common carotid artery
2. Vertebral vein
3. Inferior thyroid artery – lymphatic duct right side and thoracic duct on left side.

Posterior:

1. Transverse process of C_7 vertebra
2. Ventral rami of C_7 and C_8 nerves
3. Inferior cervical sympathetic ganglion.

Second part: Found within the foramen transversarium of C_1 to C_6 vertebra.

- Accompanied by vertebral vein and sympathetic plexus of nerves.
- It crosses the cervical spinal nerves anteriorly.

Third part: Found within sub-occipital triangle.

- Surrounded by plexus of veins and nerves.
- Lies on posterior arch of atlas.
- Between arch and artery lies C_1 nerve – dorsal rami (sub-occipital nerve).

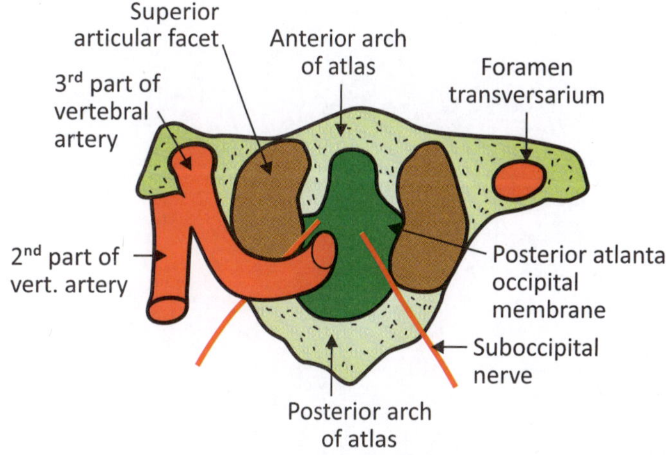

Fig. 27.14: *Third part of vertebral artery*

Fourth part: Found within the cranial cavity.

- Enters the cranium via foramen magnum.
- Lies anterior to hypoglossal nerve and medulla oblongata.
- This part of artery is present in subarachnoid space, after piercing dura and arachnoid matter in the foramen magnum.

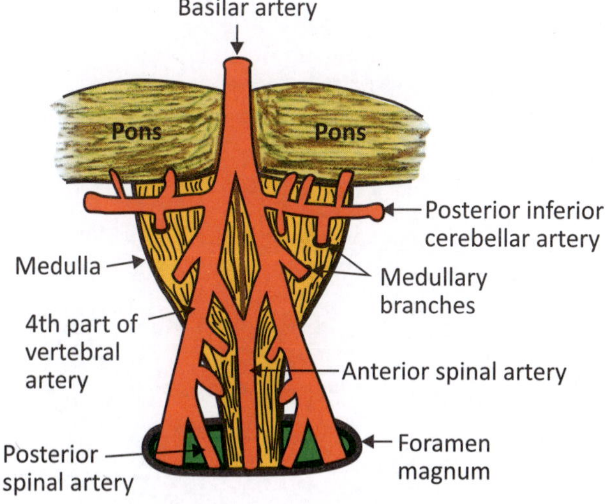

Fig. 27.15: *Fourth part of vertebral artery*

Branches of Vertebral Artery

First Part:

No branches.

Second Part:

Spinal branches to supply spinal cord, meningies and bones they enter through inter vertebral foramen.

Third Part:

Muscular branches to suboccipital muscles.

Fourth Parts:

1. Meningeal branches – to duramater of posterior cranial fossa.
2. Posterior spinal artery supplies posterior 1/3 of spinal cord.
3. Anterior spinal artery supplies anterior 2/3 of spinal cord.
4. Posterior inferior cerebellar artery.
5. Medullary branches to supply medulla oblongata.

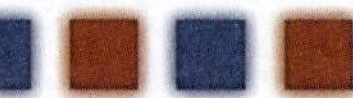

CHAPTER 28

Carotid Arteries, Internal Jugular Vein and Cervical Sympathetic Trunk

COMMON CAROTID ARTERY

- Chief artery supplying head and neck.
- There are two common carotid arteries one on right and one on left side.

Commencements:

- **Right common carotid artery:** Arises from brachiocephalic artery behind right sternoclavicular joint.
- **Left common carotid artery:** Arises from arch of aorta in the thorax behind the manubrium sterni. It crosses anterior to trachea, then left side of the trachea and reaches the neck.

Termination: Both common carotid arteries terminate at the level of upper border of thyroid cartilage which lies at intervertebral disc between C_3 and C_4 vertebra by dividing into its 2 terminal branches, i.e.,

1. External carotid artery
2. Internal carotid artery.

Terminal part of common carotid artery and beginning of internal carotid artery shows a dilatation called carotid sinus. It has a rich innervation from the glossopharyngeal and sympathetic nerves.

- It acts as a baroreceptor (pressure receptor) and regulates the Blood Pressure (B.P.).
- In carotid sinus – tunica media is thin and tunica adventia is thick and richly innervated by nerves.

CAROTID BODY

It is a small reddish brown oval structure situated just behind the bifurcation of common carotid artery.

- It receives rich nerve supply from glossopharyngeal, vagus and sympathetic nerves.
- It acts as a chemoreceptor and responds to the changes in the oxygen, carbondioxide and pH content of the blood.

Other sites of chemoreceptors are:

- Arch of aorta, right subclavian artery
- Ductus arteriosus
- All are supplied by branches of vagus nerve.

Course: In the neck both arteries have similar course.

- Each runs upwards from sternoclavicular joint to upper border of lamina of thyroid cartilage enclosed in a carotid sheath.

Carotid sheath – Encloses

- Common carotid artery and internal carotid artery
- Internal jugular vein and
- Vagus nerve (X).

Relations of Common Carotid Artery

- Lower part of the artery is deeply situated
- Upper part is superficially situated.

Superficial Relations

1. Sternocleido mastoid muscle
2. Sternohyoid
3. Sternothyroid
4. Superior belly of omohyoid.

Veins crossing the artery

1. Superior thyroid vein

2. Middle thyroid vein
3. Anterior jugular vein.

Posterior relations

1. Longus colli and capitis
2. Cervical sympathetic trunk
3. Ascending cervical artery.

Lower part of artery is posteriorly related to

1. Vertebral vessels
2. Inferior thyroid artery.

Medial Relations

1. Larynx and pharynx
2. Trachea and oesophagus
3. Inferior thyroid artery
4. Recurrent laryngeal nerve
5. Lateral lobe of thyroid gland.

Lateral relations: Internal jugular vein and vagus nerve.

BRANCHES OF COMMON CAROTID ARTERY

It gives only two terminal branches, i.e.,

1. External carotid artery
2. Internal carotid artery.

A. EXTERNAL CAROTID ARTERY

Origin: It is one of the terminal branches of common carotid artery at the upper border of lamina of thyroid cartilage.

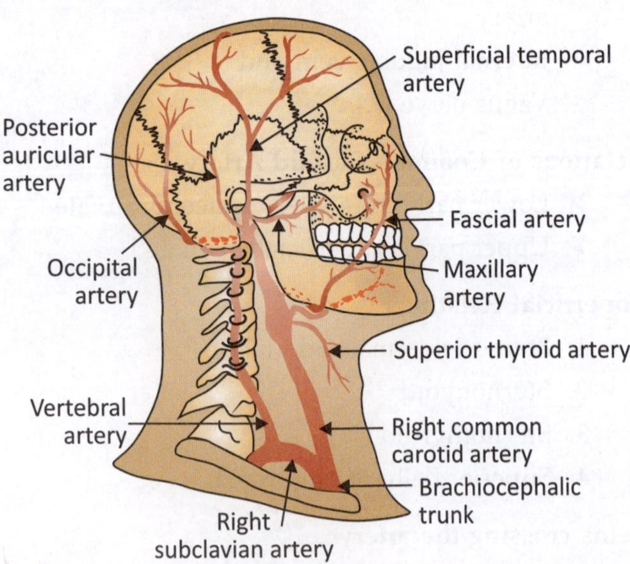

Fig. 28.1

Area of distribution: Structures present external to the skull and those in front of the neck are supplied by it.

Termination: It ends by dividing into its terminal branches behind the neck of mandible in the upper part of parotid gland.

Courses:

- External carotid artery ascends upwards in a curved manner.
- At the beginning it lies medial and anterior to the internal carotid artery.
- It crosses over it anteriorly inclining backwards to lie anterolateral to internal carotid artery.
- It then runs upwards in the deep part of parotid gland (posteromedial surface) and ends behind the neck of the mandible by dividing into its terminal branches, i.e., small superficial temporal artery and maxillary artery (larger branch).

Relations of External Carotid Artery

I. Carotid Triangle

Anterolaterally – Skin

- Superficial fascia containing platysma, cutaneous nerves and vessels.
- Investing layer of deep fascia.
- Anterior division of retro mandibular vein.
- Common facial and lingual veins.
- Hypoglossal nerve.
- Sternocleido mastoid overlaps artery.

Deep: Inferior and middle constrictors of pharynx.

- External and internal laryngeal nerves.

II. Parotid Region

Superfical: Posterior belly of digastric

- Stylohyoid muscle
- Stylo mandibular ligament
- Parotid gland
- Branches of facial nerve and retromandibular vein within the parotid gland.

Deep:

1. Structures which intervene between external and internal carotid artery.
   (a) Styloid process
   (b) Stylo glossus

(c) Stylo pharyngeus
(d) Glossopharyngeal nerve (IXth C.N.)
(e) Pharyngeal branch of vagus (Xth C.N.).

2. Internal carotid artery
3. Portion of parotid gland

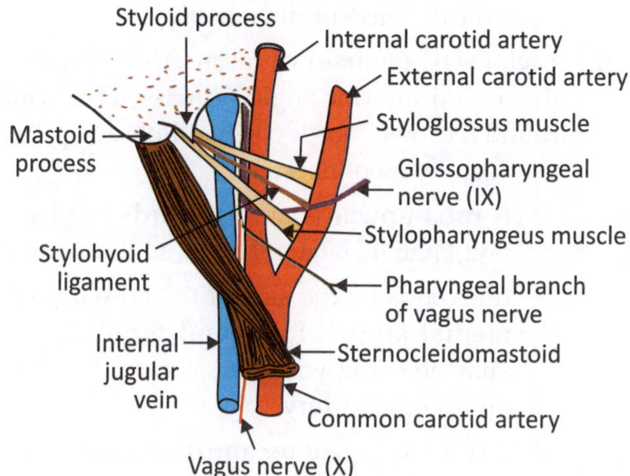

Fig. 28.2: ***Structures intervening between internal and external cartotid arteries***

Medially:

(a) Pharyngeal wall
(b) Superior laryngeal nerve.

Laterally:

(a) Internal jugular vein
(b) Vagus nerve (X).

Branches of External Carotid Artery

1. **Ascending Pharyngeal Artery:** It is a slender branch arising from medial aspect of external carotid artery near its lower end.
   - Runs vertically upwards on the sidewall of pharynx upto base of skull.
   - It gives following branches:
     (a) *Pharyngeal branches* to wall of pharynx.
     (b) *Meningeal branches:* Which traverse through jugular foramen and foramen lacerum to supply meninges of posterior and middle cranial fossa.
     (c) *Inferior tympanic branch:* Passes through inferior tympanic canaliculus situated between jugular foramen and carotid canal for supply of tympanic cavity.
     (d) *Palatine branches:* Accompany levator veli palatini muscle of palate at superior border of superior constrictor of pharynx to supply soft palate and tonsil.
2. **Superior Thyroid Artery:** Arises from anterior aspect of external carotid artery below the tip of greater cornu of hyoid bone.
   - Runs downwards and forwards parallel and superficial to external laryngeal nerve to reach the upper pole of thyroid gland.
   - Artery is close to external laryngeal nerve proximally and lies anterolateral to it. It diverges from the nerve near the thyroid gland, where artery lies superficial to upper pole of gland and nerve lies deep to it.

   Note: In thyroidectomy to avoid injury to nerve the artery should be ligated as near to the gland as possible. It's damage will lead to hoarseness of voice.

   Branches are:

   (a) *Infrahyoid branch:* Runs below hyoid bone and anastomoses with its fellow of opposite side.
   (b) *Sternocleiodmastoid branch:* To supply same muscle.
   (c) *Superior laryngeal artery:* Accompanies the internal laryngeal nerve, passes deep to thyrohyoid muscle and pierces the thyrohoid membrane to supply the larynx above vocal cords.
   (d) *Glandular branches:* To thyroid gland. Anterior branch anastomoses with its fellow of opposite side along the upper border of isthmus of gland. And posterior branch anastomoses with branches of inferior thyroid artery.
3. **Lingual Artery:** Arises from anterior aspect of external carotid artery opposite the tip of greater cornu of hyoid bone.
   - It is divided into three parts by hyoglossus muscle:
     (a) **First part:** Lies in carotid triangle and forms a characteristic loop with its convexity upwards. It is crossed superficially by hypoglossal nerve (XIIth C.N.). Loop permits free movement of the hyoid bone.
       - It gives only one branch, i.e., suprahyoid branch runs above hyoid

bone and anastomoses with its fellow of opposite side.

(b) **Second part:** Lies deep to the hyoglossus muscle runs along the upper border of hyoid bone and gives two – dorsal lingual branches – to supply dorsum of tongue and tonsil.

(c) **Third Part:** Also called arteria profunda linguae or deep lingual artery – runs upwards along the anterior border of hyoglossus muscle and then forwards on the under surface of tongue where it anastomoses with its fellow of opposite side. It gives sublingual branches to supply sublingual gland and floor of mouth.

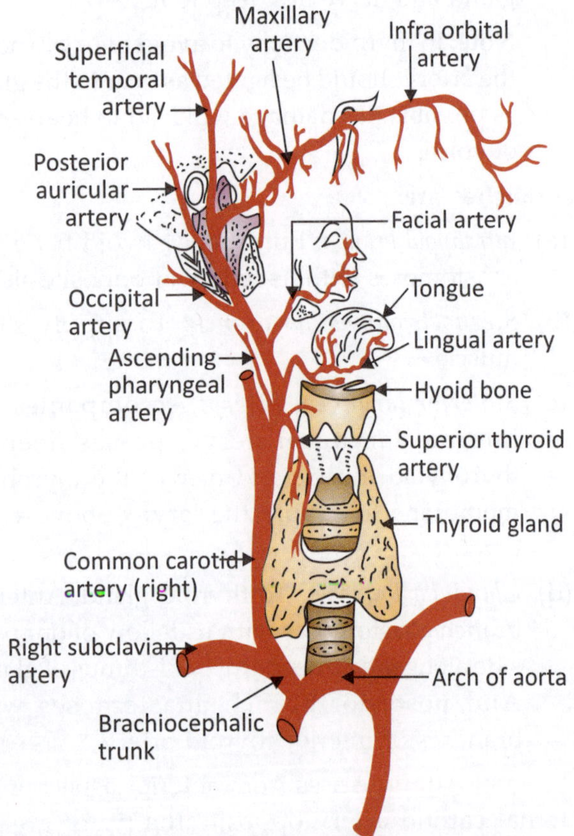

Fig. 28.3: ***External carotid artery with its branches***

4. Facial artery (external maxillary artery)

Origin: Arises from anterior aspect of external carotid artery just above the tip of the greater cornu of hyoid bone.

Termination: It terminates at the medial end of the eye as angular artery and anastomoses with the dorsal nasal artery branch of ophthalmic artery (internal carotid artery).

Course: It is divided into two parts:

(a) **Cervical part:** It ascends deep to posterior belly of digastric and stylohyoid muscles.

- Then it passes deep to ramus of mandible and grooves the posterior border of submandibular gland and then passing up over the base of the mandible.

(b) **Facial part** (course) of facial artery begins at the antero inferior angle of masseter – winds round the lower border of mandible and pierces the deep fascia of neck.

- It runs upwards and forwards to reach a point half inch lateral to the angle of mouth.
- It ascends by the side of the nose upto the medial angle of eye and terminates by anastomosing with dorsal nasal branch of ophthalmic artery.
- Artery is tortuous and this allows it to move easily over facial muscles as they contract.

Important Relations of Facial Artery:

I. In the Neck

Anterior: Posterior belly of digastric and

- Stylohyoid muscle
- Lower part of ramus of mandible.

Posterior: Stylopharyngeus

- Middle and superior constrictor of pharynx.

II. In the Face: Facial vein lies above and behind the artery.

Anterior: Branches of facial nerve

- Facial vein
- Zygomaticus major and minor muscles
- Skin and superficial fascia.

Posterior: Mandible in lower part

- Buccinator muscle
- Levator anguli oris muscle.

Branches of Facial Artery:

I. From Cervical Part

(a) **Ascending palatine artery:** Arises near origin of facial artery ascends up to accompany levator palati – passes over upper border of superior constrictor and supplies soft palate.

(b) **Tonsillar artery:** Is the main artery of the tonsil.
- Pierces superior constrictor and ends in tonsil.

(c) **Glandular branches:** To supply submandibular gland.

(d) **Submental artery:** Runs forwards on mylohyoid muscle alongwith mylohyoid nerve and supplies it, submandibular and sublingual salivary glands.

II. From the Facial Part

(a) **Inferior labial artery:** Supplies lower lip.

(b) **Superior labial artery:** Supplies upper lip.

(c) **Lateral nasal artery:** Supplies ala and dorsum of nose.

(d) **Angular artery:** Terminal part of artery at medial canthus of eye anastomoses with branches of ophthalmic artery.

(e) **Small unnamed branches:** Arise from posterior aspect of facial artery and supplies muscles, fascia and skin of face.

5. Occipital Artery

- Arises from posterior aspect of external carotid artery at the same level as facial artery.
- Runs backwards and upwards under cover of posterior belly of digastric crossing internal carotid artery, internal jugular vein and last four cranial nerves.
- It runs deep to mastoid process by making a groove medial to mastoid notch.
- Crosses apex of suboccipital triangle to reach under trapezius muscle, pierces the muscle 2.5 cm away from midline and comes to lie just lateral to the greater occipital nerve.
- Supplies most of the back of scalp.

Branches:

- Sternomastoid branches – two
- Mastoid artery
- Meningeal branches – passes through jugular foramen
- Muscular branches
- Auricular branch
- Descending branches
- Occipital branches.

Important Points

- Hypoglossal nerve hooks under the origin of occipital artery.
- Occipital arteries cross the apex of posterior triangle of neck.
- Sternocleidomastoid branch – Upper one accompanies XIIth C.N.
  - Lower one crosses XIIth C.N.

6. Posterior Auricular Artery

- Arises from posterior aspect of external carotid artery a little above occipital artery.
- It crosses superficial to stylohyoid muscle.
- Runs upwards and backwards parallel to occipital artery under cover of upper border of posterior belly of digastric deep to parotid gland.
- Becomes superficial and lies on the base of mastoid process behind the auricle which it supplies.

Branches:

- Stylomastoid artery – enters the stylomastoid foramen and supply facial nerve and middle ear.
- Auricular branch – for auricles.
- Occipital branch – for occipital area of scalp.

7. Superficial Temporal Artery

- Is a small terminal branch of external carotid artery.
- Begins behind the neck of the mandible deep to upper part of parotid gland.
- Runs vertically upwards crossing the root of zygoma. (Pulsations of the artery can be felt on zygoma.)
- About 5 cm above the zygoma it divides into anterior and posterior branches, which supply temple and scalp.

Branches:

- Transverse facial artery – runs forward below the zygomatic arch and supplies.
- Middle temporal artery – runs on temporal fossa and supplies temporalis muscle and fascia.
- Anterior and posterior terminal branches.

8. Maxillary Artery (Internal Maxillary Artery): It is the larger terminal branch of external carotid artery.

Courses:

- Begins behind the neck of mandible.
- Runs horizontally forwards deep to neck of mandible upto lower border of lower head of lateral pterygoid.
- From here it turns upwards, forwards and crosses the lower head of lateral pterygoid superficially (sometimes deep).
- After emerging between two heads, it enters the pterygo – palatine fossa by passing through the pterygo-maxillary fissure.
- Here it ends by giving its terminal branches.

Parts: Maxillary artery is divided into three parts by lower head of lateral pterygoid –

(i) First part or mandibular part

- From its origin to lower border of lateral pterygoid.
- Lies between neck of mandible laterally and sphenomandibular ligament medially.
- Auriculo temporal nerve – lies above this part.

(ii) Pterygoid part: From lower border to upper border of lower head of lateral pterygoid.

(iii) Third part or pterygo-palatine part: Lies in pterygo-palatine fossa – From upper border of lower head of lateral pterygoid, here it lies in front of pterygo palatine ganglion.

Branches of Maxillary Artery:

Ist part:

1. Deep auricular artery
2. Anterior tympanic artery
3. Middle meningeal artery
4. Accessory meningeal artery
5. Inferior alveolar artery.

IInd part:

1. Two deep temporal arteries
2. Pterygoid branches to muscles
3. Masseteric artery
4. Buccal artery.

IIIrd part:

1. Posterior superior alveolar artery
2. Infra orbital artery
3. Greater palatine artery
4. Pharyngeal artery
5. Artery of pterygoid canal
6. Spheno palatine artery.

B. INTERNAL CAROTID ARTERY

- It is the upward continuation of the common carotid artery, lies in the carotid sheath.
- It supplies structures lying within the skull and in the orbit.

Origin: It begins at the upper border of the lamina of thyroid cartilage (Disc between C_3 and C_4) and runs upwards to reach the base of skull, where it enters the carotid canal in the petrous part of temporal bone.

Termination: It enters the cranial cavity by passing through the upper part of the foramen lacerum.

In the cranial cavity it enters the cavernous – sinus and finally ends below the anterior perforated substance of the brain by dividing into the anterior cerebral and middle cerebral arteries.

Structures Passing between External and Internal Carotid Artery

1. Stylopharyngeus muscle
2. Glossopharyngeal nerve
3. Pharyngeal branch of vagus nerve
4. Styloid process
5. Deep part of parotid gland.

Course and Branches of Internal Carotid Artery

It is divided into four parts:

I. Cervical Part:

1. From its origin it ascends vertically upwards and lies infront of transverse process of upper cervical vertebrae.
2. Enclosed in the carotid sheath alongwith internal jugular vein and vagus nerve.
3. In the lower part it lies in carotid triangle.
4. Upper part is deeply located and lies deep to posterior belly of digastric, styloid process with the structures attached to it and the parotid gland.
5. At the upper end internal jugular vein lies posterior to internal carotid artery.

6. Last four cranial nerves (IXth, Xth, XIth and XIIth) lie between the internal jugular vein and internal carotid artery at the base of skull.

Branches: It gives no branches in the neck.

II. Petrous Part

1. Internal carotid artery enters the petrous part of temporal bone in the carotid canal.
2. It first runs upwards and then turns forwards and medially at a right angle.
3. It emerges in the posterior wall of foramen lacerum and passes through its upper part to enter the cranial cavity.

Branches from petrous part of internal carotid artery:

(a) Carotico tympanic branch to middle ear.

(b) Pterygoid branch – a small and inconstant branch that enters the pterygoid canal.

III. Cavernous Part:

- From the foramen lacerum the internal carotid artery ascends and enters the cavernous sinus.
- In the sinus it passes forwards along the side of sella trucica in the floor and medial wall of the sinus. It lies outside the endothelial lining of the sinus and is related to abducent nerve infero laterally.

  In the anterior part of the sinus, the artery ascends up and pierces the dural roof of the sinus between the anterior and posterior clinoid processes to reach the under surface of the cerebrum.

Branches:

(a) Carvenous branch to trigeminal ganglion.

(b) Superior and inferior hypophyseal arteries to the hypophysis cerebri or pituitary gland.

IV. Cerebral Part of Internal Carotid Artery

- After emerging from the roof of cavernous sinus artery turns backwards in the subarchnoid space along the roof of the cavernous sinus and lies below the optic nerve.
- Finally it turns upwards by side of the optic chiasma and reaches the anterior perforated substance of the brain.
- Here it ends by dividing into anterior and middle cerebral arteries.

Branches:

(a) Ophthalmic artery

(b) Anterior choroidal artery

(c) Posterior communicating artery

(d) Anterior cerebral artery

(e) Middle cerebral artery.

INTERNAL JUGULAR VEIN

- It is main venous channel of head and neck.
- Receives blood from brain, face and neck.

Extent: Begins at the base of skull in the jugular foramen as a direct continuation of the sigmoid sinus.

- It ends behind the sternal end of clavicle by joining the subclavian vein to form the brachiocephalic vein.
- The vein has two dilatations – one at its upper end – called superior bulb – lies in jugular fossa and related to floor of middle ear.
- Other at its termination called inferior bulb, it is present in the lesser supraclavicular fossa between sternal and clavicular heads of sterno cleidomastoid. Inferior bulb has bicuspid valve.

Course: The vein passes vertically down from its origin within the carotid sheath.

- It lies lateral to internal carotid artery above and to the common carotid artery below.
- Deep cervical lymph nodes are closely related to the vein.

Relations:

(a) **Antero laterally:** Skin, fascia, sternocleidomastoid muscle and parotid gland.

  - Lower part is covered by infrahyoid muscles, i.e., sternohyoid, sternothyroid and omohyoid covered with sternocleido mastoid.
  - Upper part is crossed by stylohyoid, stylopharyngeus, styloid process, posterior belly of digastric, sternomastoid branch of occipital and superior thyroid artery, inferior limb of ansa cervicalis, spinal root of accessory nerve.
  - Deep cervical lymph nodes.

(b) **Posteriorly:**

  - Transverse process of Ist cervical vertebra
  - Levator scapulae

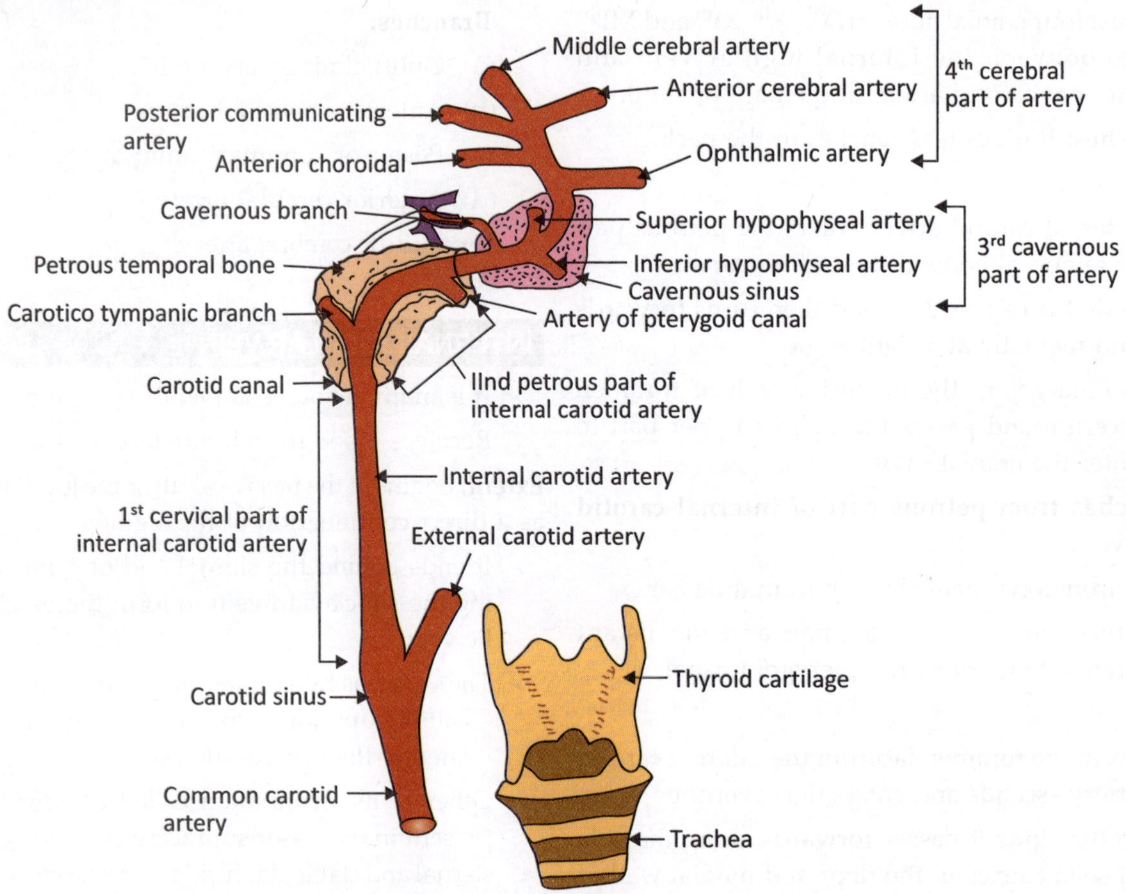

Fig. 28.4: ***Internal carotid artery and its branches***

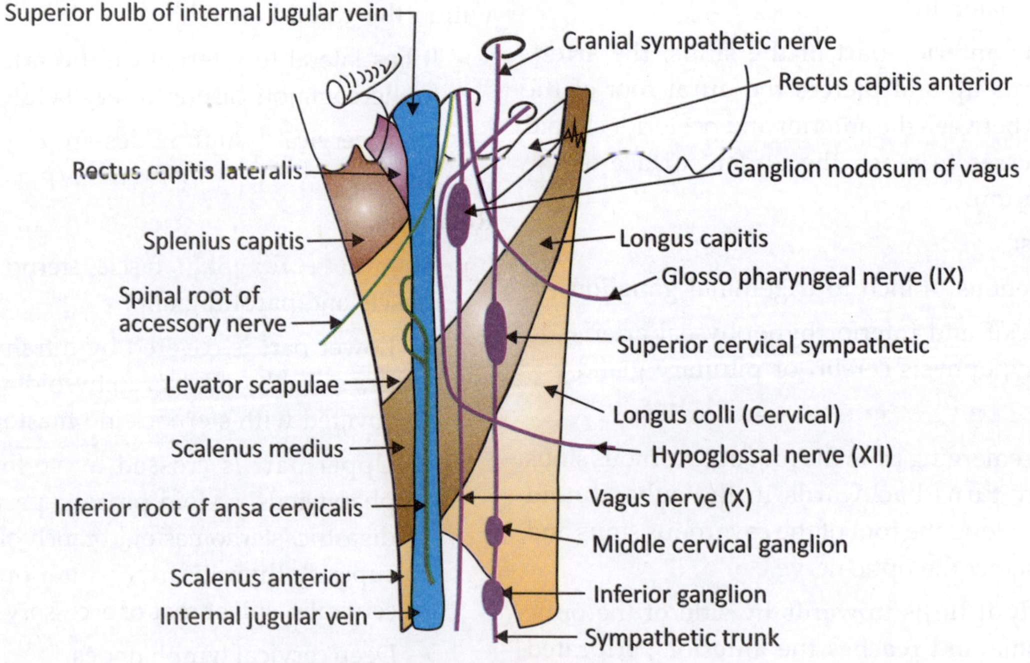

Fig. 28.5: ***Relations of internal jugular vein***

- Scalenus medius and anterior muscle
- Cervical plexus of nerves
- Phrenic nerve (C_3, C_4 and C_5)
- Thyro cervical trunk
- Ist part of subclavian artery
- Vertebral vessels
- Thoracic duct on left side and right lymphatic duct on right side.

(c) **Medial:**

- Internal carotid artery
- Common carotid artery
- Vagus nerve (Xth C.N.)

TRIBUTARIES OF INTERNAL JUGULAR VEIN

1. **Inferior petrosal sinus:** Connects cavernous sinus with superior bulb of internal jugular vein.
2. **Pharyngeal veins:** From pharyngeal venous plexus.
3. **Common facial vein:** Formed by union of facial vein and anterior division of retromandibular vein. It drains face, scalp and infra temporal fossa.
4. **Lingual vein:** Formed by union of venae commitance hypoglossi and venae commitance – linguae – drains tongue.
5. **Superior thyroid vein:** Drains upper part of thyroid gland.
6. **Middle thyroid vein:** From middle part of gland. It is a short vein passing infront of carotid sheath.
7. **Occipital vein:** Drains occipital area.
   - Thoracic duct opens at jugulo subclavian angle on left side.
   - Right lymphatic duct opens at right jugulo subclavian angle.
   - In the upper part of neck internal jugular vein communicates with the external jugular vein by the oblique jugular vein.

Applied Anatomy of Internal Jugular Vein

1. It acts as a guide for surgeons during removal of deep cervical lymph nodes (Block dissection of neck in cases of oral malignancies).
2. **In congestive heart failure:** Internal jugular vein is dilated and engorged due to increase venous pressure.
3. Central venous catheterization is done through lower part of internal jugular vein in lesser supraclavicular fossa in cases of cardiovascular collapse.

CERVICAL SYMPATHETIC TRUNK

Extent: From base of skull to the neck of first rib.

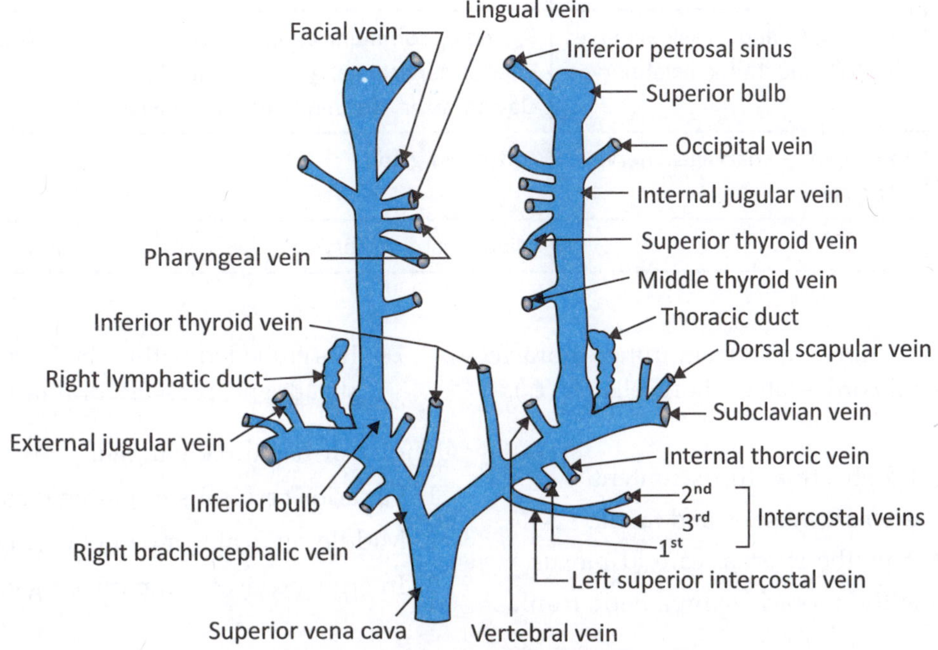

Fig. 28.6: ***Tributaries of internal jugular vein***

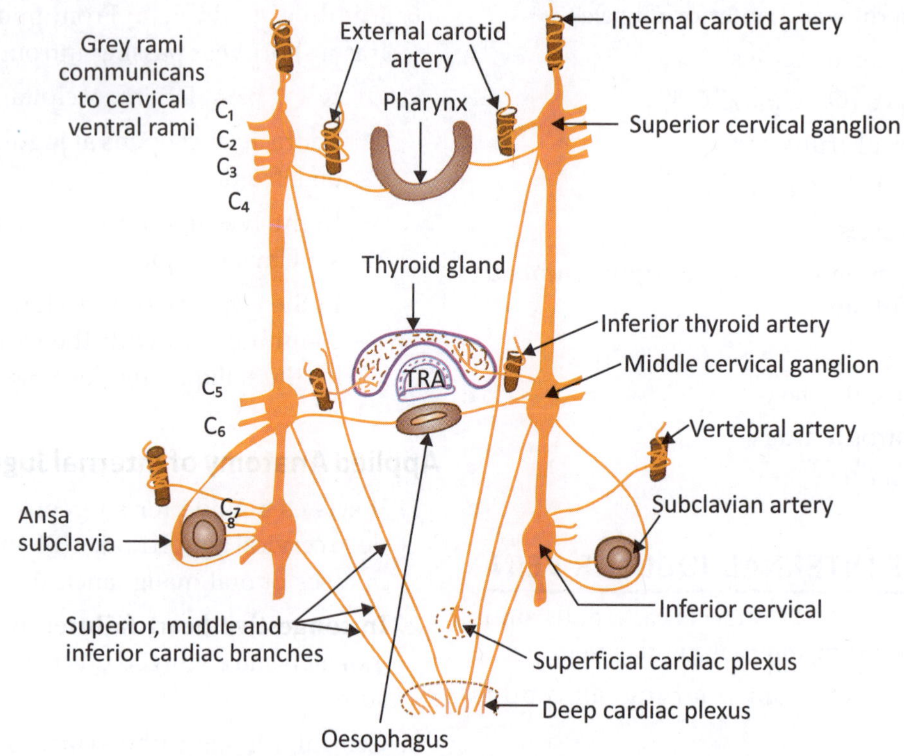

Fig. 28.7: *Cervical sympathetic trunk*

Table 28.1: *Cervical Sympathetic Trunk Branches*

Branches	Superior cervical ganglion	Middle ganglion	Inferior cervical ganglion
Arterial branches	To – Internal carotid artery – External carotid artery – Common carotid artery	Inferior thyroid artery	– Subclavian artery – Vertebral artery
Communicating branches	To C_1, C_2, C_3 and C_4 spinal nerves 9th, 10th and 11th cranial nerves	C_5 and C_6 communicating branch to inferior cervical ganglion infront of sub-clavian artery forming ansa subclavian	C_7 and C_8
Visceral branches	To Pharynx – Pharyngeal nerve – Larynx	To thyroid gland	
Cardiac branches		Middle cardiac nerve	Inferior cardiac nerve

- Preganglionic fibres arise from upper thoracic part of spinal cord – lateral horncells (T_1-T_5).

Relations:

Anterior: Carotid sheath with its content.

Posterior: Prevertebral muscles and fascia.

Superiorly: It joins the internal carotid plexus.

Inferiorly: Joins the thoracic sympathetic trunk.

- It is embeded within the fascia between carotid sheath and pre-vertebral fascia.

Ganglia: It has three ganglia:

1. Superior cervical sympathetic ganglion
2. Middle cervical sympathetic ganglion
3. Inferior cervical sympathetic ganglion.

1. **Superior cervical sympathetic ganglion**
   - Largest ganglion.
   - Situated below base of skull anterior to transverse process of C_2 and C_3 vertebra.
2. **Middle cervical sympathetic ganglion**
   - Small ganglion
   - Lies at the level of C_6 vertebra.
   - Related to loop of inferior thyroid artery.
3. **Inferior cervical sympathetic ganglion**
   - Larger than middle ganglion.
   - Lies in the interval between neck of 1st rib and transverse process of C_7 vertebra, may be fused with T_1 ganglion and forms stellate ganglion.
   - Crossed anteriorly by vertebral artery.

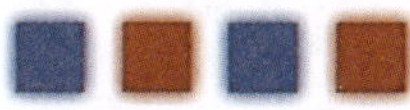

CHAPTER 29

Thyroid Gland

INTRODUCTION

- This is a large endocrine gland.
- Situated in front of the lower part of the neck and overlies 2-4th tracheal cartilages.
- Its functions are controlled by the thyroid-stimulating hormone from the anterior (adeno) hypophysis.

Developments:

- It develops from endodermal epithelial proliferation of median thyroid diverticulum.
- The "C" cells of the gland are developed from the fourth branchial pouch.

Situation:

Lower part of front of neck. The gland is situated in front of C_5, C_6, C_7 and T_1 vertebrae.

Part:

The gland has a pair of lobes united by an isthmus in the median plane.

Size:

Each lateral lobe has approximate dimensions as follows:

- **Length:** 5 to 6 cm
- **Width:** 3 cm
- **Thickness:** 2.5 cm.

Isthmus:

- Vertical length is 1.25 cm
- Transversely – 1.25 cm.
- **Weight:** About 25 to 30 gms.

LATERAL LOBE OF THYROID

(a) Apex or upper pole is pointed and extends superiorly up to the oblique line of thyroid cartilage.

(b) Lower pole is blunt and rounded, extends inferiorly up to 6th tracheal ring. Lower pole on left side is related to thoracic duct.

Borders:

(a) Anterior border is sharp and related to anterior branch of superior thyroid artery.

(b) Posterior border is blunt and rounded and is related to posterior branch of superior thyroid artery and ascending branch of inferior thyroid artery which anastomose with each other.

- It is also related to parathyroid glands.

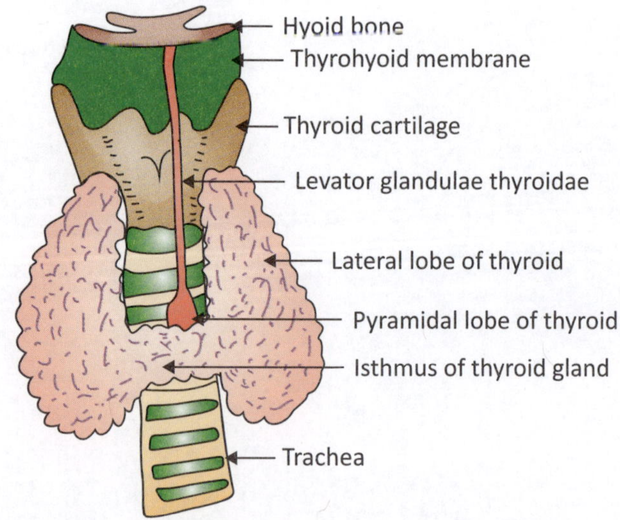

Fig. 29.1: ***Location of thyroid gland-front view***

Surfaces are:

1. Antero lateral or superficial surface

2. Postero lateral surface
3. Medial surface.

RELATIONS OF SUPERFICIAL SURFACE

This is related to:

1. Skin.
2. Superficial fascia containing platysma and cutaneous nerves and blood vessels.
3. Investing layer of deep cervical fascia (see Fig. 14.2)
4. Sternohyoid muscle.
5. Sternothyroid muscle.
6. Omohyoid muscle.
7. Sternocleido mastoid muscle.

Superiorly the lobe is limited by "insertion of sternothyroid muscle".

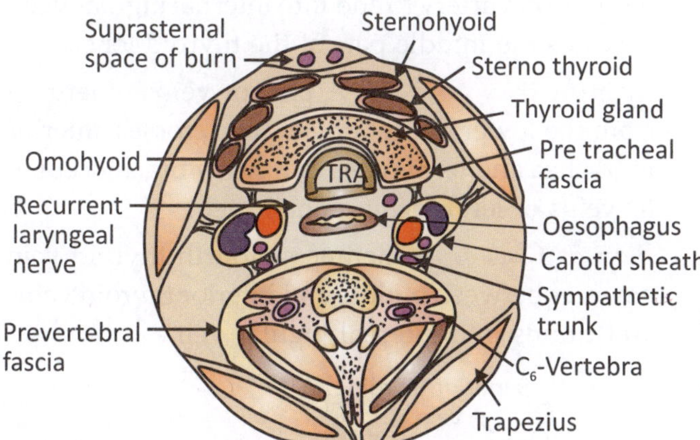

Fig. 29.2: *T.S. of neck at C6 level (Relations of thyroid gland)*

Medial Relations of Thyroid Lobe

1. **Two viscera:**
   (a) Larynx and trachea
   (b) Pharynx and oesophagus.
2. **Two muscles:**
   (a) Cricothyroid muscle
   (b) Inferior constrictor of pharynx.
3. **Two nerve:**
   (a) External laryngeal nerve (X)
   (b) Recurrent laryngeal nerve (X).
4. **Two cartilages:**
   (a) Thyroid cartilage
   (b) Cricoid cartilage.

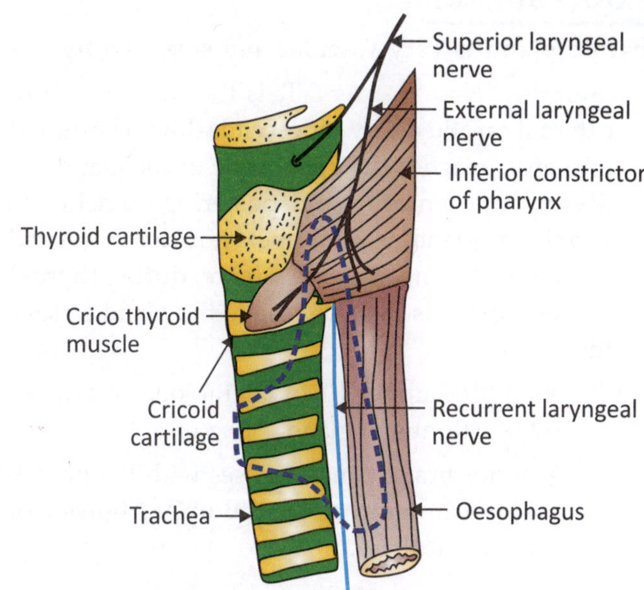

Fig. 29.3: *Medial relations of thyroid gland*

Postero Lateral Relations of Thyroid Lobe

1. **Carotid sheath and its contents:**
   - Common carotid artery
   - Internal jugular vein
   - Vagus nerve (X).
2. **Cervical sympathetic trunk with its middle ganglion.**

Isthmus: It crosses 2nd, 3rd and 4th tracheal rings.

- Upper border shows pyramidal lobe and related to anastomosis between superior thyroid arteries.
- Lower border is related to inferior thyroid vein.
- Levator glandulae thyroidea connects pyramidal lobe to hyoid bone.

CAPSULE OF THYROID GLAND

It has two capsules:

1. **False capsule:** It is formed by pretracheal fascia and is weakest posteriorly.
   - Pretracheal fascia thickens posteriorly and is attached to cricoid cartilage. This thickened band is called suspensory ligament of Berry.
2. **True capsule:** It is formed by condensation of fascia around the gland. A plexus of veins lies deep to the true capsule. Therefore, during thyroidectomy the gland is removed with its capsule to prevent bleeding.

BLOOD SUPPLY

Thyroid gland is very vascular and supplied by:

1. **Superior thyroid artery:** It is the first branch of external carotid artery. It descends downwards and forwards, reaches the upper pole of the gland – it divides into anterior and posterior branches to supply the gland near the apex. It is closely related to external laryngeal nerve. Hence, during thyroid surgery artery is ligated close to the gland to save the nerve.
   - It supplies upper 1/3 of lateral lobe and upper 1/2 of isthmus of gland.
   - Anterior branch anastomoses with the branch of opposite side along the upper border of isthmus of gland.

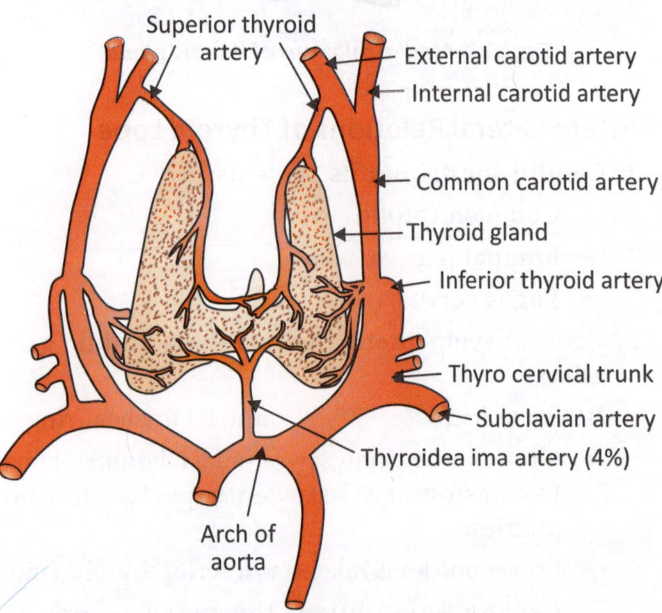

Fig. 29.4: ***Arterial supply of thyroid gland***

2. **Inferior thyroid artery:** It is a branch of thyrocervical trunk of subclavian artery. It passes deep to carotid sheath and middle cervical sympathetic ganglion, in front of vertebral vessels and reaches the posterior surface of the gland. It is accompanied by recurrent laryngeal nerve near the gland. It divides into 4 or 5 branches and supply lower 2/3 of the lateral lobe and lower half of isthmus of the gland. One branch ascends upwards along posterior border and anastomoses with the posterior branch of superior thyroid artery at the junction of upper 1/3 with lower 2/3 of the posterior border. During surgery on thyroid this artery is ligated away from the gland to save recurrent – laryngeal nerve.
3. **Thyroidea ima artery:** It is present only in 3% of individuals and is a branch from arch of aorta or brachiocephalic trunk. It runs upwards in the midline of neck to the isthmus of the gland.
4. **Accessory arteries:** Oesophageal and tracheal arteries also supply thyroid gland.

VENOUS DRAINAGE

Veins do not follow arteries:

1. **Superior thyroid vein:** Drains upper part of thyroid lobe, crosses anterior to common carotid and drains into internal jugular vein.
2. **Middle thyroid vein:** Also crosses anterior to common carotid artery to end into internal jugular vein. It drains the middle part of the thyroid lobe.
3. **Inferior thyroid vein:** A pair of veins emerging from the lower border of isthmus, crosses anterior to trachea and terminates into either brachiocephalic veins or left brachiocephalic vein.
4. **Vein of Kocker:** Sometimes a fourth thyroid vein emerges between middle and inferior thyroid veins and drains into internal jugular vein.

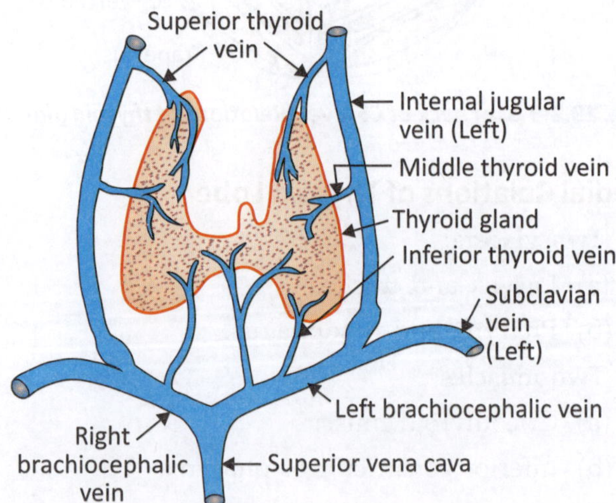

Fig. 29.5: ***Venous drainage of thyroid gland***

Lymphatic drainage into:

1. Pre-laryngeal lymph nodes
2. Pre-tracheal lymph nodes

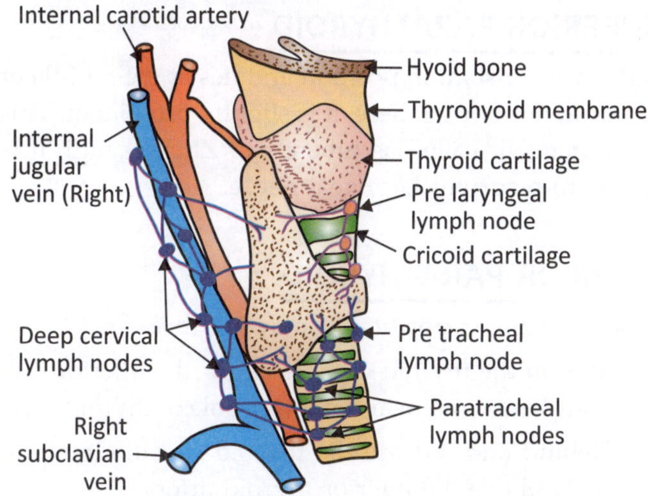

Fig. 29.6: *Lymphatic drainage of thyroid*

3. Deep cervical lymph nodes
4. Recurrent chain of lymph nodes along recurrent laryngeal nerve (para tracheal group).

NERVE SUPPLY OF THYROID GLAND

Sympathetic supply: Vasomotor in function.

- Post ganglionic fibres from the superior, middle and inferior cervical sympathetic ganglia. These fibres form plexus around the thyroid arteries.

Parasympathetic supply: Vagus and recurrent laryngeal nerves.

- The secretary functions of the gland is controlled by the T.S.H. of the anterior pituitary.

ACCESSORY THYROID (ECTOPIC THYROID TISSUE)

1. **Lingual thyroid:** Presence of thyroid tissue around the foramen caecum of the tongue.
2. Suprahyoid ectopic thyroid
3. Infrahyoid actopic thyroid
4. Mediastinal thyroid

Ectopic thyroid tissue is found along the course taken by the thyroglossal duct.

SECRETIONS OF THE GLAND

It secretes:

1. Thyroxin (T_4) or Tetraiodothyronine.
2. Tri-iodo thyronine (T_3).

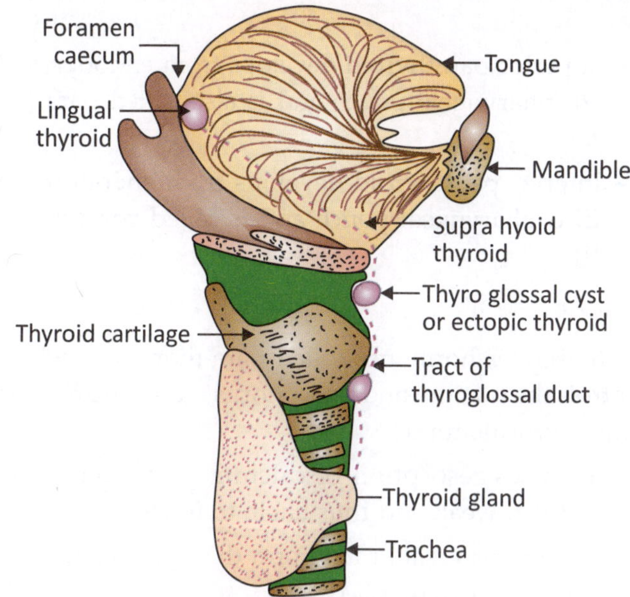

Fig. 29.7: *Descent of thyroid and sites of ectopic thyroid tissue*

- Required for normal growth and development of body and maintain B.M.R. of body. (Both psychic and somatic growth.)

3. Thyrocalcitonin – secreted by the para follicular cells ("C" cells) – helps in deposition of calcium on bones – calcium metabolism.

PARATHYROID GLANDS

- Usually 2 to 6 in number.
- Essential for life.
- Two pairs – superior and inferior parathyroid glands.
- It is a small endocrine gland.
- Lies on the posterior border of the thyroid gland within the false capsule.

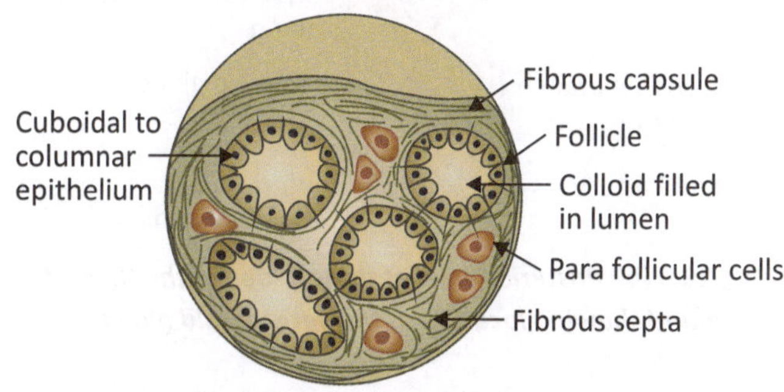

Fig. 29.8: *Microscopic structure of thyroid gland*

Developments:

- Superior parathyroid develops from endoderm of 4th pharyngeal pouch and is also called parathyroid IV.
- Inferior parathyroid develops from endoderm of IIIrd pharyngeal pouch and is called parathyroid III.

Secretion:

It secretes hormones called para-thormone, which controls the calcium and phosphorus metabolism along with thyrocalcitonin.

It causes resorption of calcium from bones and makes them weak and thus liable to fracture.

- **Shape:** Oval or lentiform (half pea shaped)
- **Size:** Approximate size
- **Length:** 6 mm
- **Width:** 3 – 4 mm
- **Thickness:** 2 mm
- **Weight:** About 50 mgm

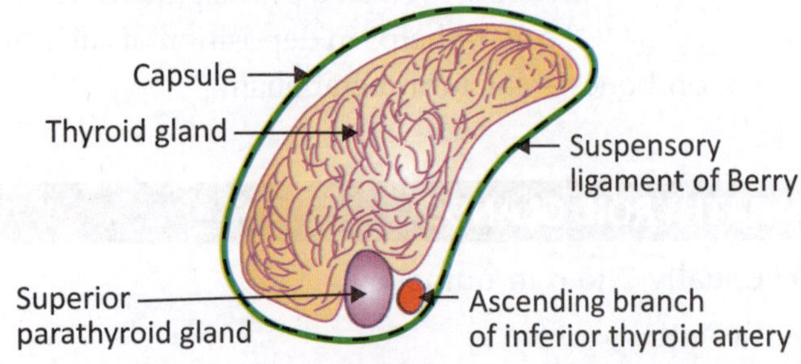

Fig. 29.9 (i): *T.S. of left lobe of thyroid gland*

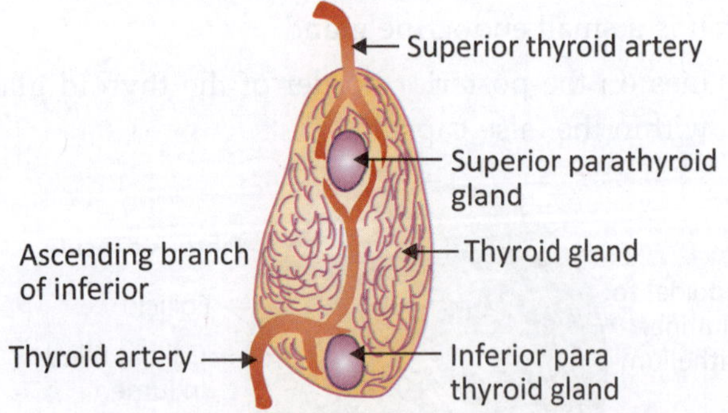

Fig. 29.9 (ii): *Posterior view of the left lobe of the thyroid gland showing location of the parathyroid glands*

SUPERIOR PARATHYROID

It is more constant in position and lies at the middle of the posterior border, here, it is slightly prominent. This prominence is called as tubercle of Zuckerkandl. It is dorsal to recurrent laryngeal nerve.

INFERIOR PARATHYROID

More variable in position. It may lie:

1. Within the thyroid capsule below the inferior thyroid artery and near the lower pole of thyroid lobe.
2. Behind and outside the thyroid capsule immediately above the inferior thyroid artery.
3. Within the substance of the thyroid lobe and ventral to recurrent laryngeal nerve.

Blood Supply:

Receives rich blood supply from inferior thyroid artery and from anastomosis between superior and inferior thyroid arteries.

Veins and lymphatics of the gland are associated with those of thyroid gland, i.e., inferior thyroid and middle thyroid vein.

- Pre and paratracheal group of lymph nodes.

Nerve Supply:

Vasomotor nerves are derived from middle and superior cervical sympathetic ganglion.

Parathyroid Activity:

It is controlled by blood calcium levels – low levels – stimulate and high level inhibit the activity of the gland.

Applied Anatomy

1. **Tumours of parathyroid glands** – lead to excessive secretion of parathermone – cause increased removal of calcium from bones making them weak and liable to fracture.
   - Hypercalcaemia and increased urinary excretion of calcium salts lead to formation of stones in urinary tract.

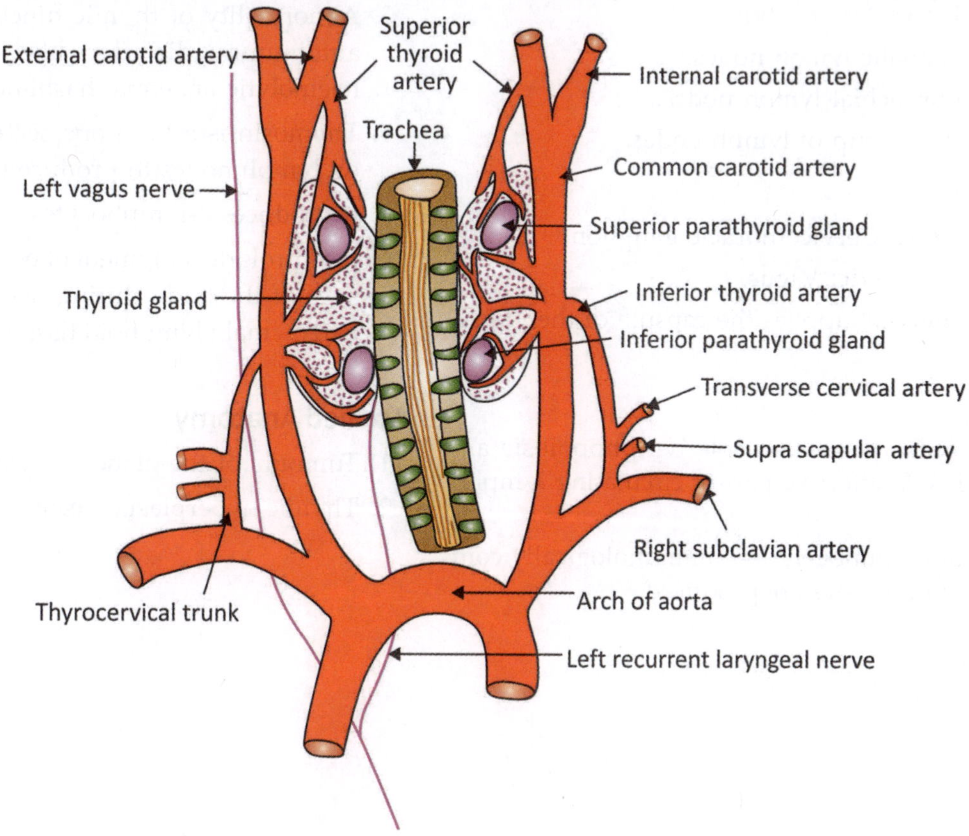

Fig. 29.10: ***Parathyroids and thyroid gland with its arterial supply***

2. Hypoparathyroidism – may occur spontaneously or from accidental removal of glands during – thyroidectomy – results in hypocalcaemia leading to increased neuromuscular irritability causing muscular spasm and convulsions (Tetany).

THYMUS GLAND

- It is an important lymphatic structure and essential for immunity of the body.
- This is well developed at birth, continues to grow upto puberty, thereafter atrophy and replaced by fat.

Development: It develops from the endoderm of the third pharyngeal pouch.

Situation: Superior mediastinum and upper part of anterior mediastinum, extending above into the lower part of the neck.

Colour: Pinkish grey.

Weight: At the time of birth – 10 to 13 gms.

- Greatest development during first two years of life.
- **At puberty:** 35 to 40 gms.
- Adult – It regresses after puberty and gets atrophied in the adult. It weighs only less than 10 gms.

Parts:

- A pair of lobes united by connective tissue.
- Cervical part of the thymus is usually rudi-mentary.
- Upper end of each lobe extends upto the thyroid gland and lower end extends upto the 4th costal cartilage. It lies anterior to great vessels, pericardium and trachea.

Blood Supply:

Anterial Supply:

1. Internal thoracic artery.
2. Inferior thyroid artery.

Venous Drainage:

1. Left brachiocephalic vein.
2. Inferior thyroid vein.
3. Internal thoracic vein.

Lymphatic Drainage of Thymus:

1. Brachiocephalic lymph nodes.
2. Tracheo bronchial lymph nodes.
3. Parasternal group of lymph nodes.

Nerve Supply:

Sympathetic: Cervicothoracic ganglion.

Para sympathetic: Vagus.

Phrenic nerve: Supplies the capsule of the gland.

Functions

1. Lymphoid organ – controls lymphopoiesis and maintains an effective part of circulating lymphocytes.
2. Organ of immunogenesis – immunologically competent lymphocytes are produced.
3. Abnormality of thymic functions may produce – autoimmune disorders like – myasthenia gravis, haemolytic anaemia, hashimotos thyroiditis.
4. Thymosin is a hormone secreted by gland – acts on lymph nodes to produce lymphocytes.
5. It produces T-lymphocytes.
6. It controls development of peripheral lymphoid tissues of the body during neonatal period. By puberty – main lymphoid tissues are fully developed.

Applied Anatomy

1. Tumours of the gland – thymoma.
2. Thymic hyperplasia – causes myasthenia gravis.

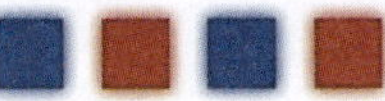

CHAPTER 30

The Pharynx

INTRODUCTION

- The pharynx is a musculo membranous tube.
- It is a common chamber for digestive and respiratory system.

Situation:

It is situated posterior to nose, mouth and larynx, but anterior to upper six cervical vertebrae.

Length: About 12 to 14 cm.

Transverse Diameter

- In the upper part about 3.5 cm.
- In the lower part about 1.5 cm.

The pharyngo oesophageal junction is the narrowest part of the alimentary system next to the vermiform appendix.

Parts of the Pharynx

1. Naso pharynx
2. Oro pharynx
3. Laryngo pharynx

Relations

- **Superiorly:** Base of skull.
- **Inferiorly:** At the level of lower border of C_6 vertebra it becomes oesophagus.
- **Anteriorly:** Nose, mouth and larynx.
- **Posteriorly:** Upper six cervical vertebrae.
- Prevertebral muscles and fascia.

Communications

(a) **Laterally:** It communicates with middle ear cavity via pharyngo tympanic tube.

(b) **Anteriorly:** Communicates with cavity of nose, mouth and larynx.

(c) **Inferiorly:** It communicates with oesophagus.

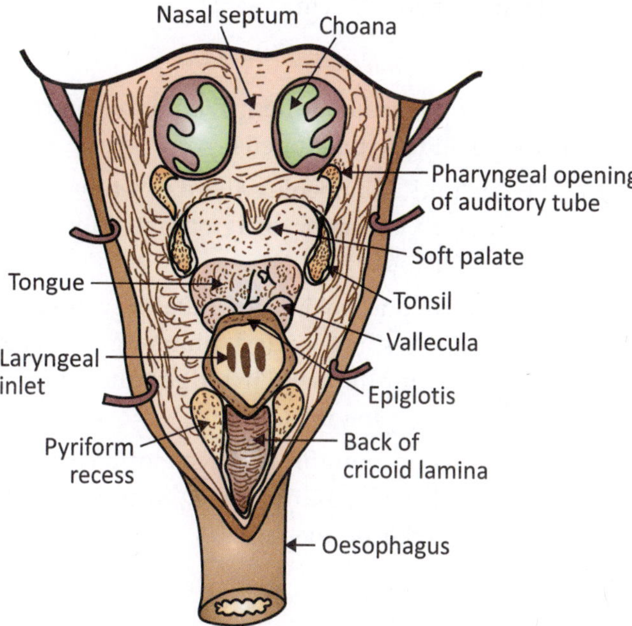

Fig. 30.1: *Anterior wall of pharynx*

Attachments of the Pharynx

From above downwards it is attached to:

1. Medial pterygoid plate.
2. Pterygo mandibular raphe.
3. Mandible.

4. Mucous membrane of the side of tongue.
5. Hyoid bone.
6. Thyroid cartilage.
7. Cricoid cartilage.

I. NASO PHARYNX

This is the upper most part of the pharynx.

Boundaries:

Superiorly: Basi sphenoid and basi occiput

Anteriorly: Through the posterior nasal aperture it communicates with the nose.

Posteriorly:

1. Arch of atlas.
2. Upper half of axis.

Inferiorly: With oropharynx through pharyngeal isthmus.

Dimensions: Anteroposteriorly – 2.5 cm.

Transversely: 3.5 cm.

Interior of the Naso Pharynx:

On the lateral wall about 1 cm behind the inferior nasal concha – auditory tube opens.

- Behind this opening there is a tubal elevation due to collection of lymphoid follicles called tubal tonsil.
- Above and behind the tubal elevation there is a depression called pharyngeal recess of Rosenmuller which lodges the pharyngeal tonsil (Adenoids).
- Mucous membrane of nasopharynx is respiratory in nature, i.e., lined by ciliated columnar epithelium.

Nerve Supply:

Sensory supply is by pharyngeal branch of pterygo palatine ganglion (maxillary nerve). These fibres are also secretomotor coming from ganglion.

II. ORO-PHARYNX

This is the middle part of pharynx.

Boundaries:

Superiorly: Soft palate.

Inferiorly: Upper border of epiglottis.

Anteriorly: Mouth, tonsillar fossa and dorsum of posterior 1/3 of the tongue.

Posteriorly: Lower 1/2 of 2nd cervical vertebra and 3rd cervical vertebra.

Communications:

Superiorly: It communicates with the naso pharynx via pharyngeal isthmus.

Anteriorly: It communicates with oral cavity via oro-pharyngeal isthmus.

Inferiorly: With laryngo pharynx.

Interior of Oropharynx:

In between palato-glossal and palato pharyngeal arches, palatine tonsil is situated, mucous membrane is of oral type means – it is lined by stratified squamous epithelium.

Nerve Supply:

Sensory, supply is via branches of glossopharyngeal nerve.

Secretomotor: Fibres coming via lesser palatine nerve branch from pterygo palatine ganglion.

III. LARYNGO PHARYNX

- This is the lowest part of the pharynx.
- It extends from upper border of epiglottis to the level of lower border of cricoid cartilage.

Communication:

Anteriorly: It communicates with larynx via laryngeal inlet.

Inferiorly: It is continuous with oesophagus.

Superiorly: Communication with oropharynx.

Relations:

Posteriorly: It is related to 4th, 5th and 6th cervical vertebra.

Anteriorly: Related to:

1. Inlet of larynx.
2. Posterior surface of arytenoid cartilage.
3. Posterior surface of cricoid cartilage.

Boundaries of Laryngeal Inlet

Antero-superior – Upper border of epiglottis.

Postero-inferior – Inter arytenoids fold of mucous membrane.

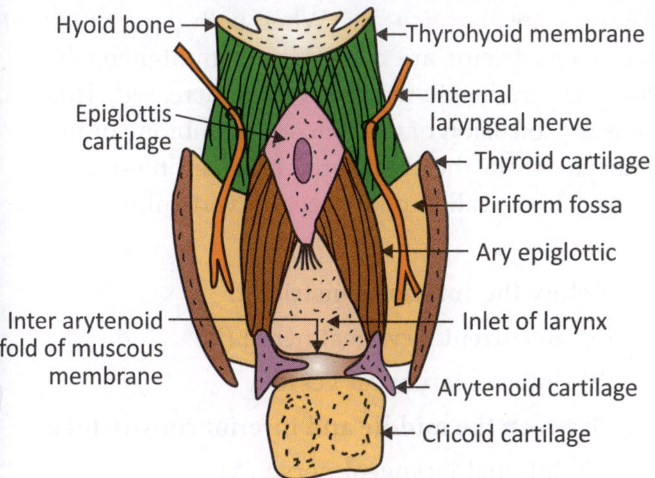

Fig. 30.2: ***Boundaries of inlet of larynx***

Laterally – ary – epiglottic fold of mucous nembrane.

Piriform – recess is a depression situated on either ;ides of laryngeal inlet.

The floor of this recess is supplied by internal aryngeal nerve (X). It is pear shaped fossa.

Boundaries of Piriform Fossa

Medially – Ary epiglottic fold.

Laterally – Inner surface of lamina of thyroid cartilage and thyrohyoid membrane.

Hard food particles may be lodged with in the fossa accidentally when an instrument is used to remove such foreign particles, it may result in injury to the nternal laryngeal nerve and causes anasthesia of the arynx, and considered as surgeons grave yard.

Nerve supply: Via internal laryngeal nerve branch of superior laryngeal nerve (X).

Muscles of Pharynx

Muscles of pharynx are of two types:

A. **Constrictors:** Superior, middle and inferior constrictor of pharynx.

They overlap each other from below upwards.

1. **Superior constrictor of pharynx:**

Origin is from:

(a) Posterior border of medial pterygoid plate.

(b) Pterygoid hamulus.

(c) Pterygo mandibular raphe.

(d) Above and behind mylohyoid line of mandible.

(e) Mucous membrane of lateral border of posterior 1/3 of tongue.

Insertion on

(a) Pharyngeal tubercle of occipital bone.

(b) Median fibrous raphe.

➤ Between the base of skull and upper border of superior constrictor muscle, there is a space called hiatus of morgagni. It is closed by thickened pharyngo basilar fascia and bucco-pharyngeal fascia.

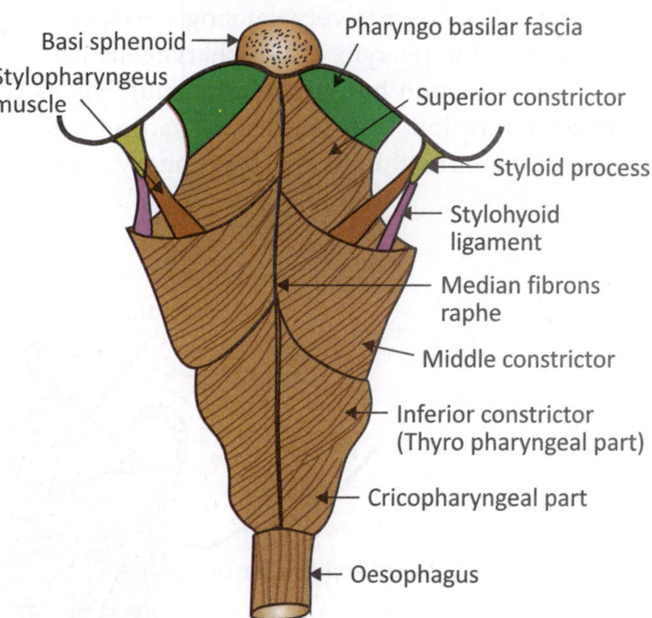

Fig. 30.3: ***Posterior view of pharynx***

2. **Middle constrictor of pharynx**

Origin is from

(a) Lower part of stylohyoid ligament.

(b) Greater and lesser horn of hyoid bone.

Insertion on – Median fibrous raphe of pharynx.

3. **Inferior constrictor of pharynx**

Origin is from

(a) Oblique line and inferior horn of lamina of thyroid cartilage.

(b) Lateral surface of cricoid cartilage.

(c) Fibrous band extending from thyroid tubercle to cricoid cartilage.

Insertion on – Median fibrous raphe.

Inferior Constrictor has two parts:

(a) **Thyropharyngeus part:** Arising from thyroid lamina is ascending upwards.

(b) **Cricopharyngeus part:** Arising from cricoid cartilage is horizontal and acts as sphincter.

The dehiscence of Killian is a weak area between these two parts of inferior constrictor.

Nerve supply of constrictors: Via pharyngeal plexus of nerves containing fibres of vagus and cranial root of accessory nerve.

Action of constrictors: During deglutition they contract and relax alternatively causing peristaltic movement of the pharynx. Thyropharyngeus has propulsive function but cricopharyngeus has a sphincteric function. Cricopharyngeal part relaxes during the contraction of the thyropharyngeal part.

Pharyngeal diverticulum: When both parts of inferior constrictor are constricted simultaneously, the pressure inside the pharynx is increased. This causes protrusion of the mucous membrane of the pharynx from the weak area between these two parts. This is called pharyngeal diverticulum.

Structures Passing between the Constrictors:

1. **Below the inferior constrictor:**
   (a) Recurrent laryngeal nerve (X)
   (b) Inferior laryngeal vessels.
2. **Between the middle and inferior constrictors:**
   (a) Internal laryngeal nerve (X)
   (b) Superior laryngeal vessels.
3. **Between the middle and superior constrictors:**
   (a) Stylopharyngeus muscle
   (b) Glossopharyngeal nerve (IX).
4. **Between the base of skull and superior constrictor:**

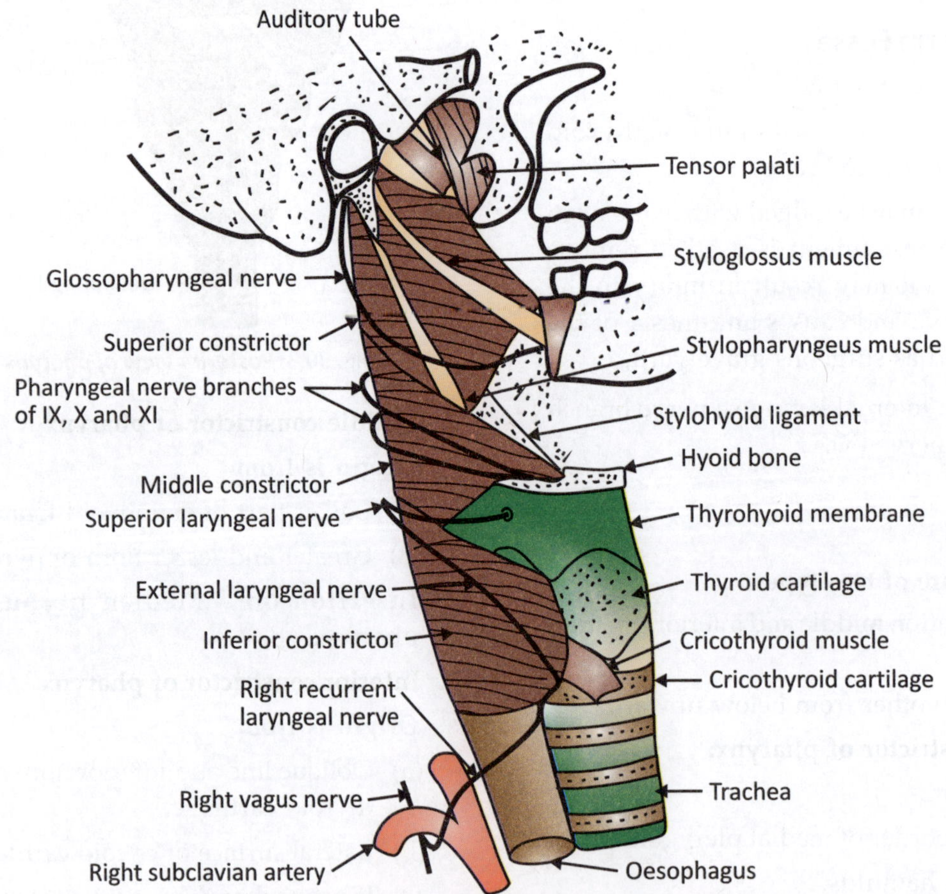

Fig. 30.4: *Lateral view of pharynx-showing constrictors*

(a) Pharyngotympanic tube
(b) Levator veli palatini
  (i) Ascending palatine artery branch of facial artery.
  (ii) Palatine branch of ascending pharyngeal artery.

B. Other Muscles of Pharynx (Longitudinal Muscles):

(a) Stylopharyngeus – arises from styloid process.

(b) Palatopharyngeus – arises from superior surface of palatine aponeurosis.

(c) Salpingopharyngeus – arises from lower part of auditory tube.

These muscles descends downward inside the constrictors and inserted on the pharyngeal wall and posterior border of lamina of thyroid cartilage.

Action: Elevation of the pharynx and larynx.

Nerve supply: Palato pharyngeus and salpingoharyngeus are supplied by pharyngeal plexus of nerves (X and XI).

Stylopharyngeus is supplied by glossopharyngeal nerve (IX).

Nerves forming pharyngeal plexus are branches of:

1. Glossopharyngeal – pharyngeal branch.
2. Vagus nerve containing fibres of cranial root of accessory.
3. Superior cervical sympathetic ganglion – pharyngeal branch.

Pharyngeal plexus of nerves – lies on the surface of middle constrictor of pharynx deep to buccopharyngeal fascia.

Blood supply of pharynx – by branches of:

(a) Dorsalis linguae artery (lingual artery).
(b) Greater and lesser palatine artery, pharyngeal and pterygoid branches of maxillary artery 3rd part.
(c) Tonsillar branch of facial artery.
(d) Ascending palatine branch of facial artery.
(e) Ascending pharyngeal artery branch of external carotid artery.

Venous drainage: Via pharyngeal venous plexus drains into internal jugular vein.

Lymphatic drainage: Lymphatics go to deep cervical and retropharyngeal group of lymph nodes.

RETROPHARYNGEAL SPACE

Retropharyngeal space is found behind the pharynx. A mid-line septum divides the space into right and left halves. Space is bounded anteriorly by buccopharyngeal fascia and pharyngeal wall. Posteriorly it is bounded by prevertebral muscles and fascia.

Contents of Retropharyngeal Space

It contains:

Retropharyngeal lymph nodes separated by a septum and drains:

(a) Posterior part of the nose.
(b) Pharynx.
(c) Pharyngo tympanic tube.
(d) Posterior part of palate and tongue.
(e) Posterior ethmoidal and sphenoidal air sinuses.

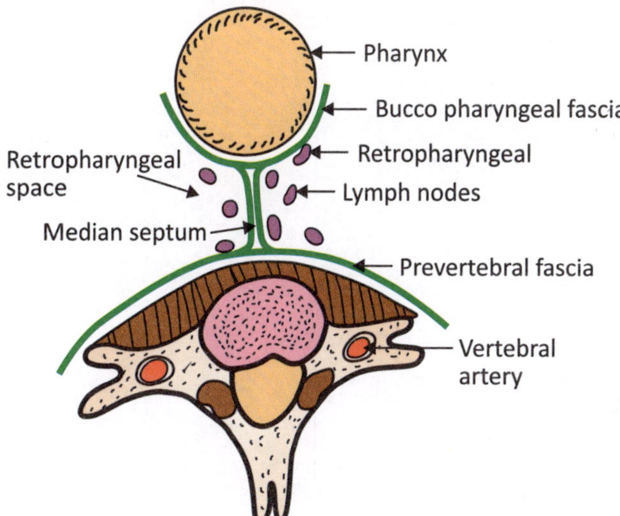

Fig. 30.5: *Contents of retropharyngeal space*

Applied Anatomy

1. Retropharyngeal abscess – due to suppuration of retro pharyngeal lymph nodes – remain unilateral due to septum.
2. Pharyngitis – inflammation of pharynx.
3. Retropharyngeal abscess from the caries of the cervical vertebrae spreads across the midline deep to pre-vertebral fascia, as there is no septum.

4. Diphtheria – occurs on the oropharynx.
5. Hypopharyngeal pouch is formed by herniation of mucous membrane through dehiscence of Killians of the posterior pharyngeal wall.
6. Pharyngeal keratosis – thickening and hardening of the mucous membrane of the pharynx.
7. Pharyngoscopy – examination of interior of pharynx via pharyngoscope.
8. Malignant tumours like – squamous cell carcinoma, lympho-epithelioma etc.

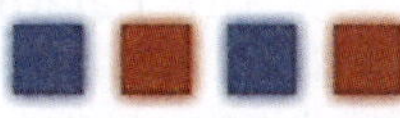

CHAPTER 31

Larynx

It is the chamber concerned with respiration and phonation.

Constitution:

It is formed by:

1. Cartilages
2. Muscles
3. Membranes.

Average Dimensions:

	Male	Female
Length	44 mm	36 mm
Transverse	43 mm	41 mm
Depth	36 mm	26 mm

Situation:

Anterior part of the neck at the level of 3rd, 4th, 5th and 6th cervical vertebrae.

- Superiorly it opens into laryngo pharynx.
- Inferiorly it is continuous with the trachea.

CARTILAGES OF THE LARYNX

Paired and unpaired.

(a) Unpaired cartilages are:

(i) Thyroid cartilage.

(ii) Cricoid cartilage.

(iii) Epiglottis.

(b) Paired cartilages are:

(i) Arytenoid cartilage.

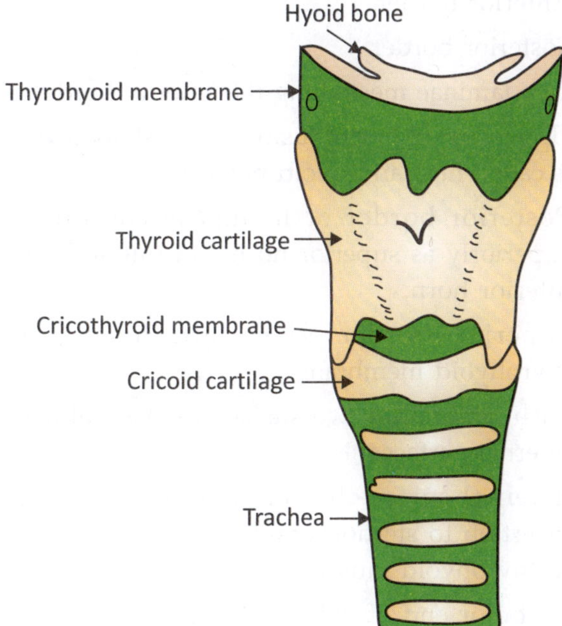

Fig. 31.1: *Anterior surface of larynx*

(ii) Corniculate cartilage.

(iii) Cuneiform cartilage.

UNPAIRED CARTILAGES

Thyroid Cartilage

- It is the largest cartilage of the larynx.
- **Histologically:** It is hyaline cartilage.

Parts:

It has a pair of laminae.

Lamina has four borders:

1. Superior border.
2. Inferior border.

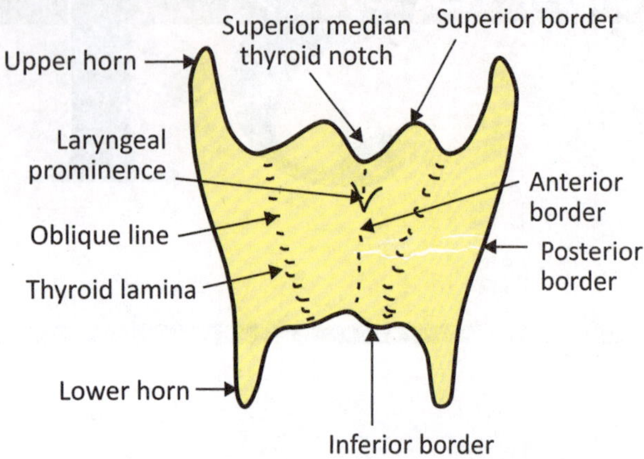

Fig. 31.2: *Thyroid cartilage front view*

3. Anterior border.
4. Posterior border.

- Two laminae meet along the anterior border.
- Upper part of line of fusion is "V" shaped and is called median thyroid notch.
- Posterior border of lamina is continued superiorly as superior horn and inferiorly as inferior horn.
- Superior border gives attachment to thyrohyoid membrane.
- Each lamina has two surfaces – external and internal surfaces.
- External surface has oblique line, it gives insertion to sternothyroid muscle and origin to thyrohyoid muscle.
- Posterior end of oblique line gives origin to inferior constrictor of pharynx.
- Near the lower border cricothyroid muscle is inserted.

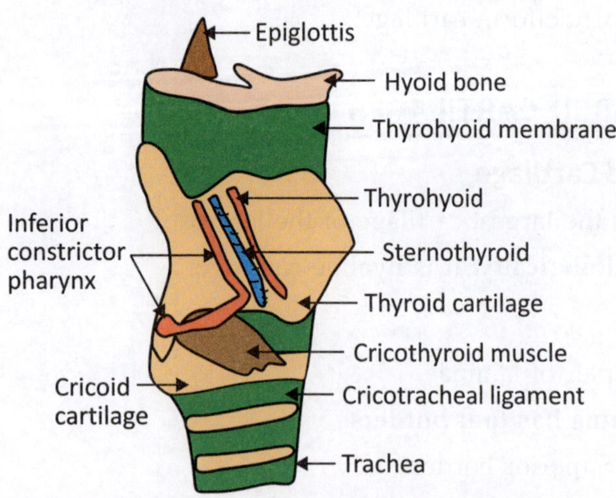

Fig. 31.3: *Lateral view of thyroid cartilage*

- Inner surface of laminae of thyroid cartilage bounds the larynx – in the midline epiglottis is attached.
- Inner surface gives attachment to cricothyroid membrane – upper border of this membrane forms the vocal cord.
- Laterally inner surface is related to Piriform fossa – in the floor of the fossa internal laryngeal nerve is situated.

Cricoid Cartilage

- It is a variety of hyaline cartilage.
- It is the only cartilage of larynx, that forms a complete ring (signet ring shaped).

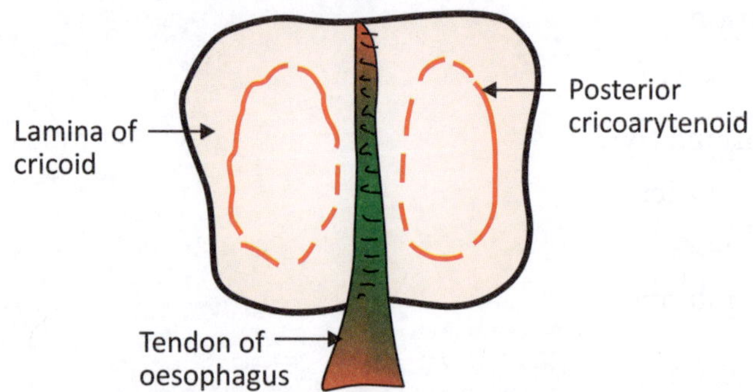

Fig. 31.4: *Posterior view of cricoid cartilage*

Parts of the Cricoid Cartilage:

1. Narrow arch is present anteriorly.
2. Broad lamina is present posteriorly.
   - Upper border of lamina articulates with arytenoid cartilages.
   - Upper border of arch gives attachment for the cricothyroid membrane. The lower border of arch is connected to trachea by cricotracheal ligament.

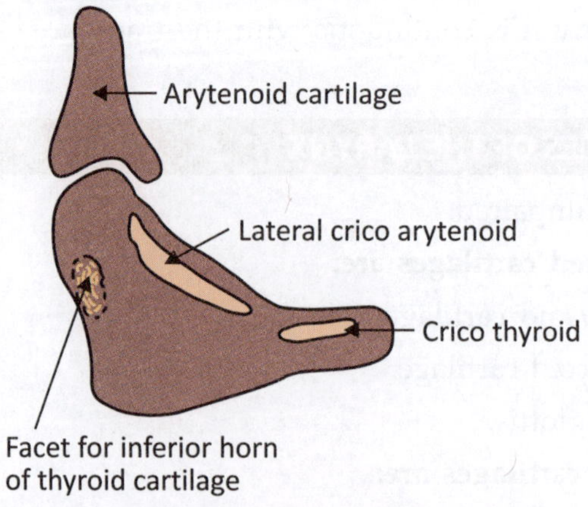

Fig. 31.5: *Lateral view of cricoid cartilage*

- Midline of the posterior surface of lamina gives attachment for the tendon of oesophagus. On either side of the midline posterior surface of lamina gives origin for the posterior crico arytenoids muscle. Lateral aspect of lamina has a facet for articulation with the inferior horn of thyroid cartilage.

Epiglottis

- It is made up of elastic cartilage and is leaf shaped, broader above and narrow below.
- Situated posterior to the tongue and connected anteriorly to it by a median and lateral glossoepiglottic folds.
- It is connected to the hyoid bone by hyoepiglottic ligament.
- Lower end is pointed and attached to angle between two laminae of thyroid cartilage by thyroepiglottic ligament.
- Right and left margins give attachment to aryepiglottic folds.
- Posterior surface is covered with mucous membrane and present a tubercle in the lower part.

PAIRED CARTILAGES

Arytenoid Cartilage

Arytenoid cartilage is pyramidal shaped, lying on the upper border of lamina of cricoid cartilage.

Parts:

1. Apex – Situated above.
2. Base – Situated below.
3. Vocal process – Directed forwards from the base, gives attachment to vocal ligament.
4. Muscular process – Projects laterally from the base and gives attachment to muscles of larynx.

Joint formed:

- Apex articulates with the corniculate cartilage.
- Base articulates with cricoid cartilage and forms crico arytenoid joint – synovial variety.
- Surfaces are antero lateral, medial and posterior.

Corniculate Cartilages

Corniculate cartilages are small pea shaped, paired cartilage.

- Situated along the apex of arytenoids cartilage, found within the aryepiglottic fold.
- Elastic in nature.

Cuneiform Cartilage

Cuneiform cartilage – Two small rod shaped pieces of cartilage placed in aryepiglottic folds.

- Elastic in nature.

MUSCLES OF THE LARYNX

Classified into extrinsic and intrinsic muscles.

A. **Extrinsic muscles:** Moves the larynx up and down during swallowing.

(a) **Muscles that elevates the larynx are:**

(i) Stylohyoid
(ii) Digastric
(iii) Mylohyoid
(iv) Middle constrictor and thyropharyngeus part of inferior constrictor of pharynx.
(v) Thyrohyoid.

(b) **Muscles that depress the larynx are:**

(i) Sternothyroid
(ii) Sternohyoid
(iii) Omohyoid.

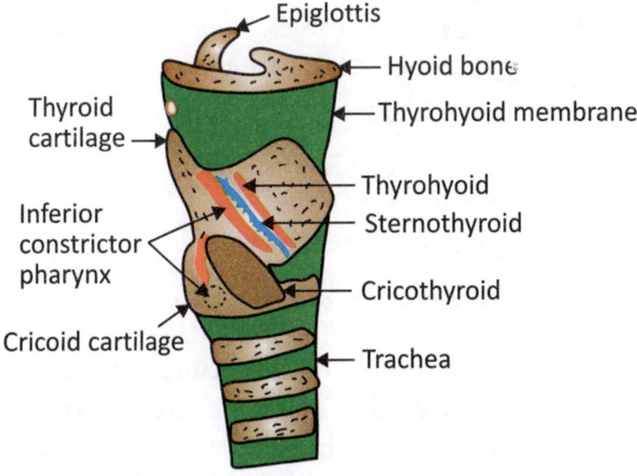

Fig. 31.6: *Lateral view of larynx*

B. Intrinsic muscles are of two varieties:

1. Muscles of controlling the inlet of larynx.
2. Muscles controlling the vocal cord.

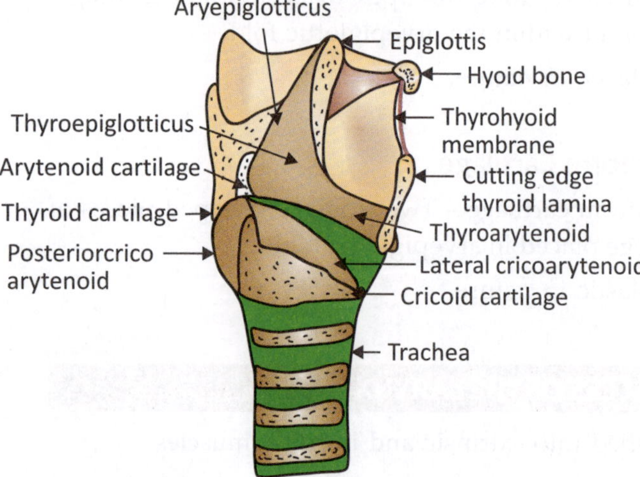

Fig. 31.7: ***Intrinsic muscles of larynx***

1. Muscles acting on inlet of larynx:

(a) Oblique arytenoid muscle

Origin: From muscular process of arytenoid cartilage of one side.

Insertion: Apex of opposite arytenoid cartilage.

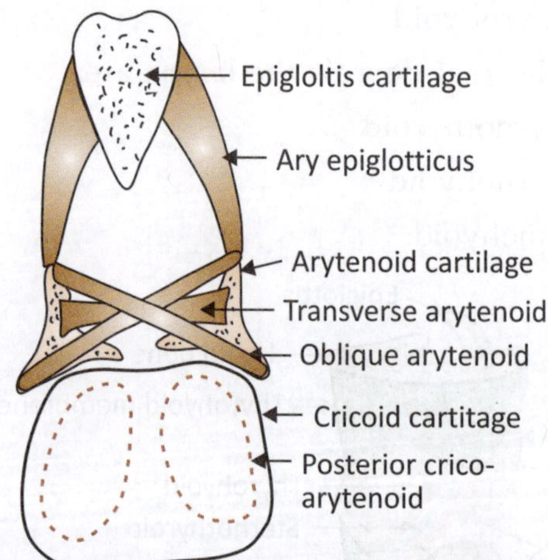

Fig. 31.8: ***Muscles acting of inlet of larynx***

(b) Ary epiglottic muscle: Some fibres of obique arytenoids enter the aryepiglottic fold and form this muscle.

Action: Contraction of both sides of muscles reduces the size of laryngeal inlet (closing).

Nerve supply: Recurrent laryngeal nerve.

(c) Thyro epiglotticus: Arises from thyroid angle, fibres run backwards and upwards for insertion into the aryepiglottic fold to reach the edge of epiglottis.

Action: Opening of laryngeal inlet.

Nerve supply: Recurrent laryngeal nerve.

2. Muscles controlling the movement of vocal cords:

(a) **Cricothyroid** is tensor of vocal cords.
(b) **Posterior cricoarytenoid** is abductor of vocal cords.
(c) Transverse arytenoids.
(d) Thyro arytenoids.
(e) Lateral cricoarytenoids.

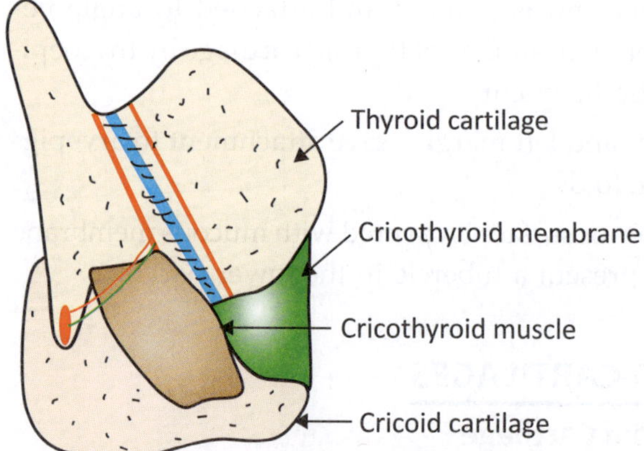

Fig. 31.9: ***Cricothyroid muscle***

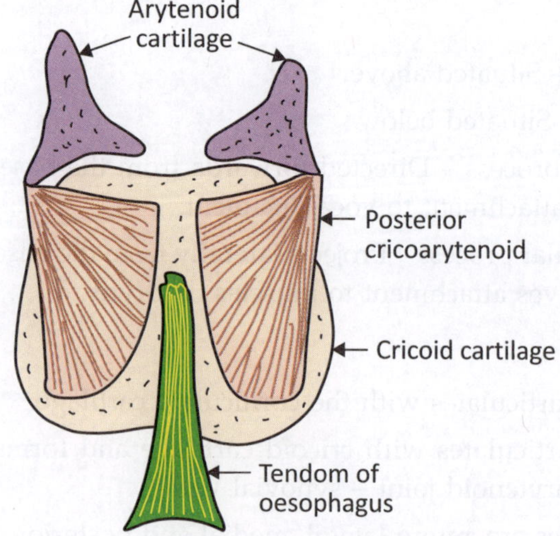

Fig. 31.10: ***Posterior cricoarytenoid muscle***

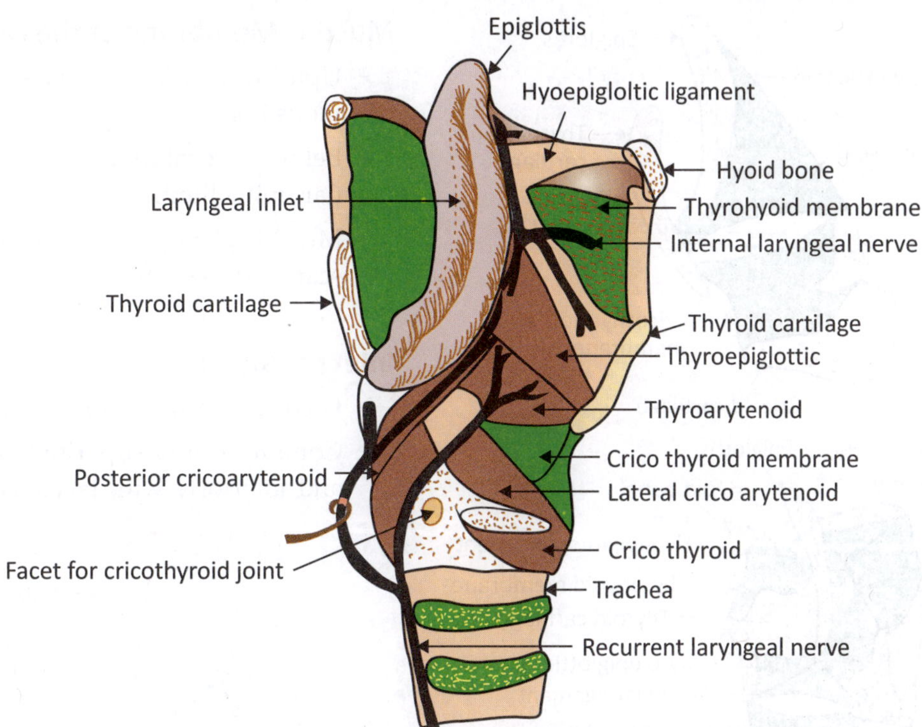

Fig. 31.11: *Intrinsic muscles of larynx-with its nerve supply*

Table 31.1: *Intrinsic Muscles Acting on Vocal Cords of Larynx*

S.No.	Muscles	Origin	Direction of fibres	Insertion	Action	Nerve supply
1.	Cricothyroid	Lateral surface of arch of cricoid cartilage	Backwards and upwards	Lower border and inferior horn of thyroid cartilage	Tensor of vocal cords	External laryngeal nerve (X)
2.	Posterior-cricoarytenoid	Posterior surface of lamina of cricoid cartilage	Upwards and laterally	Muscular process of arytenoid	Abductor of vocal cords	Recurrent laryngeal nerve (X)
3.	Lateral crico-arytenoid	Upper border of arch of cricoid (lateral part)	Upwards and backwards	Muscular process of arytenoid	Adductor of vocal cords	Recurrent laryngeal nerve
4.	Transverse-arytenoid	Posterior surface of one arytenoid	Transverse	Posterior surface of another arytenoid	Adductor of vocal cords	Recurrent laryngeal nerve
5.	Thyroarytenoids	Thyroid angle	Backwards and upwards	Antero-lateral surface of arytenoid	Relaxor of vocal cords	Recurrent laryngeal nerve

MEMBRANES AND LIGAMENTS OF LARYNX

1. Thyrohyoid membrane
2. Cricothyroid ligament
3. Cricotracheal ligament
4. Hyoepiglottic ligament
5. Thyroepiglottic ligament
6. Vestibular ligament
7. Vocal ligament
8. Quadrate membrane.

Interior of the Larynx

There are two mucosal folds present within the larynx. Vestibular folds and vocal folds. These folds divide the cavity of larynx into three parts:

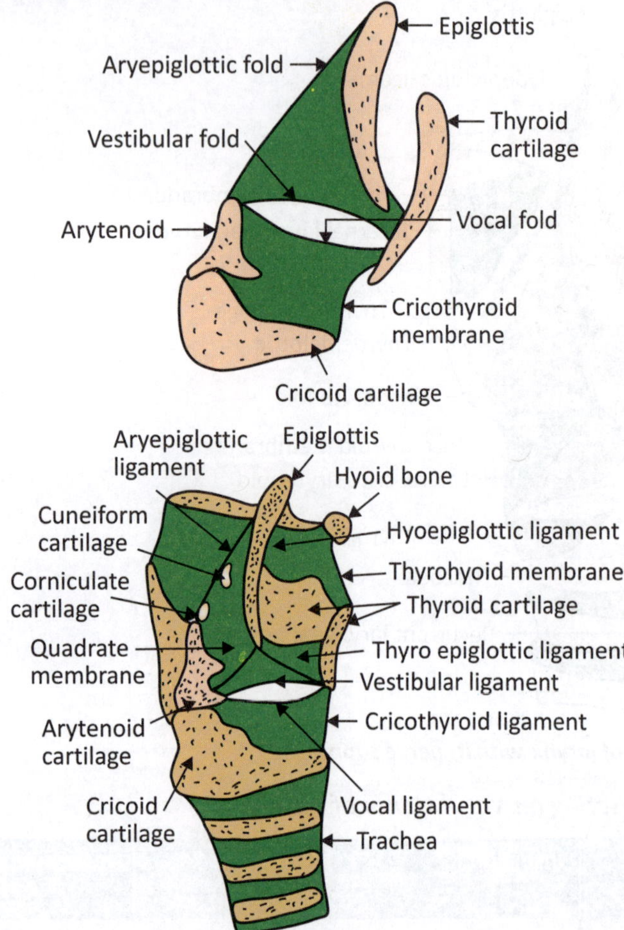

Fig. 31.12: *Internal framework of larynx on median section showing ligaments and membranes along with its cartilages*

1. **Vestibule:** Lies between laryngeal inlet and vestibular fold (false vocal cords)
2. **Ventricle of the larynx:** It is a space between vestibular folds and vocal folds. The sinus is a recess situated between these folds. Saccule is the anterior ascending part of the sinus. Saccule contains numerous mucous glands, secretion of these glands lubricate the vocal folds.
3. **The infra glottic portion:** It extends from vocal cord to the lower border of cricoid cartilage.

Rima vestibuli: It is the space between two vestibular folds.

Rima glottids: It is the space between two vocal folds (true vocal cords). It has an anterior intramembranous portion and posterior intra cartilaginous portion. It is the narrowest part of the larynx.

Mucous Membrane of the Larynx

- Upto vocal folds – larynx is lined by stratified squamous epithelium.
- Below to vocal folds – it is lined by ciliated columnar epithelium.
- Mucous glands – are absent over vocal cords and scattered over the rest of the larynx.

Inlet of Larynx

- Directed upwards and backwards.
- Communicated superiorly with laryngo pharynx and inferiorly with laryngeal cavity.

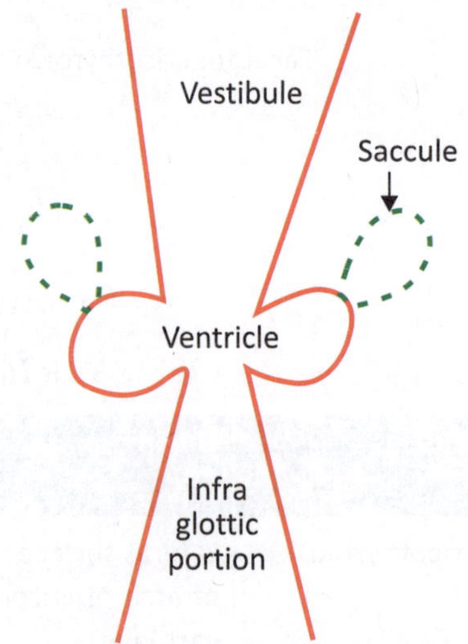

Fig. 31.13: *Inferior of the larynx*

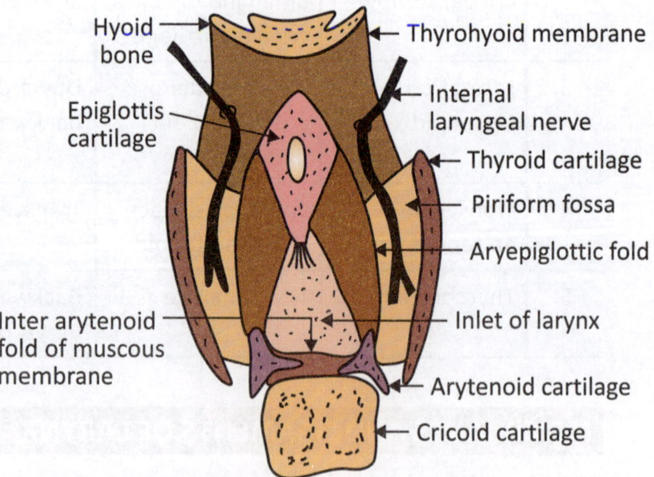

Fig. 31.14: *Boundaries of inlet of larynx*

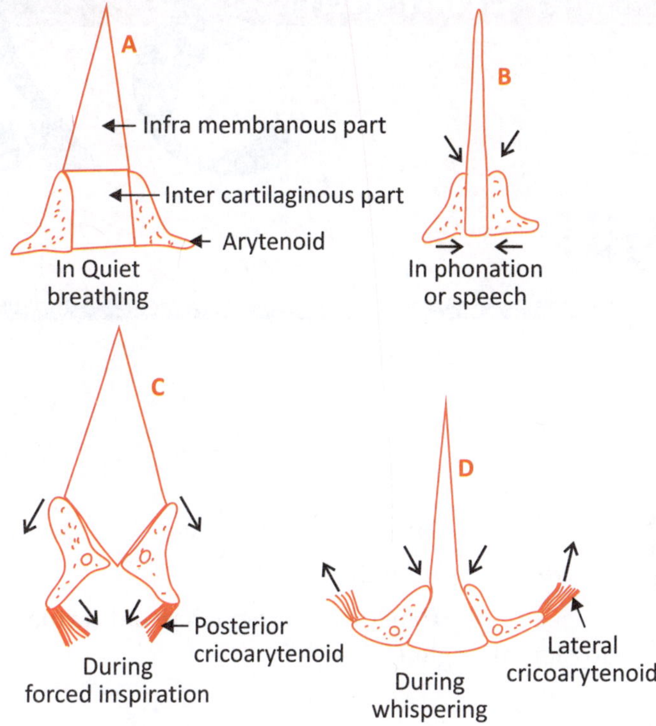

Fig. 31.15: ***Movements of Rima glottids***

Boundaries:

- Antero superiorly – upper border of epiglottis.
- Laterally – Aryepiglottic folds.
- Postero-inferiorly – inter arytenoids fold.
- Joints of the larynx – are synovial variety – crico-thyroid joint and cricoarytenoids joint.

BLOOD SUPPLY OF LARYNX

1. Superior laryngeal branch of superior thyroid artery.
2. Inferior laryngeal branch of inferior thyroid artery.
3. Cricothyroid artery.

Lymphatic Drainage:

- Above vocal cords – drained into pre-epiglottic and upper deep cervical lymph nodes.
- Below vocal cords – drained into pre-laryngeal lymph nodes.
- Pre and para-tracheal group of lymph nodes.
- Lower deep cervical group of lymph nodes.
- In the glottis lymphatics are absent practically; hence lymphatic spread of carcinoma of vocal cord is late.

Nerve supply:

1. **Sensory supply** is by vagus nerve.

   Above vocal cords: Internal laryngeal branch of superior laryngeal nerve (X).

   Below vocal cords: Recurrent laryngeal nerve (X).
2. **Motor supply:** All the muscles of the larynx are supplied by recurrent laryngeal nerve (X) except cricothyroid – supplied by external laryngeal nerve (X).

FUNCTIONS OF LARYNX

1. **Closure of laryngeal inlet:** During swallowing, cough reflex – expels any foreign body-entering trachea.
2. **Phonation:** Exhaled air forces the adducted vocal cords apart and vibrate them – to produce voice – pitch depends on number of vibration per second, changes in the length and tension of vocal cord.

   Quality of Voice is due to resonators like nose, pharynx, oral cavity and para nasal air sinuses.

   Volume of voice is controlled by intensity of air pressure generated by the lung.
3. **Respiratory function.**
4. **Fixation of chest:** During strenuous work, larynx closes and thoracic cage becomes fixed, which helps in the performance like climbing, straining for stools, parturition etc.

Applied Anatomy

1. Laryngitis.
2. Laryngeal diphtheria.
3. Congenital laryngeal web.
4. Singer's nodes (vocal nodule) – develops due to misuse or overuse of voice.
5. Laryngocele is a bulbs air containing prolongation of the ventricle and saccule – it may herniate outside or inside of larynx.
6. Layngoscopy – examination of larynx by laryngoscope.

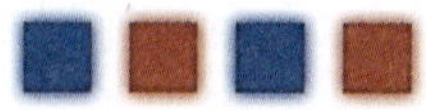

CHAPTER 32

Trachea and Oesophagus

TRACHEA

Trachea (wind pipe) is part of lower respiratory passage – only air passes through this tube.

STRUCTURE

There are 16 to 20 tracheal rings formed by 'C' shaped cartilages which are posteriorly filled by smooth muscle fibres called trachealis. Tracheal rings are connected with each other by tracheal ligaments. Internally it is lined by ciliated columnar epithelium containing mucous and serous glands and externally these are covered by pre-tracheal fascia.

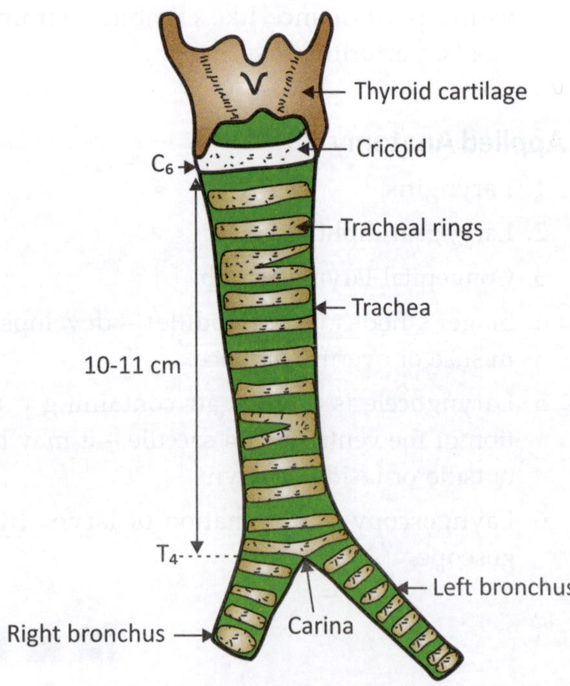

Fig. 32.1: *Trachea*

Length – Approximately – 10 cm

Breadth – 12 mm

Extent – From lower border of cricoid cartilage (C_6) to sternal angle (T_4).

PARTS

- **Cervical part:** This is upper half of the trachea and lies in neck.
- **Thoracic part:** The lower half lies in the upper part of thorax.

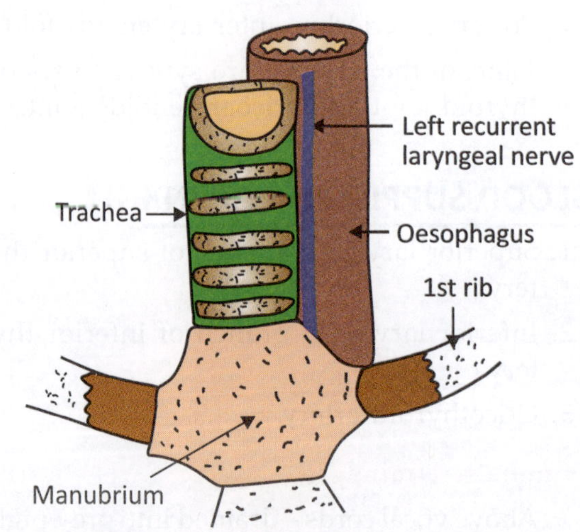

Fig. 32.2: *Cervical part of trachea*

RELATIONS OF TRACHEA

I. Cervical Part:

Anteriorly:

1. Skin, superficial and deep fascia of neck.
2. Isthmus of the thyroid gland.

3. Inferior thyroid veins.
4. Anterior jugular venous arch.
5. Pretracheal lymph nodes.
6. Superior thyroid vessels.

Laterally:

1. Recurrent laryngeal nerves.
2. Carotid sheath with its contents – common carotid artery, internal jugular vein and vagus nerve.
3. Para tracheal group of lymph nodes with lobes of thyroid gland.
4. Inferior thyroid vessels.

Posteriorly: It is related to body of 7th cervical vertebra separated by prevertebral muscles, fascia and oesophagus.

II. Thoracic Part:

Anteriorly:

1. Sternum.
2. Thymus gland.
3. Left brachiocephalic vein.
4. Origins of brachiocephalic and left common carotid artery.
5. Arch of aorta.

Posteriorly: Oesophagus and left recurrent laryngeal nerve.

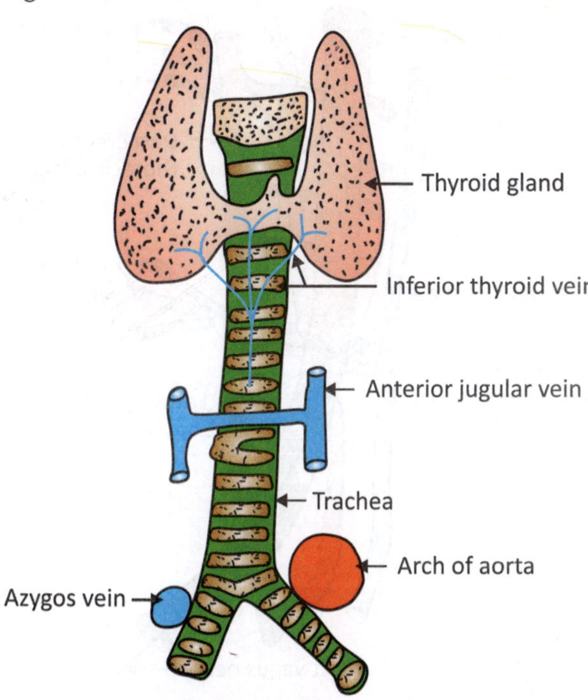

Fig. 32.3: *Anterior relations of trachea*

LATERAL RELATIONS OF TRACHEA IN THE THORAX (SUPERIOR MEDIASTINUM)

Right side	Left side
– Azygos vein – Right vagus nerve – Pleura	– Arch of Aorta – Left common carotid artery – Left subclavian artery – Left vagus nerve – Left phrenic nerve – Pleura

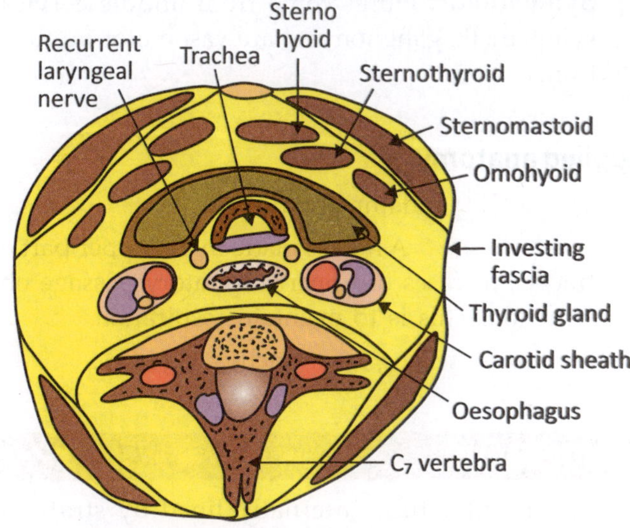

Fig. 32.4: *Relations of cervical trachea T.S. neck at C_7*

BLOOD SUPPLY OF TRACHEA

A. **Cervical part:** Branches of inferior thyroid and superior thyroid artery.

B. **Thoracic part:** Tracheal and oesophageal branches of descending thoracic aorta.

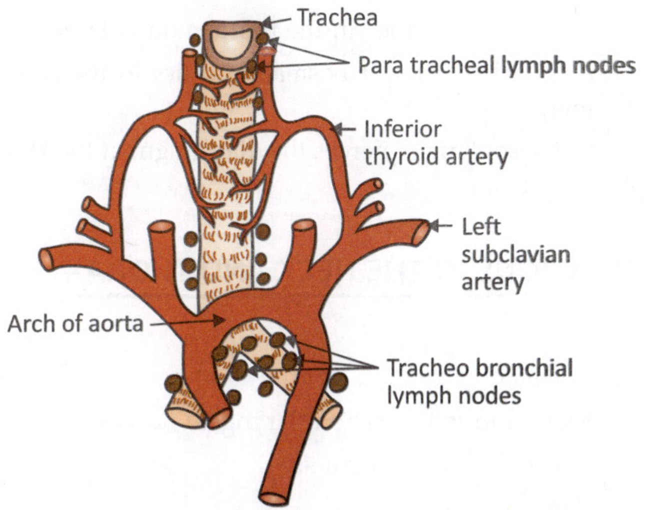

Fig. 32.5: *Blood supply and lymphatic drainage of trachea*

Veins: Drain into brachiocephalic vein – via inferior thyroid veins.

Lymphatics: Goes to pre and para tracheal group of lymph nodes.

- Lower deep cervical group of lymph nodes.

Nerve supply:

- Vagus nerve via its recurrent laryngeal branch supplies trachealis muscle and mucous membrane both sensory and secretomotor fibres.

  Sympathetic: Fibres come from middle cervical sympathetic ganglion and are vasomotor in function.

Applied anatomy

1. **Tracheaitis:** Inflammation of trachea.
2. **Tracheostomy:** A hole is made in the upper part of trachea in cases of upper respiratory passage obstruction. This is to maintain respiration.
3. **Tumours:** Arising from trachea, e.g., CA.

OESOPHAGUS

It is a muscular tube internally lined by stratified squamous epithelium. The length of oesophagus is about 10 cm or 25 cm and this extends from the pharynx, i.e., lower border of C_6 vertebra to the stomach, i.e., T_{11} vertebra. It's upper 5 cm lies in the neck.

PARTS

1. **Cervical part:** Lies in the neck and is small.
2. **Thoracic part:** Lies in the thorax and is large.
3. **Abdominal part:** It is small and lies in the abdomen.

The oesophagus pierces the diaphragm at the level of T_{10} vertebra.

RELATIONS IN THE NECK AND THORAX

Anterior:

1. Trachea.
2. Right and left recurrent laryngeal nerves.
3. Left principal bronchus.
4. Pericardium.

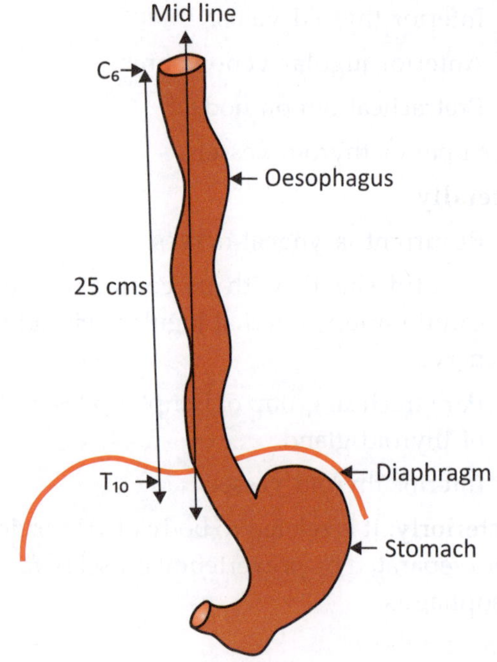

Fig. 32.6: ***Curvatures of oesophagus***

Posterior:

1. Pre-vertebral muscles and fascia.
2. Vertebral column – C_7, T_1 to T_{11} vertebra.
3. Thoracic duct.
4. Azygos vein.
5. Right posterior intercostal nerves and vessels.
6. Descending thoracic aorta.

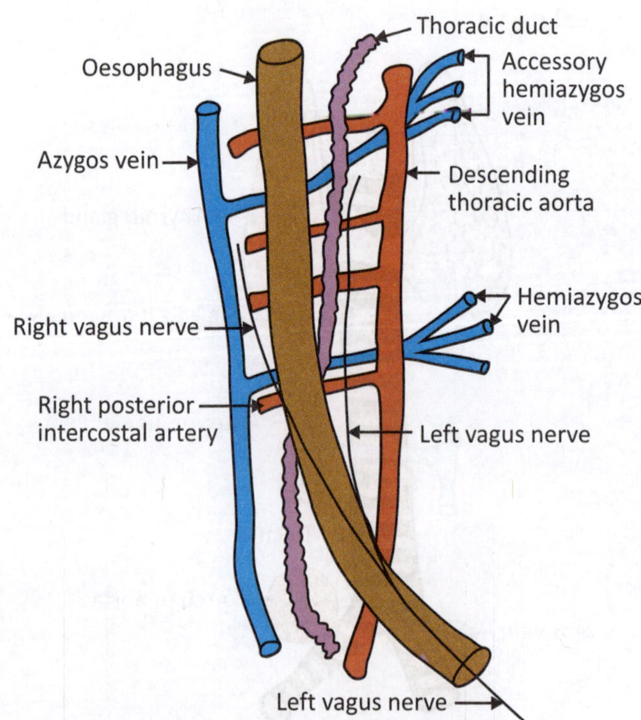

Fig. 32.7: ***Relations of oesophagus***

Later:

1. Thyroid lobes.
2. Carotid sheath with its contents (common carotid artery, internal jugular vein and vagus nerve).

   Right side: Mediastinal pleura.

   Left side:

   — Left subclavian artery, aortic arch.

   — Thoracic duct and mediastinal pleura.

OESOPHAGEAL CONSTRICTIONS

These are at four places:

1. At its origin – C_6 vertebral level in the neck.
2. At the level of arch of aorta – between T_2 and T_3 (Thorax).
3. At the site of tracheal bifurcation – T_4 and T_5 (Thorax).
4. At its passage through diaphragm – T_{10} level.

Applied Anatomy

1. **Oesophagitis:** This is inflammation of oesophageal wall.
2. **Oesophageal varices:** Dilated veins at the site of porto caval anastomosis.
3. **Carcinoma of oesophagus:** Commonest site is middle 1/3.

Table 32.1: ***Blood supply, nerve supply and lymphatics of oesophagus***

Parts of Oesophagus	Arterial Supply	Venous Drainage	Nerve Supply	Lymphatics
Upper 1/3 of oesophagus	Inferior thyroid artery	Inferior thyroid veins	Recurrent laryngeal nerve (X) and sympathetic from middle cervical ganglion	Lower deep cervical group of lymph nodes
Middle 1/3 of oesophagus	Oesophageal branches of descending thoracic aorta	Azygos vein	Branches of vagus nerve and sympathetic from thoracic ganglion	Superior and posterior mediastinal group of lymph nodes
Lower 1/3 of oesophagus	Branches of left gastric artery	Through left gastric vein blood drains into portal vein	Branches of vagus nerve and sympathetic from coeliac ganglion	Lymph nodes along left gastric vein goes to coeliac group of lymph nodes

CHAPTER 33

Ear

This is an organ of hearing and balancing. This is concerned with maintaining equilibrium of the body.

The ear consists three parts:

1. External ear.
2. Middle ear (tympanic cavity).
3. Internal ear (labyrinth).

EXTERNAL EAR

This is formed by:

1. Auricle or pinna.
2. External acoustic meatus.

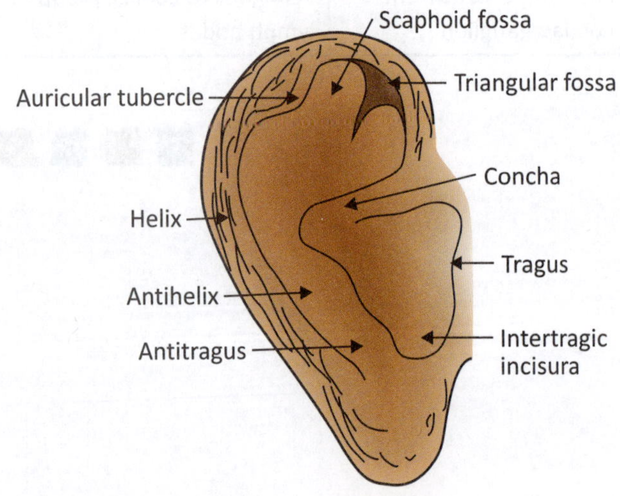

Fig. 33.1: *External ear*

I. AURICLE

Formed by yellow elastic, single crumpled plate of cartilage, covered by skin.

- Lowest part is soft and consists only of connective tissue covered by skin called lobule.
- Large depression is called concha which leads into external auditory meatus.

Developed: The ear develops as six tubercles around the first branchial cleft.

Parts: Helix, antihelix, scaphoid and triangular fossa concha, tragus, anti-tragus and incisura terminalis.

Nerve Supply of Pinna

1. Great auricular nerve (C_2 and C_3) – supplies lower 1/3 of pinna both sides.
2. Lesser occipital nerve (C_2) – upper 2/3 of posterior – surface of pinna.
3. Auriculo temporal nerve – upper 2/3 of anterior surface of pinna.
4. Auricular branch of vagus – This supplies root of auricle

Blood Supply

1. Superficial temporal vessels supply anterior surface of pinna.
2. Posterior auricular vessels supply posterior surface of pinna.

Lymphatic Drainage

1. **Anterior surface:** This is drained by pre-auricular group of lymph nodes.
2. **Posterior surface:** This is drained by posterior auricular or mastoid group of lymph nodes.
3. **Superficial cervical:** Group of lymph nodes.

Muscles of Auricle

These are extrinsic and intrinsic.

1. **Extrinsic muscles:** Move the auricle as a whole, e.g.,
   - Auricularis anterior
   - Auricularis superior
   - Auricularis posterior.
2. **Intrinsic muscles:** Alter the shape of the auricle, e.g.,
   - Helicis major and minor
   - Tragicus and anti-tragicus
   - Transversus auriculae
   - Oblique auriculae.

Ligaments of Auricle

1. **Extrinsic ligaments:** These connect the auricle with temporal bone.
2. **Intrinsic ligaments:** These connect various cartilages of the pinna.

EXTERNAL AUDITORY MEATUS

Development: First branchial cleft.

Length: About 2.5 cm.

Extent: From concha to tympanic membrane.

Parts:

Cartilagineous part: This is outer 1/3 of external auditory meatus.

Bony part: This is inner 2/3 of external meatus.

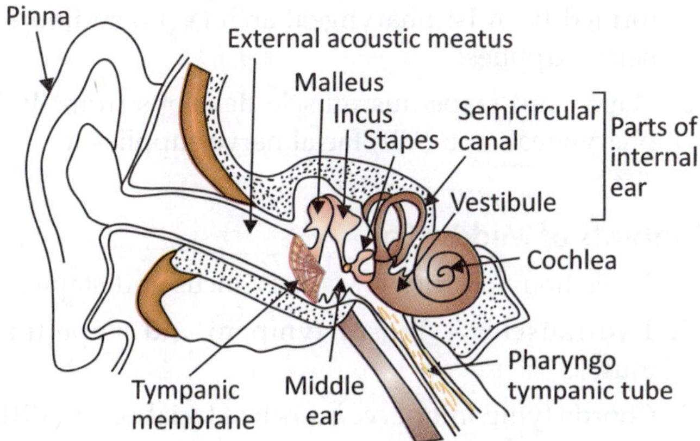

Fig. 33.2: *Ear showing three parts*

Direction: Canal is "S" shaped.

Ist directed — medially, upwards and forwards.

Then directed — medially, backwards and upwards.

Finally directed — medially, forwards and downwards.

Narrowest part of the canal is isthmus – This is 5 mm lateral to the tympanicc membrane.

During examination — Pinna is pulled upwards and backwards.

Functions: It conducts the sound waves to the tympanic membrane.

Relations:

Anteriorly – Temporo-mandibular joint.

Posteriorly – Mastoid air cells and mastoid antrum.

Superiorly – Middle cranial fossa.

Inferiorly – Parotid gland (parotid abscess may burst into external auditory meatus).

Inflammation of external auditory meatus causes painful opening of the mouth – Trismus.

Anterior wall of the canal is longer than posterior wall.

Bony part is narrower than the cartilagenous part.

Cartilagenous part: Formed by "C" shaped cartilage.

In the floor – fissures of santorini is present, filled by fibrous tissue, they permit free mobility of pinna and abscess burst through these fissures into external auditory meatus.

Bony part: "C" shaped tympanic plate of temporal bone forms, squamous part completes the deficiency in bony part.

Skin lining the external auditory meatus has – sebaceous glands, modified sweat gland called ceruminous glands and hair.

Blood Supply

1. Superficial temporal artery
2. Posterior auricular artery.

Lymphatic Drainage

- Pre-auricular lymph nodes
- Post-auricular lymph nodes
- Infra auricular lymph nodes.

Nerve Supply

1. Auriculo temporal nerve supplies anterior ½ of meatus.
2. Auricular branch of vagus (Arnolds' nerve) – supplies posterior half of meatus. Stimulation of this nerve causes ear cough and even vaso vagal symptoms.

Applied Anatomy

1. Pre-auricular sinus – formed due to incomplete fusion of auricular tubercles.
2. Partial or total agenesis of pinna.
3. Accessory auricles.
4. Bat's ear (protruding ears)
5. Peri chondritis of pinna.
6. Cauliflower ear – Permanent deformity due to organized haematoma under perichondrium (Boxers).
7. Rodent ulcer (Basal cell CA).
8. Blaindile's ear – Congenital asymmetry of ears.
9. Cagot's ear – Congenital absence of lobule of ear.
10. Treacher – Collin's syndrome – poor development of external and middle ear, eyes, zygomatic, maxillary and mandible bone.

MIDDLE EAR CAVITY

- It is an air conditioning chamber, situated with in the petrous part of the temporal bone – slit like cavity.
- Connects external ear with internal ear.
- Communicates with nasopharynx through auditory tube anteriorly and posteriorly communicates with mastoid antrum via aditus.

Shape

Biconvex: Antero posterior – 15 mm.

- **Vertical diameter:** 15 mm.
- **Transverse diameter:**
  - Upper part – 6 mm
  - Central part – 2 mm
  - Lower part – 4 mm

Parts of Middle Ear

Three parts:

1. **Epi-tympanum:** Situated above tympanic membrane also known as attic part of cavity.

   Contains: Head of malleus and body of incus with its short process.
2. **Meso-tympanum or tympanic cavity proper:** Situated behind the tympanic membrane.

   Contains: Handle of malleus and long process of incus parallel to handle and stapes.
3. **Hypo-tympanum:** Situated below tympanic membrane.

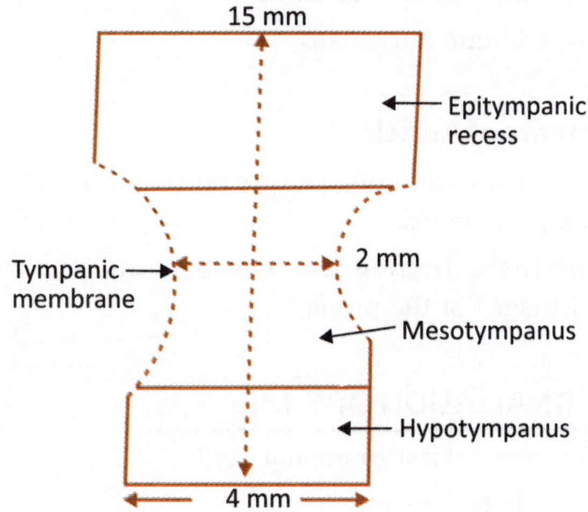

Fig. 33.3: *Parts and dimensions of middle ear*

Development of Middle Ear

Develops from:

1. Tubo tympanic recess.
2. Malleus, incus, and tensor tympani muscle are formed from Ist pharyngeal arch (V_3) mandibular nerve supplies.
3. Stapes and stapedius muscle develops from IInd pharyngeal arch (VII) facial nerve supplies it.

Contents of Middle Ear

1. Three bony ossicles – Malleus, incus and stapes.
2. Two muscles – Tensor tympani and stapedius muscle.
3. Chorda tympanic nerve branch of facial nerve (VII).
4. Tympanic plexus of nerves.
5. Blood vessels and lymphatics of middle ear.
6. Air fills the cavity.

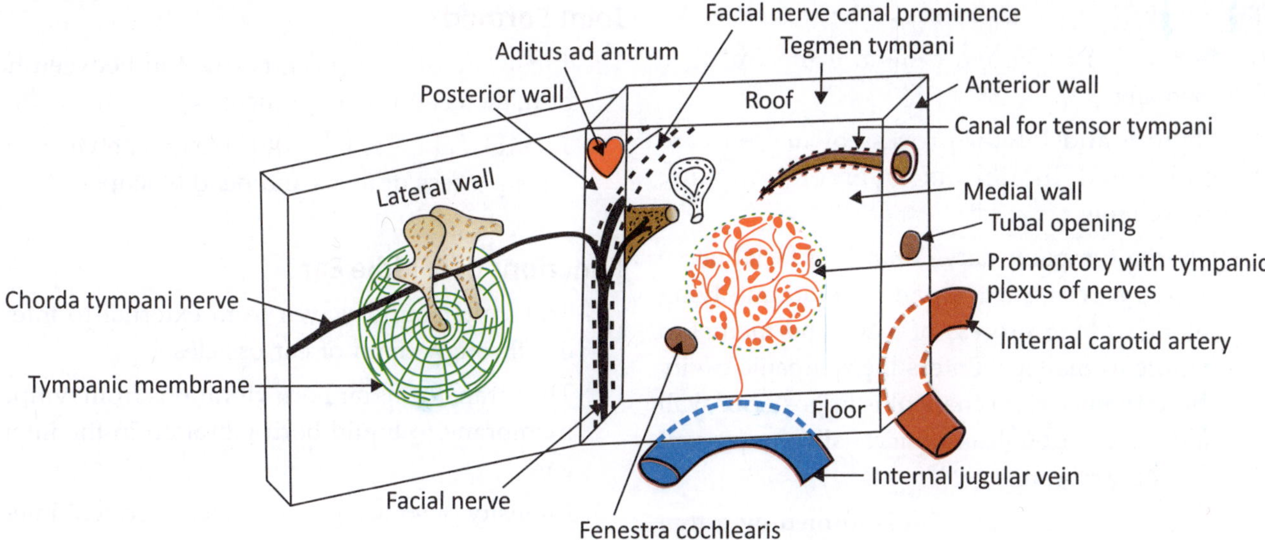

Fig. 33.4: ***Schematic view of middle ear and its contents***

All these structures are covered by mucous membrane.

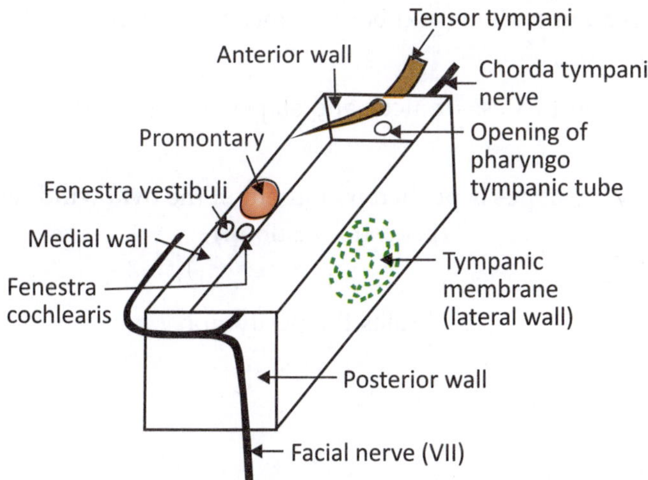

Fig. 33.5: ***Schematic diagram of the middle ear***

Boundaries of Middle Ear Cavity

It is like a six sided box having – anterior, posterior, medial and lateral walls with a roof and a floor.

I. **Anterior wall or carotid wall:** Having openings of:

1. Anterior canliculus for chorda tympani nerve.
2. Canal for tensor tympani muscle.
3. Opening of pharyngo tympanic tube (from above downwards).

II. **Posterior wall or mastoid wall:** Having following features:

1. Upper part has an opening – leading to aditus to mastoid antrum.
2. Pyramid – Is a thin bony elevation has an opening at its apex – through this tendon of stapedius passes.
3. Facial nerve prominence (facial nerve canal).
4. Posterior canaliculus – for chorda tympani nerve.
5. Fossa Incudis is a shallow depression – lodging short process of incus.

III. **Medial wall or labyrinthine wall:** Having following features:

1. Prominence caused by lateral semicircular canal.
2. Impression of facial nerve canal (prominence).
3. Promontary – smooth rounded elevation formed by basal turn of cochlea. Tympanic plexus of nerves lies on it.
4. Fenestra vestibuli – The opening is closed by foot piece of stapes and annular ligament. It transmits sound waves from ear ossicles to the perilymph of scala vestibuli. Situated above and behind the promontary.
5. Fenerstra cochlearis – This is the round window situated below and behind promontary – closed by secondary tympanic membrane. It accommodates the pressure waves transmitted to the perilymph of scala tympani.
6. Sinus tympani is a small depression situated behind the promontary between fenestra vestibuli and fenestra cochlearis.
   - Deep to it ampulla of posterior semi-circular canal is situated.

IV. Lateral wall or membranous or tympanic wall

(a) Formed by tympanic membrane buldges medially.

(b) Handle and lateral process of malleus are embedded in fibrous layer of tympanic membrane.

(c) Chorda tympanic nerve branch of facial nerve passes across the tympanic membrane lying lateral to long process of incus and medial to handle of malleus. Enters the tympanic cavity through posterior canaliculus in posterior wall and leaves through anterior canaliculus present in anterior wall.

V. Roof of middle ear cavity: It is formed by a thin plate of bone known as tegmen tympani. This separates middle ear from middle cranial fossa.

VI. Floor or jugular wall: Related to superior bulb of internal jugular vein.

Tympanic branch of glossopharyngeal nerve enters through a canaliculus present in the posterior part of the floor.

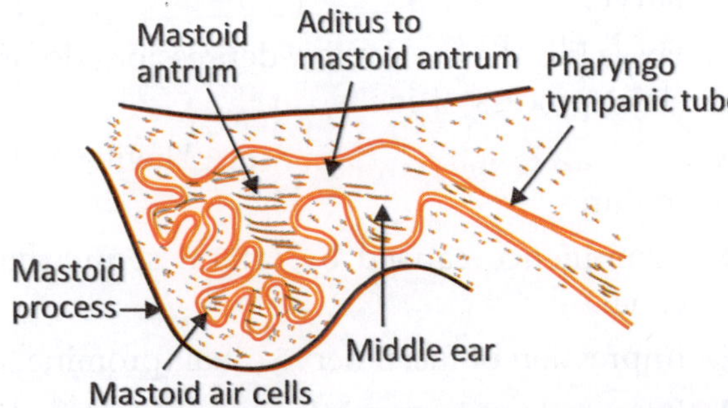

Fig. 33.6: ***Mastoid antrum and middle ear cavity***

Joint Formed

1. **Incudo malleolar joint:** Formed in between head of malleus and body of incus.
2. **Incudo stapedial joint:** It is formed between lentiform process of incus and head of stapes.

Functions of Middle Ear

1. Transmits sound waves from external to internal ear through chain of ear ossicles.
2. Thus transforms air born vibrations from tympanic membrane to liquid born vibration in the internal ear.
3. Intensity of sound waves is increased ten times by ossicles.
4. Chain of ear ossicles moves as a whole:

Handle of malleus moves inwards

Head of malleus and body of incus moves outwards

↓

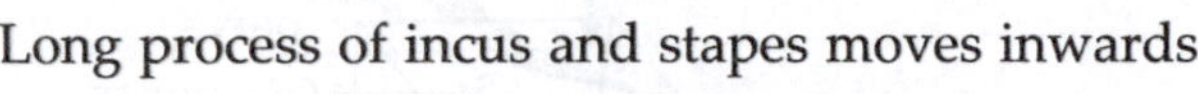

Long process of incus and stapes moves inwards

↓

Base of stapes is pushed in and out of the oval window (Fenestra Vestibuli)

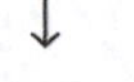

It vibrates the perilymph

Table 33.1: ***Bony Ossicles of Middle Ear***

Features	Malleus	Incus	Stapes
Development	Ist Pharyngeal arch	Ist Pharyngeal arch	Second pharyngeal arch
Shape	Hammer shaped	Anvil shaped	Stirrup shaped
Length	8-9 mm	10 mm	4 mm
Parts	Head, neck, manubrium, process (handle), anterior and lateral process	Body, Short process, Long process, (lentiform process)	Head, neck, Anterior, and Posterior crura Foot piece
Muscles attached	Tensor tympani is inserted into neck	No muscle	Stapedius muscle is inserted into neck

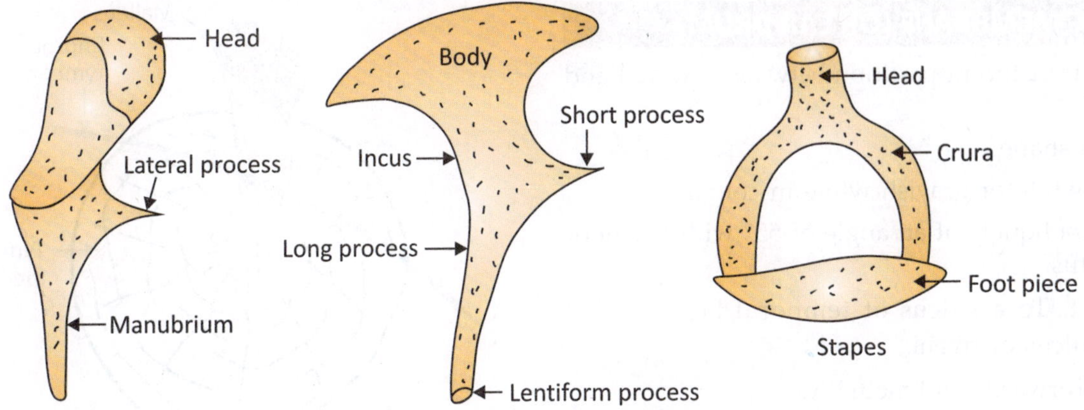

Fig. 33.7: *Ear ossicles-three bones*

Joints of Middle Ear

1. **Incudo malleolar joint:** Saddle type synovial joint between head of malleus and body of incus.
2. **Incudo stapedial joint:** Ball and socket, synovial type joint formed between long process of incus and head of stapes.

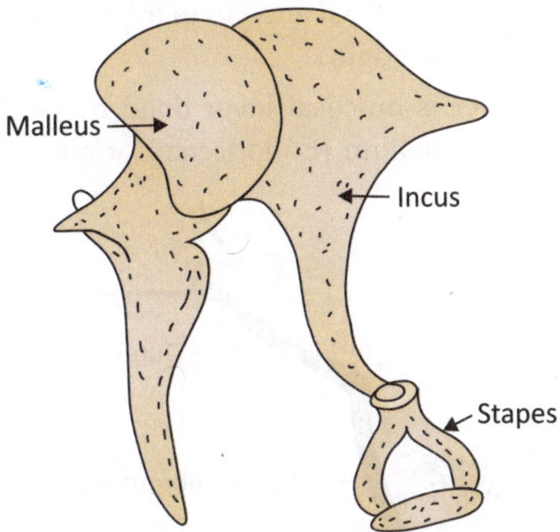

Fig. 33.8: *Ear ossicles*

3. Foot piece of stapes is fixed to oval window by annular ligament.

Muscles of Middle Ear

1. **Tensor tympani:** Arises from bony and cartilaginous part of auditory tube.

   Insertion: Into handle of malleus.

   Nerve supply: Branch from mandibular nerve (medial pterygoid nerve).

   Action: Damping the sound waves reaching the internal ear.

2. **Stapedius:** Arises from internal wall of pyramid present in posterior wall of middle ear.

   Insertion: Into neck of stapes.

   Nerve supply: Branch of facial nerve.

   Action: Damping the sound waves reaching middle ear.

Blood Supply of Middle Ear

1. Anterior tympanic artery – branch of maxillary artery.
2. Posterior tympanic artery – branch of stylomastoid artery branch of posterior auricular artery.
3. Petrosal branch of middle meningeal artery.
4. Superior tympanic artery branch of middle meningal artery.
5. Inferior tympanic artery branch of ascending pharyngeal artery.
6. Artery of pterygoid canal.
7. Tympanic branch of internal carotid artery.

Venous Drainage:

1. Pterygoid venous plexus
2. Superior petrosal sinus.

Lymphatic Drainage:

Retro pharyngeal group of lymph nodes.

Nerve Supply

Tympanic plexus is formed by:

1. Tympanic branch of glossopharyngeal nerve (sensory).
2. Carotico tympanic nerve (sympathetic) from plexus around internal carotid artery.

TYMPANIC MEMBRANE (OR EAR DRUM)

It is a thin, translucent partition between external and middle ear.

- Oval in shape.
- Pearly white or grayish white in colour.
- Placed obliquely at an angle of 55° with the floor of meatus.

Attachment: To a sulcus of temporal bone, called tympanic sulcus of riveni.

Direction: Forwards and medially.

Dimensions:

Vertically – 10 mm

Transverse – 8 mm.

Parts of the Membrane

There are two parts:

1. Pars tensa and
2. Pars flaccida.

Surfaces

Medial and lateral surface.

- Lateral surface is concave.
- Medial surface is convex, maximum convex point is called Umbo – Handle of malleus is attached to the inner surface of umbo.

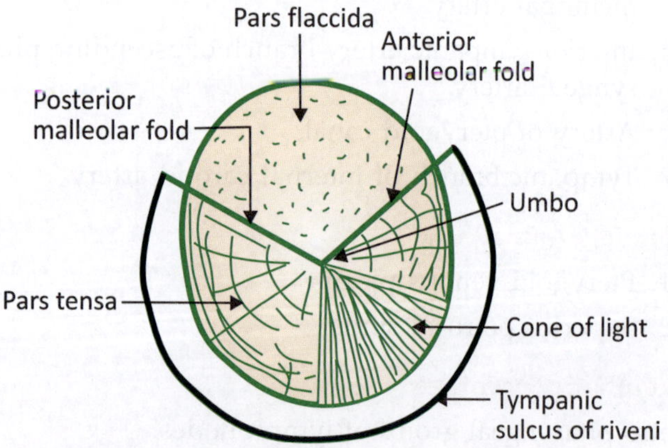

Fig. 33.9: *Lateral surface of tympanic membrane*

Cone of light is light reflex area present along antero-inferior part of membrane.

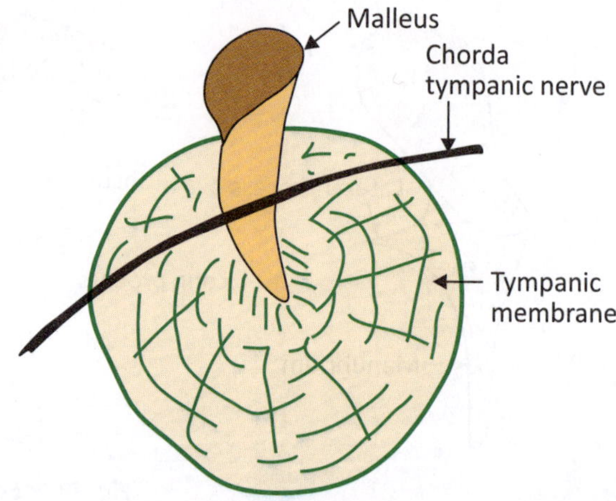

Fig. 33.10: *Medial surface of tympanic membrane*

Structure

These are layers:

1. Outer layer is cuticular – formed by skin epithelium (Ectodermal in origin).
2. Middle layer is fibrous – consisting of radial fibres which are superficial and circular fibres lies – deep (Mesodermal origin).
3. Inner layer is mucosal layer lined by ciliated columnar epithelium (Endodermal origin).

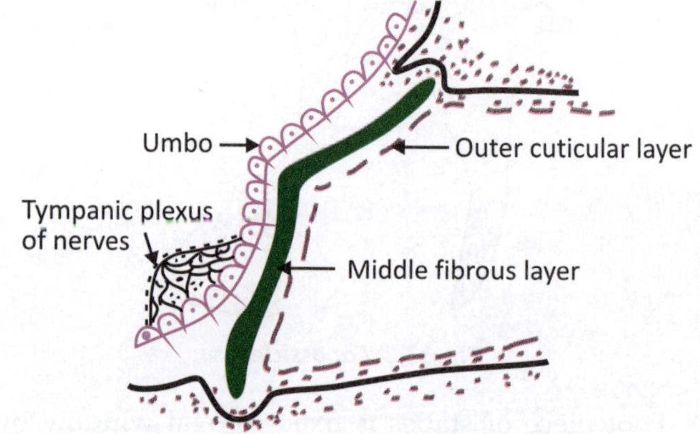

Fig. 33.11: *Structure of tympanic membrane and its curvatures*

Blood Supply

1. **External surface:** Deep auricular artery
2. **Internal surface:**
   - Anterior tympanic branch of maxillary artery.
   - Posterior tympanic branch of stylomastoid artery, branch of posterior auricular artery.

Venous Drainage

1. **External surface:** Into external jugular vein.
2. **Internal surface:** Into transverse sinus and venous plexus of pharyngo tympanic tube.

Lymphatic Drainage:

1. **External surface:** Into posterior auricular lymph node.
2. **Internal surface:** Into retro pharyngeal lymph node.

Nerve Supply

I. **External surface** is supplied by
   1. Auriculo temporal nerve – anterior half.
   2. Auricular branch of vagus – posterior half.

II. **Internal surface** is supplied by tympanic plexus, formed tympnic branch of glossopharyngeal nerve.

Applied Anatomy

1. **Myringitis:** Inflammation of tympanic membrane, it becomes reddish.
2. **Perforation of tympanic membrane** due to Acute Suppurative Otitis Media (ASOM) usually – antero inferior quadrant is perforated.
3. **Myringotomy:** Tympanic membrane is incised to drain the pus in middle ear.
4. **Tympanoplasty:** Reconstruction of tympanic membrane and ossicular chain after treating disease of middle ear.
5. Congenital atresia of meatus.
6. **Ear wax:** May close meatus and causes deafness.
7. **Otorrhoea:** In head injury, C.S.F. or blood leaks from ear.
8. **Foreign bodies:** Insects, maggots, peas, grains, pearl and stones etc.
9. **Inflammatory stenosis:** Causes deafness.
10. **Otoscope** is an instrument used for ear examination (for external auditory meatus and tympanic membrane).

MASTOID PROCESS

It is one of the five parts of temporal bone:

1. Squamous part
2. Mastoid part
3. Petrous part
4. Tympanic part
5. Styloid part.

Mastoid Part

It is situated postero inferiorly. It has two surfaces:

1. External surface
2. Internal surface.

There are two borders:

- Superior border
- Posterior border.

It is the downward prolongation of external surface of temporal bone – rough and convex in nature, gives insertion for the following muscles – superior to inferior.

1. Sternocleido mastoid
2. Splenius capitis
3. Langissimus capitis.

- Superior to insertion of sternocleidomastoid it gives origin to:
  - Auricularis posterior.
  - Occipital belly of occipito frontalis muscle.
  - Mastoid process is a nipple shaped projection.
  - It is absent in foetus, so facial nerve is very much superficially situated.
  - Along the medial surface of the process – mastoid notch is found – gives origin to posterior belly of digastric muscle.
  - Medial to the notch groove for occipital artery is situated.

Internal surface: Bounds the posterior cranial fossa. It is grooved by sigmoid sinus.

Borders

1. **Superior border** is thick and serrated, it articulates with inferior border of parietal bone at the mastoid angle.
2. **Posterior border** is thick and serrated, it articulates with the squamous part of occipital bone.
   - Mastoid air cells and mastoid antrum are found in the mastoid part. They communicate with

the middle ear through aditus to mastoid antrum, when mastoid air cells are not developed the mastoid process is solid and sclerotic.

MASTOID ANTRUM

Mastoid antrum is a small air filled space situated in the posterior part of petrous temporal bone.

Shape: Circular

Diameter: 10 mm

Capacity: 1 ml.

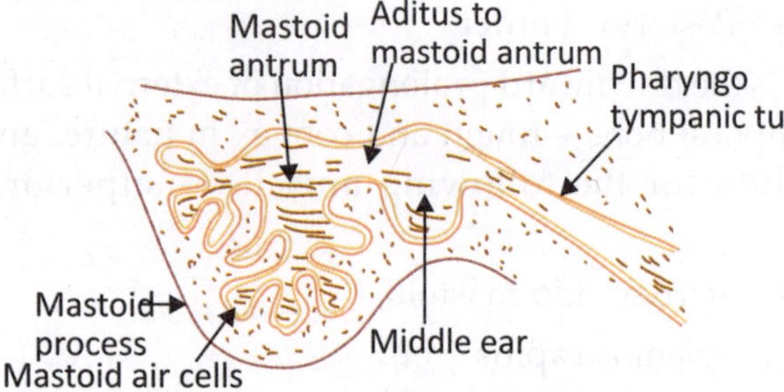

Fig. 33.12: *Mastoid antrum*

Boundaries:

Superior: Tegmen tympani (2 mm thick).

Inferior: Mastoid process and air cells.

Anterior:

1. Medial part of external auditory meatus.
2. Epitympanic recess of middle ear.

Aditus is related to VIIth nerve above and behind.

Posterior: Thin plate seprates the antrum from:

1. Sigmoid sinus and
2. Cerebellum.

Medial:

1. Facial nerve canal.
2. Lateral semi circular canal.
3. Posterior semi circular canal.

∴ Infections affecting medial wall damages VIIth nerve or semi circular canals.

Lateral: Cortex of mastoid bone medial to supra-meatal triangle.

- **In new born:** Lateral wall thickness is about 2 mm and increases 1 mm per year. (Antrum is of adult size at birth – size of small pea.)
- **In adult:** About 15 mm (no increase after puberty) thick.

Communications:

Anteriorly: Epitympanic recess.

Postero inferiorly: Mastoid air cells.

Mastoid air cells: These are variable in size and arrangement:

- Situated in mastoid antrum.
- Communicate with middle ear.

Classification: According to the site:

1. Zygomatic cells
2. Subdural cells
3. Cells of petrosal angle
4. Peri sinus cells
5. Tip cells
6. Facial cells.

Types of Mastoid Process

According to air cells:

1. **Cellular mastoid process:** Air cells are larger in size and numerous in number – found in 80%.
2. **Diploic mastoid process:** Air cells are smaller in size and less in number.
3. **Sclerotic mastoid process:** No air cells are found 20%.

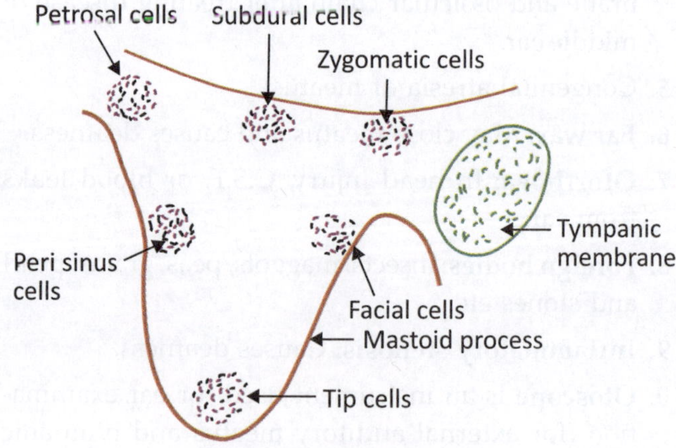

Fig. 33.13: *Mastoid air cells*

Blood Supply (Arterial Supply)

Posterior tympanic artery arises from stylomastoid artery branch of posterior auricular artery.

Venous Drainage of Mastoid Antrum

1. Mastoid emissary vein
2. Sigmoid sinus
3. Posterior auricular vein.

Lymphatic Drainage

Posterior auricular nodes.

Nerve Supply

1. Tympanic plexus (IX)
2. Nervi spinosus (V_3).

Supra Meatal Triangle of Macewen

Surgical exposure of mastoid antrum is done through this triangle.

It is bounded:

- **Superiorly:** Supra mastoid crest.
- **Posteriorly:** Perpendicular line drawn from supra-mastoid crest to the posterior border of external auditory meatus.
- **Antero inferiorly:** Superior and posterior borders of external auditory meatus.
  - On the surface of triangle – supra meatal spine of Henla is found.

Applied Anatomy

1. Congenital absence of mastoid process.
2. At the time of birth mastoid antrum is well developed, mastoid air cells are rudimentary. Only by 2nd year mastoid process develop, and only by 4th year mastoid air cells enter the process. At puberty mastoid air cells are fully grown. In 20% mastoid has no air cells (Sclerotic).
3. **Mastoiditis:**
   - May cause labyrinthitis or facial palsy.
   - Sigmoid sinus thrombosis, subdural abscess etc.

Applied Anatomy of Middle Ear

1. **A.S.O.M. (Acute Suppurative Otitis Media):** Perforation of tympanic membrane at antero inferior quadrant.
2. **C.S.O.M. (Chronic Infection Otitis Media):** Tympanic membrane ruptured at:
   - Pars flaccida or
   - Pars tensa.
3. **Haemotympanum:** Blood is present in tympanic cavity – head injury.
4. **Otosclerosis:** Fixation of stapes at oval window due to new bone formation – causes conductive deafness.
5. **Hyper acousia:** Paralysis of stapedius muscle after VIIth nerve injury – severe hizzing noise in ear present.
6. **Tympano sclerosis:** Due to C.S.O.M. depostition of chalky white patches on tympanic membrane and on ear ossicles.

AUDITORY TUBE OR PHARYNGO TYMPANIC TUBE OR EUSTACHIAN TUBE

It is a trumpet shaped tube which connects the middle ear cavity with naso pharynx.

Develops: From medial part of tubo tympanic recess.

In children: Tube is shorter, wider and straighter.

Length: About 3.6 to 4 cm.

Direction: Downwards, forwards and medially.

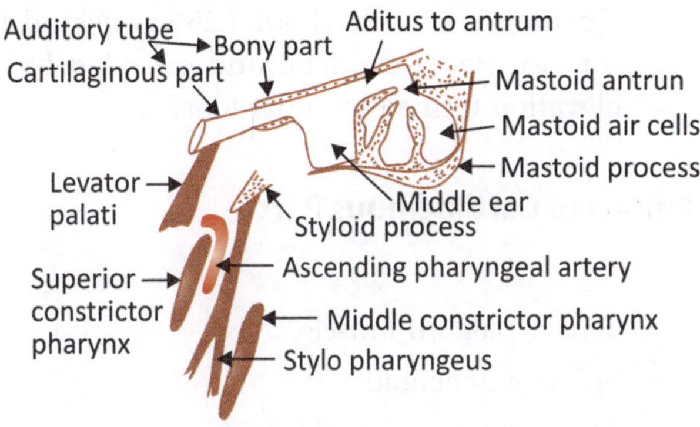

Fig. 33.14: *Coronal section showing auditory tube*

Parts

- Posterior 1/3 – Bony part – 12 mm long, lies in petrous temporal bone.
- Anterior 2/3 – Cartilagenous part – 25 mm long lies in sulcus tube (a groove between greater wing of sphenoid and apex of petrous temporal).

Isthmus is the junction of anterior 2/3 and posterior 1/3.

- Oval on cross-section.

Relations of Bony Part

Superior: Canal for tensor tympani muscle.

Inferiorly: Tympanic plate of temporal bone.

Medial: Carotid canal.

Laterally: Chorda tympani nerve.

- Spine of sphenoid
- Temporo mandibular joint
- Lower portion of tegmen tympani.

Cartilagenous part of tube (Anterior 2/3 = 25 mm).

A triangular cartilage forms – superior and medial walls of the tube–lateral wall and floor is completed by fibrous membrane.

- Cartilagenous part is attached to the anterior part of bony tube.
- Passes through the space above the upper border of superior constrictor of pharynx (i.e., sinus of Morgagni).
- It pierces the pharyngobasilar and buccopharyngeal fascia and opens into the lateral wall of naso-pharynx.
- Opening is present about 1.25 cm behind the inferior nasal choncha and guarded by an elevation formed by tubal tonsil.

Relations of Cartilaginous Part

Antero-laterally:

- Tensor palatini muscle.
- Spine of sphenoid.
- Mandibular nerve with its branches.
- Otic ganglion and chorda tympani nerve.
- Middle meningeal artery.
- Medial pterygoid plate.

Postero-medially:

- Apex of petrous temporal bone.
- Levator palati.

Muscles Acting on Tube: Tensor palati, levator palati and salpingopharyngeus – dilates the tube.

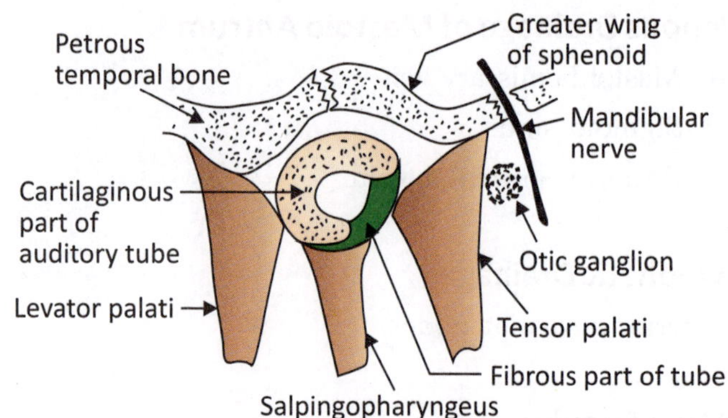

Fig. 33.15: ***Relations of auditory tube***

Muscles attached on inferior surface of tube are:

- Portion of levator palati and
- Slapingopharyngeus.

Blood Supply

- Artery of pterygoid canal.
- Middle menigeal artery branches.
- Branches of ascending pharyngeal artery.

Veins: Drain into:

- Pterygoid venous plexus and
- Pharyngeal venous plexus.

Lymphatics: Go to retropharyngeal group of lymph nodes.

Nerve Supply

- Pharyngeal branch of pterygo palatine ganglion (maxillary nerve) at ostium.
- Cartilaginous part by nervi spinosus (mandibular nerve).
- Bony part by tympanic plexus (Glossopharyngeal nerve).

Function

It communicates middle ear cavity with exterior, thus ensuring equal air pressure on both sides of tympanic membrane.

- Tube is usually closed.
- It opens during swallowing, yawning and sneezing by the action of tensor and levator palati.

Applied Anatomy of Auditory Tube

1. Infection from throat may pass to middle ear via tube, common in children because tube is shorter, straighter and wider.
2. When tympanic membrane is ruptured, fluid entering the external ear enters the pharynx through middle ear and then through auditory tube.
3. Inflammation of tube is known as salpingitis.
4. Valselva's test.
5. Eustachian catheterization.
6. Eustachian catarrah – Allergic condition.

INTERNAL EAR OR LABYRINTH

- Lies in petrous part of temporal bone.
- Consists of a bony labyrinth within which lies a membranous labyrinth.
- Membranous labyrinth is filled with fluid called endolymph.
- Membranous labyrinth is separated from bony labyrinth by another fluid called perilymph.

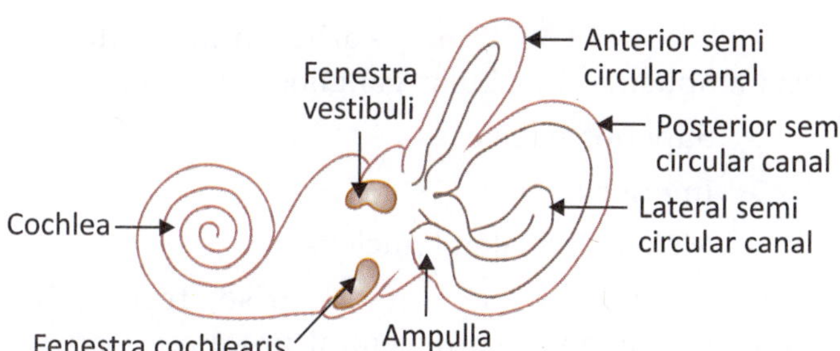

Fig. 33.16: *Internal ear bony labyrinth*

BONY LABYRINTH

Consists of three parts:

1. Cochlea – anteriorly
2. Vestibule – in the middle
3. Semicircular canals posteriorly:
   (a) Anterior semicircular canal.
   (b) Posterior semicircular canal.
   (c) Lateral semicircular canal.

1. Cochlea

Has a conical central axis. Modiolus around which cochlear canal makes two and three quarter turns.

- A spiral bony ridge called spiral lamina projects from modiolus and divides the cochlear canal partially into scala vestibuli above and scala tympani below. Division is completed by basilar membrane.
- Scala vestibuli communicates with scala tympani at the apex of cochlea – Helicotrema.

2. Vestibule

Vestibule is the middle part of internal ear.

- Laterally related to middle ear.
- Fenestra vestibuli communicates vestibule with the middle ear.
- Medial wall of vestibule has an opening for aqueduct of vestibule. It opens through a fissure on posterior surface of petrous temporal bone and is closed by ductus endolymphaticus.

3. Semicircular Canals

Three in number:

- Arranged as anterior, posterior and lateral.
- Situated above and behind the vestibule.
- Canals are arranged at right angles with each other.
- Dilated lower ends called ampullae.
- Crus commune is the site of fusion of posterior end of anterior semicircular canal with anterior end of posterior semicircular canal.
- Anterior canal is also known as superior canal.

MEMBRANOUS LABYRINTH

A closed system of inter communicating membranous sacs and ducts within the bony labyrinth and is filled with endolymph.

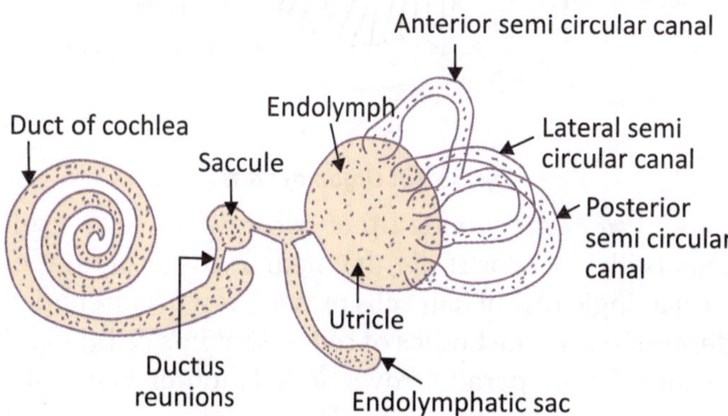

Fig. 33.17: *Membranous labyrinth*

Parts

- Duct of cochlea, utricle, saccule and
- Semicircular ducts.

Parts of epithelium of membranous labyrinth are specialized to form sensory receptors for sound.

1. **Organ of corti:** Present in duct of cochelea anteriorly.

   With in vestibule lies utricle and saccule – lined by specialized neuro epithelium called maculae is responsible for linear acceleration and gravitational pull. For static balance – thickend neuro epithelium on medial wall of saccule and utricle is responsible.

2. **In semicircular ducts:** Specialized neuro epithelium is present in ampula – as cristae is responsible for kinetic balance – angular acceleration and caloric stimulation.

Duct of Cochlea or Scala Media

Situated in between scala vestibuli and scala tympani. Floor of duct is formed by vestibular membrane, on the upper surface of basilar membrane the duct of organ of corti is arranged.

Organ of corti is an end organ formed by neuro epithelium of auditory function. Peripheral processes of spiral ganglion cells supply the organ of corti and central processes become the cochlear nerve Endolymph is secreted by stria vascularis situated on the outer wall.

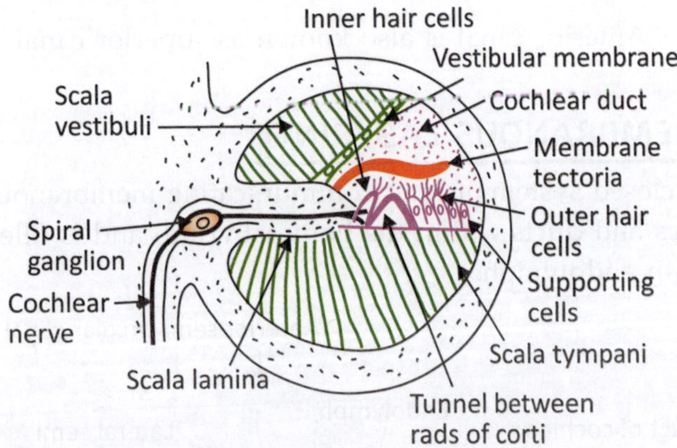

Fig. 33.18: *Organ of corti*

Tunnel of corti is made up of two rows of cells – still cells (Pillars of corti), on the medial side of tunnel of corti a single row of hair cells present, rest in cup shaped depressions in the bodies of cells – Deitier's cells lateral to tunnel four parallel rows of cells (outer hair cells) supported by Henson cells.

Tectorial membrane is made up of jelly like material.

- About 3,500 inner hair cells.
- About 20,000 outer hair cells present.
- Arrangement of cells on the upper surface of basilar membrane from medial to lateral are:
  1. Border cells.
  2. Inner hair cells.
  3. Inner phalangeal cells.
  4. Outer phalangeal cells and outer hair cells
  5. Cells of Henson → cells of Claudius or supporting cells.

Utricle: Is connected with saccule via – Ductus utriculo – saccularis, utricle has a lining of neuro epithelium called macula → end organ → responding to gravitational pull and linear acceleration.

Saccule has a patch of neuro epithelium called macula – responding to gravitational pull and linear acceleration (static balance).

Semicircular ducts: Floating in perilymph, ampullae contain → crista ampularis → hair present get displaced during movements of endolymph respond to angular accelaration and caloric stimulates (kinetic balance).

Vestibular part of VIIIth nerve arises form macula and crista ampularis, vestibular ganglion – having –

- Superior nucleus
- Inferior nucleus
- Medial and lateral nucleus.

Chochlear part of VIIIth nerve arises from spiral ganglion of organ of corti, central processes – arising from

- Ventral cochlear nucleus.
- Dorsal cochlear nucleus.

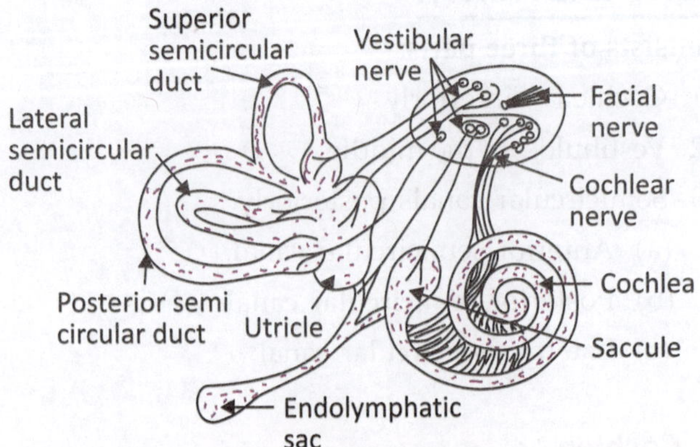

Fig. 33.19: *Distribution of vestibular and cochlear nerve to membranous labyrinth*

Endolymph is secreted by stria vascularis.

I. **Spiral duct of cochlea:** Organ of hearing (organ of corti).

II. (a) **Utricle and saccule:** Organ of static balance (Maculae).

(b) **Semicircular ducts:** Organ of kinetic balance (Cristae Ampularis).

Blood Supply of Labyrinth

1. Labyrinthine branch of basilar artery accompanies vestibulo cochlear nerve.
2. Stylomastoid branch of posterior auricular artery.

Venous Drainage

Into superior and inferior petrosal sinus or transverse sinus and internal jugular vein.

Applied Anatomy

1. Changes in secretion and absorption of endolypmph results in Mennier's disease with vertigo and deafness.
2. Certain drugs, e.g., Streptomycin, quinine may affect cochlear nerve and causes deafness.
3. **Vestibular nerve involvement produces:**
   - Vertigo
   - Nystagmus
   - Nausea and vomiting, tachycardia.
4. **Cochlear nerve involvement:**
   - Tinnitus
   - Deafness
   - Hearing scotoma (deafness for certain pitches)
   - Word deafness (sensory aphasia).
5. Fracture of petrous part of temporal bone may involve VIIth and VIIIth nerve.
6. Acoustic neuroma is a tumour affecting (VIII) vestibulo cochlear nerve – cochlear part especially.

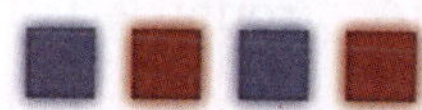

CHAPTER 34

Cranial Cavity

INTRODUCTION

This is a bony highest placed cavity of the body containing vital organs like brain enclosed in tough membranous coverings – called meninges. The cranium protects these vital structures and is formed by bones.

Bony features: Out of 22 bones of skull 8 bones take part in formation of cranial cavity.

A. Frontal – 1
B. Parietal – 2
C. Occipital – 1
D. Temporal – 1
E. Sphenoid – 1
F. Ethmoid – 1.

For descriptive purpose we divide cranial cavity into:

I. **Skull cap or calvaria:** This forms roof of cranial cavity.

II. **Internal surface of base of skull:** This forms lateral wall and floor of cavity.

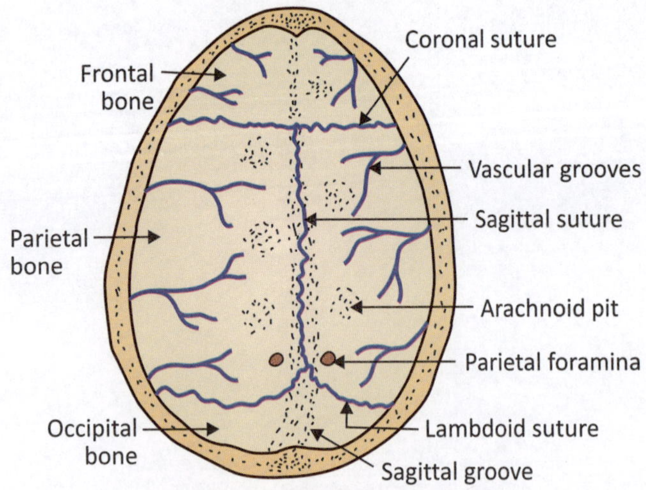

Fig. 34.1: *Skull cap or calvaria (interior)*

Contents

Cranial cavity contains:

1. Brain with meninges.
2. Venous dural sinuses.
3. **Arteries:**
   (a) Internal carotid arteries
   (b) Vertebral arteries
   (c) Middle meningeal arteries
   (d) Accessory meningeal arteries.
4. Roots of 12 cranial nerves and their meningeal branches.
5. **Four petrosal nerves:**
   (a) Deep petrosal nerve
   (b) Greater petrosal nerve
   (c) Lesser petrosal nerve
   (d) External petrosal nerve.

CRANIAL FOSSAE

The interior of the base of skull is divided into three fossae:

1. Anterior cranial fossa
2. Middle cranial fossa
3. Posterior cranial fossa.

They are arranged above downwards.

I. ANTERIOR CRANIAL FOSSA

It is the highest among the cranial fossae.

Boundaries:

Anterior and sides – Frontal bone.

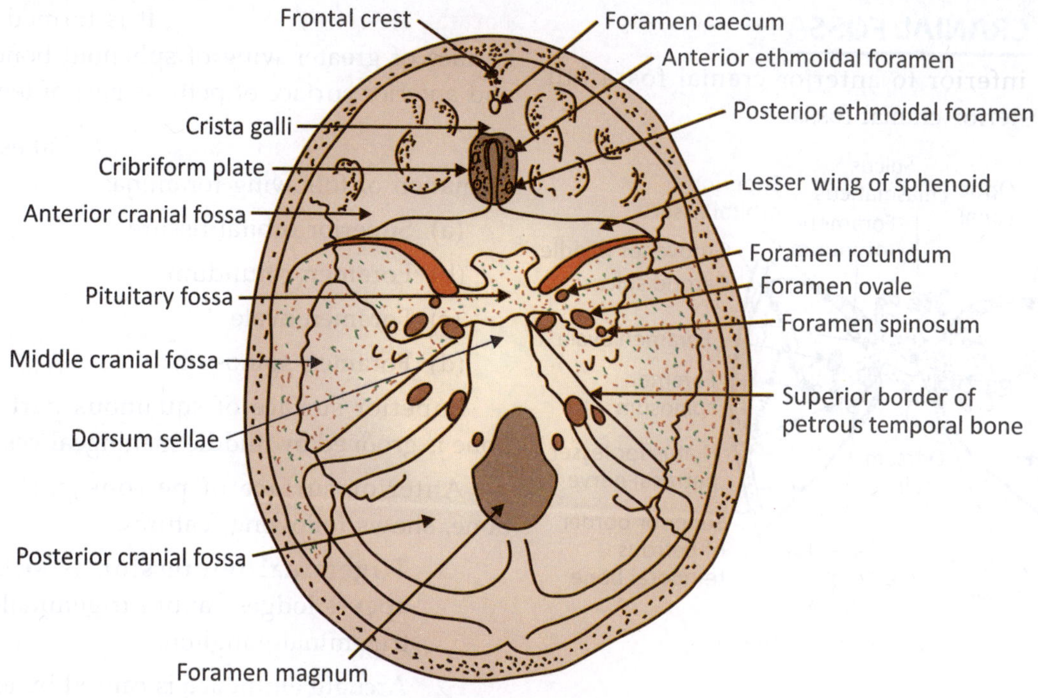

Fig. 34.2: ***Supeior surface of base of skull***

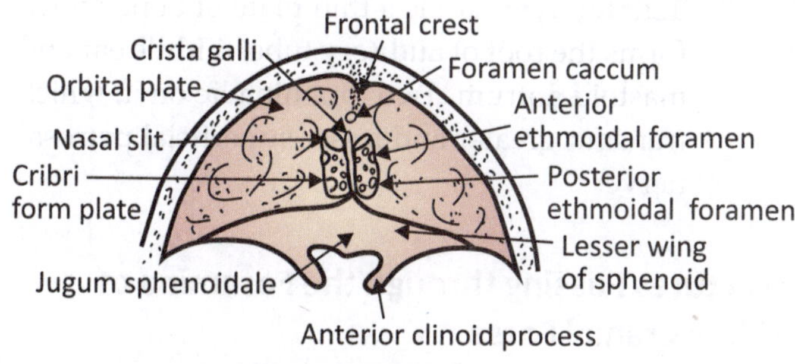

Fig. 34.3: ***Anterior cranial fossa***

Posterior:

- Lesser wing and body of sphenoid bone.
- Lesser wing projects postero medially to form the anterior clinoid process.

Floor:

1. Orbital plate of frontal bone.
2. Cribriform plate of ethmoid bone.
3. Lesser wing of sphenoid and anterior portion of body of sphenoid bone.

Anteriorly in the midline – median frontal crest is situated.

Characteristic Features of the Fossa are:

1. **Foramen caecum** is present between median frontal crest and crista galli of the ethmoid bone.

   In foetus an emissary vein passes through this foramen, which connects olfactory venous plexus with superior sagittal sinus. After birth it obliterates and disappears.
2. **Crista galli** is an upward projection of perpandicular plate of ethmoid bone. It gives attachment to falx cerebri (Dural fold).
3. **Anterior and posterior ethmoidal foramina** are found along the sides of ethmoid bone. Anterior ethmoidal foramen transmits the anterior ethmoidal nerve and vessels from the orbit to the nose.
   - Posterior ethmoidal foramen transmits only posterior ethmoidal artery.
4. **Cribriform plate** is situated on ether side of crista galli. Through this 15 to 20 olfactory nerves passes from the nose to the anterior cranial fossa to join the olfactory bulb.
5. **Jugum sphenoidale** is situated anterior to the sulcus chiasmaticus sulcus lodges – optic chiasma.
6. **Orbital plate of frontal bone** has impressions caused by gyri and sulci of frontal lobe of cerebrum.
7. Posterior border of lesser wing of sphenoid is related to spheno-parietal sinus.
8. The anterior clinoid process gives attachment for free border of the tentorium cerebelli.

II. MIDDLE CRANIAL FOSSA

It is situated inferior to anterior cranial fossa but superior to posterior cranial fossa.

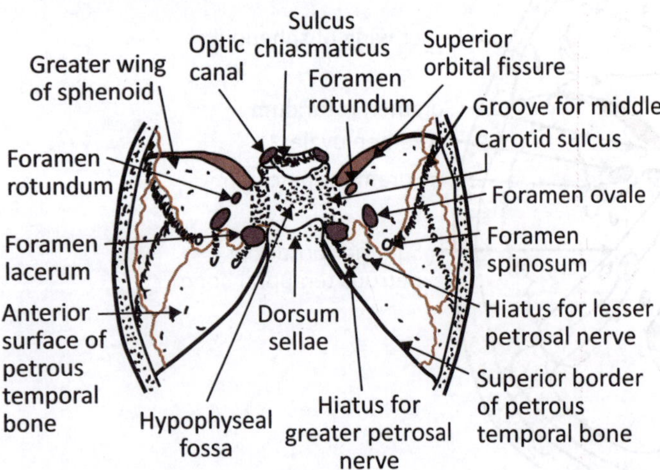

Fig. 34.4: *Middle cranial fossa*

Boundaries:

Anterior – Posterior border of lesser wing of sphenoid.

Posterior – Superior border of petrons part of temporal bone.

Dorsum sellae of sphenoid bone.

Lateral – Squamous part of temporal bone.

Greater wing of sphenoid bone.

Antero inferior angle of the parietal bone.

Floor

- Body of sphenoid.
- Greater wing of sphenoid bone.
- Petrous part of temporal bone.

Characteristic features are:

- In the middle of this fossa sella tursica is situated. It is a depression on the body of sphenoid and lodges pituitary gland.
- Behind sella tursica – dorsum sellae is situated. Lateral sides of dorsum sellae projects upwards and forms posterior clinoid processes, it gives attachment to attached border of tentorium cerebelli.
- Petrosal process is a spicular process projects laterally below the posterior clinoid process, it connects the apex of petrous temporal bone by the petroclinoid ligament of Gruber.
- On either of sella tursica – carotid grooves are situated – lodges internal carotid artery with sympathetic plexus of nerves around it.

Lateral aspect of the fossa: It is formed by superior surface of greater wing of sphenoid bone, squamous and anterior surface of petrous part of temporal bone.

Greater wing of sphenoid bone: Takes part in the formation of following foramina:

(a) Superior orbital fissure
(b) Foramen rotundum
(c) Foramen ovale
(d) Foramen spinosum.

Superior surface of squamous part of temporal bone is grooved by middle meningeal vessels.

Anterior surface of petrous part of temporal bone, shows following features:

1. **Trigeminal impression is situated at the apex** – lodges cavum trigeminale containing trigeminal ganglion.
2. **Arcuate eminence** is caused by anterior semicircular canal of internal ear.
3. **Tegmen tympani** is a thin plate of bone which forms the roof of auditory tube, middle ear and mastoid antrum. Two foramina lie on it, which transmit greater and lesser superficial petrosal nerve.

Structures Passing through the Foramina of Middle Cranial Fossa

1. **Optic foramen:**
   (a) Optic nerve with meninges.
   (b) Ophthalmic artery with its sympathetic plexus of nerves around it.
2. **Superior orbital fissure** is an oblique cleft, forms the apex of orbit.

   Boundaries:
   - Superiorly – Lesser wing of sphenoid.
   - Inferiorly – Greater wing of sphenoid.
   - Medially – Body of sphenoid.
   - A common tendinous ring divides the fissure into three compartments.

   (a) Structures passing lateral to the common tendinous ring
   1. Lacrimal nerve.
   2. Frontal nerve.
   3. Trochlear nerve.

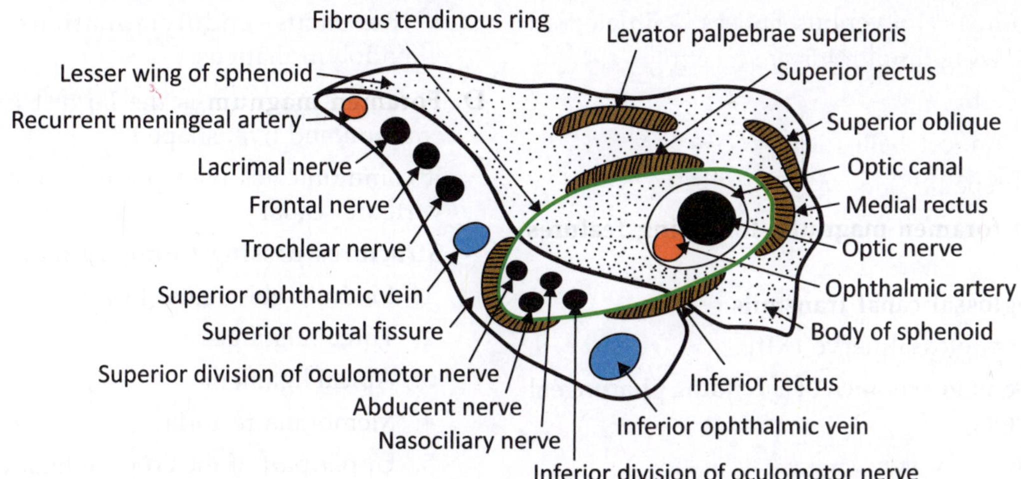

Fig. 34.5: ***Structures passing through superior orbital fissure and optic canal***

4. Superior ophthalmic vein.
5. Recurrent branch of lacrimal artery is the lateral most structure.
6. Lacrimal branch of middle meningeal artery.

(b) Structures passing within the common tendinous ring

1. Superior and inferior division of oculomotor nerve (III).
2. Naso ciliary nerve (V_1).
3. Abducent nerve (VI).

(c) Structures passing medial to the common tendinous ring

— Inferior ophthalmic vein.

3. Foramen rotundum

Transmits: Maxillary division of trigeminal nerve (V_2).

4. Foramen ovale

(a) Motor and sensory roots of mandibular nerve (V_3).
(b) Accessory middle meningeal artery.
(c) Emissary vein – connects pterygoid venous plexus with cavernous sinus.
(d) Lesser superficial petrosal nerve.

5. Foramen spinosum

(a) Middle meningeal artery.
(b) Nervi spinosus (meningeal nerve) (V_3).

6. Emissary sphenoidal foramen of vesalius – not always present. When present it transmits emissary vein connecting pterygoid venous plexus with cavernous sinus.

7. Foramen lacerum

(a) Meningeal branch of ascending pharyngeal artery.
(b) Emissary vein – connecting cavernous sinus with pharyngeal plexus of veins.

8. Carotid canal

(a) Internal carotid artery with sympathetic plexus of nerves around it.
(b) Emissary vein – from pharyngeal plexus to cavernous sinus.

III. POSTERIOR CRANIAL FOSSA

It is the deepest cranial fossa.

Boundaries:

Anterior:

1. Dorsum sellae.
2. Body of sphenoid.
3. Basilar part of occipital bone.
4. Posterior surface of petrous part of temporal bone.

Posterior: Squamous part of occipital bone.

Laterally:

1. Mastoid part of temporal bone.
2. Condylar part of occipital bone.

Characteristic Features of the Fossa are:

A. Internal occipital protuberance is situated in the centre of inner aspect of squamous part of occipital bone. Confluence of venous sinuses is situated on it and following dural folds are meeting:

1. Falx cerebri
2. Tentorium cerebelli
3. Falx cerebelli.

B. Lateral to foramen magnum, following features are seen:

1. **Hypoglossal canal transmits**
   (i) Hypoglossal nerve (XII).
   (ii) Meningeal branch of ascending pharyngeal artery.
   (iii) Emissary vein.
2. **Jugular tubercle** is situated above the hypoglossal canal and projects into jugular foramen. It is grooved by rootlets of IXth, Xth and XIth neves.
3. **Jugular foramen transmits:**
   (i) Terminal part of sigmoid sinus and commencement of internal jugular vein.
   (ii) IXth, Xth and XIth cranial nerves.
   (iii) Emissary vein
   (iv) Inferior petrosal sinus
   (v) Meningeal branch of ascending – pharyngeal artery.
4. **Posterior condylar canal:** This is not always present, when present it transmits an emissary vein connecting occipital venous plexus with sigmoid sinus.

C. Posterior surface of petrous part of temporal bone, shows following features:

1. Upper border is grooved by superior petrosal sinus.
2. Posterior and inferior aspect is grooved by sigmoid sinus.
3. Antero inferior aspect is grooved by inferior petrosal sinus.
4. **Internal acoustic meatus transmits**
   (i) Facial nerve (VII).
   (ii) Vestibulo-cochlear nerve (VIII).
   (iii) Labyrinthine artery.
5. Subarcuate fossa is a shallow depression situated postero-lateral to internal acoustic meatus.
6. Aqueduct of vestibule is a slit like opening behind the internal acoustic meatus. It lodges the sacus endolymphaticus and ductus endolymphaticus.

D. Foramen magnum is the largest foramen of the cranium and oval shaped.

It communicates with posterior cranial fossa and vertebral canal.

Structures passing through this are:

1. Medulla oblongata (lower end)
2. Three meninges
3. Apical ligament
4. Membrana tectoria
5. Upper part of the cruciate ligament
6. Right and left vertebral arteries
7. Spinal root of accessory nerves
8. Sympathetic plexus of nerves around vertebral arteries
9. Anterior spinal artery
10. Posterior spinal arteries
11. Veins accompanying the arteries
12. Tonsil of the cerebellum.

Meninges: Membranes covering the brain and spinal cord are Duramater or patchy meninx.

- Arachnoid mater and Pia mater or Leptomeninges.

DURAMATER OR PATCHY MENINX

Double layered tough covering of brain:

(i) Endosteal layer – outer
(ii) Meningeal layer – inner one.

Both layers are closely held, together except at Dural Venous sinuses.

1. **Endosteal layer** is connected to skull by sutural ligaments and anchored to borders of foramina at base of skull.
   - Outer layer is crossed by meningeal vessels.

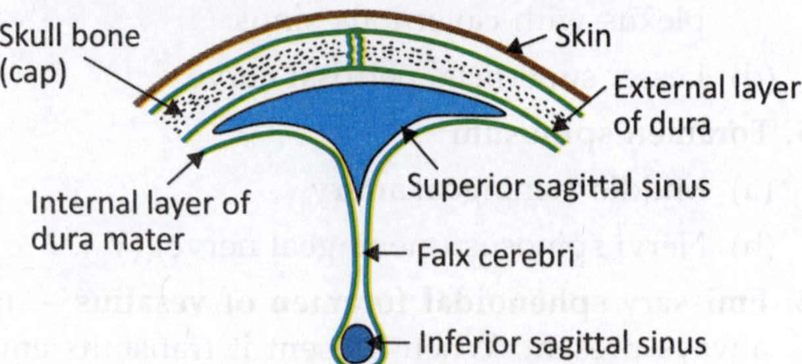

Fig. 34.6: *Fold of duramater-encephali*

2. **Meningeal layer:** Reduplicated at certain places to form folds
   (a) **Vertical folds**
      (i) Falx cerebri
      (ii) Falx cerebelli.
   (b) **Horizontal folds**
      (i) Tentorium cerebelli
      (ii) Diaphragm sellae.
      - These folds divide the cranial cavity into compartments to lodge various parts of brain.

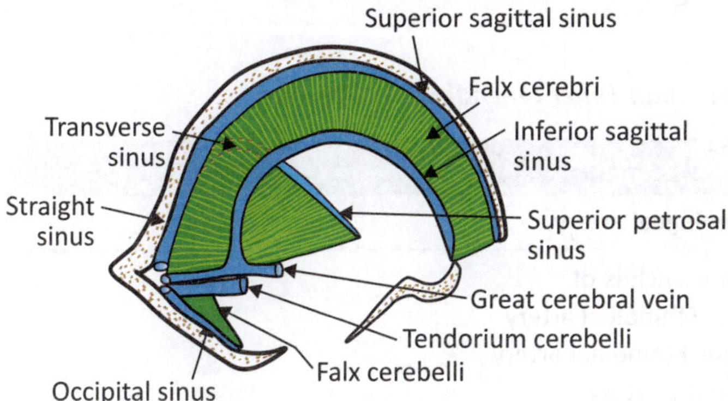

Fig. 34.7: *Sagittal section showing folds of duramater*

Falx Cerebri:

Sickle shaped fold.

- Present in midline between median fissure of brain.
- Separates two cerebral hemispere.

Attachment:

Anteriorly:

- Crista galli and
- Median frontal crest.

Posteriorly and inferiorly – joins tentorium cerebelli.

Structure enclosed:

1. Superior sagittal sinus – upper border.
2. In lower border – inferior sagittal sinus and straight sinus.

Tentorium Cerebelli

Present in posterior cranial fossa and forms roof.

- Separates cerebrum from cerebellum.
- Has attached and free border.

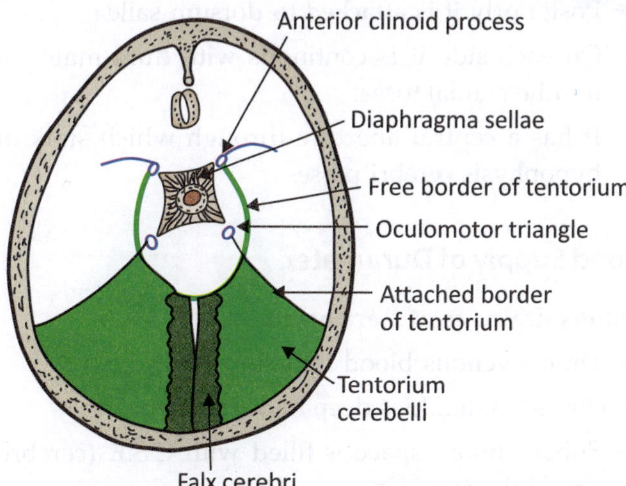

Fig. 34.8: *Tentorium cerebelli*

Attached border: Posterior to internal occipital protuberence is attached and also to lips of transverse sulcus.

Anteriorly and laterally attached to upper border of petrous temporal and posterior clinoid process.

Free border is concave and forms – Tentorial notch which lodges – mid-brain.

- Attached to anterior clinoid process between free and attached border is a triangular space called oculomotor triangle.
- Below free border (trochlear) – IVth cranial nerve passes.

Relations:

Superiorly – Cerebrum and Falx cerebri.

Inferiorly – Cerebellum and Falx cerebelli.

Anteriorly – Mid- brain.

Venous sinuses: Related are –

- Straight sinus
- Confluence of sinuses
- Transverse sinuses (right and left)
- Superior petrosal sinuses (right and left)
- Cavum trigeminale – lodges trigeminal ganglion.

Diaphragma Sellae

- It is a small circular, horizontal fold of dura mater forming the roof of hypophyseal fossa.
- Anteriorly it is attached to tuberculum sallae.

- Posteriorly it is attached to dorsum sallea.
- On each side it is continous with dura mater of middle cranial fossa.
- It has a central aperture through which stalk of hypophysis cerebri passes.

Blood Supply of Duramater

Venous drainage of duramater:

- Drains venous blood into sinuses.

Arachnoid mater: Lies deep to duramater.

- Subarachnoid space is filled with C.S.F. (cerebro spinal fluid).
- Dilated subarchnoid spaces are called cisterns, e.g.
  - Cisterna pontis – space anterior to pons and medulla.
  - Inter peduncular cistern – space anterior to mid-brain peduncles.
  - Cerebello – Medullary cistern – space posterior to cerebellum and medulla.
- Subarachnoid space lodges blood vessels to supply brain.

Piamater is a thin vascular membrane which closely invests the brain, dipping into various sulci and other irregularities of its surface.

Table 34.1: ***Outer layer is Vvery Vascular than Inner One which is Fibrous***

S. No.	Area of Distribution	Artery of Supply
1.	Vault or dura of supra tentorial space	1. Middle meningeal artery
2.	Dura of anterior cranial fossa	2. Meningeal branches of – Anterior Ethmoidal artery – Posterior Ethmoidal artery – Ophthalmic artery
3.	Dura of middle cranial fossa	3. Middle meningeal artery of – Accessory meningeal artery – Internal carotid artery – Meningeal branch of ascending pharyngeal artery
4.	Dura of posterior cranial fossa	4. Meningeal branches of – Vertebral artery IVth part – Occipital artery – Ascending-pharyngeal artery

Table 34.2: ***Nerve Supply of Duramater***

S. No.	Area	Nerves (Meningeal branch)
1.	Dura of vault	1. Ophthalmic division of Trigeminal nerve
2.	Dura of anterior cranial fossa	2. Anterior Ethmoidal Nerve V_1 – Maxillary Nerve V_2
3.	Middle cranial fossa	3. Maxillary Nerve V_2 – Mandibular Nerve V_3 – Trigeminal ganglion
4.	Posterior cranial fossa	4. Recurrent branches of C_1, C_2 and C_3 spinal nerves. – Meningeal branches of IXth, X^{th} (vagus) and 12th cranial nerves. – Sympathetic – meningeal branch from superior cervical ganglion.

VENOUS SINUSES (DURAL VENOUS SINUSES)

- Venous spaces present between two layers of duramater, lined by endothelium.
- No muscle in their walls and have no valves.
- **Receives venous blood from:**
  - Brain
  - Meninges
  - Skull bones
  - Excess of C.S.F. is poured into them.
- Communicate with veins outside the skull through emissary veins – helps in keeping the pressure of blood constant in the sinuses.
- Venous sinuses are 23 in number:
  - Paired – 8
  - Unpaired – 7

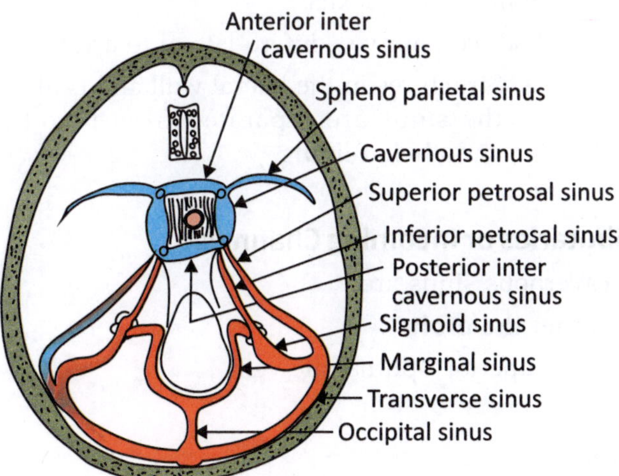

Fig. 34.9: ***Dural venous sinuses***

Paired cranial venous sinuses: These are on right and left side:

1. Cavernous sinus
2. Superior petrosal sinus
3. Inferior petrosal sinus
4. Transverse sinus
5. Sigmoid sinus
6. Spheno parietal sinus
7. Petro squamous sinus
8. Middle meningeal sinus/veins.

Unpaired sinuses: They are in median position:

1. Superior sagittal sinus
2. Inferior sagittal sinus
3. Straight sinus
4. Occipital sinus
5. Basilar plexus of veins
6. Anterior inter cavernous sinus
7. Posterior inter cavernous sinus.

CAVERNOUS SINUS

Situation:

- Large paired venous sinus, present in the middle cranial fossa on the sides of body of sphenoid.

Size:

2 cm long and 1 cm wide.

- Space is divided into multiple small spaces by means of trabeculae giving honeycomb appearance – called caverns.

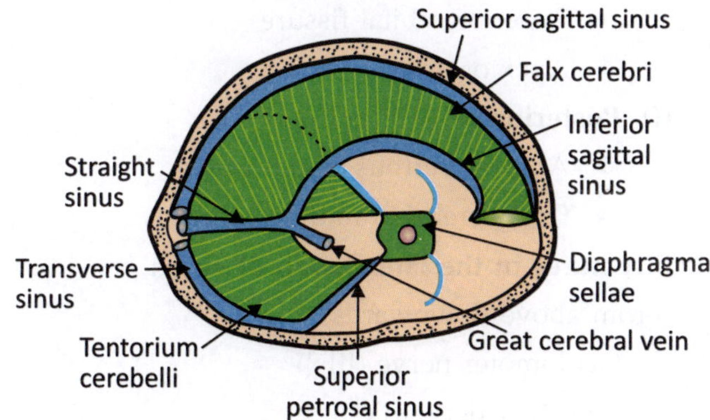

Fig. 34.10: ***Folds of duramater and dural venous sinuses***

Extent:

Anteriorly: It extends upto medial end of superior orbital fissure.

Posteriorly: Extends upto apex of petrous temporal bone.

- Cavity is lined by endothelium.

Development:

Primitive head vein.

- Floor of the sinus is formed by endosteal duramater.
- Lateral wall, roof and medial wall are formed by meningeal duramater.

Relations of Cavernous Sinus

I. Structures outside the sinus

(a) Superiorly

- Optic tract

- Optic chiasma
- Olfactory tract
- Internal carotid artery
- Anterior perforated substance.

(b) Inferiorly

- Foramen lacerum
- Junction of body and greater wing of sphenoid.

(c) Medially

- Hypophysis cerebri
- Sphenoidal air sinus in the body of sphenoid.

(d) Laterally: Temporal lobe with uncus (cerebrum).

(e) Anteriorly

- Superior orbital fissure
- Apex of orbit.

(f) Posteriorly:

- Apex of petrous temporal
- Crus cerebri of mid-brain.

II. Structures in the lateral wall of sinus

(From above downwards)

1. Oculomoter nerve (IIIrd)
2. Trochlear nerve (IVth)
3. Ophthalmic nerve with its branches (V_1)
4. Maxillary nerve (V_2)
5. Trigeminal ganglion with its dural cave project into posterior part of lateral wall of sinus.

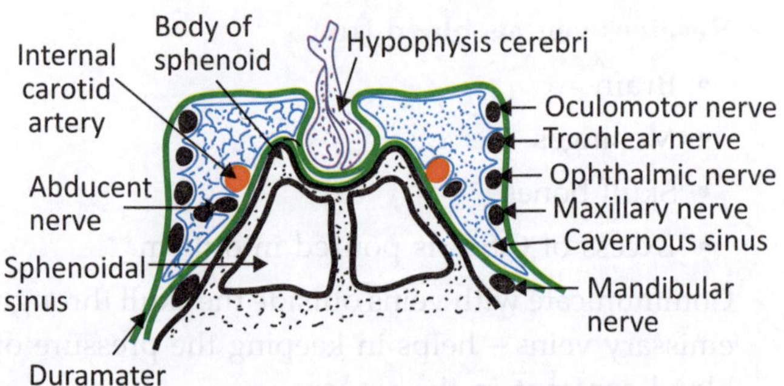

Fig. 34.11: *Coronal section-showing relations of cavernous sinus*

III. Structures passing through Centre of sinus

1. Internal carotid artery – with venous and sympathetic plexus.
2. Abducent nerve – infero-lateral to artery.
   - Structures in the lateral wall and centre of the sinus are separated from blood by endothelial lining.

Tributaries or Incoming Channels

To cavernous sinus are:

A. From the orbit:

- Superior ophthalmic vein

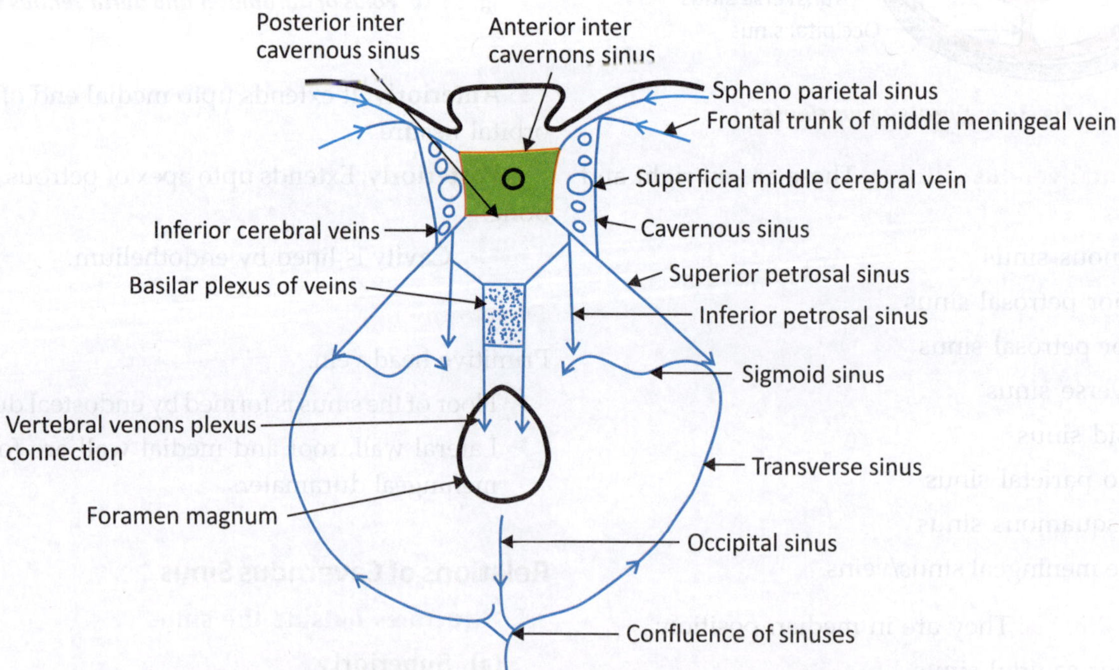

Fig. 34.12: *Tributaries of cavernous sinus incoming and draining channels*

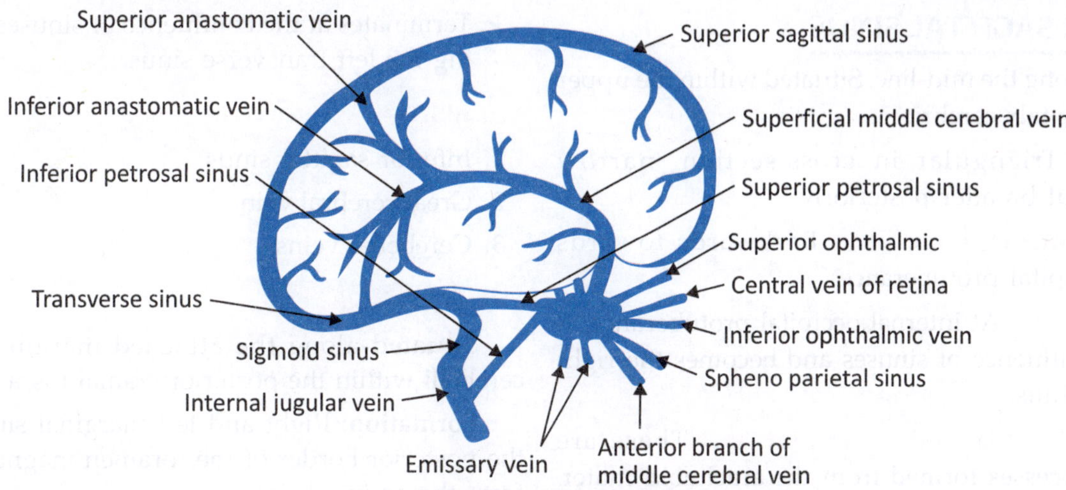

Fig. 34.13: *Tributaries of cavernous sinus*

- Inferior ophthalmic vein
- Central vein of retina.

B. From brain:
- Superficial middle cerebral vein
- Anterior branch of middle meningeal vein either directly or through spheno parietal sinus.
- Inferior cerebral veins

C. From hypophysis cerebri: Hypophyseal veins.

D. From skull bones: Diploic veins.

Draining channels of cavernous sinus: (communications) Drains its venous blood into:

1. Transverse sinus – through superior petrosal sinus.
2. Interal jugular vein – through inferior petrosal sinus.
3. Pterygoid plexus of veins – via emissary veins.
4. Facial vein via communication with superior ophthalmic vein.
5. Through basilar plexus of veins into vertebral vein.

Factors helping expulsion of blood from sinus:

1. Expansile pulsation of internal carotid artery within the sinus.
2. Gravity.
3. Position of the head.

Circular Sinus

It is formed by both sides of cavernous and inter cavernous sinuses.

Applied Anatomy of Cavernous Sinus

1. Nerves related to cavernous sinus are affected during thrombosis. Features are:
   - Pain around orbit and forehead
   - Eyelid swelling
   - Chemosis
   - Proptosis
   - Pupillary dilatation
   - Ophthalmoplegia
   - Papilloedema.
2. Fracture of middle cranial fossa involves cavernous sinus and internal carotid artery → Arterio venous anastomosis → Pulsating exophathalmia.
3. Cavernous sinus thrombosis – due to infection from orbit, face, para nasal air sinuses, middle ear infections.
   - Septae dividing the sinus into many compartments retard blood circulation within the sinus.

Roof of the sinus is crossed by:

1. Oculomotor nerve (III)
2. Trochlear nerve (IV).

Roof is pierced by:

1. Internal carotid artery
2. Oculomotor nerve
3. Trochlear nerve.

Structures passing within the sinus:

1. Internal carotid artery and
2. Abducent nerve (VIth C.N.).

SUPERIOR SAGITTAL SINUS

It is found along the mid-line. Situated within the upper border of the falx cerebri.

Shape: Triangular in cross-section, narrow anteriorly but broader posteriorly.

Direction of blood flow: Backwards towards internal occipital protuberance.

Termination: At internal occipital protuberance, it joins the confluence of sinuses and becomes the right transverse sinus.

Arachnoid villi and granulations: These are tortuous processes formed from the arachnoid mater. It invaginates into the superior sagittal sinus. The arachnoid villi are covered by specialized mesothelial cells called meningocytes. They filter the cerebro spinal fluid into the superior sagittal sinus. Collection of arachnoid villi constitute arachnoid granulations – found only in adults.

Tributaries:

1. A pair of parietal emissary veins from the scalp.
2. Superior cerebral veins.
3. Meningeal veins.
4. Emissary vein from nose passing through foramen caecum.

INFERIOR SAGITTAL SINUS

Situated:

- Within lower border of falx cerebri.
- It terminates by forming the straight sinus by joining the great cerebral vein, at the junction between falx cerebri and tentorium cerebelli.

Tributaries:

1. Great cerebral vein,
2. Meningeal veins, and
3. Cerebral veins.

STRAIGHT SINUS

- Situated along the junction of falx cerebri and tentorium cerebrelli.
- It is formed by the union of inferior sagittal sinus and great cerebral vein.
- Terminates at the confluence of sinuses by becoming the left transverse sinus.

Tributaries:

1. Inferior sagittal sinus
2. Great cerebral vein
3. Cerebellar veins.

Occipital Sinus:

Situated along the attached margin of the falx cerebelli within the posterior cranial fossa.

Formation: Right and left marginal sinuses along the posterior border of the foramen magnum unite to form the occipital sinus.

Termination: Confluence of sinuses.

TRANSVERSE SINUS

Right transverse sinus is the continuation of the superior sagittal sinus and left transverse sinus is formed from the straight sinus.

Course: Passes within the transverse sulcus along the posterior attached border of the tentorium cerebelli.

Terminates: By becoming sigmoid sinus together forms the lateral sinus.

Tributaries:

1. Superior petrosal sinus
2. Inferior cerebral veins
3. Inferior cerebellar veins
4. Inferior anastomotic vein.

SIGMOID SINUS

It is the continuation of the transverse sinus at mastoid angle.

It runs within the sigmoid groove of temporal and occipital bones and enters the posterior compartment of the jugular foramen.

Terminates: By becoming the internal jugular vein.

Tributaries:

1. Labyrinthine veins
2. Cerebellar veins
3. Condylar emissary vein
4. Mastoid emissary vein.

Applied Anatomy

1. Infections from middle ear and mastoid antrum may spread into sigmoid sinus and causes thrombosis.
2. Extra cranial infections from scalp, nose or occipital venous plexus may go to intra cranial sinuses and infects them causing serious problems like thrombosis, meningitis, encephalitis etc.

THE EMISSARY VEINS

These are small veins connecting extra cranial veins with intra cranial dural venous sinuses. They do not have valves. For example,

1. Emissary vein of foramen caecum – communicates the veins of nose with superior sagittal sinus. These veins carries extra cranial nasal infections intra cranially.
2. Mastoid emissary veins – communicates scalp veins with superior sagittal sinus.
3. Mastoid emissary vein – communicates posterior auricular vein and sigmoid sinus.
4. Emissary veins passing through foramen ovale, foramen vesalius and foramen lacerum are communicating the cavernous sinus with the pterygoid venous plexus.
5. Ophthalmic vein connects the facial vein and cavernous sinus.
6. Sigmoid sinus is connected with internal jugular vein by an emissary vein passing through hypoglossal canal.
7. Suboccipital plexus of veins and sigmoid sinus are connected by an emissary vein passing through posterior condylar canal.

Importance:

Emissary veins convey extra cranial infections intra cranially, e.g., infection from dangerous area of face enter the cavernous sinus through emissary communications. This leads to meningitis or encephalitis.

HYPOPHYSIS CEREBRI (PITUITARY GLAND)

- Is a small endocrine gland and known as Master of Endocrine orchestra.
- Lies in Hypophyseal fossa situated in middle cranial fossa, in relation to base of brain – suspending from the floor the third ventricle.

Shape is oval

Size: Antero-posteriorly 8 mm

Transversely: 12 mm

Weight: About 500 to 600 mgm

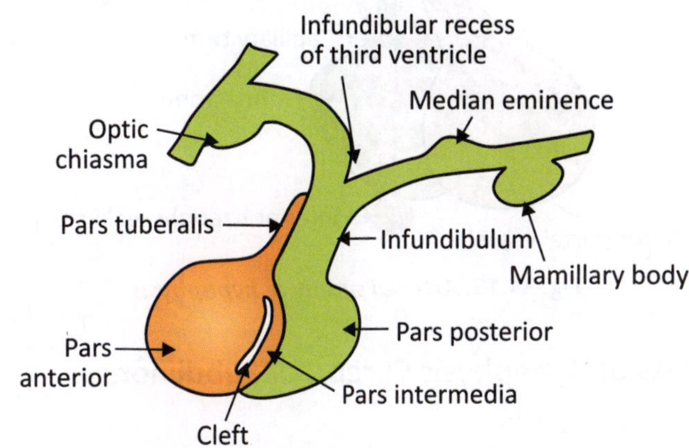

Fig. 34.14: ***Parts of hypophysis cerebri***

Development

- **Anterior lobe:** From buccal epithelium an upward growth arises becomes Rathkes pouch and forms of anterior lobe.
- **Posterior lobe:** Diencephalic diverticulum – descends downward and forms posterior lobe.

Relations

1. **Superiorly**
   - Diaphragm sellae
   - Optic chiasma
   - Tuber cinerium
   - Infundibular recess of IIIrd ventricle.
2. **Inferiorly:**
   - Irregular venous plexus
   - Dura lining the floor of fossa
   - Pituitary fossa
   - Sphenoidal air sinus.
3. **On each side laterally:**
   - Cavernous sinus with its contents.
4. **Anteriorly:** Anterior – Inter-cavernous sinus.
5. **Posteriorly:** Posterior – Inter-cavernous sinus.

Arterial Supply

- Superior and inferior hypophyseal artery branch of internal carotid artery.

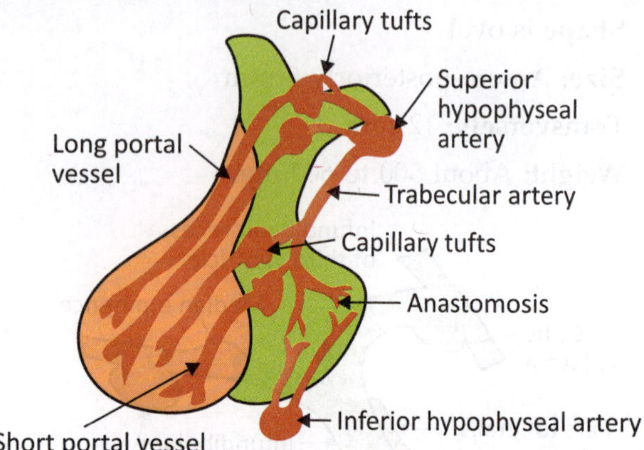

Fig. 34.15: *Arterial supply of hypophysis*

Parts of Hypophysis Cerebri or Subdivions

It has two parts:

- Adenohypophysis
- Neurohypophysis.

They differ embryologically, morphologically and functionally.

I. Adenohypohysis: It develops as an upward growth from ectodermal roof of stomodeum (Buccal epithelium) called Rathke's pouch – forms –

- Anterior lobe – pars anterior
- Intermediate lobe – pars inter-media
- Tuberal extension called pars tuberalis – it extends upwards around the sides of infundibulum.

A cleft is present between anterior and inter-mediate lobe.

It has cells arranged in cords around sinusoids.

Cell are:

- Acidophilic or alfa cells (chromophils and chromophobe)
- Basophilic (chromophils)
  - Beta cells
  - Delta cells.

Beta cells: Secrete – T.S.H. (Thyroid Stimulating Hormone) and A.C.T.H. (Adreno Cortico Trophic Hormone).

Delta cells: Secrete – F.S.H. (Follicle Stimulating Hormone), Luitinising Hormone and I.C.S.H. (Interstitial Cell Stimulating Hormone).

Alfa cells: Secrete – growth hormone and lactogenic hormone (prolactin).

Chromophobes are precurssor cells (stem cells)

Intermediate lobe – has plenty of chromophobes and chromophil cells – which secrete M.S.H. (Melanocyte Stimulating Hormone).

Arterial supply of anterior and intermediate lobe is through:

- Superior hypophyseal artery – which forms superior and inferior capillary tuft from which long and short portal vessels arise – carry hormone releasing factor from hypothalamus.

Venous drainage: Into neighbouring dural sinuses–

- Cavernous and inter cavernous sinuses.
- Short veins carry hormones secreted by glandular cells.

II. Neurohypophysis: Develops as downward growth from floor of diencephlon and is connected to hypothalamus by neural pathways (axons).

It has:

- Neuroglial cells or tissue
- Neurons – called pituicytes
- Axon – forms hypothalmo-hypophyseal tract.

Parts: It forms – posterior lobe, infundibular stem and median eminence of tubercinerium.

Functions:

1. It provides neural pathway which controls secretary activity of anterior lobe.
2. Vassopressin (A.D.H.) – Antidiuretic hormone acts on kidney and tubules.
3. Oxytocin – Acts on smooth muscles of uterus and breast – causes contraction – both hormones are secreted by neurons of hypothalamus and reaches to posterior lobe.

INTERNAL CAROTID ARTERY

It begins in the neck as one of the terminal branches of the common carotid artery, at the level of upper border of thyroid cartilage.

Parts: They are four parts:

1. Cervical part

(a) Lies within carotid sheath in the neck.

(b) Gives no branch.

2. Petrous part: Lies within petrous part of the temporal bone, i.e., in the carotid canal.

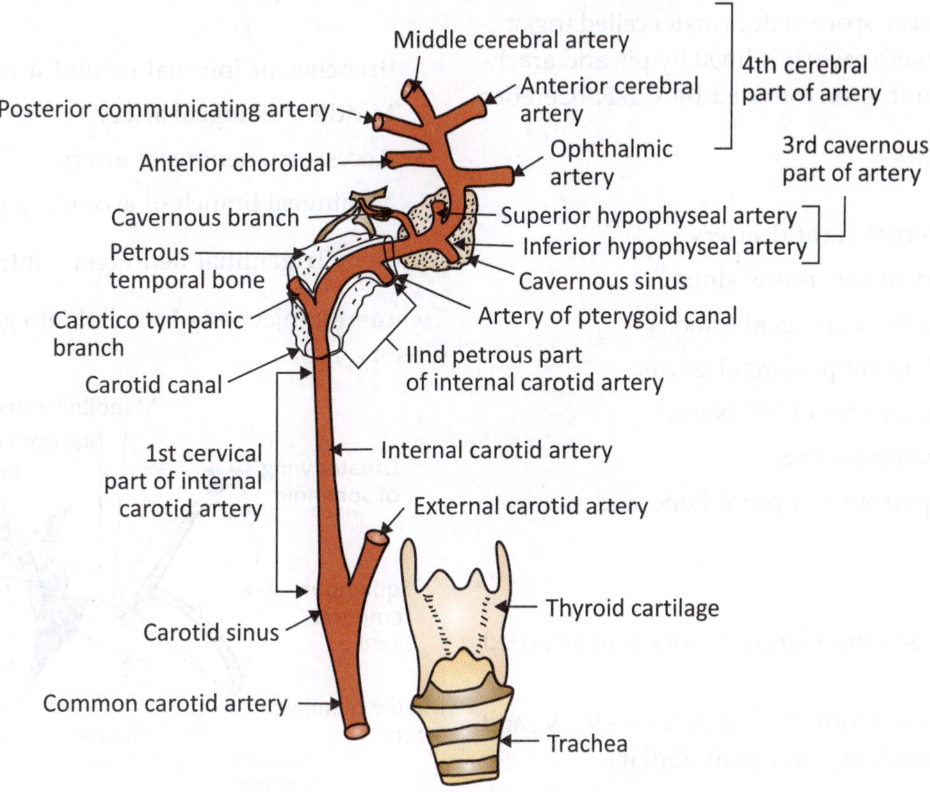

Fig. 34.16: *Internal carotid artery and its branches*

Branches:

(a) Carotico tympanic branch to middle ear cavity.

(b) Artery of pterygoid canal.

3. **Cavernous part of internal carotid artery:** Lies within the cavernous sinus. It gives:

(a) Cavernous branch to trigeminal ganglion.

(b) Superior hypophyseal branch to hypophysis cerebri.

(c) Inferior hypophyseal branch to hypophysis cerebri.

4. **Cerebral part of internal carotid artery:** Lies at the base of brain.

Branches are:

(a) Ophthalmic artery to orbit

(b) Anterior cerebral artery

(c) Middle cerebral artery

(d) Posterior communicating branch

(e) Anterior choroidal artery

➤ Curvatures of petrous, cavernous and cerebral part of internal carotid artery together form an 'S' shaped figure (carotid siphon of angiograms).

TRIGEMINAL GANGLION

It is a sensory ganglion of Vth cranial nerve made up of pseudounipolar nerve cells with a 'T' shaped arragement of their processes.

One process arises from cell body → it divides into a central and a peripheral process.

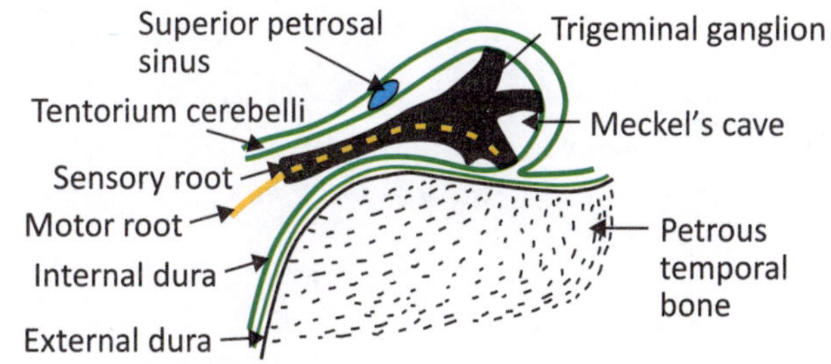

Fig. 34.17: *Trigeminal ganglion*

Shape is cresantric or semilunar and three divisions arise from its convexity.

Concavity: Receives sensory root of the nerve.

Situation and Meningeal Relations

➤ Lies on trigeminal impression on the anterior surface of petrous temporal bone near its apex.

- Occupies a special space of dura mater called trigeminal cave (Meckel's cave) it is lined by pia and arachnoid mater so it is surrounded by C.S.F. (Cerebro Spinal Fluid).

Relations

Medially: Internal carotid artery.

Posterior: Part of cavernous sinus.

Laterally: Middle meningeal artery.

Superiorly: Para hippocampal gyrus.

Inferiorly: Motor root of Vth Nerve.

- Greater petrosal nerve
- Apex of petrous temporal bone and foramen lacerum

Root and Branches:

Central processes form large sensory root attached to pons.

Peripheral process form three divisions – V_1, V_2 and V_3 (ophthalmic, maxillary and mandibular).

Motor root is also attached to pons and joins V_3 (mandibular) nerve.

Blood supply by:

- Branches of internal carotid artery
- Middle meningeal artery
- Accessory meningeal artery
- Meningeal branch of ascending pharyngeal artery.

Applied: Trigeminal neuralgia – intractable pain.

Treatment: Injection of alcohol into ganglion or cutting sensory root.

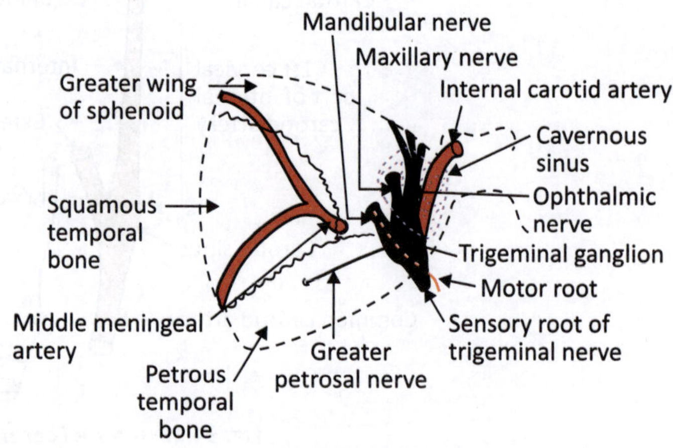

Fig. 34.18: *Some contents of middle cranial fossa-trigeminal ganglion*

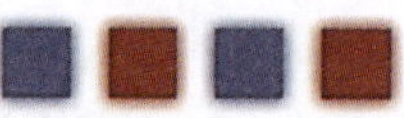

CHAPTER 35

Cranial Nerves

INTRODUCTION

- There are twelve pairs of cranial nerves.
- They leave the brain and pass through foramina in the skull.
- All the nerves are distributed in the head and neck, except vagus (X), which supplies structures in the thorax and abdomen.

CRANIAL NERVES

1. Olfactory – sensory – sense of smell
2. Optic – sensory – vision
3. Oculomotor – motor
4. Trochlear – motor
5. Trigeminal – sensory root and motor root – mixed
6. Abducent – motor
7. Facial – sensory root and motor root – mixed
8. Vestibulo cochlear – sensory – hearing and balancing
9. Glossopharyngeal – sensory and motor – mixed
10. Vagus – sensory and motor – mixed
11. Accessory – motor
12. Hypoglossal – motor.

NUCLEI OF CRANIAL NERVES

(a) First and second nerves are attached to Fore-Brain.

(b) Mid-brain – nucleus of third and fourth nerve lies in it are attached to it.

(c) Hind brain – consists – pons and medulla.

(i) **Pons** – has nucleus of 5th, 6th, 7th and 8th nerves, which are attached to it.

(ii) **Medulla** – 9th, 10th, 11th and 12th cranial nerves are attached to it and having their nuclei inside the medulla.

Note: Several cranial nerves are connected to more than one nucleus and that same nuclei contribute fibres to more than one nerve.

1. OLFACTORY NERVE

Nerve of smell (sensory)

Commencement:

- Arises from central process of bipolar olfactory receptor nerve cells (neurons) present in the olfactory mucous membrane, situated in the upper part of the nasal cavity above the level of the superior concha.
- About 15 to 20 nerves arise from olfactory plexus of nerves and pass through the openings of cribriform plate of ethmoid bone to enter the olfactory bulb in the anterior cranial fossa.
- Olfactory bulb is connected to the olfactory area of cerebral cortex by olfactory tract.
- Carry smell sensation from the nose to the brain.

Termination: Glomerulus of the olfactory bulb.

Olfactory Pathway:

First order neuron
(Present in olfactory epithelium)
Olfactory nerve
↓
Second order neuron
(Present in olfactory bulb)
↓
Olfactory tract
↓
Ends in pre-piriform and piriform cortex
(Primary olfactory cortex)
Receives smell sense
↓
Uncus and para hippocampus
(Secondary olfactory cortex)
↓
Receives smell sense

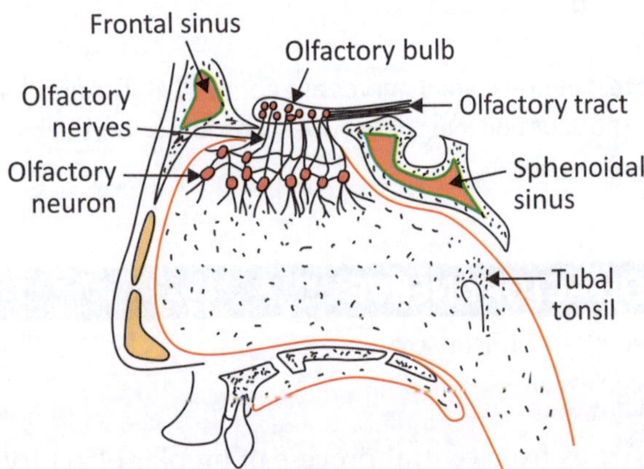

Fig. 35.1: ***Olfactory nerves***

Applied Anatomy

1. **During fracture of anterior cranial fossa:** Olfactory nerves may separate from olfactory bulb and Cerebrospinal Fluid (C.S.F.) leaks through nose – Rhinorrhoea.
2. **Anosmia:** Loss of smell sensation, e.g., in Rhinitis.
3. **Parosmia:** Perverted sense of smell.
4. **Caprosmia:** Unpleasent odour due to decomposition of the tissue of the individual – bad smell is felt during expiration.
5. **Clinically:** Each nostril must be tested separately either from clove oil or rose water.

2. OPTIC NERVE

Nerve of sight and is second cranial nerve.

- It is a tract having more than one million nerve fibres.
- Surrounded by three layers of meninges.

Development: Develops as a diverticulum from the diencephalon – optic stalk.

Commencement: From central process of the cells present in the ganglionated cell layer of retina.

Courses:

- Fibres pierce the choroid and sclera, emerges through the lamina cribrosa situated 3 mm medial to central pole of the sclera.
- Nerve passes via retrobulbar compartment of the orbit, enters the optic canal via optic foramen and reaches the anterior cranial fossa.

Termination: Joins the optic nerve of the opposite side to form optic chiasma – where nasal fibres cross and temporal fibres do not cross.

Length – is about 40 mm.

Parts:

1. Intra orbital part – 25 mm long
2. Part of nerve within the optic canal – 5 mm long
3. Intra cranial part – 10 mm long.

Relations in the orbit: Nerve is longer than the space, so it is tortuous and surrounded by orbital pad of fat and muscles of eyeball.

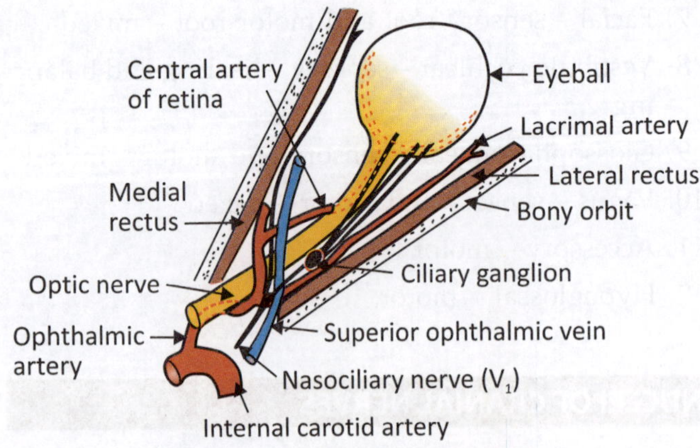

Fig. 35.2: ***Relations of optic-nerve***

Crossed superiorly: From lateral to medial side by:

1. Superior ophthalmic vein

2. Ophthalmic artery
3. Nasociliary nerve.

Laterally:
1. Ciliary ganglion
2. Lateral rectus muscle.

Medially: Central artery of retina – pierces the optic nerve 1 cm behind the eyeball.

Posteriorly: Nerve is surrounded by origin of recti-muscles.

Inferiorly: Nerve to medial rectus.

Relations within the optic canal: 5 mm long.

Infero-laterally: Ophthalmic artery.

Medially:
- Sphenoidal air sinus.
- Posterior ethmoidal air sinus.

Relations of intra cranial part: – 10 mm long.

Superior: Anterior cerebral artery.

Posterior: Hypophysis cerebri.

Lateral: Internal carotid artery.

Blood supply:
1. Central artery of retina
2. Superior hypophyseal artery
3. Ophthalmic artery
4. Posterior ciliary artery.

Venous drainage: Central vein of retina drains into cavernous sinus.

Structure:
1. Nerve is covered by dura, arachnoid and piamaters.
2. Piamater enters into the nerve as septulae – which divides the nerve into many compartments.

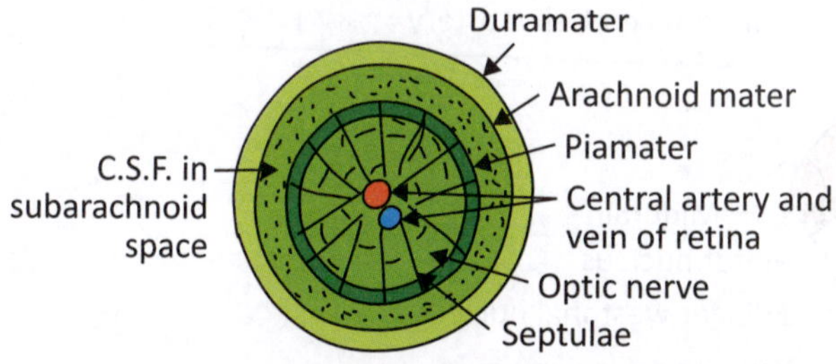

Fig. 35.3: ***Structure of optic nerve***

3. In the centre of the nerve – central artery and vein of retina are situated.

Applied Anatomy

1. Infection from brain and meninges may spread to optic nerve.
2. Injury of one optic nerve results in complete loss of vision of that side.
3. When intra cranial pressure is increased – optic nerve head in the retina is swollan – called papilloedema.

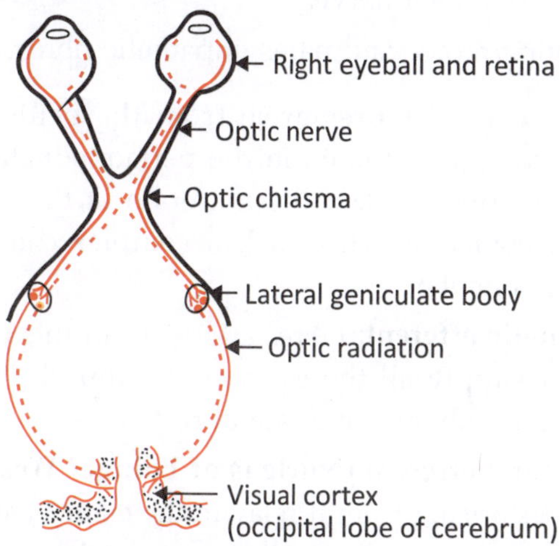

Fig. 35.4: ***Connections of optic nerve (IInd)***

Visual Pathway

Visual receptors (Rods and Cones)

↓

Bipolar cells (Primary neurons)

↓

Ganglionated cells (Secondary neurons)

↓

Optic nerve

↓

Optic chiasma (Nasal fibres cross and temporal do not cross)

↓

Optic tract

↓

Lateral geniculate body (Tertiary neuron)

↓

↓

Optic Radiation

↓

Visual area in the occipital cortex (area – 17)

↓

Visual interpretation is given at visuopsychic area (area – 18)

3. OCULOMOTOR NERVE (MOTOR)

Is the third cranial nerve.

- Having motor and parasympathetic fibres.

Nuclear origin: Fibres arise from the oculomotor nuclear complex situated in the periaqueductal grey matter of upper part of the midbrain at the level of superior colliculus. This nuclear complex consists of two components:

1. **Somatic efferent:** Fibres arising from this component supply all the extra ocular muscles except superior oblique and lateral rectus.
2. **Visceral efferent (Nucleus of Edinger Westphal):** Fibres arising from it relay in the ciliary ganglion.

From there postganglionic – parasympathetic fibres arise supply the sphincter pupillae and ciliaris muscle.

- After arising from the nuclear complex, the fibres run forwards through the substance of the midbrain to emerge on the anteromedial side of the cerebral peduncle.

Course:

- Nerve emerges as a single trunk from oculomotor sulcus of midbrain runs infront of crus cerebri between posterior cerebral and superior cerebellar arteries, lies in interpeduncular cistern.
- It pierces the arachnoid and runs forwards and laterally to the oculomotor triangle between the free and attached margins of the tentorium cerebelli.
- Passes lateral to posterior clinoid process and pierces the duramater to enter the roof of the cavernous sinus. Here, it runs forwards in the lateral wall of the sinus.
- In the anterior part of the cavernous sinus, nerve divides into upper and lower divisions, which enter the orbit by passing through the superior orbital fissure within the common tendinous ring.

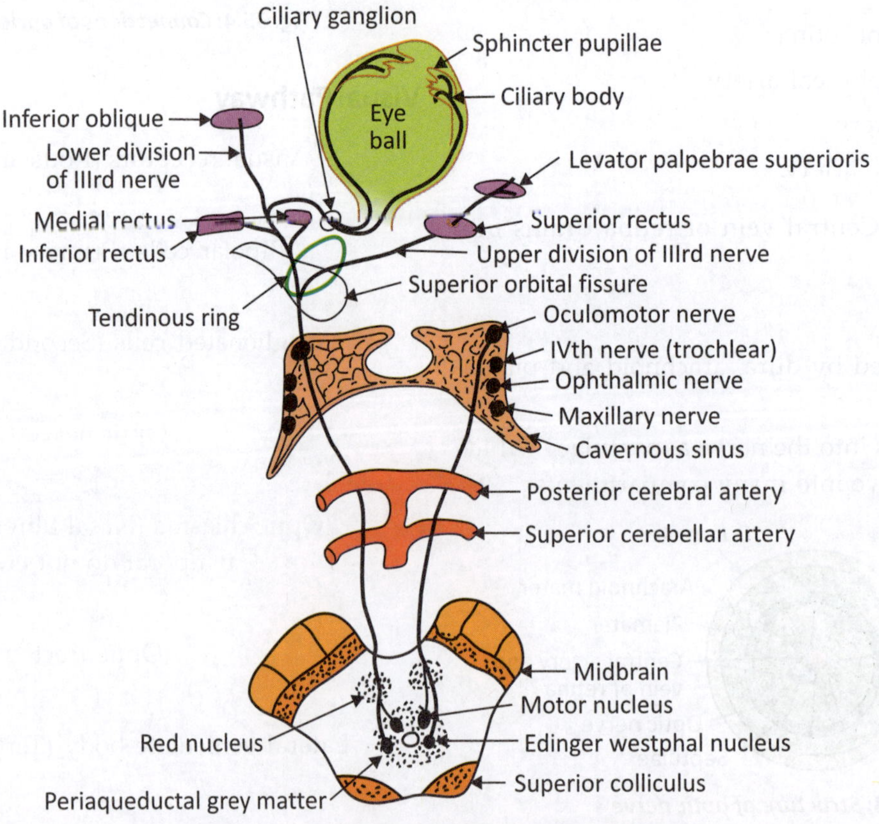

Fig. 35.5: *Oculomotor nerve and its distribution*

Distributions:

1. Smaller superior division passes upwards on the lateral side of the optic nerve to supply superior rectus, it pierces the muscle and reaches the levator palpebrae superiors to supply it on its inner aspect.
2. **Large inferior division divides into three branches:**
   (a) One branch passes below the optic nerve and supplies medial rectus.
   (b) Second branch supplies inferior rectus muscle.
   (c) Third branch passes between inferior rectus and lateral rectus to supply inferior oblique muscle.

Nerve to inferior oblique gives a motor root to the ciliary ganglion. From ganglion short ciliary nerves arise and supply the ciliary muscle and sphincter pupillae. These are parasympathetic fibres coming from Edinger Westphal nucleus.

4. TROCHLEAR NERVE (MOTOR)

It is the fourth cranial nerve. It is most slender nerve and the only one, which arises from the dorsal aspect of the midbrain.

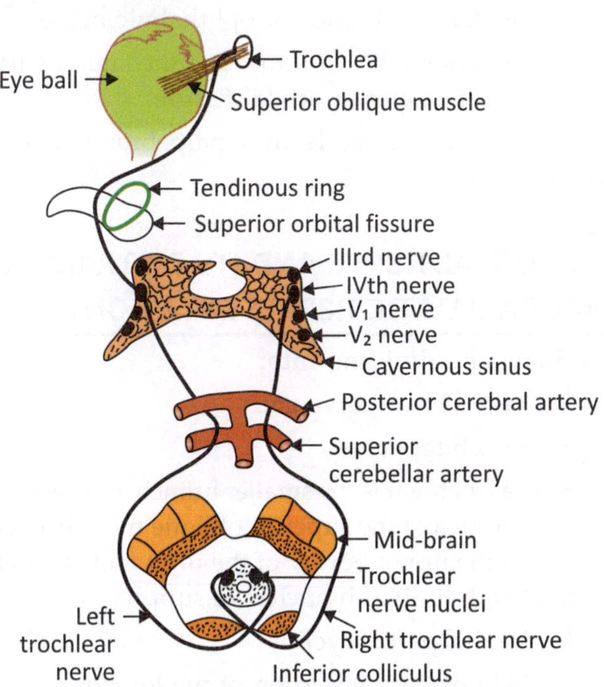

Fig. 35.6: ***Trochlear nerve***

Nuclear Origin:

- Trochlear nucleus lies in the ventro medial part of the central grey mater around the cerebral aqueduct, situated in the lower part of midbrain at the level of inferior colliculus.
- Fibres arise, wind backwards around the central grey mater and decussate with the nerve fibres of the opposite side in the superior medullary velum.
- It emerges on the dorsal surface of brain as a single trunk one on either side of the frenulum.

Courses:

- Each trochlear nerve passes laterally crossing the superior cerebellar peduncle.
- It winds forward between the temporal lobe and cerebral peduncle.
- Now it passes between posterior cerebral and superior cerebellar arteries and appears in the triangular area of duramater in front of the crossing of the attached and free margins of the tentorium cerebelli.
- It pierces the duramater lateral to the posterior clinoid process and passes forward in the lateral wall of cavernous sinus below the oculomotor nerve.
- The nerve enters the orbit through the lateral part of superior orbital fissure.
- In the orbit nerve passes forwards and medially above the levator palpebrae superioris and supplies the superior oblique muscle from its orbital surface.

Distribution: It supplies the superior oblique muscle only.

Peculiarity of the Trochlear Nerve:

1. Only cranial nerve, emerges from the dorsal aspect of brain stem.
2. It is the only nerve that undergoes complete decussation with the nerve of opposite side before emerging.

Applied Anatomy

1. Injury to 4th nerve causes paralysis of superior oblique muscle – person cannot look downward and laterally. Hence, during descending a stair – difficulties are noted and head is tilted as a compensatory adjustment.
2. During cavernous sinus thrombosis 3rd, 4th and 6th cranial nerves may be paralysed.
3. Brain tumour, syphilis, meningitis, encephalitis and

cavernous sinus thrombosis involves IIIrd, IVth and VIth cranial nerves.

Fracture of superior orbital fissure may involve these nerves in cases of head injuries.

5. TRIGEMINAL NERVE

It is the fifth cranial nerve, containing both sensory and motor roots, i.e., mixed nerve.

Nuclei

Motor and sensory both nuclei are situated in the pons.

(i) **Motor nucleus of trigeminal:** Lies medial to sensory nucleus in the pons. It supplies muscles of mastication, anterior belly of digastric, mylohyoid, tensor tympani and tensor palati muscles.

(ii) **Superior sensory nucleus of trigeminal:** Lies lateral to motor nucleus in the pons. Inferior to this nucleus lies the nucleus of the spinal tract of the trigeminal nerve. It receives sensory impulses from the face, conjunctiva, nose and mouth etc.

(iii) **Mesencephalic nucleus** is situated in between the sensory and motor nuclei present in the pons. It superiorly extends into the mid-brain. It receives proprioceptive impulses from muscles of mastication, face and eye.

Course: The nerve leaves anterior aspect of the pons as a small motor root and a large sensory root.

- Passes forwards from the posterior cranial fossa to the apex of the petrous temporal in middle cranial fossa.
- Large sensory root expands to form trigeminal ganglion (crescentric shaped).
- From the convex anterior border of the ganglion three divisions arise:
  1. **Ophthalmic nerve** – purely sensory – divides into – Lacrimal, frontal and nasociliary branches.
  2. **Maxillary nerve** – sensory.
  3. **Mandibular nerve** – mixed.

Ophthalmic Nerve

Purely sensory, runs in lateral wall of cavernous sinus below the trochlear nerve. Reaching the anterior part of the sinus nerve divides into three branches:

(i) Lacrimal,
(ii) Frontal, and
(iii) Nasociliary nerves.

They enter into the orbit through superior orbital fissure.

Ophthalmic nerve via its branches may supply:

(i) Anterior quadrant of scalp
(ii) Cornea
(iii) Conjunctiva
(iv) Eye ball
(v) Eye lids
(vi) Nose
(vii) Frontal and ethmoidal air sinuses
(viii) Lacrimal gland.

(i) **Lacrimal Nerve:** It passes through the lateral most aspect of the superior orbital fissure and enters the orbit. It runs forwards and laterally to supply:

(a) Lateral portion of eyelids
(b) Palpebral conjunctiva
(c) Lacrimal gland

(ii) **Frontal Nerve:**

- Largest branch of ophthalmic nerve.
- Enters the orbit through the lateral part of the superior orbital fissure.

It passes above the levator palpebrae superioris muscle.

TRIGEMINAL NERVE AND ITS DISTRIBUTION (DIAGRAMMATIC REPRESENTATION)

Terminates by dividing into:

1. Supra trochlear nerve and
2. Supra orbital nerve.

1. Supra trochlear is the smaller branch, passes round the trochlea of the superior oblique muscle, curves round the upper border of the orbit and enters the forehead. It gives branches to supply:

(i) Medial part of eyelids
(ii) Skin of central portion of the forehead.

2. Supra orbital nerve: Passes through supra orbital foramen or notch, runs in the forehead and scalp to supply:

(i) Conjunctiva

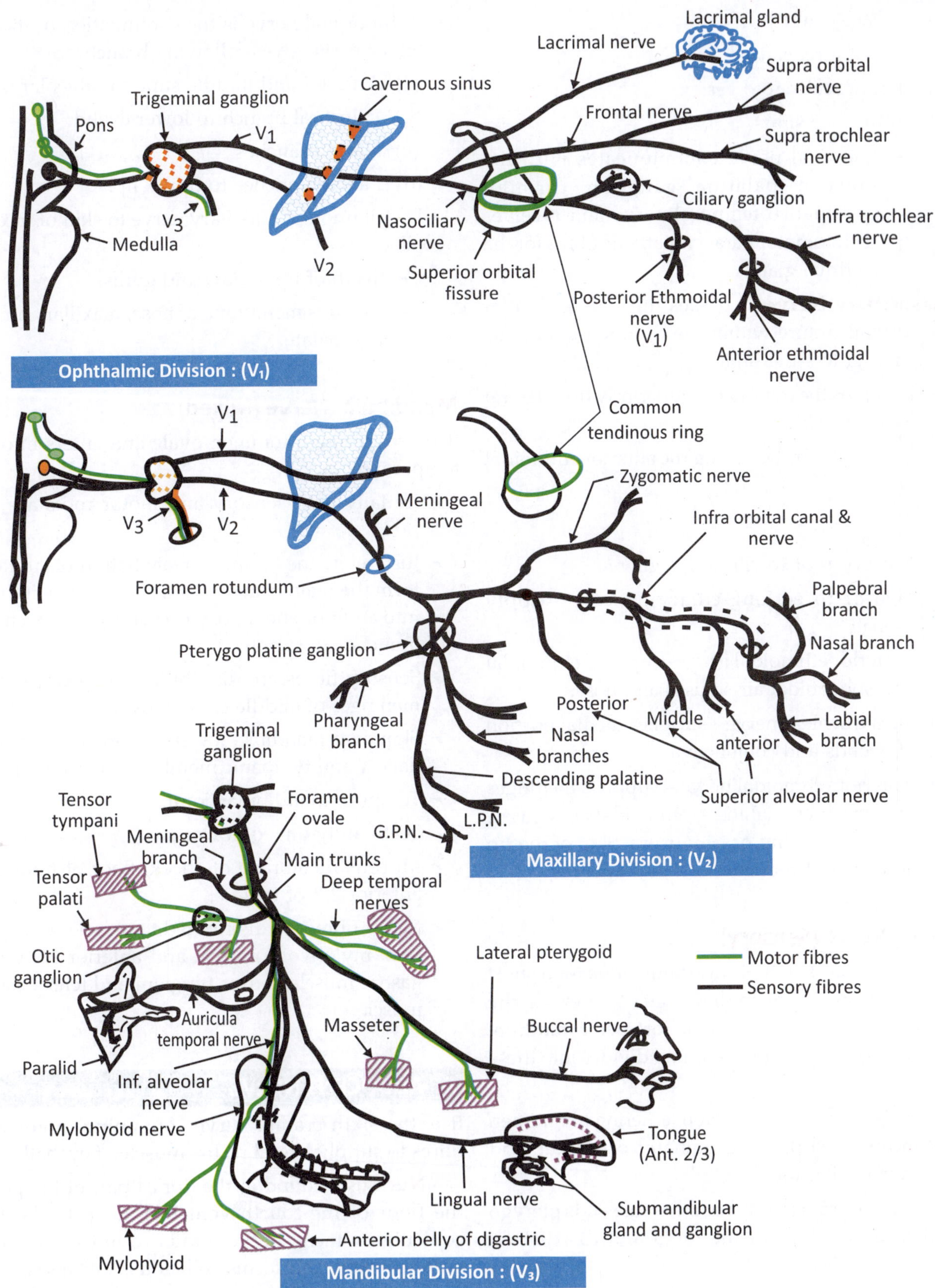

Fig. 35.7: ***Trigerminal nerve and its distribution***

(ii) Upper eyelid
(iii) Skin of forehead
(iv) Skin of scalp upto vertex
(v) Frontal air sinus.

- Lacrimal nerve communicates with the pterygo palatine ganglion through zygomatico temporal nerve and receives secretomotor parasympathetic fibres for the lacrimal gland.

3. **Nasociliary Nerve:** It passes through the superior orbital fissure within the common tendinous ring and enters the orbit.
   - It crosses the optic nerve superiorly from lateral to medial side.
   - Terminates by becoming the anterior ethmoidal nerve.

Branches:

(a) Sensory root to ciliary ganglion.
(b) Two or three long ciliary nerves – supply eyeball.
(c) Posterior ethmoidal nerve – supplies ethmoidal and sphenoidal air sinuses and nose.
(d) Infra trochlear nerve – supplies medial portion of eyelids and conjunctiva.
(e) Anterior ethmoidal nerve – supplies meninges of anterior cranial fossa, ethmoidal air sinuses, frontal sinus and nasal mucosa. Skin of the tip and around the anterior nasal opening.

Maxillary Nerve (Sensory)

It runs in the lateral wall of cavernous sinus for a short distance below the opthalmic nerve, pierces the duramater and passes through the foramen rotundum. Enters into pterygopalatine fossa and divides into these branches:

1. Meningeal branch arise before entering to foramen rotundum it supplies duramater of middle and anterior cranial fossa.
2. Ganglionic branches two or three suspends pterygo palatine ganglion in the fossa and distributed through its branches.
3. Zygomatic branch is divides into zytomatico temporal and zygomatico facial branch.
4. Posterior superior alveolar nerve.
5. Infra orbital nerve is the continuation of the maxillary nerve gives following branches:
   (a) Anterior and middle superior alveolar nerves.
   (b) Palpebral branch to lower eyelid.
   (c) Nasal branches.
   (d) Labial branches to upper lip.

Distribution of maxillary nerve to skin of face over maxilla.

- Teeth of upper jaw and gums.
- Mucous membrane of nose, maxillary air sinus and palate.

Mandibular Nerve (Mixed)

It passes through foramen ovale and enters into infra temporal fossa.

- Initially both sensory and motor roots are separate.
- Just below the foramen ovale both roots unite and form the main trunk, after a short course it divides into anterior and a posterior divisions which gives branches to supply.
- Sensory fibres are distributed to – skin of cheek, meninges of middle cranial fossa.
- Skin over mandible, lower lip, side of head, external ear and tympanic membrane, mastoid antrum.
- Temporo-mandibular joint.
- Teeth and gums of lower jaw.
- Mucous membrane of cheek, floor of mouth and anterior 2/3 of tongue.
- Motor fibres are distributed to muscles of mastication, mylohyoid muscle and anterior belly of digastric muscle, tensor tympani and tensor palatini muscle.

6. ABDUCENT NERVE

It is the sixth cranial nerve containing motor nerve fibres to supply lateral rectus muscle of eyeball.

Nucleus is found in the dorsal part of the pons in the floor of the fourth ventricle, deep to the facial colliculus – facial nerve winds round the abducent nerve nucleus and forms colliculus. VIth nerve passes forwards within the tegmentum of the pons.

Emergence from the pons: It leaves between upper border of pyramid and lower border of pons.

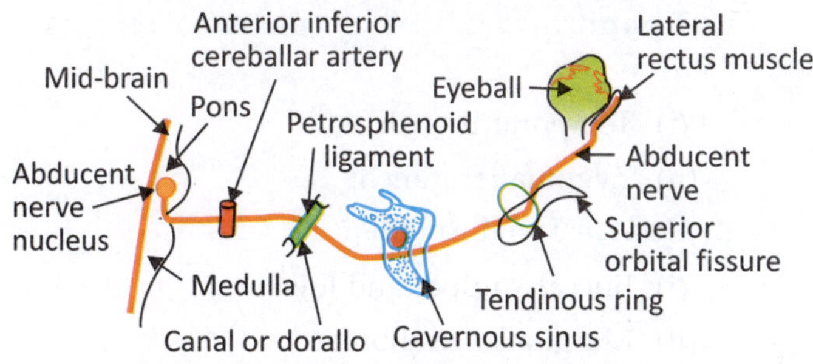

Fig. 35.8: *Abducent nerve and its distribution*

Course: Passes forwards and laterally pierces the duramater lateral to dorsum sellae, passes via canal of Dorallo and enters the cavernous sinus. Here, it lies infero lateral to internal carotid artery and passes through the superior orbital fissure within the common tendinous ring and enters the orbit.

Termination: It terminates by supplying the proximal part of medial surface of the lateral rectus muscle.

Applied Anatomy

1. Fracture of base of skull involve VIth nerve.
2. Carvernous sinus thrombosis – VIth nerve is affected compressed and paralysed.
3. Brain tumours.
4. Meningitis, encephalitis may involve VIth nerve.

7. FACIAL NERVE (VIITH CRANIAL NERVE)

- It is a mixed cranial nerve.
- Nerve of IInd pharyngeal arch.

Nuclei of Facial Nerve

They are situated in the dorsal part of pons.

1. Motor nucleus – for muscles of face, ear and scalp, posterior belly of digastric and stylohyoid.
2. Sensory nucleus (for taste) – nucleus of tractus solitarius
   - Sensory root is also called nervous intermedius.
3. **Parasympathetic nucleus:**
   (a) Superior salivatory nucleus – for supply of submandibular and sublingual glands.
   (b) Lacrimatory nucleus – for lacrimal gland.
4. Upper part of nucleus of spinal tract of trigeminal (for general sensation).

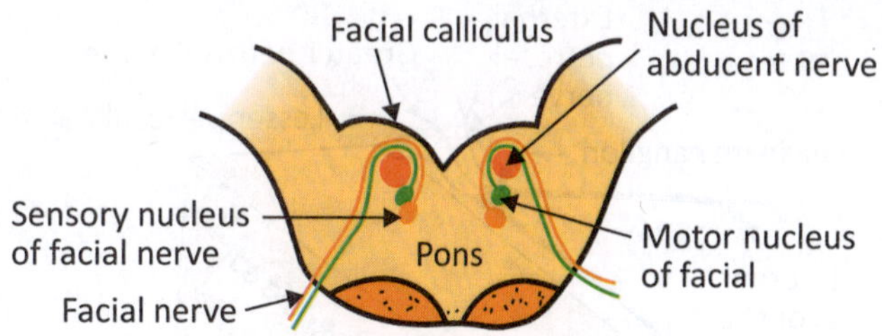

Fig. 35.9: *Facial nerve nucleus*

Course within the pons: Motor and sensory roots winds round the abducent nerve nucleus to form facial colliculus. They pass forwards and leave the pons – between lower border of pons and upper border of olive of medulla oblongata.

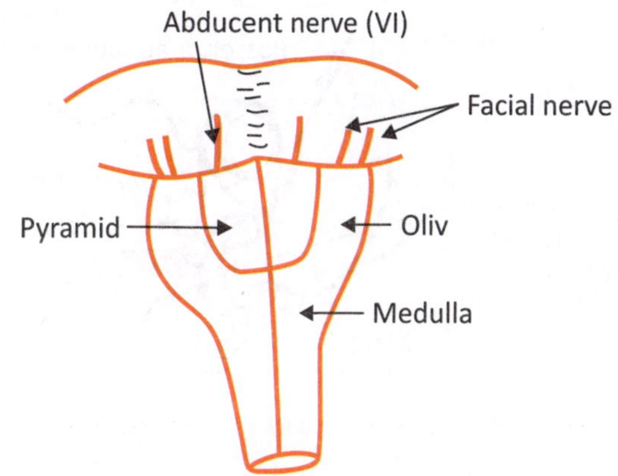

Fig. 35.10: *Emergence of facial nerve*

Course outside the pons (VIIth N.): Intra petrous course

- Two roots of VIIth nerve pass laterally and enter the internal auditory meatus – accompanied by VIIIth nerve.
- Two roots unite to form geniculate ganglion and from the ganglion-trunk of facial nerve is formed.
- Now the nerve is passing through facial canal or canal of fallopei.
- On reaching the medial wall of middle ear it runs posteriorly – situated superior to the promontary of middle ear.

Passes behind the posterior wall and runs vertically downwards to the stylomastoid foramen.

Extra cranial course of facial nerve:

After emerging through stylomastoid foramen it runs forwards and crosses the styloid process of temporal bone and enters the postero-medial surface of parotid gland. Within the gland it crosses laterally to retromandibular vein and external carotid artery.

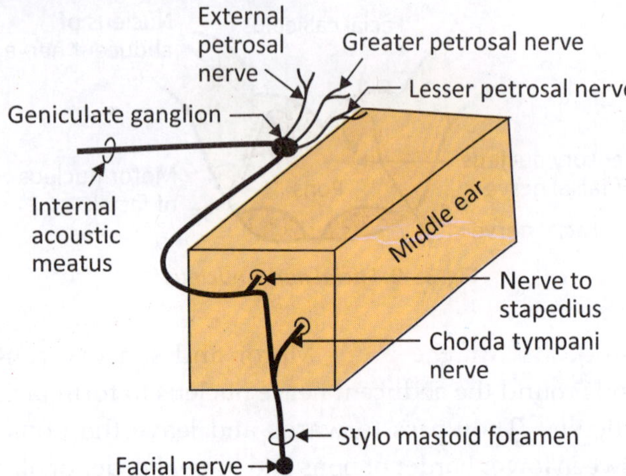

Fig. 35.11: *Intra petrous course of facial nerve*

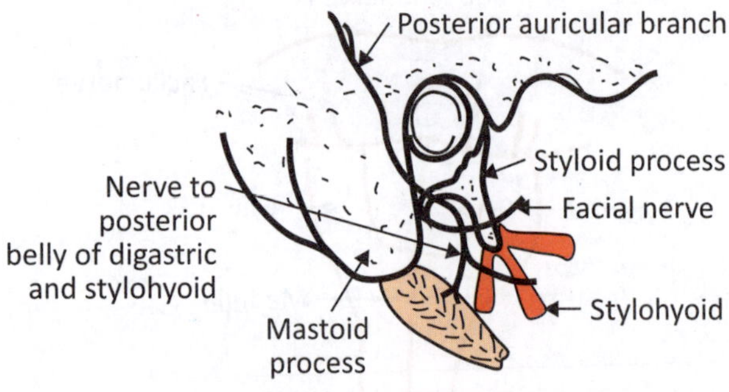

Fig. 35.12: *Relation with styloid process*

Termination: It terminates by dividing into temporo facial and cervico facial branches.

- Temporo facial divides into temporal and zygomatic branch.
- Cervico facial divides into buccal, marginal mandibular and cervical branches.

Branches of Facial Nerve

1. **Branches in the facial nerve canal:**
   (a) Nerve to stapedius
   (b) Chorda tympani nerve.
2. **Branches immediately below the stylomastoid foramen:**
   (a) Posterior auricular nerve
   (b) Nerve to posterior belly of digastric gives a branch to stylohoid.
3. **Branches on the face:** Supplies all the muscles of facial expression except levator palpebrae superioris which is supplied by oculomotor nerve.

1. **Temporo-facial or zygomatico temporal division:**
   (i) Temporal branch
   (ii) Zygomatic branch.
2. **Cervico facial division:**
   (i) Buccal – upper and lower
   (ii) Marginal mandibular
   (iii) Cervical branch.

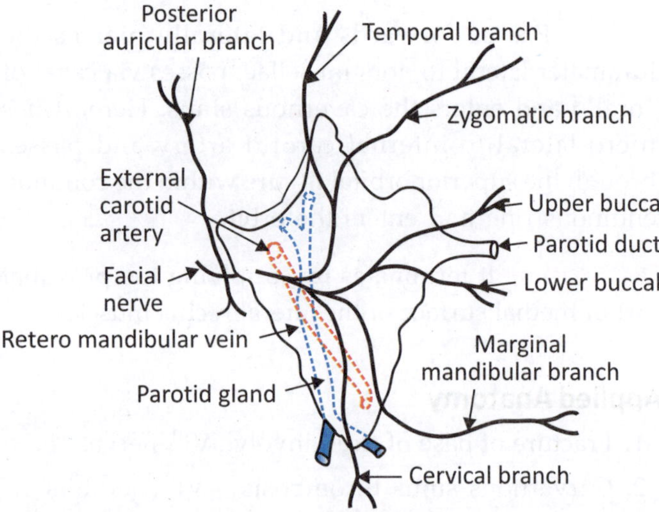

Fig. 35.13: *Relation of facial nerve within the parotid gland*

Communications of VIIth Nerve:

1. Communicating branch to VIIIth nerve within internal acoustic meatus.
2. Communicating branch at geniculate ganglion
   (a) External petrosal to middle meningeal plexus.
   (b) Lesser superficial petrosal nerve – otic ganglion.
   (c) Greater superficial petrosal nerve – pterygo palatine ganglion.
3. At facial nerve canal – communicates with auricular branch of vagus.
4. Just below stylomastoid foramen – communicates with IXth, Xth, auriculo temporal and great auricular nerves.
5. In face – it communicates with branches of trigeminal nerve (Vth).

8. VESTIBULO COCHLEAR NERVE

- It is the eighth cranial nerve – purely sensory.
- Also called as stato acoustic nerve.

- It performs the functions of hearing and balancing of the body.

Cochlear Nerve (the nerve of hearing) – The spiral ganglion of the spiral organ has bipolar cells.

- The peripheral processes of these cells end in the organ of corti.
- The central processes of these cells form the cochlear nerve.

Vestibular Nerve: (the nerve of balance) Vestibular ganglion of the vestibule of internal ear is made up of bipolar cells.

- The peripheral processes of these cells pass to the neuro-epithelium of the semicircular canals (crista ampularis), utricle and saccule (Maculae).
- The central processes of these bipolar cells collect to form the vestibular nerve.

Course of vestibulo cochlear nerve:

The cochlear nerve and vestibular nerve are passing through the internal acoustic meatus. They run along with the facial nerve and enter the posterior cranial fossa reaching at ponto-medullary junction.

Termination:

A. The cochlear nerve: End in the dorsal and ventral cochlear nuclei. From cochlear nuclei fresh fibres originate and go to the trapezoid body and lateral lemniscus. From the lateral lemniscus these fibres enter the medial geniculate body. From the medial geniculate body via auditory radiation they ultimately end in the auditory cortex.

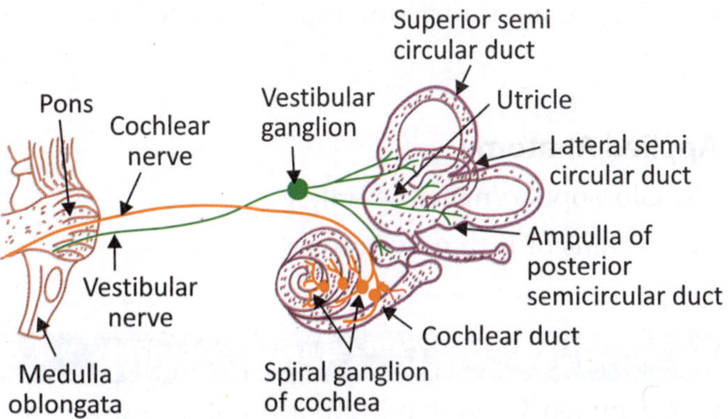

Fig. 35.14: ***Distribution of vestibulo cochlear nerve to membranous labyrinth***

B. The Vestibular Nerve

- Terminates within the superior, inferior, medial and lateral vestibular nuclei, these fibres go to the cerebellum.
- From the lateral vestibular nucleus fibres go to the spinal cord via vestibulo-spinal tract.
- From superior and medial nuclei fibres go to those nuclei innervating eye muscles.
- Medial longitudinal bundle connects this nucleus with other motor cranial nerve nuclei.

Applied Anatomy

1. Certain drugs like streptomycin, quinine may affect the cochlear nerve.
2. **Vestibular nerve involvement has the following features:**
   (a) Vertigo
   (b) Nystagmus
   (c) Nausea and vomiting
   (d) Tachycardia.
3. **Cochlear nerve involvement has the following features:**
   (a) Tinnitus
   (b) Deafness
   (c) Hearing scotoma (deafness for certain pitches)
   (d) Word deafness (sensory aphasia).
4. Fractures of petrous part of temporal bone may involve facial and vestibulo cochlear nerve.

9. GLOSSOPHARYNGEAL NERVE (IXTH CRANIAL NERVE)

- It is a mixed cranial nerve.
- Embroylogically, it is the nerve of the third pharyngeal arch.

Nuclei are situated within the medulla oblongata.

(a) Motor nucleus is a part of nucleus ambiguuas.
(b) Sensory nucleus is a part of nucleus of the tractus solitarius.
(c) Para sympathetic nucleus is the inferior salivatory nucleus.

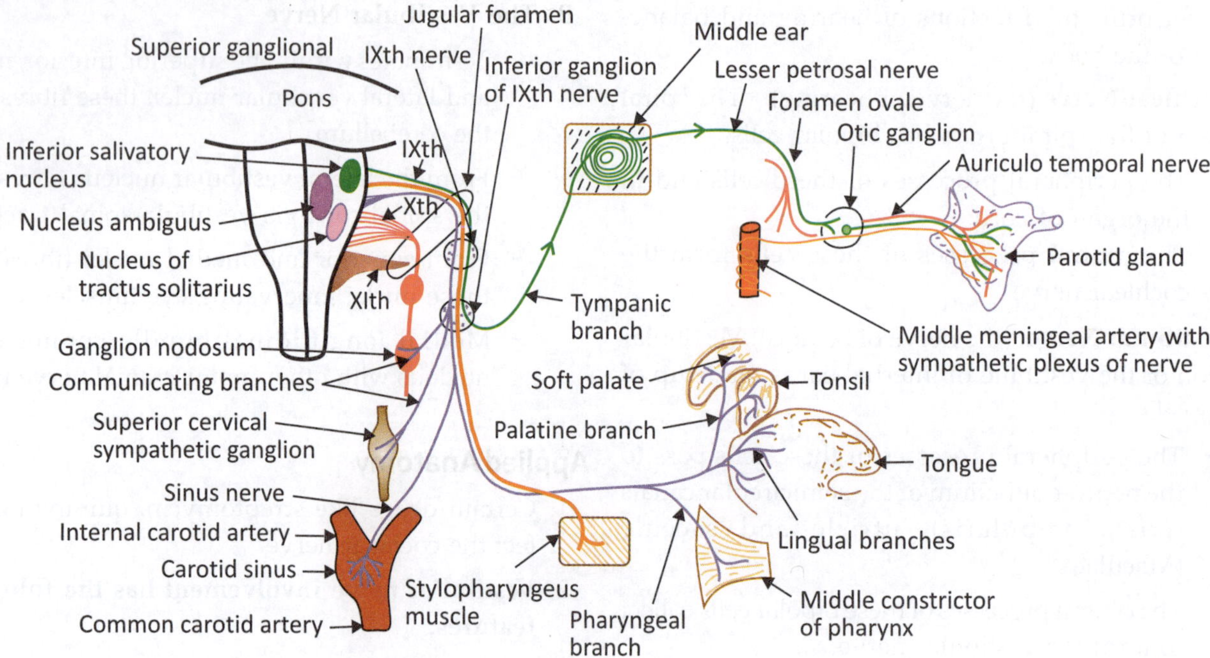

Fig. 35.15: *Glossopharyngeal nerve and its distribution*

Emergence from the medulla oblongata – about 8 to 10 root lets emerge through the postero lateral sulcus of medulla oblongata superior to the vagus and accessory nerves.

Courses:

- All roots unite to form the nerve trunk. It passes through middle part of jugular foramen and leaves the cranial cavity.
- At jugular foramen it has a pair of ganglia, i.e., superior and inferior ganglia.
- It descends between internal carotid artery and internal jugular vein, passes forwards between internal and external carotid arteries, lies deep to the styloid process. It hooks round the stylopharyngeus muscle and passes in the interval between the superior and middle constrictors of the pharynx.

Termination:

It terminates by supplying the posterior 1/3 of the tongue, tonsil, pharynx and glands of the mouth.

Branches:

1. Tympanic branch (Jacobson's nerve) is carrying para-sympathetic fibres to supply the parotid gland.
2. Carotid sinus nerve (nerve of herring) to supply the carotid sinus and carotid body.
3. Pharyngeal branches to join pharyngeal plexus of nerves.
4. Muscular branch to supply stylopharyngeus.
5. Tonsillar branch for palatine tonsil and soft palate.
6. Lingual branches to supply posterior 1/3 to tongue. It carries general sensation and taste sensation from posterior 1/3 of tongue.

Parasympathetic Component: Inferior salivary nucleus → glossopharyngeal nerve → tympanic branch → tympanic plexus → lesser superficial petrosal nerve → otic ganglion → auricuotemporal nerve → parotid gland.

Applied Anatomy

1. Glossopharyngeal neuralgia.
2. Lesions of IXth nerve causes loss of gag reflex.

10. VAGUS NERVE (XTH CRANIAL NERVE)

It is a mixed nerve having both motor and sensory fibres.

Nuclei:

1. Dorsal nucleus
2. Nucleus ambigus

3. Nucleus of the tractus solitarius
4. Spinal tract of trigeminal nerve.

All nuclei of vagus nerve lies in medulla oblongata.

Dorsal nuclei is situated in the floor of 4th ventricle, supplies motor muscles of the thoracic and abdominal viscera.

Nucleus ambiguus: Fibres supply muscles of larynx and constrictor muscles of pharynx.

Nucleus of tractus solitarius: It receives taste sensation from the epiglottis and root of tongue (vallecula).

Spinal tract of trigeminal: It receives sensory fibres from the external ear and tympanic membrane.

Emergence from medulla oblongata 8 to 10 rootlets emerge from postero lateral sulcus of medulla oblongata between glossopharyngeal and cranial part of accessory nerve.

Course: It leaves the cranial cavity through the intermediate compartment of jugular foramen.

Ganglia of vagus: Within the jugular foramen – superior ganglion and below the jugular foramen inferior ganglion are situated. The cranial root of accessory nerve fuses with the vagus just below the inferior ganglion.

The nerve enters the carotid sheath and passes vertically downwards, at the root of neck it crosses anterior to the first part of subclavian artery and enters the thorax.

Right vagus nerve: In the superior mediastinum it lies on the right side of trachea but postero medial to the right brachiocephalic vein and superior vena cava. It is crossed by the arch of azygos vein and descends behind the root of right lung. After giving pulmonary branches it passes behind the oesophagus, joins the oesophageal plexus and passes through the oesophageal opening of the diaphragm as posterior vagal trunk and ends by supplying the pyloric end of the stomach.

Left vagus nerve:

- From the neck it enters the superior mediastinum, passes deep to left brachiocephalic vein between the left common carotid and left subclavian arteries.
- It crosses the left side of the arch of aorta, passes posterior to the root of left lung, gives branches

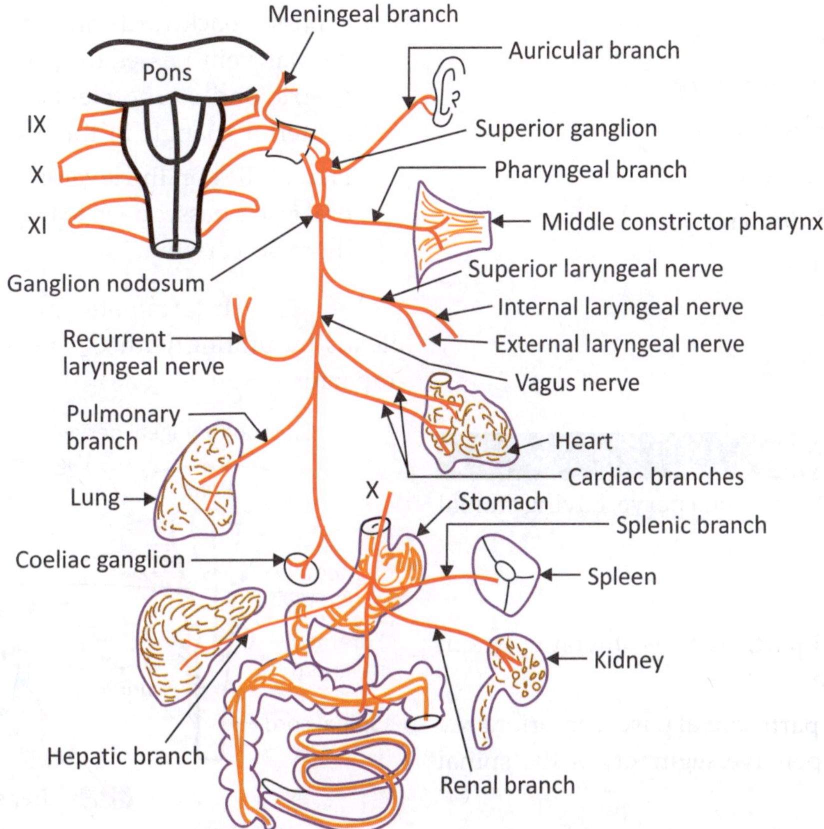

Fig. 35.16: ***Vagus nerve and its distribution***

to left pulmonary plexus and passes anterior to oesophagus.

- Enters the abdomen through oesophageal opening in the diaphragm as anterior vagal trunk.

Branches:

(a) From the jugular ganglion (superior ganglion)

1. Meningeal nerve.
2. Auricular nerve (Alderman's nerve or Arnold's nerve).

(b) From ganglion nodosum (inferior ganglion)

1. Communicating branches to:
   (i) Cervical plexus
   (ii) Superior cervical sympathetic ganglion
   (iii) Hypoglossal nerve.
2. Pharyngeal branches.
3. Superior laryngeal nerve.

(c) From trunk of vagus nerve in the neck

1. Right recurrent laryngeal nerve.
2. Superior cervical cardiac nerve.

(d) Branches in thorax

1. Cardiac nerves
2. Left recurrent laryngeal nerve
3. Pulmonary branches
4. Oesophageal branches.

(e) Branches in the abdomen

1. Gastric branch
2. Coeliac branch
3. Hepatic branch.

11. ACCESSORY NERVE

It is a motor nerve and XIth cranial nerve, having cranial part and spinal part.

Nuclei:

1. **Nucleus of cranial part:** Nucleus ambiguus lies in medulla oblongata.
2. **Nucleus of spinal part:** Lateral part of anterior grey column of the upper five segments of the spinal cord.

Emergence: Cranial part emerges from postero-lateral sulcus of medulla below IXth and X^{th} nerve.

Spinal part emerges from the lateral surface of the upper five cervical segments of the spinal cord.

Courses:

- Cranial part passes forwards and laterally to the jugular foramen.
- Within the jugular foramen both cranial and spinal roots unite to form main trunk of accessory nerve.
- In the lower part of the foramen, both roots separate.
- The cranial part joins the inferior ganglion of vagus and fibres are distributed with vagus nerve branches, e.g., pharyngeal, laryngeal and cardiac branches.

Spinal part: Has five roots:

1. Unite to form spinal accessory passes upwards through foramen magnum and enters the posterior cranial fossa.
2. Passes laterally towards jugular foramen and unites with cranial part.
3. At lower part of foramen it separates and leaves the foramen.
4. It passes backwards and laterally deep to internal jugular vein passes deep to posterior belly of digastric and sterno-cleidomastoid and enters the posterior triangle of the neck.
5. Here, it lies on the levator scapulae and pre-vertebral fascia passes deep to trapezius muscle upto 12th thoracic vertebra.

Termination: It terminates by forming sub-trapezoid plexus by uniting with C_3 and C_4 nerves and supply trapezius.

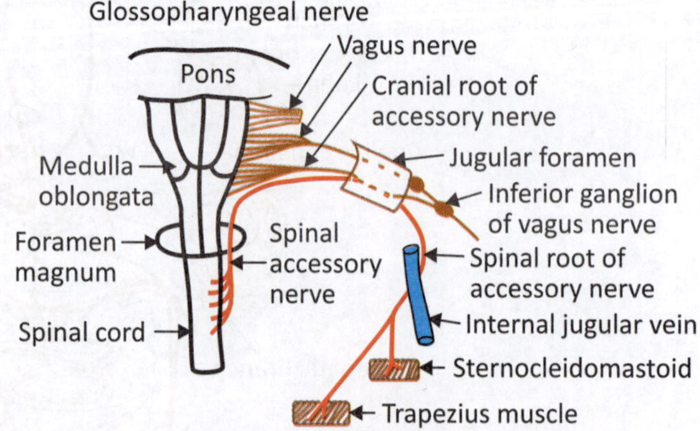

Fig. 35.17: *Accessory nerve*

Branches:

1. Muscular branches to sternocleido mastoid and trapezius muscle.
2. Communicating branches to C_3, C_4 and C_5 nerves.

Applied Anatomy

1. Spinal accessory may be irritated by enlarged lymph nodes of posterior triangle of neck and causes spasmodic torticollis.
2. During bilateral paralysis of accessory nerve, there is difficulty in rotating the neck on raising the chin, head drops forwards, trapezius atrophy and results in flat shoulder.
3. Cervical lymph glands are enlarged and compress the accessory nerve.

12. HYPOGLOSSAL NERVE (MOTOR CRANIAL NERVE)

- It is the XIIth cranial nerve.
- Emerging from anterior part of medulla oblongata just like ventral root of a spinal nerve emerges from the spinal cord (i.e., Antero-lateral sulcus of medulla).

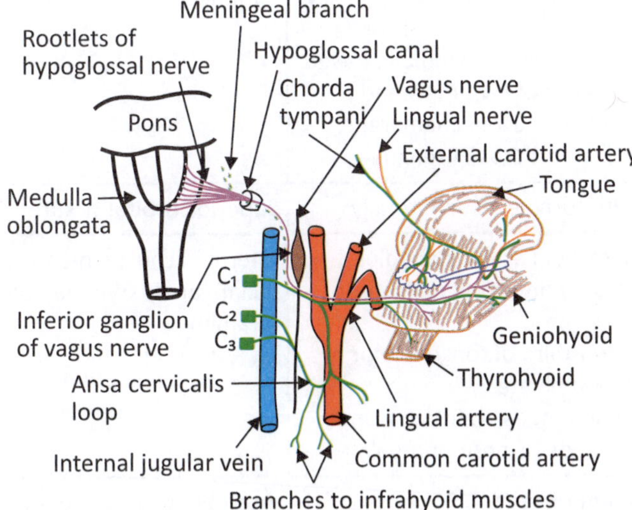

Fig. 35.18: *Hypoglossal nerve*

Nucleus: 2 cm long nucleus present in medulla oblongata in the floor of the 4th ventricle.

Emergence from brain stem – about 10 rootlets emerge from lateral sulcus of medulla in between pyramid and olive.

Courses:

- Passes forwards and laterally towards hypoglossal canal. Here, fibres unite to form two nerve bundles.
- Pierce the duramater and two bundles unite to form a single nerve and leaves the cranial cavity.
- It winds round the inferior ganglion of vagus nerve.
- It runs vertically downwards between internal jugular vein and internal carotid artery.
- Passes deep to posterior belly of digastric and reaches the carotid triangle.
- At the level of the angle of the mandible it passes forwards and crosses superficial to:
  - Internal carotid artery
  - External carotid artery
  - Loop of lingual artery.
- It is superficially crossed by common facial vein.
- It runs on the outer surface of hyoglossus muscle and accompanied by vene commitence hypo-glossi.
- The nerve is related superiorly to deep part of submandibular gland, submandibular ganglion, submandibular duct and lingual nerve.

Termination: It passes deep to mylohyoid muscle and ends by supplying all the muscles of the tongue except palato glossus muscle – supplied by pharyngeal plexus.

Communications:

1. Superior cervical sympathetic ganglion.
2. C_1 fibres join the hypoglossal nerve and leaves it as the superior limb of ansa cervicalis.
3. Pharyngeal plexus.
4. Lingual nerve.

Branches:

1. Meningeal branch – nervi spinosus
2. Superior limb of ansa carvicalis
3. Nerve to thyrohyoid and geniohyoid
4. Muscular branches to supply muscles of tongue
   (a) Styloglossus
   (b) Hyoglossus
   (c) Genioglossus
   (d) All the intrinsic muscles of the tongue.

Applied Anatomy

1. When hypoglossal nerve is injured unilaterally the affected side of the tongue is swollen. When protruded it deviates towards the affected side.
2. Bilateral injury of XIIth nerve causes:
   (a) Immobile tongue
   (b) Sticky speech
   (c) Difficulty in swallowing

   The tongue may fall back and closes the glottis, this produces suffocation.

Table 35.1: ***Cranial Nerves***

Name of Nerve	Components	Function	Opening in Skull
I. Oflactory	Sensory	Smell	Opening in cribri form plate of ethmoid
II. Optic	Sensory	Vision	Optic canal
III. Oculomotor	Motor	Lifts upper eyelid, turns eyeball upward, downward, and medially; constricts pupil; and accommodates eye	Superior orbital fissure
IV. Trochlear	Sensory	Assists in turning eyeball downward and laterally	Superior orbital fissur
V. Trigeminal Ophthalmic division	Mixed Sensory	Cornea, skin of forehead, scalp, eyelids, and nose; also mucous membrane of paranasal sinuses and nasal cavity	Superior orbital fissure
Maxillary division	Sensory	Skin of face over maxilla and the upper lip; teeth of upper jaw; mucous membrane of nose, the maxillary air sinus and palate	Foramen Rotundum
Mandibular division	Motor + Sensory] Mixed	Muscles of mastication, mylohoid, anterior belly of digastric, tensor veli palatini, and tensor tympani skin of cheek; skin over mandible, lower lip, and side of head; teeth of lower jaw and temporomandibular joint; mucous membrane of mouth and anterior two-thirds of tongue	Foramen ovale
VI. Abducent	Motor	Lateral rectus muscle: turns eyeball laterally	Superior orbital fissure
VII. Facial	Motor Sensory Secretomotor parasympathetic	Muscles of face, cheek, and scalp; stapedius muscle of middle ear; stylohyoid; and posterior belly of digastric Taste from anterior two-third of tongue, floor of floor of mouth and hard palate Submandibular and sublingual salivary glands, lacrimal gland, and glands of nose and palate	Internal acoustic meatus, facial canal, stylomastoid foramen
VIII. Vestibulocochlear – Vestibular – Cochlear	Sensory Sensory	Position and movement of head Hearing	Internal acoustic meatus
IX. Glossopharyngeal	Mixed-motor Secreto motor Parasympathetic Sensory	Stylopharyngeus muscle: Assists swallowing Parotid salivary gland General sensation and taste from posterior one-third of tongue, and pharynx; carotid sinus and carotid body	Jugular foramen

Name of Nerve	Components	Function	Opening in Skull
X. Vagus	Motor Sensory	Constrictor muscles of pharynx and intrinsic muscles of larynx; involuntary muscle of trachea and bronchi, heart, alimentary tract from pharynx to splenic flexure of colon; liver and pancreas Taste from epiglottis and vallecula and afferent fibres from structures named above	Jugular foramen
XI. Accessory – Cranial root – Spinal root	Motor Motor	Muscles of soft palate, pharynx and larynx Sternocleidomastoid and trapezius muscles	Jugular foramen
XII. Hypoglossal	Motor	Muscles of tongue controlling its shape and movement (except palatoglossus)	Hypoglossal canal

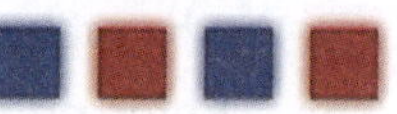

Review of Head and Neck

1. What is the root value of cervical plexus and name the branches of cervical plexus?

Ans.: Refer pg no. 186, chapter 27.

2. Name the branches of subclavian artery?

Ans.: Refer pg no. 190, chapter 27.

3. Name the branches of vertebral artery?

Ans.: Refer pg no. 192, chapter 27.

4. What are boundaries of suboccipital triangle?

Ans.: Refer pg no. 94, chapter 12.

5. What are the boundaries of parotid bed?

Ans.: Refer pg no. 129, chapter 16.

6. What are structures present within parotid gland?

Ans.: Refer pg no. 131, chapter 16.

7. What is nerve supply of parotid gland?

Ans.: Refer pg no. 132, chapter 16.

8. What is mumps?

Ans.: This is a viral infection of the parotid gland and involves both sides.

9. Enumerate bones forming skull?

Ans.: Refer pg no. 45, chapter 9.

10. What is bregma?

Ans.: Junction between two parietal and frontal bone is called Bregma. It is the point at which coronal and sagittal sutures meet.

11. What is lambda?

Ans.: Lambda is the meeting point of two parietal and occipital bone, i.e., junction of sagittal and lambdoid suture. In the foetal skull it is represented as the posterior fontenelle.

12. What is pterion?

Ans.: It is the meeting point of greater wing of sphenoid, parietal bone, frontal and temporal bones. It is deeply related to middle meningeal vessels.

13. What is asterion?

Ans.: Asterion is the meeting point of parietomastoid, occipitomastoid and lambdoid sutures. In infant it is the site of postero lateral fontanelle.

14. What is anterior fontanelle?

Ans.: Refer pg no. 51, chapter 9.

15. What are layers of scalp and explain its nerve supply?

Ans.: Refer pg no. 74, chapter 10.

16. Which is the dangerous layer of scalp?

Ans.: **Loose areolar tissue** is dangerous layer of scalp because emissary veins lies in this layer. Extra cranial infection can spread intra canially due to presence of emissary veins or *vice-versa.*

17. What is caput succedanum?

Ans.: Heeping up of scalp in foetus occurs during labour due to over lapping of skull bones and collection of fluid in the loose areolar tissue due to forces of labour and poor venous and lymphatic return.

18. Explain mandible?

Ans.: Refer pg no. 52, chapter 9.

19. What is suprameatal triangle?

Ans.: Refer pg no. 48, chapter 9.

20. What is arterial supply of pituitary gland?

Ans.: Refer pg no. 253, chapter 34.

21. What temporal fossa?

Ans.: Refer pg no. 76-77, chapter 10.

22. What is chalazion?

Ans.: It is a chronic granulomatous inflammation of the Meibomian gland (Tarsal glands).

23. What is levator palpebrae superioris?

Ans.: Refer pg no. 79, chapter 11.

24. What is central artery of retina?

Ans.: Refer pg no. 104, chapter 13.

25. What is papilloedema?

Ans.: When intra cranial pressure is increased – optic nerve head in the retina is swollen – called papilloedema.

26. What is accommodation?

Ans.: Refer pg no. 112, chapter 13.

27. What is cataract?

Ans.: Refer pg no. 112, chapter 13.

28. Explain dural venous sinuses?

Ans.: Refer pg no. 249, chapter 34.

29. Explain sigmoid sinus?

Ans.: Refer pg no. 252, chapter 34.

30. What are emissary veins?

Ans.: Refer pg no. 253, chapter 34

31. Explain submandibular gland?

Ans.: Refer pg no. 135-139, chapter 17.

32. What is cutaneous nerve supply of neck and what are layers of deep cervical of neck?

Ans.: Refer pg no. 113, chapter 14.

33. Name the triangle of neck?

Ans.: Refer pg no. 117, chapter 14 and pg no. 123-128, chapter 15.

34. Name the branches of maxillary artery?

Ans.: Refer pg no. 146, chapter 18.

35. Name the branches of external carotid artery?

Ans.: Refer pg no. 195-198, chapter 28.

36. What is Waldeyer's ring?

Ans.: Refer chapter 25.

37. What is the boundaries of piriform fossa?

Ans.: Refer pg no. 213, chapter 30.

38. What is the Eustachian tube?

Ans.: Refer pg no. 237, chapter 33.

39. Classified muscles of the tongue and larynx?

Ans.: Muscles of tongue (Refer pg no. 165, chapter 23)
Muscles of larynx (Refer pg no. 219, chapter 31)

40. What is characteristic features of tonsils?

Ans.: Refer pg no. 171-172, chapter 25.

41. Enumerate the cranial nerves.

Ans.: Refer pg no. 217, chapter 35.

42. Name the branches of mandibular nerve?

Ans.: Refer pg no. 147-149, chapter 18.

43. Name the branches of maxillary nerve?

Ans.: Refer pg no. 154, chapter 20.

44. Name the branches of glossopharyngeal nerve?

Ans.: Refer pg no. 268, chapter 35.

45. Name the branches of vagus nerve in head and neck

Ans.: Refer pg no. 270, chapter 35.

46. What are the parts of tooth?

Ans.: Refer pg no. 158, chapter 21.

47. What are timings of eruption of teeth?

Ans.: Refer pg no. 157, chapter 21.

48. What are muscles of tongue?

Ans.: Refer pg no. 165, chapter 23.

49. What is the sensory supply of tongue?

Ans.: Refer pg no. 167, chapter 23.

50. Name the branches of hypoglossal nerve?

Ans.: Refer pg no. 271, chapter 35.

SELF ASSESSMENT QUESTIONS

1. Describe scalp in detail with its applied.
2. Describe deep fascia of neck in detail.
3. Describe posterior triangle of neck.
4. Describe parotid gland in detail.
5. Describe submandibular gland.
6. Describe muscles of masticate in a tabular form.

7. Describe T.M.J. with its applied.
8. Describe mandibular nerve.
9. Describe soft palate with its applied.
10. Describe para nasal air sinuses.
11. Describe external carotid artery.
12. Describe thyroid gland with its development.
13. Describe intracranial dural sinus.
14. Describe facial nerve.
15. Describe mandibular nerve
16. Write short notes on:
    - Facial artery
    - Sensory nerve supply of face
    - Orbicularis oculi
    - Orbicularis oris
    - Buccinator
    - Lacrimal apparatus
    - Extra ocular muscles
    - Ophthalmic artery
    - Optic nerve
    - Trapezius
    - Levator scalpulae
    - Sub occipital triangle
    - Submental triangle
    - Digastric triangle
    - Carotid triangle
    - Otic ganglion
    - Chorda tympani nerve
    - Maxillary artery
    - Pterygo palatine ganglion
    - Maxillary nerve
    - Cleft palate
    - Structure of tooth
    - Waldayer's lymphatic ring
    - Palatine tonsil
    - Maxillary air sinus
    - Lateral wall of nose
    - Scalene mass
    - Scalene mars
    - Vertebral triangle
    - Styloid apparatus
    - Vertebral artery
    - Lingual artery
    - Superior thyroid artery
    - Facial artery
    - Internal jugular vein
    - Cervical sympathetic trunk
    - Hyoglossus
    - Sternocleido mastoid
    - Mylohyoid
    - Digastric
    - Development of tongue
    - Development of teeth
    - Pharynx
    - Thyroid cartilage
    - Structure of larynx
    - Tympanic cavity
    - Ear ossicles
    - Tympanic membrane
    - Labyrinth
    - Cervical plexus of nerves
    - Brachial plexus of nerves
    - Ansa cervicalis
    - Ansa subclavia
    - Subclavian artery
    - Phrenic nerve
    - Cavernous sinus
    - Trigeminal ganglion
    - Pituitary gland
    - Superior orbital fissure
    - Maxillary nerve
    - Nasociliary nerve
    - Optic nerve
    - Oculomotor nerve
    - Trochlear nerve
    - Abducent nerve
    - Glossopharyngeal nerve
    - Hypoglossal nerve
    - Accessory nerve
17. Make diagrams of:
    - T.S. neck of C6
    - T.S. at parotid region
    - Sensory nerve supply face
    - Lymphatic drainage of tongue
    - Hemioglossus with its relations
    - Hyoglossus with its relations
    - Structure of tooth

PART 3

BRAIN

THE CHAPTERS ARE:

36. Brain

37. Mid Brain (Mesencephalon)

38. Cerebellum

39. Pons

40. Medulla Oblongata

41. Spinal Cord

CHAPTER 36

Brain

INTRODUCTION

The nervous system is the most complex system of the body. It controls all the activities of the body directly or indirectly that includes physical, psychological and intellectual. It is responsible for judgement, intelligence and memory. It is highly evolved at the cost of regeneration. It is the chief controlling and co-ordinating system of the body. It adjusts the body to the surroundings and regulates all bodily activities both voluntary and involuntary.

DIVISIONS OF NERVOUS SYSTEM

It is divided into two parts:

A. **Central Nervous System (C.N.S.):** Includes Brain and spinal cord.

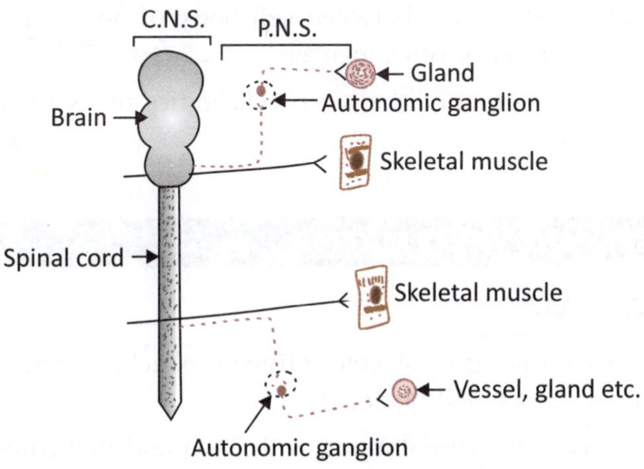

Fig. 36.1: *Parts of nervous system*

B. **Peripheral Nervous System (P.N.S.):** Peripheral nerves supply body wall and skeletal muscles (spinal and cranial nerves) and associated ganglions of autonomic nervous system, both sympathetic and parasympathetic system which suppliy smooth muscles of viscera, gland and blood vessels.

Parts of brain:

1. Cerebrum
2. Cerebellum
3. Mid Brain
4. Pons
5. Medulla.

Brain stem – includes mid-brain + pons + medulla

↓

Spinal cord → spinal nerves

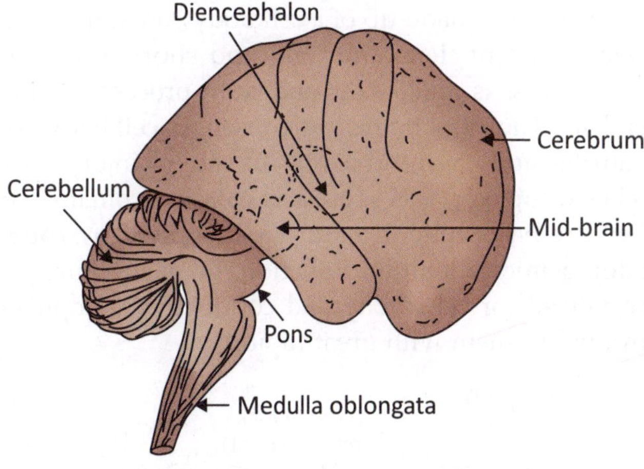

Fig. 36.2: *Parts of brain*

Peripheral nerves attached to brain are cranial nerves.

The nerves supply body wall and limbs are called cerebrospinal nerves.

C. **Autonomic Nervous System (A.N.S.):** The nerves supplying viscera alongwith parts of brain and spinal cord related to them constitute A.N.S.

A.N.S.: It has two parts:

(a) Sympathetic and

(b) Para sympathetic.

NERVOUS TISSUES

Two types of cells are found in nervous system:

1. **Neurons:** These are specialized cells of nervous system and main cells concerned with functioning of nervous system.
2. **Neuroglia:** This is special connective tissue present in nervous system. Various types of neuroglial cells are:

   Astrocytes: These are concerned with the nutrition of the nervous tissue.

   Microglia: These are macrophages of C.N.S.

   Ependymal cells: These are columnar cells lining the cavities of C.N.S.

   Oligodendrocytes: These myelinate the tracts. Proliferation of glial cells is called gliosis. C.N.S. lesions heal by gliosis and form scar in nervous system.

NEURON

Each neuron is made-up of a cell body containing nissl substance, a nucleus and long and short processes. Long process is called axon and short process is called dendrite. The Nissl bodies are present in cell body and dendrites and absent in axons. In case of injury these bodies disappear, this process is called chromatolysis. They are basophilic in nature and formed by rough endoplasmic reticulum. Functionally each neuron is specialized for sensitivity and conductivity. Impulses can flow in them with great rapidity.

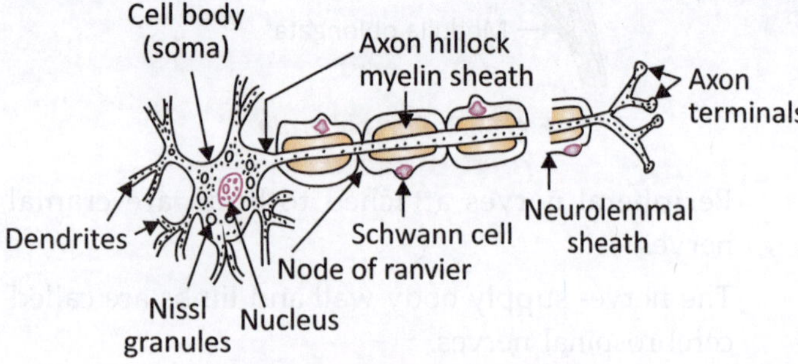

Fig. 36.3: ***Structure of a neuron***

PERIPHERAL NERVES

These are collections of nerve fibres (axon).

SYNAPSE

The junction between two neurons is called synapse. They are connected to each other by their process, forming long chains along which the impulses are conducted. Contacts between neurons is by contiguity and not by continuity. The impulse is transmitted across a synapse through biochemical neurotransmitters.

Axon

Terminates by meeting another neuron in brain.

- Outside the central nervous system – it may end
  - in muscle
  - in gland or
  - neuron in ganglion at peripheral region.

Types of Synapse

It may be:

1. Axo-axonic – between two axons.
2. Axo-dendritic – between axon of one neuron and dendrite of another neuron.
3. Dendrodendritic – between two dendrites.
4. Somo-dendritic – between cell body of one neuron and dendrite of another neuron.
5. Somo-axonic – between cell body of one neuron and axon of other neuron.
6. Somo-somatic – between cell bodies of two neurons.

GREY AND WHITE MATTER

GREY MATTER

Have a darker greyish colour due to collection of nerve cells (dark stained nucleus).

- Neurons present along with axon and dendrites
- Axon are unmyelinated.

WHITE MATTER

- Whitish in colour.

- Axons are – Myelinated fibres due to reflection of light from myelin give whitish look.

BRAIN

Brain is divided into three parts:

I. Forebrain (Prosencephalon)	1. Cerebrum 2. Diencephalon
II. Mid brain (Mesencephalon)	1. Mid brain
III. Hind brain (Rhombancephalon)	1. Pons 2. Medulla 3. Cerebellum

In brain grey matter lies out side and white matter lies inside while in spinal cord grey matter lies around the central canal and white matter lies at periphery.

FOREBRAIN (PROSENCEPHALON)

It is constituted by:

I. Cerebrum

II. Diencephalon.

I. Cerebrum

It is made-up of two large cerebral hemispheres which are incompletely separated by the median longitudinal fissure. Two hemispheres are connected to each other across the median plane by the corpus collosum. Each hemisphere has a cavity called lateral ventricle. The presence of sulci and gyri on the surface of hemisphere increases the surface area of the brain to accommodate many neurons without increasing the size of the brain. There are specific areas on the brain for specific functions.

External features:

Each cerebral hemisphere has three surfaces:

1. **Superolateral surface** is convex and related to cranial vault.
2. **Medial surface** is flat and vertical, falx cerebri separates it from other hemisphere.
3. **Inferior surface** is irregular and divided into an anterior part – orbital surface and a posterior part – tentorial surface. Two parts are separated by – a deep cleft called stem of lateral sulcus.

Borders are three:

1. **Supero medial border:** It separates supero-lateral surface from medial surface.
2. **Infero lateral border:** Separates superolateral surface from the inferior surface.
3. **Infero medial border divided into two parts:**
   (a) **Medial orbital border:** Separates medial surface from orbital surface.
   (b) **Medial occipital border:** It separates medial surface from tentorial surface.

Poles are three:

1. Frontal pole – present at anterior end.
2. Occipital pole – present at posterior end.
3. Temporal pole – lies laterally at the anterior end of the temporal lobe.

The surface of the cerebrum is made into elevations and depressions. The elevations are called gyri and depressions are called sulci.

Types of Sulci: They are classified into:

1. **Limiting sulcus:** They are separating two functionally different areas, e.g., Central sulcus – it separates sensory and motor areas.
2. **Complete sulcus:** They are deep sulci – make elevations in the floor of the lateral ventricle, e.g., Calcarine sulcus and collateral sulcus.
3. **Axial sulcus:** Develops in the long axis of a rapidly growing homogenous area, e.g., Post-calcarine sulcus.
4. **Operculated sulcus:** Separates by its lips two areas and contains a third area in the walls of the sulcus, e.g., Lunate sulcus.

Central sulcus (the fissure of Rolando): It is situated in the superolateral surface. Anterior to this sulcus the motor cortex and posterior to the sulcus the sensory cortex are situated.

(a) It commences from the supero medial border about 1 cm posterior to mid-point between frontal and occipital poles.

(b) It is directed downwards, forwards and laterally.

(c) It is situated in the centre of three parallel sulci.

(d) In front of the central sulcus is the frontal lobe and behind the sulcus is the parietal lobe.

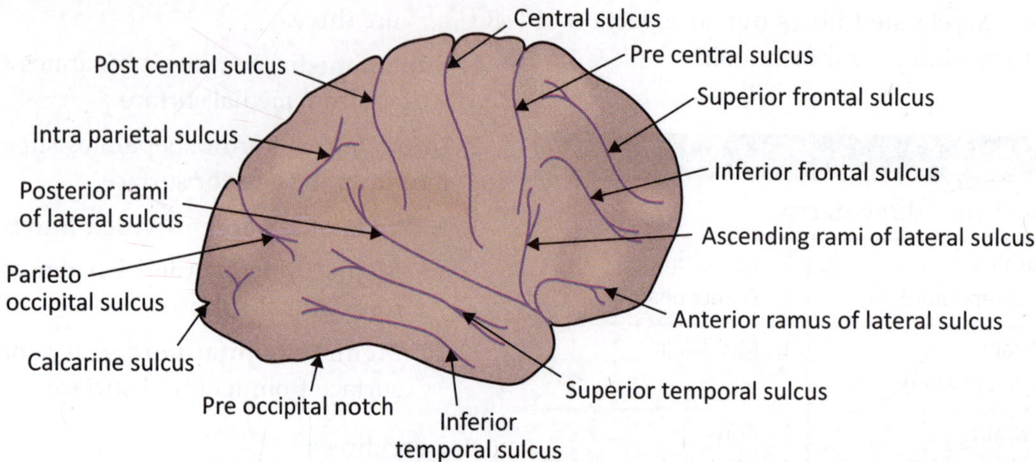

Fig. 36.4: ***Sulci of the superolateral surface of cerebrum***

Lobulation of the Cerebrum

It has four lobes are bounded as follows:

S. No.	Boundaries	Frontal lobe	Parietal lobe	Temporal lobe	Occipital lobe
1.	Anteriorly	Frontal pole	Central sulcus	Temporal pole between	Imaginary line drawn between parieto-occipital sulcus and preoccipital notch
2.	Posteriorly	Central sulcus	Imaginary line drawn between parieto occipital sulcus and preoccipital notch	Imaginary line drawn between parieto occipital sulcus and preoccipital notch	Occipital pole
3.	Superiorly	Supero medial border	Supero medial border	Posterior ramus of lateral sulcus and imaginary line drawn backwards.	Supero medial border
4.	Inferiorly	Super-ciliary border and posterior ramus of lateral sulcus	Posterior ramus of lateral sulcus and imaginary line drawn backwards	Inferolateral border	Inferolateral border

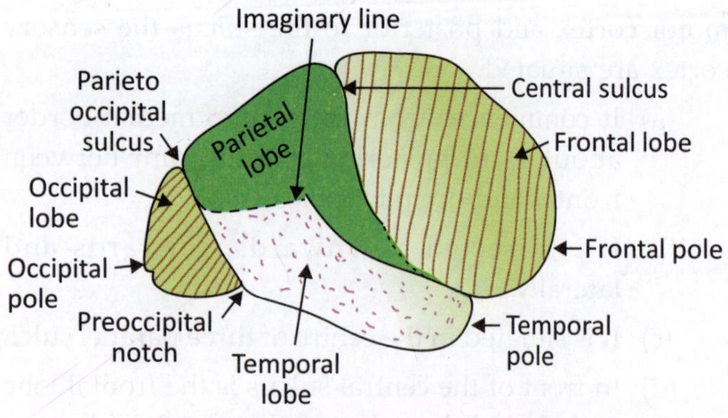

Fig. 36.5: ***Lobulation of the cerebrum***

Lateral sulcus (Sylvian Sulcus): It commences in the inferior surface of the cerebrum has following parts:

1. Stem
2. Anterior ramus
3. Ascending ramus
4. Posterior ramus.

Note: The parieto occipital sulcus is situated 5 cm anterior to the occipital pole in the supero medial border. Preoccipital notch is situated 5 cm anterior to the occipital pole in the inferolateral border.

1. **Frontal Lobe:** It is situated anterior to the central sulcus. Its features are:

(a) Anterior to central sulcus the pre central gyrus is situated. It is motor cortex of the opposite half of the body. Body is represented upside down.

(b) Anterior to pre central gyrus – pre central sulcus is situated.

(c) Infront of the pre central sulcus – superior and inferior frontal sulci are running antero posteriorly.

(d) Superior to superior frontal sulcus the superior frontal gyrus is situated.

(e) The middle frontal gyrus is found between superior and inferior frontal sulci.

(f) Below the inferior frontal sulcus the inferior frontal gyrus is found.

(g) The inferior frontal gyrus is traversed by anterior and ascending rami of lateral sulcus. They divide the inferior frontal gyrus into three parts:

(i) **Pars orbitalis** is situated inferior to the anterior ramus of lateral sulcus.

(ii) **Pars triangularis** is situated between anterior and ascending rami of lateral sulcus.

(iii) **Pars opercularis** lies posterior to ascending ramus.

➢ These three areas together form Motor speech area of Broca.

Functions of frontal lobe:

➢ Pre central gyrus is motor cortex for opposite half of the body.

➢ Pre frontal area lies anterior to pre central gyrus is concerned with the development and maintenance of personality, behaviour, intelligence and adjustment with the social environment.

➢ Hindsight, insight and foresight are the functions performed by pre frontal area.

➢ Orbital surface of frontal lobe is concerned with emotion and behaviour.

➢ Learning and development of memory pattern are also concerned with the frontal lobe.

➢ In the posterior part of middle frontal gyrus the area of frontal eyefield is situated.

2. **Parietal lobe:** Lies posterior to central sulcus. Its features are:

(a) Behind the central sulcus post central gyrus is situated. It is the sensory areas of the opposite half of the body. Body is represented upside down.

(b) Behind the post central gyrus – post central sulcus is situated.

(c) Intra parietal sulcus arises from the middle of the post central sulcus and runs backwards. It divides the parietal lobe into superior and inferior parietal lobule.

(d) Inferior parital lobule is subdivided by the entry of:

(i) Posterior ramus of lateral sulcus

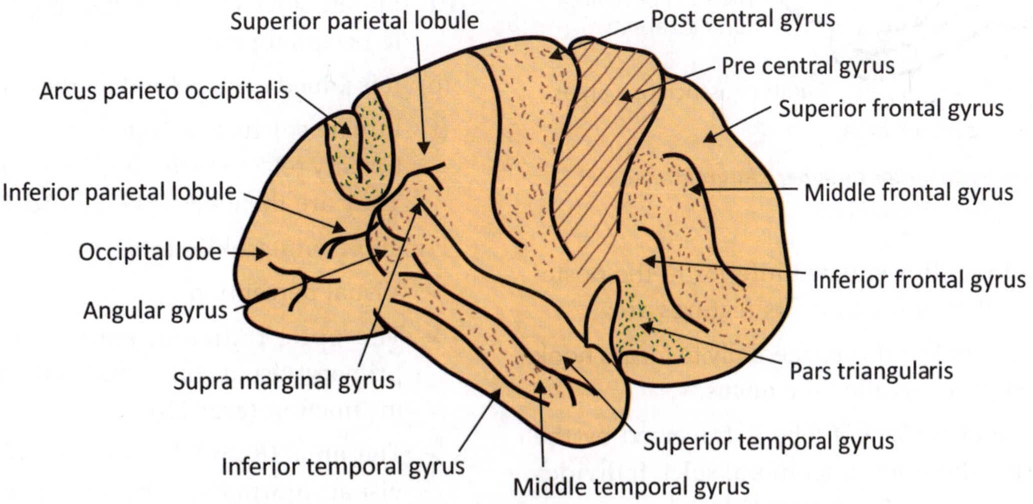

Fig. 36.6: *Gyrus of the supero-lateral surface of cerebrum*

(ii) Superior temporal sulcus

(iii) Inferior temporal sulcus.

- The part of inferior parietal lobule surrounding posterior ramus of lateral sulcus is called supra marginal gyrus.
- The part surrounding the superior temporal sulcus is called angular gyrus.
- The part surrounding the inferior temporal sulcus is called posterior parietal lobule.

Functions of parietal lobe:

- Primary sensory cortex of the opposite half of the body.
- Touch, pressure, temperature, joint sense and vibrations are appreciated.
- Special recognition of the body, e.g., position and movements of the body and limbs.
- Tactile localization and discrimination are done by this lobe.
- The parietal speech centre – sensory speech area is formed by supra marginal and angular gyrus.
- Parietal operculum of the insula has taste area.
- Stereognostic function, i.e., tridiamentional memory is done in this lobe.

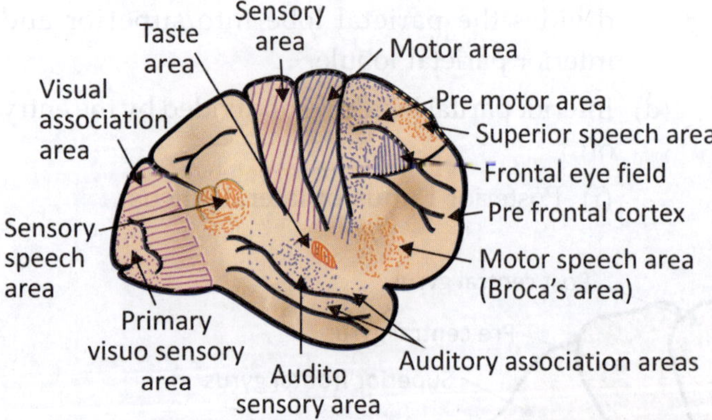

Fig. 36.7: *Functional areas on supero lateral surface of cerebrum*

3. Temporal lobe: It is situated inferior to the posterior ramus of lateral sulcus. Its features are:

(a) Temporal pole is turned medially to form a hook shaped process called the uncus.

(b) The lateral surface of lobe is traversed by the superior and inferior temporal sulci. It divides the surface into three gyri:

(i) **Superior temporal gyrus** – lies above superior temporal sulcus.

(ii) **Middle temporal gyrus** – lies between superior and inferior temporal sulcus.

(iii) **Inferior temporal gyrus** – lies below the inferior temporal sulcus.

(c) The middle of the superior temporal gyrus and anterior transverse temporal gyri together form the principal auditory area.

(d) The audito psychic area is situated in the superior, middle and inferior temporal gyri.

Functions of temporal lobe

- Auditory area is present in superior temporal and anterior transverse gyrus. Auditory fibres project bilaterally into the cortex.
- Audito-psychic function.
- Storage of memory.
- Smell sensation – center lies in uncus.
- Temporal lobe helps in the articulated speech.

4. Occipital lobe: It is situated posterior to an imaginary line between parieto occipital sulcus and pre occipital notch. Its features are:

(a) Arcus parieto occipital is a gyrus encircling the parieto occipital sulcus.

(b) Just behind the arcus parieto occipitalis, the transverse occipital sulcus descends from supero-medial margin.

(c) The lateral occipital sulcus is antero posteriorly situated in the occipital lobe. It divides the lobe into superior and inferior occipital gyri.

(d) Lunate sulcus is semi lunar shaped, lies anterior to occipital pole.

(e) It is joined from behind by the calcarine sulcus.

(f) Lunate sulcus is an operculated sulcus – functionally related to the areas of visual perception. They are the areas – 17, 18 and 19.

Functions of occipital lobe

- Visual perception.
- The optic radiation enters into the area 17 primary visual cortex and is the visuo psychic in function (area 18).
- The area 18 and 19 are able to correlate the visual informations in recognizing an object.

Medial Surface of the Cerebrum

It lies between the infero medial border and supero medial border. In this surface there is a white band called corpus callosum is situated. It has following parts – rostrum, genu, body and splenium.

- Rostrum is connected to the optic chiasma by lamina terminalis. Below the corpus callosum lateral ventricle lies. Above the corpus callosum – callosal sulcus is situated.
- Cingulate sulcus commences below and anterior to corpus callosum. It runs above upwards, forwards and then backwards to corpus callosum. Terminal part of this sulcus passes towards supero medial border.
- Cingulate gyrus lies between cingulate and callosal sulcus.
- Above the cingulate sulcus median frontal gyrus lies, posterior part of the gyrus is called para central lobule.

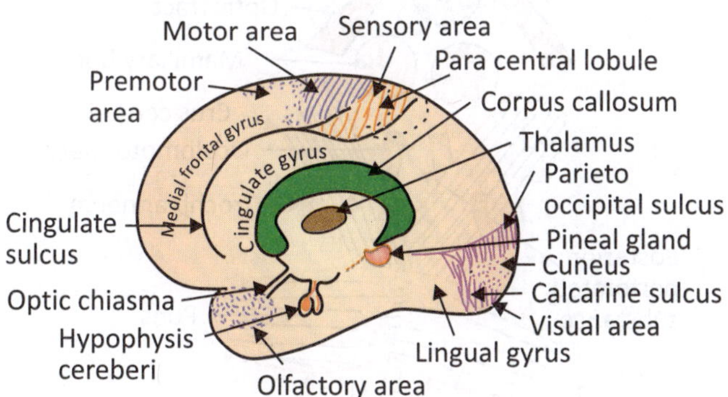

Fig. 36.8: *Medial surface of cerebrum*

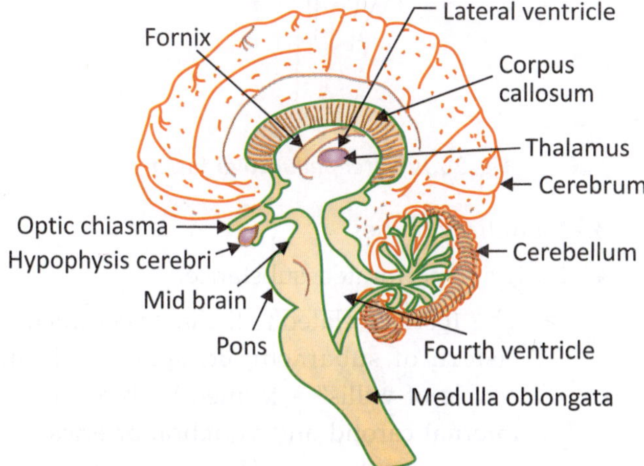

Fig. 36.9: *Medial surface of the brain*

Functionally: Para central lobule controls defaecation, micturition and parturition.

Posterior to the upturned part of cingulated sulcus – pre cuneus gyrus lies, which is limited posteriorly by parieto occipital sulcus. Below and behind this sulcus cuneus lies.

- The calcarine sulcus is situated postero inferior to the cuneus. Anteriorly it unites with the parieto occipital sulcus.
- Below the gyrus – lingual gyrus is situated.
- The lingual gyrus, cuneus and floor of calcarine sulcus are having visual functional areas.

Inferior Surface of the Cerebrum

Boundaries:

1. Laterally – Super ciliary border
2. Infero lateral border.

Medially:

1. Median orbital border
2. Median occipital border.

Parts:

It has two parts:

1. Anterior part is called orbital surface.
2. Posterior part is called tentorial surface.

1. **Orbital surface** is formed by:
   - Frontal lobe and is concerned with emotion and behaviour.
   - Along the medial border of this surface lies gyrus rectus. Lateral to this gyrus is olfactory sulcus which it, lodges olfactory bulb, receiving olfactory nerves from nose.
   - Lateral to olfactory sulcus a "H" shaped orbital sulcus is present which divides the surface into:
     (a) Anterior orbital gyrus
     (b) Posterior orbital gyrus
     (c) Lateral orbital gyrus
     (d) Medial orbital gyrus.

   Orbital surface is related to the roof of the orbit.
2. **Tentorial surface** is formed by occipital and temporal lobes, related to tentorium – cerebelli. There are two sulci present on this surface.
   (a) Collateral sulcus
   (b) Occipito temporal sulcus – lies laterally.

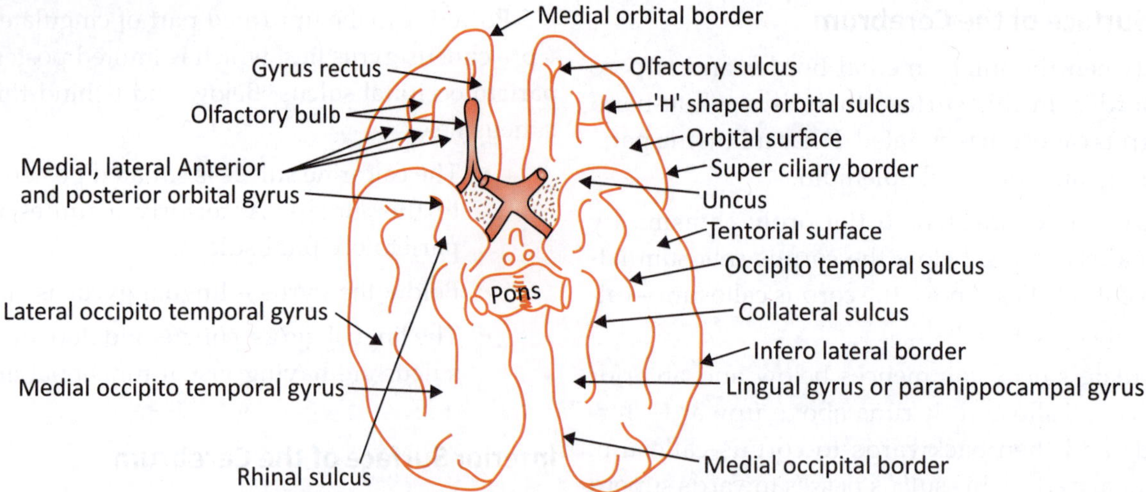

Fig. 36.10: *Inferior surface of the cerebrum*

These two sulci divide this surface into three gyri:

(i) Lateral occipito temporal gyrus

(ii) Medial occipito temporal gyrus

(iii) Para hippocampal gyrus: In the inferior surface just behind the orbital surface, lies the stem of the lateral sulcus. It commences from the triangular shaped area called anterior perforated substance.

Boundaries of Anterior Perforated Substance

- Anterior – Medial and leteral olfactory striae.
- Posteriorly – Uncus of the temporal lobe.
- Medially – Optic chiasma.

Anterior perforated substance has many openings through which central branches of the middle and anterior cerebral artery are passing.

Inter Peduncular Fossa: On the inferior surface between the two cerebral hemispheres there is hexagonal shaped inter peduncular fossa.

Boundaries of inter peduncular fossa:

Anteriorly – optic chiasma

Antero laterally – optic tract

Postero laterally – crus cerebri

Posteriorly – Upper border of the pons.

Floor is formed by the structures anterior to posterior.

1. Tuber cinereum
2. Infundibulum of the pituitary gland

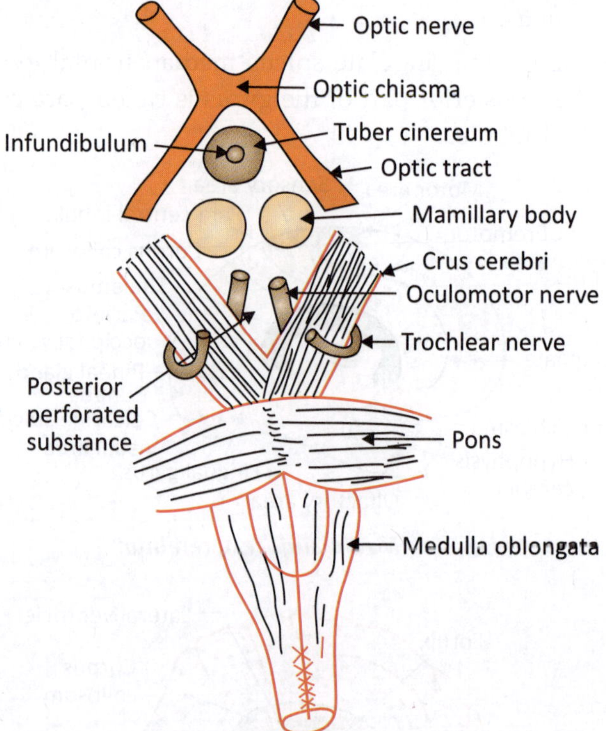

Fig. 36.11: *Inter peduncular fossa*

3. Mamillary bodies
4. Posterior perforated substance.

- This fossa is related to the inter peduncular cistern of subarachnoid space, lodging "circle of willis" – formed by branches of internal carotid and vertebral arteries.
- Oculomotor nerve emerges into this fossa medial to crus cerebri.

Veins of Cerebrum

Veins of cerebrum are classified into superficial and deep veins.

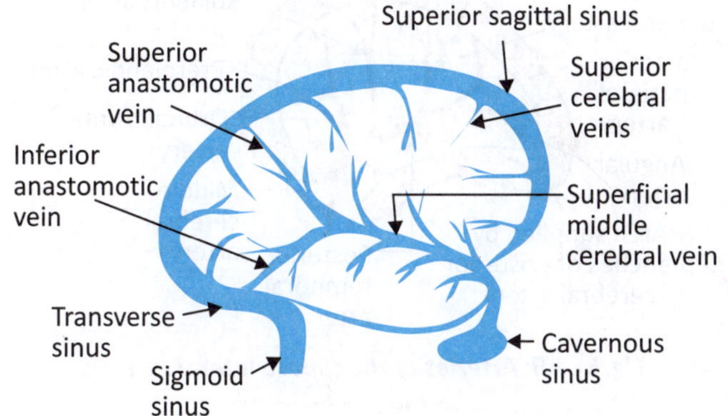

Fig. 36.12: *Superficial veins of the cerebrum*

Characteristics of Veins

1. Walls are devoid of muscles.
2. No valves (valveless thin walled running into subarachnoid space).
3. To maintain patency some of them open into venous sinuses, e.g., superior cerebral veins draining into superior sagittal sinus.
4. Superficial middle cerebral vein drains into cavernous sinus and at times into spheno parietal sinus. Through superior and inferior anastomatic veins it communicates with superior sagittal and transverse sinus.
5. Inferior cerebral veins – drain into cavernous sinus and superior – sagittal sinus.
6. Anterior cerebral veins and deep middle cerebral vein drains into basal vein – formed by union of anterior cerebral vein, striate veins and deep middle cerebral vein. Basal vein drains its blood into great cerebral vein.

II. Diencephalon

It is a middle structure embedded in cerebrum and therefore hidden from the surface. Cavity forms IIIrd ventricle. Hypothalamic sulcus extending from inter ventricular foramen to cerebral aqueduct, divides each half of diencephalon into dorsal and ventral parts.

1. Dorsal part of diencephalon is formed by:

(a) Thalamus.
(b) Metathalamus – including medial and lateral geniculate bodies.
(c) Epithalamus – including pineal body and habenula.

2. Ventral part of diencephalon is formed by:

(a) Hypothalamus
(b) Subthalamus.

BLOOD SUPPLY TO THE BRAIN

- Brain requires continuous supply of blood for its normal metabolic functions.
- 20% of the cardiac output enters the brain.
- Loss of blood supply for 4 minutes causes irreversible damage of brain tissues.
- Brain cells will die, when its blood supply is lost for more than 8 minutes.
- Brain receives its blood supply by internal carotid and vertebral arteries.
- These arteries anastomose with each other at the base of brain to form circle of Willis.

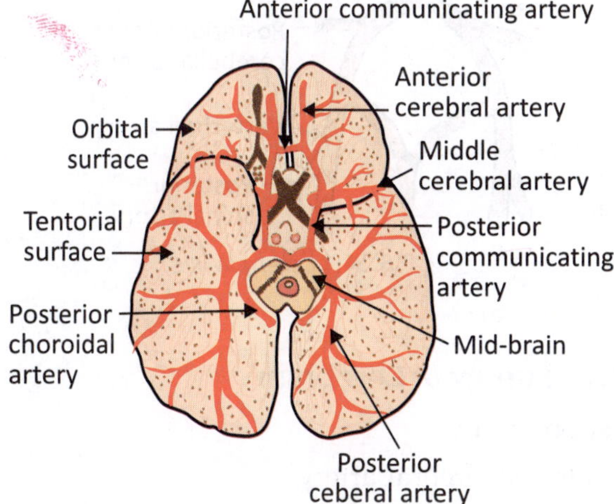

Fig. 36.13: *Arterial supply of inferior surface of cerebrum*

FORMATION OF "CIRCLE OF WILLIS"

1. Vertebral arteries enter the posterior cranial fossa through foramen magnum. Both vertebral arteries unite along the lower border of pons to form basilar artery.
2. Basilar artery terminally divides into a pair of posterior cerebral arteries.
3. Internal carotid artery enters the cranium through the carotid canal – passes through the cavernous sinus after emerging from the sinus it gives anterior cerebral and middle cerebral arteries.

4. Middle cerebral and posterior cerebral arteries are connected by posterior communicating artery.
5. Two anterior cerebral arteries are communicated by anterior communicating artery.
6. Thus an arterial network – called circle of Willis is formed within the subarachnoid space present in the inter peduncular fossa at the base of brain.

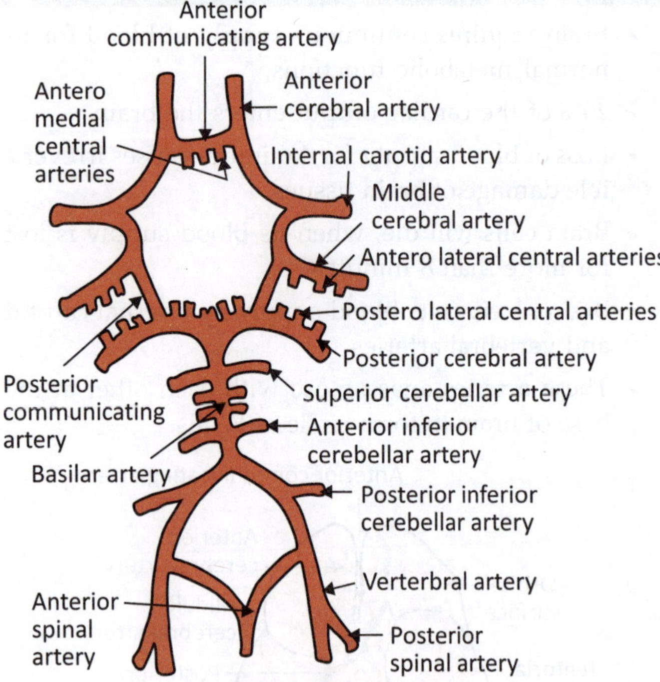

Fig. 36.14: *Circle of Willis*

Arterial Supply of Cerebrum

It is supplied by:

1. Anterior cerebral artery
2. Middle cerebral artery
3. Posterior cerebral artery

I. Arterial supply of supero lateral surface: It is supplied by branch of anterior, middle and posterior cerebral arteries.

(a) **Occipital lobe and inferior temporal gyrus** are supplied by posterior cerebral artery, i.e., visual cortex mainly.

(b) **Anterior cerebral artery** supplies sensory and motor areas of the leg and perineum, i.e., a gyrus breadth along the supero medial border upto the parieto occipital sulcus.

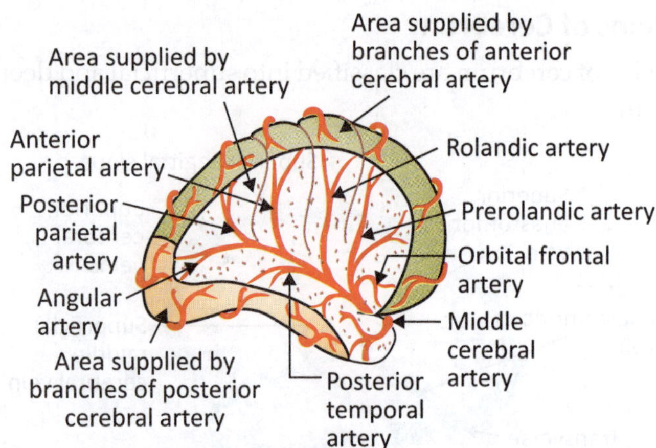

Fig. 36.15: *Arteries of the supero lateral surface of the cerebrum*

(c) **Middle cerebral artery supplies:**

(i) Motor and sensory cortex of the opposite half of the body except the area of leg and perineum.

(ii) Motor speech area.

(iii) Auditory area.

(iv) Stereognostic area.

(v) Pre frontal area.

Middle cerebral artery also supplies supero lateral surface except occipital lobe, inferior temporal gyrus and finger breadth along the superior medial border.

II. Arterial supply of inferior surface of the cerebrum:

(i) Medial part of the orbital surface is supplied by anterior cerebral artery.

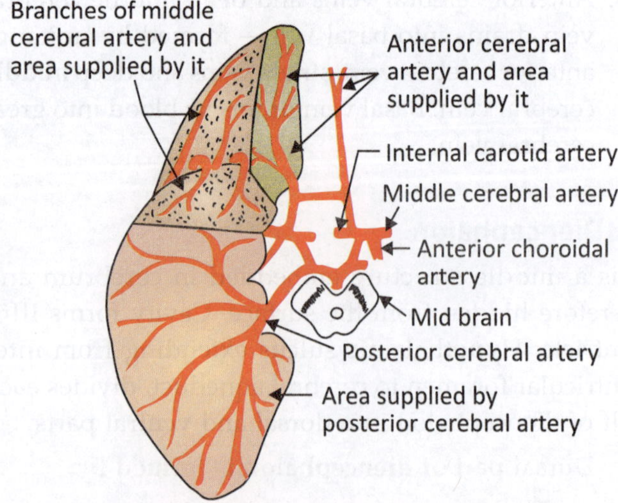

Fig. 36.16: *Arterial supply of inferior surface of cerebral hemisphere*

(ii) Lateral part of orbital surface is supplied by middle cerebral artery. It also supplies the anterior part of temporal lobe inferiorly.

(iii) Posterior part of temporal lobe is supplied by posterior cerebral artery. It also supplies the inferior surface of the occipital lobe.

III. Arterial supply of medial surface of cerebrum:

(i) Posterior cerebral artery supplies – medial surface of occipital lobe and para hippocampus.

(ii) Anterior cerebral artery supplies medial surface above the corpus callosum upto parieto occipital sulcus.

(iii) Middle cerebral artery supplies uncus.

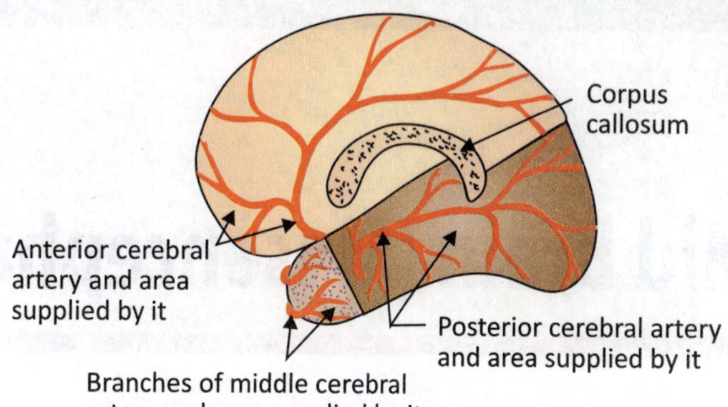

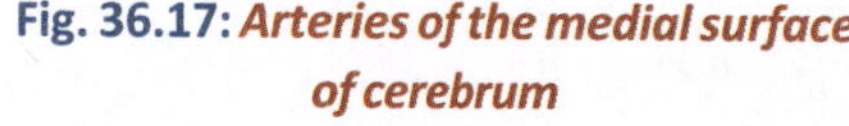

Fig. 36.17: ***Arteries of the medial surface of cerebrum***

CHAPTER 37

Mid Brain (Mesencephalon)

INTRODUCTION

It is a small part which connects the forebrain with hind brain.

Situation: Lies in posterior cranial fossa, superior to pons and it is found within the tentorial notch.

Length is about 2 cm.

Cerebral aqueduct is a canal which traverses the mid-brain, and connects third and fourth vertricles.

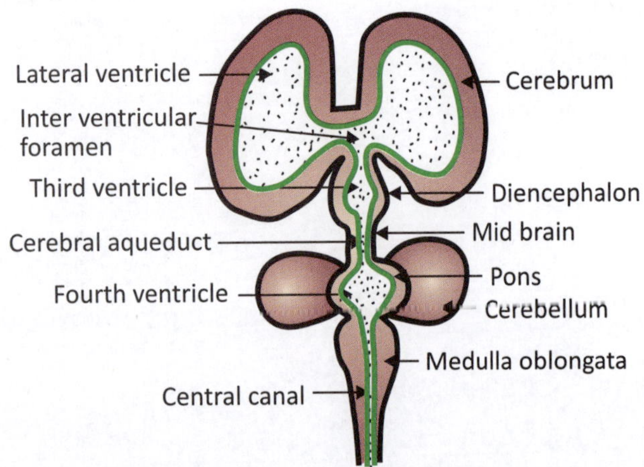

Fig. 37.1: ***Parts of brain***

Parts: A transverse section of mid brain shows following parts:

1. Tectum – dorsally situated.
2. Cerebral peduncles – ventrally situated.
   - Each cerebral peduncle is divided into crus cerebri and tegmentum by the substantia nigra.
   - Crus cerebri is the anterior part of the mid brain and forms posterior boundary of the inter peduncular fossa. Here, it is related to the posterior perforated substance.

The crura are separated by a median sulcus, through this sulcus the oculomotor nerve enters the inter peduncular fossa. The lateral surface of the crus is crossed by the trochlear nerve.

Colliculi

Colliculi (tectum) are situated on the dorsal surface of the tegmentum. Colliculi are four in number, arranged into a pair of superior colliculi and a pair of inferior colliculi. They are separated from each other by a cruciform shaped sulcus.

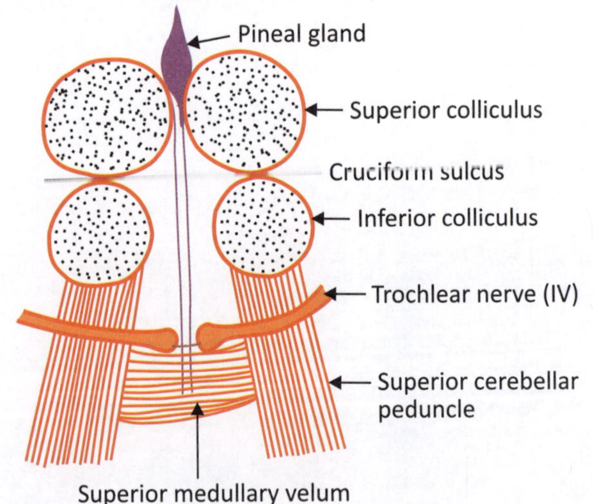

Fig. 37.2: ***Colliculi of mid brain***

Superior Colliculi

Superior colliculi are larger and darker than the inferior colliculi and are associated with the reflex activities of the visual pathway. It is made up of collection of neurons present in different layers.

Superior colliculus is connected to the lateral geniculate body by a rope like structure called superior brachium.

Inferior Colliculi

Inferior colliculi are smaller, associated with reflex activities of auditory pathway and is connected with medial geniculate body by the inferior brachium.

STRUCTURE OF MID BRAIN

I. Transverse section of mid-brain at the level of superior colliculus

Structures can be identified are:

1. Crus cerebri – contains fibres:
   (a) Lateral 1/5 – temporo pontine fibres
   (b) Medial 1/5 – fronto pontine fibres
   (c) Middle 3/5 – cortico spinal tract

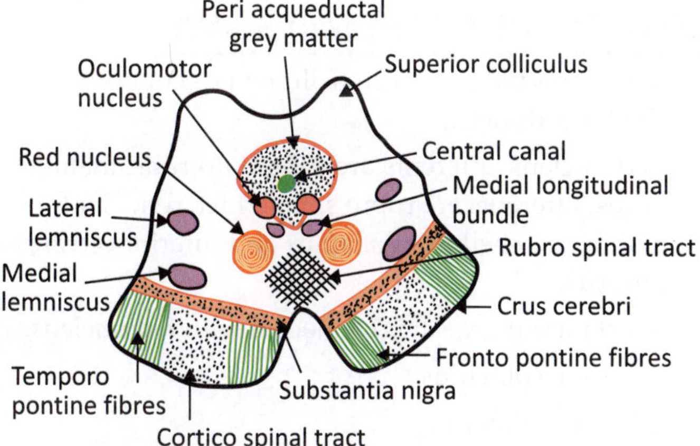

Fig. 37.3: ***Mid brain at superior colliculus level (T.S.)***

2. Substantia nigra – Band of grey matter situated in between the tegmentum and crus cerebri.
3. Red nucleus is situated anterior to the peri aqueductal grey matter.
4. Oculomotor nucleus is a nuclear complex situated with in the anterior part of peri aqueductal grey at the level of superior colliculus. It has many components namely:
   (a) Dorsal nucleus
   (b) Ventral nucleus
   (c) Ventrimedial nucleus
   (d) Intermediate nucleus
   (e) Caudal central nucleus
   (f) Edinger Westphal nucleus.

➤ Oculomotor nerve arises from this nuclear complex. Edinger Westphal nucleus is parasympathetic part of the oculomotor nucleus. It supplies sphincter pupillae and ciliaris muscles.

5. Inter peduncular nucleus
6. Pre tectal nucleus
7. Superior colliculus
8. Medial lemniscus
9. Trigeminal lemniscus
10. Dorsal tegmental decussation
11. Ventral tegmental decussation.

II. Transverse section of mid brain at the level of the inferior colliculus. Following structures can be identified:

1. Crus cerebri
2. Lateral lemniscus
3. Medial lemniscus
4. Spinal lemniscus
5. Trigeminal leminscus
6. Superior cerebellar penduncles decussate medial to the medial lemniscus. It connects the mid-brain with cerebellum.
7. Rubrospinal tract.
8. Nucleus of trochlear nerve – lies ventral to the cerebral aqueduct but within the peri aqueductal grey matter.

➤ The fibres of the trochlear nerve pass dorsally and decussate with the nerve of the opposite side. This is the only cranial nerve emerging from the dorsal surface of the brain. Inferior brachium connects the inferior colliculus with the medial geniculate body.

➤ **Substantia nigra:** Grey matter between crus cerebri and tegmentum. It is divided into thickly arranged dorsal portion and sparsely arranged ventral portion. The ventral portion contain nerve fibres and neurons.

CONNECTIONS

Afferents are received from:

1. Motor cortex
2. Sensory cortex
3. Red nucleus

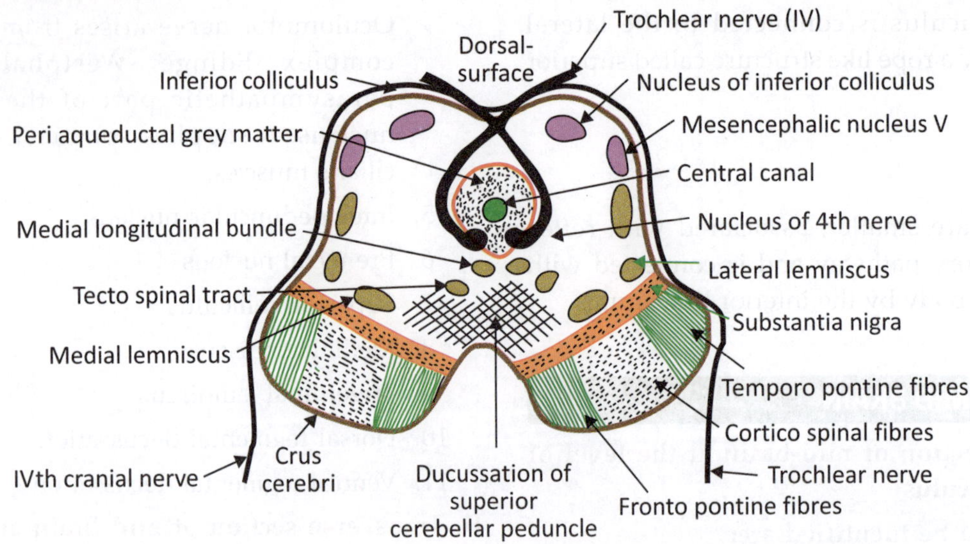

Fig. 37.4: ***Parts of the mid brain at inferior colliculus (T.S.)***

4. Lentiform nucleus
5. Reticular formation.

Efferents are received from:

1. Superior colliculus
2. Amygloid body
3. Ventro lateral thalamic nucleus
4. Caudate nucleus
5. Lentiform nucleus
6. Cingulate gyrus.

Functions of Substantia Nigra

The neuro transmitter substance found within the substantia nigra is called dopamine. It forms a part of extra pyramidal system. Lesions – cause – Parkinsonian's disease.

CONNECTIONS OF THE MID BRAIN

1. It is connected to the cerebellum via – superior cerebellar peduncle.
2. Red nucleus, afferents are – dendato rubrothalmic fibres. Efferents are rubro spinal tract, reticular formation, cerebellum, thalamus and inferior olivary nucleus.
3. Substantia-nigra – It is connected with red nucleus.
4. Superior colliculus.
5. Inferior colliculus.

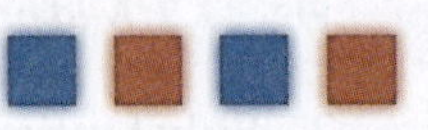

CHAPTER 38

Cerebellum

INTRODUCTION

It is the largest part of the hind brain.

Parts: Consists of two large lateral parts called cerebellar hemisphere – connected in the middle by a narrow central region called Vermis.

Situation: It lies below the tentorium cerebelli in the posterior cranial fossa.

Weight – about 150 gm.

EXTERNAL FEATURES

The surface of the cerebellum is divided into innumerable leaves called folia cerebelli. Each hemisphere has:

A. Two surfaces:
- (a) Superior and
- (b) Inferior surface.

B. Two borders
- (a) Anterior border and
- (b) Posterior border.

C. Two notches
- (a) Anterior cerebellar notch and
- (b) Posterior cerebellar notch.

Surface shows fissures:
1. Horizontal fissure
2. Fissura prima
3. Post lunate fissure
4. Post pyramidal fissure.

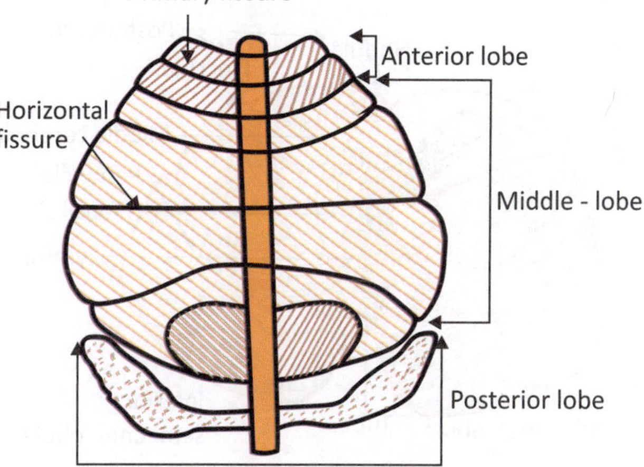

Fig. 38.1: *Parts of cerebellum*

Parts of Vermis

A. Superior vermis has:
- (a) Lingula
- (b) Central lobule
- (c) Culmen
- (d) Declive
- (e) Folium.

B. Inferior vermis has:
- (a) Tuber
- (b) Pyramid
- (c) Uvula
- (d) Nodule.

- Grey matter of the cerebellum is highly folded to accommodate millions of neurons in a small area – arrangement is called "Arborvitae" means vital tree of life.

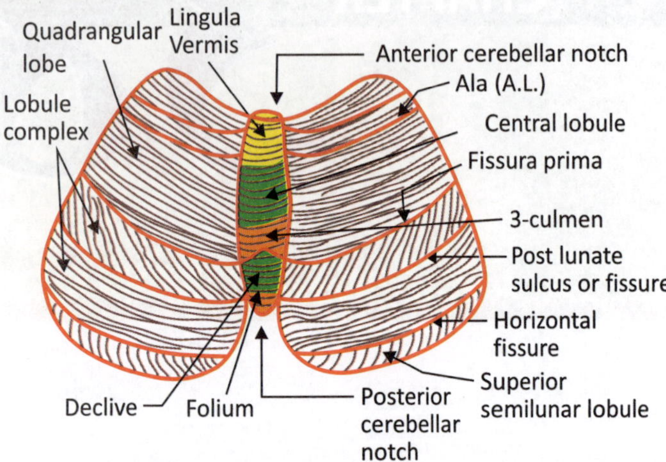

Fig. 38.2: *Superior surface of cerebellum*

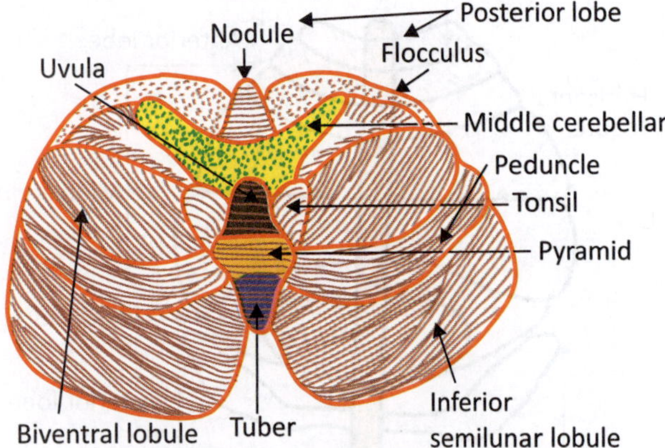

Fig. 38.3: *Inferior surface of cerebellum*

Table 38.1: *Lobulation: It is divided into – Anterior, middle and posterior lobes*

Lobe	Vermis	Cerebellar Hemisphere
Anterior	– Lingula – Central lobule – Culmen	– Ala – Quadrangular lobule
Middle	– Declive – Folium – Tuber – Pyramid – Uvula	– Lobule simplex – Superior semilunar lobule – Inferior semilunar lobule – Biventral lobule – Tonsil
Posterior	Nodule	Flocculus

Relations

Anteriorly: Forth ventricle, medulla and pons.

Posteriorly: Concavity of occipital bone.

Laterally: Sigmoid sinus, mastoid antrum and mastoid air cells.

Superiorly: Tentorium cerebelli.

PEDUNCLES OF CEREBELLUM

It is connected to other parts of the brain by peduncles, e.g.,

1. **Superior cerebellar peduncle:** Connects it with midbrain, efferent fibres pass through it.
2. **Middle cerebellar peduncle:** Connects the dorsum of pons with cerebellum, afferent fibres pass through it.
3. **Inferior cerebellar peduncle:** Connects the medulla oblongata dorso lateral aspect and cerebellum, both afferent and efferent fibres pass through it.

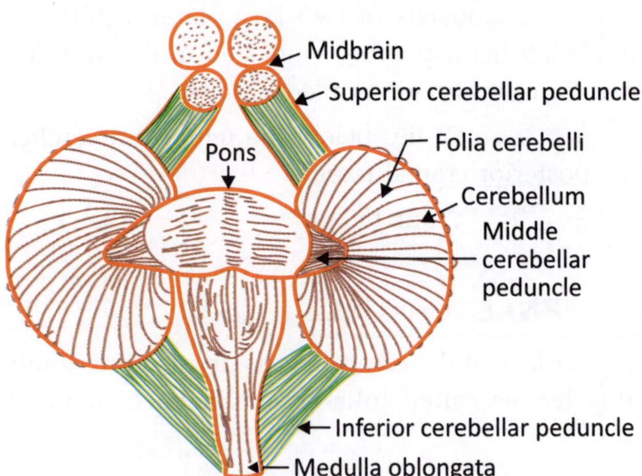

Fig. 38.4: *Peduncles of the cerebellum*

FUNCTIONS OF CEREBELLUM

It is responsible for:

1. Muscular co-ordination.
2. Maintenance of equilibrium, muscle tone and posture.
3. Controls all voluntary movements.
4. It exerts synergic control.
5. The control of cerebellum is ipsilateral.

BLOOD SUPPLY OF CEREBELLUM

Arterial supply:

1. Superior cerebellar artery.
2. Anterior inferior cerebellar artery.
3. Posterior inferior cerebellar artery.

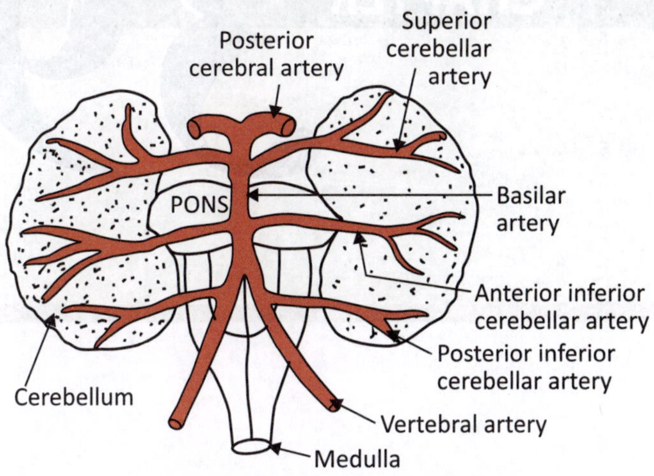

Fig. 38.5: *Blood supply of cerebellum*

Venous drainage:

Into near by dural venous sinuses like – transverse sinus, sigmoid sinus and occipital sinus etc.

CONNECTIONS OF CEREBELLUM

It receives information from following sources:

1. Vestibular part of VIIIth nerve (vestibulo cochlear nerve)
2. Spinal cord
3. Tectum of mid brain
4. Cerebral cortex.

Afferents and efferents pass to concerned areas through three pairs of cerebellar peduncles — superior, middle and inferior cerebellar peduncles.

Applied Anatomy

Each half of the cerebellum exerts its influence chiefly on the same side. Injury of cerebellum produces.

1. **Disturbances of posture, e.g.,**
   (a) **Atonia:** Loss of tone of muscles on the same side of lesion.
   (b) **Atitude:** Face is rotated to the opposite side and leg is abducted.
   (c) **Static tremor:** Slight oscillation of the head and trunk due to irregular contraction of muscles.
   (d) **Nystagmus:** Eyes tend to deviate from the central postion 10-30° to the opposite side.
   (e) **Vertigo:** Giddiness.
2. **Disturbances of movements, e.g.,**
   (a) **Asthenia:** Weakness of movement.
   (b) **Ataxia:** In co-ordination of movements.
   (c) **Asynergia:** Proper co-ordination between agonists and antagonists is lost.
   (d) **Dysdiadochokinesis:** Irregular halting in any alternating movements zig-zag gait or staggering gait.
   (e) **Dysarthria:** Slurring speech.

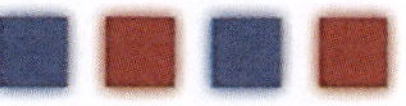

CHAPTER 39

Pons

INTRODUCTION

Pons is the bridge between mid brain and medulla.

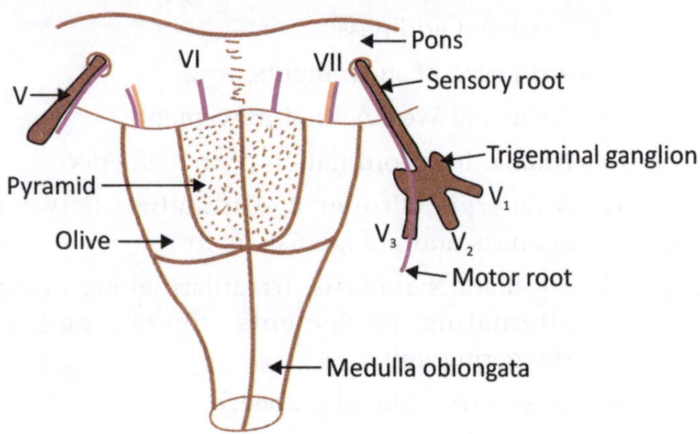

Fig. 39.1: *The pons*

Development: Rhomben cephalon.

Situation: Posterior cranial fossa on dorsum sellae.

Relations

Superiorly: Mid brain.

Inferiorly: Medulla oblongata.

Anteriorly: Pontine cistern, basilar artery, dorsum sellae.

- Basilar part of occipital bone.

Posteriorly: IVth ventricle and cerebellum.

Laterally: Middle cerebellar peduncle – connects pons with cerebellum.

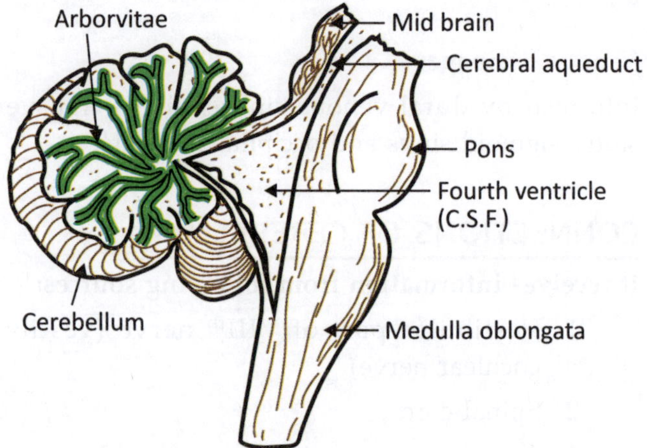

Fig. 39.2: *Relations of the pons*

EXTERNAL FEATURES

Two surfaces – dorsal and ventral surface.

I. Ventral Surface of Pons

This shows following features:

1. Transversely running fibres.
2. **Basilar sulcus:** This is present in mid line and lodges basilar artery.
3. On either sides of sulcus an eminence is present. This is due to underlying cortico spinal tract.
4. Laterally the ventral surface leads to the middle cerebellar peduncle.
5. Between pons and middle cerebellar Peduncle emerges out roots of (Vth) trigeminal nerve. The

nerve has medial motor root and lateral sensory root.

6. The lower border of ventral surface is related to pyramid and olive of medulla.
7. Between pons and pyramid – (VIth) Abducent nerve is present is emerging out here.
8. Between pons and olive – (VIIth) or facial nerve emerges out.
9. At lower border of pons – basilar artery is formed by union of right and left vertebral artery.
10. Along the lower border and lateral to the emergence of facial nerve, emerges out vestibulo cochlear nerve VIIIth cranial nerve.

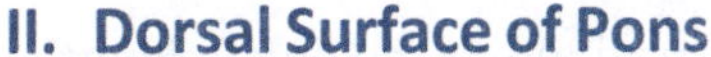

II. Dorsal Surface of Pons

Forms floor of upper part of IVth ventricle.

PARTS OF PONS

T.S. of pons shows two parts:

1. **Basilar part** is situated anterior to the emergence of trigeminal nerve.
   Neurons called – nuclei pontis are present with nerve fibres which are arranged in longitudinal direction, e.g., cortico spinal, cortico nuclear and cortico pontine tracts and transverse fibres are ponto cerebellar tract.
2. **Tegmentum:** Tracts present and is situated posterior to the emergence of trigeminal nerve.

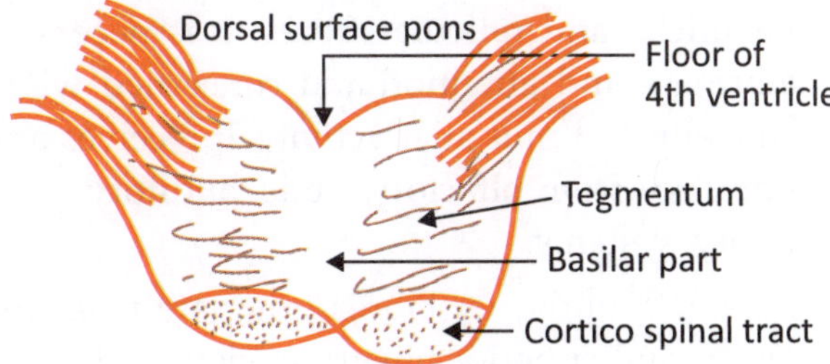

Fig. 39.3: *Parts of the pons*

BLOOD SUPPLY OF PONS

1. Basilar artery
2. Anterior inferior cerebellar artery
3. Posterior inferior cerebellar artery
4. Superior cerebellar artery.

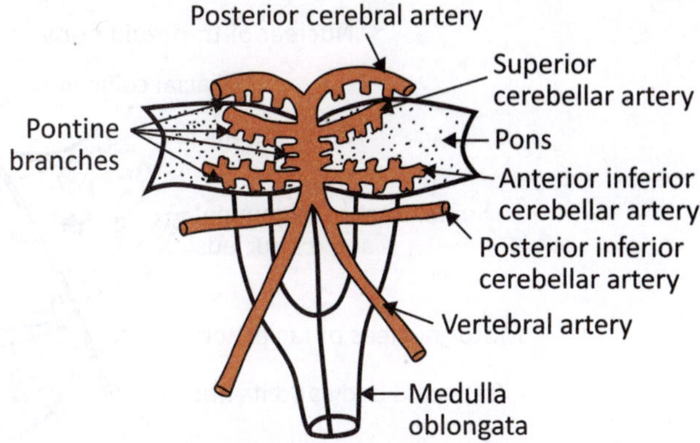

Fig. 39.4: *Blood supply of pons*

INTERNAL STRUCTURE OF PONS

Transverse section of pons:

I. **At the level of facial colliculus:** This is the upward continuation of the medulla oblongata. It contains following:

(a) **Nuclei**
- (i) Abducent nucleus
- (ii) Motor nucleus of facial nerve
- (iii) Superior salivatory nucleus
- (iv) Superior olivary nucleus
- (v) Vestibular nuclei.

(b) **Fibre tracts**
- (i) Medial longitudinal bundle
- (ii) Tecto spinal tract
- (iii) Medial lemniscus
- (iv) Lateral lemniscus
- (v) Trapezoid body
- (vi) Ventral trigeminal lemniscus.

II. **At the level of motor nucleus of trigeminal nerve:** Shows basilar and tegmental parts of the pons.

(a) **Basilar part shows – following tracts:**
- (i) Cortico spinal tract
- (ii) Cortico nuclear tract
- (iii) Cortico bulbar tract.

(b) **Tegmentum shows following nuclei:**
- (i) Motor nucleus of trigeminal
- (ii) Superior sensory nucleus of trigeminal
- (iii) Mesencephalic tract of trigeminal – lies between motor and sensory nucleus of Vth nerve. Superiorly it extends into mid brain.

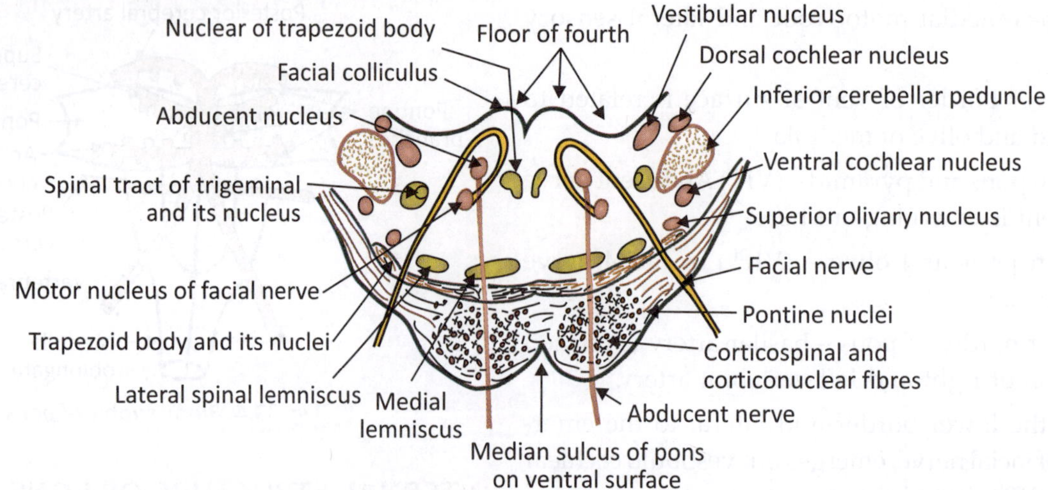

Fig. 39.5: ***T.S. through lower part of pons***

Tegmentum shows following tracts:

Fibre Tracts:

1. **Medial longitudinal bundle:** Lies lateral to mid-line.

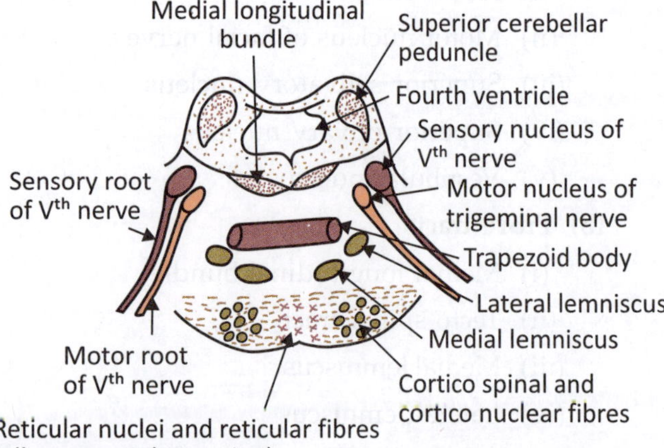

Fig. 39.6: ***T.S. of pons at the upper level of trigeminal nuclei***

2. **Tecto spinal tract:** Lies just anterior to medial longitudinal bundle.
3. **Medial lemniscus:** It is a sensory tract lies at the junction of basilar part and tegmentum.
4. **Trigeminal lemniscus** situated lateral to medial lemniscus. It ends at the thalamus.
5. **Spinal lemniscus** found along the entire length of pons. Situated lateral to medial lemniscus.
6. **Trapezoid body** is formed by transversely running fibres of auditory pathway – present in the ventral tegmentum. In the midline of trapezoid body neurons are present forms nucleus of trapezoid body.
7. **Middle cerebellar peduncle (Brachium pontis):** It connects the pons and cerebellum and carries ponto cerebellar and reticulo cerebellar fibres.
8. **Superior cerebellar peduncle:** Connects mid-brain and cerebellum.
9. **Inferior cerebellar peduncle:** Connects medulla oblongata and cerebellum.
10. **Reticular formation:** This is a network present in the central part of the brain stem – contains reticular nuclei and reticular fibres. It is necessary for alertness and attention and concerned with specific effect of muscular activity. It receives afferent impulses from olfactory, optic, auditory and gustatory systems.
11. **Lateral lemniscus:** Fibres originate from the cochlear and superior olivary nucleus. It is a part of the auditory pathway, medial geniculate body.

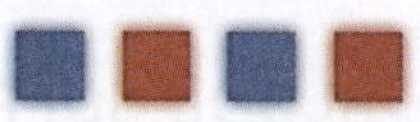

CHAPTER 40

Medulla Oblongata

INTRODUCTION

It is the lowest part of the brain stem.

Situated: In the posterior cranial fossa.

Development: Myelencephalon (Rhomben-cephalon).

Extent: Lower border of pons to the upper border of posterior arch of atlas. Superiorly it is continuous with the pons and inferiorly it is continuous with the spinal cord.

Shape: Piriform.

Measurements:

Length – 3 cm

Width – 2 cm in widest part

Thickness – 1.25 cm.

Relations:

Anterior:

1. Basilar part of occipital bone
2. Odontoid process of axis.

Posterior:

1. Cerebellar hemispheres
2. Fourth ventricle.

MEDULLA OBLONGATA

It has a lower closed part and an upper open part on its dorsal aspect.

EXTERNAL FEATURES

1. It has two surfaces:

(a) Anterior surface

(b) Posterior surface.

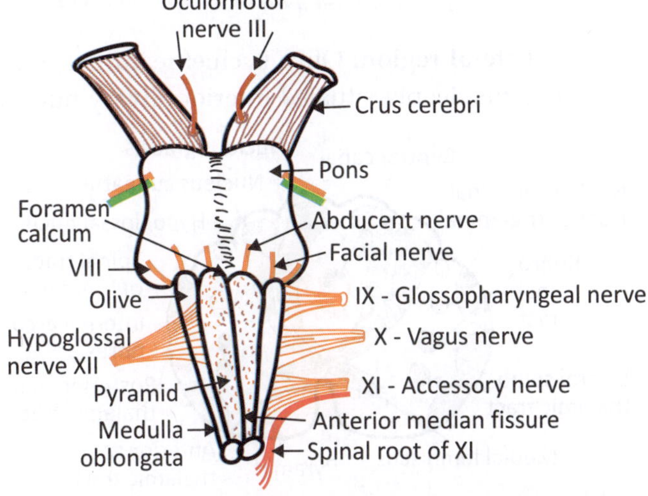

Fig. 40.1: *Cranial nerves related to ponto medullary junction*

2. **Anterior median fissure:** Upper end meets the lower border of pons at foramen caecum. It is the upward continuation of the anterior median fissure of the spinal cord.

   Anterior median fissure is crossed by decussation of pyramidal tract.

   (a) **Posterior median sulcus:** It is shallow and narrow only present at the closed part of medulla. It is the upward continuation of the posterior median sulcus of the spinal cord.

   (b) **Postero lateral sulcus:** Rootlets of IXth, Xth and XIth cranial nerves are emerging. It is lateral to the posterior median sulcus.

   (c) **Antero lateral sulcus:** Rootlets of XIIth cranial nerve are emerging. It is found lateral to the anterior median fissure.

These sulci divide medulla into three regions:

(a) **Anterior region:** Pyramid over lies cortico spinal tract.

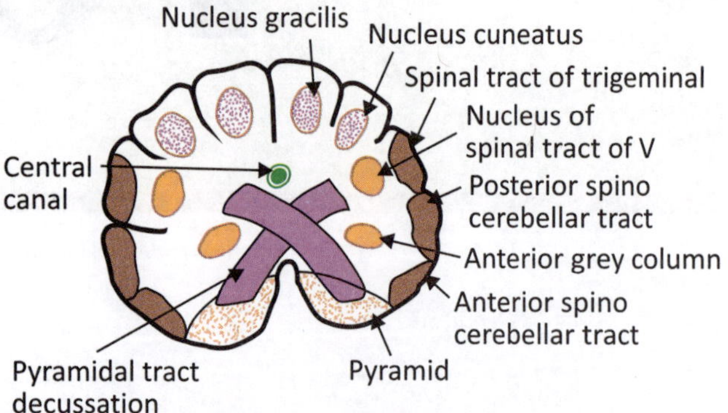

Fig. 40.2: *T.S. of medula oblongata at pyramidal decussation*

(b) **Lateral region:** Olive is chief feature. It represents deeply situated inferior olivary nucleus.

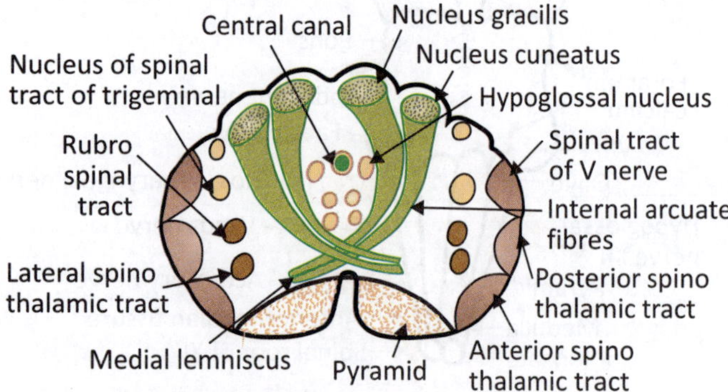

Fig. 40.3: *T.S. of medulla oblongata at senory decussation*

(c) **Posterior regions:**

- Upper part forms floor of IVth ventricle and is open.
- Lower part is closed.
- Inferior cerebellar peduncles arise from medulla and connected to cerebellum efferent and afferent fibres pass to spinal cord.
- In the floor of IVth ventricle – VIIIth, IXth, Xth and XIIth cranial nerve nuclei are present.

BLOOD SUPPLY

1. Right and left vertebral arteries – medullary branches.
2. Anterior spinal artery.
3. Right and left posterior spinal artery.
4. Posterior inferior cerebellar artery.

Veins: Drain the medulla oblongata – accompany arteries.

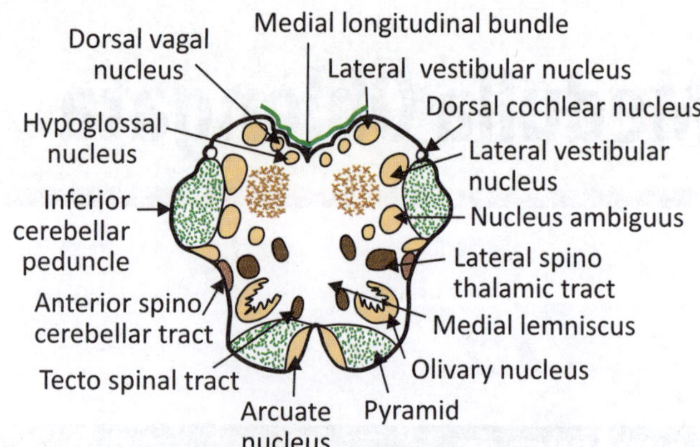

Fig. 40.4: *Olivary level of medulla oblongata*

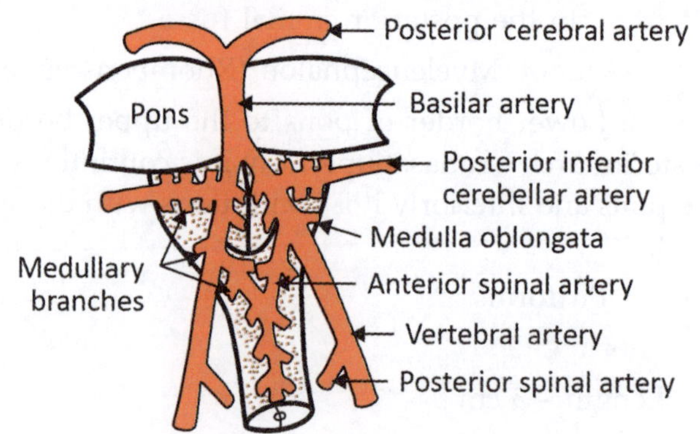

Fig. 40.5: *Blood supply of medulla oblongata*

CEREBRO-SPINAL FLUID (C.S.F.)

- It is a modified tissue fluid.
- Contained in the ventricular system of brain and subarachnoid space around the brain and spinal cord.
- C.S.F. replaces lymph in C.N.S.

Formations

1. Formed by choroid plexuses of lateral ventricles, IIIrd and IVth ventricles.
2. By capillaries on the surface of brain and spinal cord.

   Total quantity of C.S.F. is about 150 cc.

   Formed at rate of about 20 ml/hour or 500 ml/day.

   Normal pressure of C.S.F. is 60 to 100 mm of water.

Circulation

From lateral ventricle to → IIIrd ventricle via inter ventricular foramen of monro → IVth ventricle through median and lateral apertures of IVth ventricle. C.S.F. passes in the subarachnoid space on the surface of brain and drained into venous sinuses by archnoid villi and granulations.

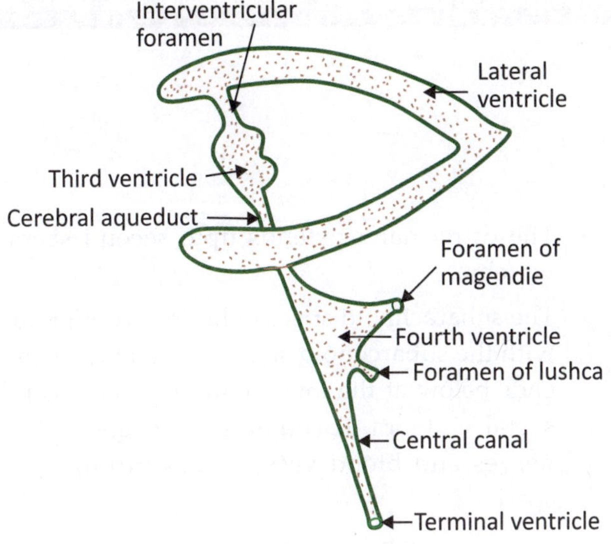

Fig. 40.6: *Ventricular system of brain*

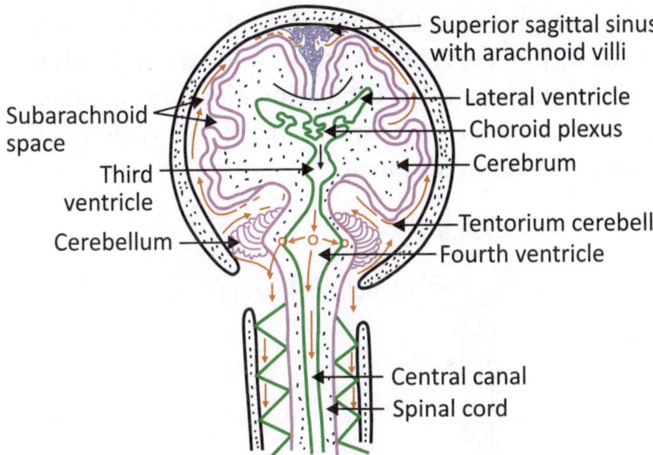

Fig. 40.7: *Circulation of cerebro spinal fluid*

Composition

- Proteins – 20-40 mg/100 cc
- Chlorides – 720-750 mg%
- Sugar – 50-75 mg%
- Cells – 0-5/cu.mm

Absorption

Done by:

1. Arachnoid villi and granulations and drained into cranial venous sinuses.
2. Perineural lymphatics around 1st, 2nd, 7th and 8th cranial nerves.
3. Veins related to spinal nerves.

Functions

- Protective
- Nutritive
- Pathway for excretion from C.N.S. (Metabolities)
- Acts as shock absorber
- Transport hormones
- Provides a stable chemical environment for neurons of C.N.S.

Applied Anatomy

1. **C.S.F. can be obtained by:**
   (a) Lumbar puncture
   (b) Cisternal puncture
   (c) Ventricle puncture.
   - Biochemical analysis of C.S.F. is of diagnostic value in various diseases, e.g., tubercular meningitis, haemorrhage etc.
2. **Excess accumulation of C.S.F. – Hydrocephalus caused by:**
   (a) Obstruction to C.S.F. circulation.
   (b) Excessive production of C.S.F.
   (c) Interference with its absorption, e.g., cerebral meningitis or haemorrhage in subarchnoid space, due to fibrosis.

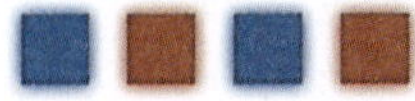

CHAPTER 41

Spinal Cord

INTRODUCTION

Spinal cord is downward continuation of medulla oblongata.

Situation: Within the upper 2/3rd of vertebral canal.

Length is about 45 cm in adult men and 42 cm in women.

Extent: From upper border of atlas vertebra to the lower border of L_1 vertebra.

The position of lower end may be variable.

It may extend to lower border of T_{12} vertebra or downwards to lower border of L_2 vertebra.

- Spinal cord is covered by meninges, i.e., dura mater, arachnoid mater and pia mater.
- The dura mater extends upto second sacral vertebra.
- The subarchnoid space of brain is continuous with the subarchnoid space of spinal cord and ends below at the lower border of the second sacral vertebra. It contains C.S.F. and spinal nerves and blood vessels pass through the space.

EXTERNAL FEATURES

The spinal cord is not having an uniform diameter. It has an upper cervical swelling and lower lumbar swelling. The lower end is tapering and conical, called the conus medullaris. The apex of the conus is continued down as the filum terminale.

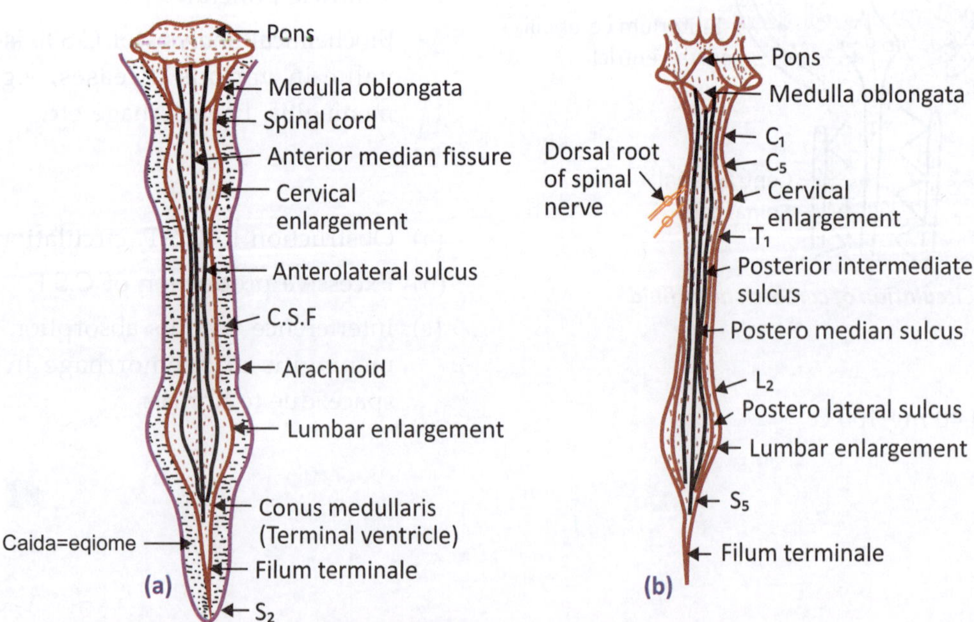

Fig. 41.1: *(a) Anterior aspect of spinal cord, (b) Posterior aspect of spinal cord*

The spinal cord gives of 31 pairs of spinal nerves:

- Cervical nerves – 8
- Thoracic nerves – 12
- Lumbar nerves – 5
- Sacral nerves – 5
- Coccygeal nerve – 1.

Cervical Swelling

It is situated where nerves of upper limb are attached. It extends between 3rd cervical to the 2nd thoracic segment of the spinal cord.

Lumbar Swelling

It is situated where nerves of the lower limb are attached. It lies between L_1 to S_3 segment of spinal cord ($T_9 - T_{12}$ vertebral level).

The spinal cord is much shorter than the length of the vertebral column. The spinal segments do not lie opposite the corresponding vertebrae. A vertebral spine is always lower than the corresponding spinal segment. It may be stated that in the cervical region there is a difference of one segment in the upper thoracic regions there is a difference of two thoracic segments, and in the lower thoracic region there is a difference of three segments.

Fissures and Sulci

The anterior median fissure and posterior median sulcus divide the spinal cord into two halves. They extend along the entire length of the cord. The antero lateral sulcus is found along the attachment of the anterior root of the spinal nerve. The postero lateral sulcus gives attachment to dorsal nerve root of spinal cord.

Spinal Nerve

The nerves are attached to the spinal cord by motor ventral and sensory dorsal roots. The dorsal root has a dorsal root ganglion which is sensory in function.

- Near the spinal cord dorsal root divides into medial and lateral divisions and enters the spinal cord. The lateral division carries pain and temperature sensations while medial division carries touch and pressure.
- The dorsal and ventral roots unite to form spinal nerve.

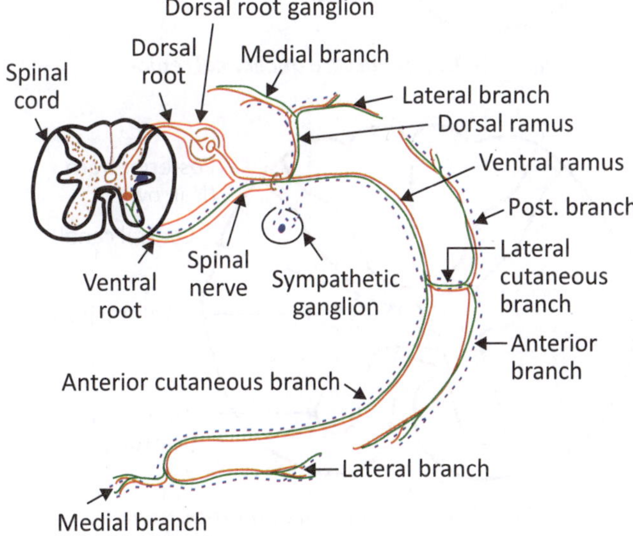

Fig. 41.2: *Typical spinal nerve*

Table 41.1: *Appearance of the Cross Section of the Spinal Cord at Various Levels*

S. No.	Segments of spinal cord	White matter	Section	Grey matter	Posterior horn	Lateral horn	Anterior horn
1.	Cervical	Plenty	Large and circular	Plenty	Slender	Absent	Broader for supply of upper limbs
2.	Thoracic	Reduced	Small and oval	Increased	Slender	Present for thoraco lumbar outflow	Slender
3.	Lumbar	Reduced	Large and circular	Greatly increased	Bulbous and broad	Present only in L_1 and L_2 segment	Bulbous for supply of lower limbs
4.	Sacral	Very much reduced	Circular and small	It is oval on each side	Thick	Present in sacral 2-4 segments for sacral outflow	Bulbous for supply of lower limbs

Cauda Equina

The lumbar, sacral and coccygeal nerves arise from conus medullaris–running vertically downwards. It resembles like a tail of a horse. Nerves are situated around the filum terminale and leave the cauda equina at respective foramina to pass through them.

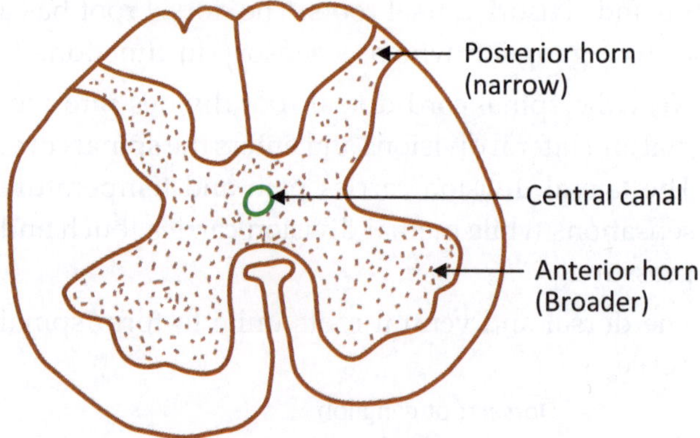

Fig. 41.3: *T.S. spinal cord at cervical region*

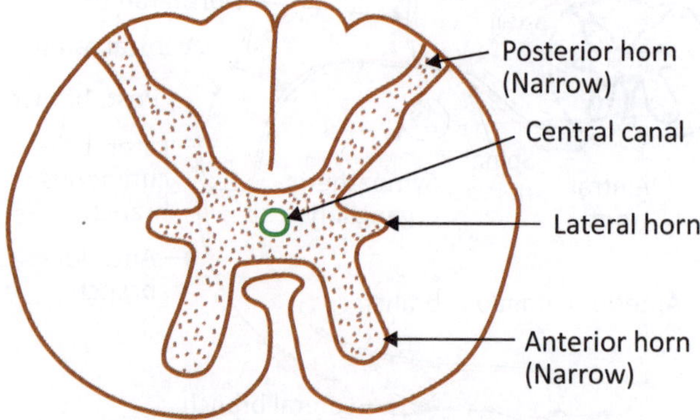

Fig. 41.4: *T.S. of spinal cord at thoracic region*

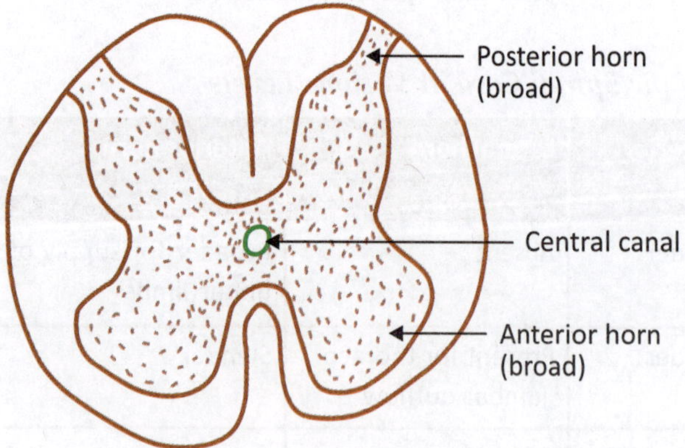

Fig. 41.5: *T.S. of spinal cord at lumbar region*

INTERNAL STRUCTURE OF SPINAL CORD

A cross-section will show:

1. White matter – situated at periphery.
2. Grey matter – situated near the center.

Grey Matter of Spinal Cord

It forms an 'H' shaped mass divisible into:

1. Anterior grey column or horn and
2. The posterior grey column or horn.
   - Lateral horns are situated only in the spinal segments of T_2 to L_1.

Anterior horn: Is directed forwards and laterally. It has a head and base – does not reach the surface of spinal cord. Neurons are motor in function. Axon of these neurons join and form the ventral root of spinal cord.

Posterior horn: It is directed backwards and laterally extend nearer to the surface and separated from the surface by the dorsi lateral tract.

It has – base, neck, head and apex.

- Apex is covered by substantia gelatinosa. Neurons are seonsory in function.

Lateral horn: Neurons are sympathetic in function situated in the spinal segments of T_2 to L_1.

Grey Commissure and Central Canal

It connects the right and left halves of grey matter and is traversed by the central canal, which is superiorly continuous with the fourth ventricle. Inferiorly canal dialates to form the terminal ventricle in the conus medullaris. It is surrounded by substantia gelatinosa centralis and canal is filled with C.S.F. and is lined by a membrane called ependyma.

White Matter of Spinal Cord

It is divided into funiculi, situated around the grey matter. They are classified into:

1. **Anterior funiculus:** It is found between anterior median fissure and ventral root of the spinal nerve.
2. **Lateral funiculus:** It is situated between ventral root and posterior lateral sulcus.

3. **Posterior funiculus:** It is situated between the postero lateral sulcus to the posterior median septum.

Tracts of the spinal cord are bundles of white matter found within the funiculi. These are classified into ascending tracts and descending tracts.

The ascending tracts are sensory tracts and descending tracts motor tracts.

CERVICAL LEVEL

(a) Section appears large

(b) Anterior horn is broader than posterior horn.

BLOOD SUPPLY

Anterial supply:

1. Anterior spinal artery (one)
2. Posterior spinal arteries (two)
3. **Spinal branches of:**
   - Vertebral arteries
   - Deep cervical artery
   - Posterior intercostal arteries
   - Lumbar arteries.

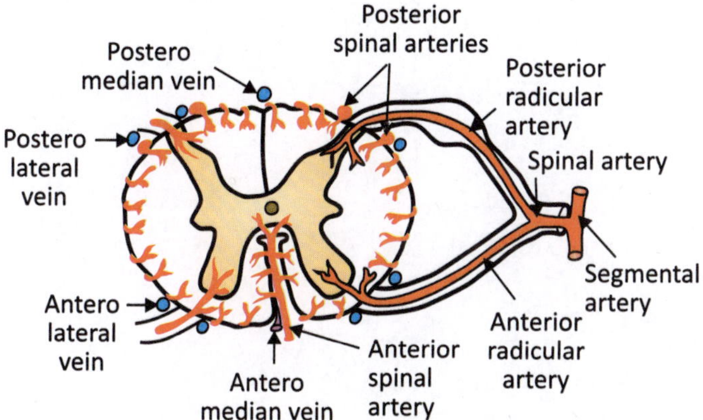

Fig. 41.6: *Blood supply of spinal cord*

1. **Anterior Spinal Artery** is a branch from 4th part of vertebral artery. It passes downwards and joins with its fellow of opposite side and forms anterior spinal arterial trunk, which descends along the anterior median fissure and is reinforced by the anterior radicular branches of vertebral, deep cervical, ascending cervical, posterior intercostal and lumbar arteries. It supplies:
   - Anterior funiculus
   - Right and left lateral funiculus
   - Anterior 2/3 of the grey column.
2. **Posterior Spinal Artery** is a branch from 4th part of vertebral artery. It divides into two collateral arteries along the medial and lateral sides of the dorsal nerve roots and forms the posterior arterial trunks. Each trunk is reinforced by posterior radicular artery braches of vertebral, deep cervical, ascending cervical, posterior intercostal and lumbar arteries. It supplies:
   1. Posterior 1/3 of grey column
   2. Posterior funiculus
   3. A small part of the lateral funiculus.

VENOUS DRAINAGE

These are six veins found on the surface of spinal cord.

- One vein along the anterior median fissure.
- One vein along the posterior median sulcus.
- One pair of veins on each side of the ventral nerve roots.
- One pair of veins on each side of the dorsal nerve roots.

These veins are directly communicating with each other and form a network of veins around the spinal cord.

These veins superiorly communicate with the dural venous sinuses of the posterior cranial fossa. Venous plexus is present in subarachnoid space and communicates with the internal vertebral venous plexus and external vertebral venous plexus.

These veins are not provided with valves.

CLINICAL SEGMENTATION OF THE SPINAL CORD

A spinal segment is formed by a portion of the spinal cord with a pair of spinal nerves.

As the spinal cord stops at the lower border of L_1 vertebra, the vertebral levels do not correspond with the spinal segments.

To understand the level segmentation is done by:

- Add one to the number of cervical vertebra. For example, C_3 spine corresponds with C_4 segment.
- Add two to the number of upper six thoracic vertebrae. For example, T_4 spine corresponds with T_6 segment.

- Add three to $T_7 - T_{10}$ spines. For example, T_7 spine corresponding with T_{10} segment.
- Add six to T_{12} spine. So that T_{12} corresponds with S_1 segment of the spinal cord.
- The sacral and coccygeal segments are situated at the level of L_1 spine.

Applied Anatomy

1. **Spinal shock:** Loss of reflexes after the transaction of the spinal cord. All the body segments below the level of transaction become paralysed and ansesthetic.
2. **Tabes dorsalis:** Due to syphilitic infection of the spinal cord.
3. **Acute polio myelitis:** Due to viral infection of cells of anterior horn of spinal cord, especially at cervical and lumbar swellings of the spinal cord.
4. **Syringo myelia:** Dilatation of the central canal of the spinal cord.
5. Fracture or dislocation of vertebra, prolapse of the intervertebral discs, tumours of meninges or secondary deposits may produce spinal cord lesions.

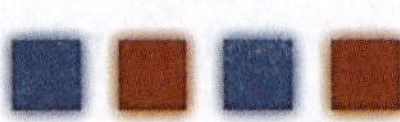

Review of Brain

1. **Explain nervous system.**

Ans.: Refer pg no. 279, chapter 36.

2. **Name the parts of brain?**

Ans.: Refer pg no. 279, chapter 36.

3. **What is neuron? Draw structure of neuron.**

Ans.: Refer pg no. 280, chapter 36.

4. **What is the function of neuron?**

Ans.: Neuron is the structural and functional unit of nervous system. It responsible for integration, interpretation, association, conduction, transformation, reception and analysis of impulses.

5. **Explain lobulation of the cerebrum.**

Ans.: Refer pg no. 282, chapter 36.

6. **What is medial and inferior surface of the brain?**

Ans.: Refer pg no. 285, chapter 36.

7. **What is the blood supply to the brain?**

Ans.: Refer pg no. 287, chapter 36.

8. **Explain formation of "Circle of Willis".**

Ans.: Refer pg no. 287-288, chapter 36.

9. **Define mid brain (Mesencephalon) and its structure.**

Ans.: Refer pg no. 290-291, chapter 37.

10. **Explain connections of the mid brain.**

Ans.: Refer pg no. 292, chapter 37.

11. **Define cerebellum.**

Ans.: Refer pg no. 293, chapter 38.

12. **Explain blood supply of cerebellum.**

Ans.: Refer pg no. 295, chapter 39.

13. **What is pons. Explain external features and internal structure of pons.**

Ans.: Refer pg no. 296-297, chapter 39.

14. **What is Cerebrospinal Fluid (CSF)?**

Ans.: Refer pg no. 300, chapter 40.

15. **Explain medulla oblongata.**

Ans.: Refer pg no. 299, chapter 40.

16. **What is spinal cord? Explain external and internal structure of spinal cord.**

Ans.: Refer pg no. 302-304, chapter 41.

17. **What is cauda equina**

Ans.: Refer pg no. 304, chapter 41.

18. **Explain blood supply of spinal cord?**

Ans.: Refer pg no. 305, chapter 41.

19. **What is spinal shock?**

Ans.: Refer pg no. 306, chapter 41.

20. **Give examples for disturbances of posture and movements.**

Ans.: Refer pg no. 295, chapter 38.

SELF ASSESSMENT QUESTIONS

1. Describe circulation of CSF (Cerebrospinal Fluid).
2. Describe external surface of cerebrum with its blood supply.
3. Describe ventricular system of brain.
4. Write short notes on:
   - Circle of Willis

- Neuron
- Hypophysis cereberi
- Inter peduncular fossa
- Superficial veins of cerebrum

5. Make diagram of:
   - T.S. mid brain at superior calliculus
   - T.S. mid brain at inferior calliculus
   - T.S. through lower part of pons
   - T.S. pons at level of trigeminal nuclei
   - Typical spinal nerve
   - T.S. of spinal cord at different levels
   - Blood supply of spinal cord

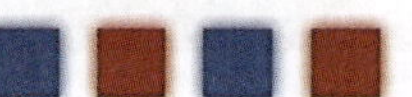

National Board Type Questions

MATCH THE FOLLOWING

1. Match the foramen in the skull on the left with the bone in which it is located on the right:

1. Optic canal	(a) Sphenoid bone
2. Carotid canal	(b) Occipital bone
3. Foramen spinosum	(c) Temporal bone
4. Hypoglossal	(d) Temporal bone
5. Foramen Rotundum	(e) None of the above
6. Facial nerve canal	
7. Foramen magnum	

Ans.: 1. — (a), 2. — (c), 3. — (a), 4. — (b), 5. — (a), 6. — (c), 7. — (b)

2. Match the cranial nerves listed on the left with the appropriate openings in the skull listed on the right, through which each nerve exits from the cranial cavity.

1. Mandibular division of trigeminal nerve	(a) Superior orbital fissure
2. Vagus nerve	(b) Foramen rotundum
3. Abducent nerve	(c) Foramen ovale
4. Ophthalmic division of trigeminal nerve	(d) Jugular foramen
5. Maxillary division of trigeminal nerve	(e) None of the above
6. Oculomotor nerve.	

Ans.: 1. — (c), 2. — (d), 3. — (a), 4. — (a), 5. — (b), 6. — (a)

3. For each joint listed on the left, give the most appropriate classification out of the list on the right.

1. Joint between vertebral bodies	(a) Synovial joint
2. Inferior tibiofibular joint	(b) Cartilaginous
3. Sutures between bones of vault of skull	(c) Fiberous
4. Wrist joint	(d) None of the above

Ans.: 1. — (b), 2. — (c), 3. — (c), 4. — (a)

4. For each type of synovial joint listed on the left, give an appropriate example from the list of joints on the right.

1. Hinge joint	(a) Metacarpo pharyngeal joint of index finger
2. Condyloid joint	(b) Shoulder joint
3. Ball and socket joint	(c) Wrist joint
4. Saddle joint	(d) Carpometacarpal joint of thumb
	(e) None of the above

Ans.: 1. — (e), 2. — (a), 3. — (b), 4. — (d).

5. For each joint listed on the left, indicate which type of movement it is associated with on the right.

1. Sternoclavicular joint	(a) Flexion
2. Superior radioulnar joint	(b) Gliding
3. Ankle joint	(c) Both (a) and (b)
	(d) Neither (a) nor (b)

Ans.: 1. — (b), 2. — (d), 3. — (a).

6. Match each structure listed on the left with a structure or occurrence listed on the right with which it is most closely associated. Each lettered answer may be used more than once.

1. Superficial fascia	(a) Divides up interior of limbs
2. Deep fascia	(b) Adipose tissue
3. Skeletal muscle	(c) Tendon spindles
	(d) None of the above

Ans.: 1. — (b), 2. — (a), 3. — (c).

7. Each type of blood vessel listed on the left, select an appropriate definition from the list on the right.

1. Arteriole	(a) A vessel that connects two capillary beds.
2. Portal vein	(b) A vessel whose terminal branches do not anastomose with branches or arteries supplying adjacent areas.
3. Anatomical end artery	(c) A vessel that connects large veins to capillaries.
4. Venule	(d) An artery less than 0.1 mm in diameter
	(e) A thin walled vessel that has an irregular cross diameter.

Ans.: 1. — (d), 2. — (a), 3. — (b), 4. — (c).

8. For each type of muscle action listed on the left, select the most appropriate definition from the list on the right.

1. Prime mover	(a) A muscle that contracts isometrically to stabilize the origin of another muscle.
2. Fixator	(b) A muscle that opposes the action of a flexor muscle.
	(c) A muscle that is chiefly responsible for a particular movement.
3. Synergist	(d) A muscle that prevents unwanted movements in an intermediate joint so that another muscle can cross that joint and act primarily on a distal joint.
4. Antagonist	(e) A muscle that opposes the action of a prime mover.

Ans.: 1. — (c), 2. — (a), 3. — (d), 4. — (e).

9. For each of the lymphatic structures listed on the left, select an appropriate structure or function listed on the right.

1. Lymph capillary	(a) Present in the central nervous system.
2. Thoracic duct directly	(b) Drains lymp from the tissues.
3. Right lymphatic duct	(c) Contains lymphatic tissue and has both afferent and efferent vessels.
4. Lymph node	(d) Drains lymph from the right side of the head and neck, right upper limb and right side of the thorax.
	(e) Drains lymph from the right side of abdomen.

Ans.: 1. — (b), 2. — (e), 3. — (d), 4. — (c).

10. Match the structures on the left with their related structures on the right.

1. Somatic afferent nerve	(a) Vestibulo-cochlear
2. Special somatic afferent	(b) Trigeminal
3. Special visceral efferent	(c) Oculomotor
4. Somatic efferent	(d) Accessory

Ans.: 1. — (b), 2. — (a), 3. — (d), 4. — (c).

11. Special features of the parts of brain:

1. Olivary nucleus	(a) Cerebellum
2. Dentate nucleus	(b) Midbrain
3. Facial colliculus	(c) Pons
4. Substantia nigra	(d) Medulla oblongata

Ans.: 1. — (b), 2. — (a), 3. — (d), 4. — (c).

MULTIPLE CHOICE QUESTIONS (MCQ'S)

1. When testing the sensory innervation of the face, it is important to remember that the skin of the lip of the nose is supplied by:

(a) Zygomatic branch of the facial nerve
(b) Maxillary division of the trigeminal nerve
(c) Ophthalmic division of the trigeminal nerve
(d) External nasal branch of the facial nerve
(e) Buccal branch of the mandibular division of the trigeminal nerve.

Ans.: (c)

2. Concerning the face:

(a) A boil on the side of the nose is potentially dangerous because of the possibility of spread of infection from the facial vein to the cavernous venous sinus via the superior ophthalmic vein.
(b) The entire skin of the face is innervated by the three divisions of the trigeminal nerve.

Ans.: (a)

3. Which of the following statements is (are) correct?

(a) The temporomandibular joint cannot be felt from the surface, because it is covered by the masseter muscle.
(b) Mastoid process of the temporal bone cannot be palpated in the newborn.

Ans.: (b)

4. Which of the following statements is (are) correct?

(a) Anterior division of the middle meningeal artery lies beneath the anterior inferior angle of the parietal bone, i.e., $1^1/_2$ inches above the midpoint of the zygomatic arch.
(b) The anterior fontanelle can easily be palpated in a baby and lies between the squamous part of the temporal bone, parietal bone, and the greater wing of the sphenoid.

Ans.: (a)

5. A patient who is standing in the anatomical position is:

(a) Facing laterally
(b) Has the palms of the hands directed medially
(c) Has the ankles several inches apart
(d) Is standing on his toes
(e) Has the upper limbs by the sides of the trunk.

Ans.: (e)

6. The lines of Cleavage or Langer's lines are:

(a) Finger prints
(b) Skin creases over joints
(c) Lines representing the interface between the superficial and deep layers of fascia
(d) The direction of the rows of elastic fibres in the dermis
(e) The direction of the rows of collagen fibers in the dermis.

Ans.: (e)

7. Inversion of the foot is the movement so that the sole faces:

(a) Downward and posteriorly
(b) Medially
(c) Laterally
(d) Downward
(e) Downward and laterally

Ans.: (b)

8. A patient is performing the movement of flexion of the hip joint when she:

(a) Moves the lower limb away from the midline in the coronal plane.
(b) Moves the lower limb posteriorly in the paramedian plane.
(c) Moves the lower limb anteriorly in the paramedian plane.
(d) Rotates the lower limb so that the anterior surface faces medially.
(e) Moves the lower limb toward the median sagittal plane.

Ans.: (c)

9. Maxillary sinus is supplied by which nerve?

(a) Maxillary (b) Ophthalmic

(c) Mandibular (d) Trigeminal

Ans.: (a)

10. Circle of willis is formed by

(a) Vertebral arteries

(b) Internal carotid arteries

(c) Both internal and external carotids

(d) Vertebral and internal carotid

Ans.: (d)

11. Which of the following tracts contains primary afferent neuron fibres

(a) Fasciculus gracilis and cuneatus

(b) Anterior spinothalamic

(c) Lateral spinothalamic

(d) Dorsal spinocerebellar

Ans.: (a)

12. Foramen magnum is present in which bone:

(a) Frontal (b) Maxilla

(c) Parietal (d) Occipital

Ans.: (d)

13. Vertebral artery passes through:

(a) Optic foramen

(b) Foramen magnum

(c) Superior orbital fissure

(d) Vertebral foramen

Ans.: (b)

14. Which muscle forms oral diaphragm?

(a) Geniohyoid (b) Myelohyoid

(c) Stylohyoid (d) Hyoglossus

Ans.: (b)

15. Pterygoid process is the part of:

(a) Vomer (b) Ethmoid

(c) Sphenoid bone (d) Maxilla

Ans.: (c)

16. All the muscles of mastication are affected to:

(a) Mandible (b) Temporal bone

(c) Sphenoid (d) Maxilla

Ans.: (a)

17. Styloid process is the part of:

(a) Maxilla (b) Occipital

(c) Mandible (d) Temporal

Ans.: (d)

18. Jugular process is the part of:

(a) Occipital (b) Frontal

(c) Sphenoid (d) Vomer

Ans.: (a)

19. Superior orbital border is formed by:

(a) Nasal bone (b) Lacrimal bone

(c) Maxilla (d) Frontal

Ans.: (d)

20. Ophthalmic artery is a branch of?

(a) External carotid (b) Internal carotid

(c) Common carotid (d) Maxillary

Ans.: (b)

21. Lower end of duramater is attached to spine of which vertebrae?

(a) T12 (b) S2

(c) L2 (d) All of the above

Ans.: (b)

22. Optic nerve is a:

(a) Motor nerve (b) Mixed nerve

(c) Parasympathetic (d) Sensory nerve

Ans.: (d)

23. Secretions of thyroid gland is controlled by?

(a) Sensory fibers (b) Parasympathetic

(c) Sympathetic (d) TSH

Ans.: (d)

24. Facial nerve supplies:

(a) Muscles of facial expression

(b) Muscles of mastication

(c) Muscles of soft palate

(d) Tongue muscles

Ans.: (a)

25. All the muscles of the tongue are supplied by:

(a) Hypoglossal (b) Mandibular nerve

(c) Lingual nerve (d) Glossopharyngeal

Ans.: (a)

26. Oral diaphragm is formed by:

(a) Hyoglossus (b) Mylohyoid

(c) Geniohyoid (d) Genioglossus

Ans.: (b)

27. Stylomastoid foramen transmits:

(a) Occipital artery (b) Trigeminal nerve

(c) Facial nerve (d) Optic nerve

Ans.: (c)

28. Muscles of mastication develops from mesoderm of:

(a) First pharyngeal arch

(b) Second arch

(c) Third arch (d) Fourth arch

Ans.: (a)

29. Nucleus receiving impulses of taste is:

(a) Dorsal nucleus of vagus

(b) Spinal nucleus of trigeminal

(c) Nucleus ambigus

(d) Nucleus of tractus solitaries

Ans.: (d)

30. Long buccal nerve is branch of:

(a) Ophthalmic nerve (b) Maxillary nerve

(c) Mandibular nerve (d) Glossopharyngeal

Ans.: (c)

31. Forehead is the part of:

(a) Scalp (b) Face

(c) Both (a) and (b) (d) Neck

Ans.: (c)

32. Thyroid gland is a:

(a) Sebaceous gland (b) Salivary gland

(c) Sweat gland (d) Endocrine gland

Ans.: (d)

33. Face receives its sensory fibers from which nerve?

(a) Facial (b) Vagus

(c) Trigeminal (d) Oculomotor

Ans.: (c)

34. Motor nerves supplies:

(a) Cardiac muscles (b) Smooth muscles

(c) Skeletal muscles (d) None of the above

Ans.: (a)

35. Recurrent laryngeal nerve supplies all the muscles of larynx except:

(a) Lateral crico arytenoid

(b) Crico thyroid

(c) Posterior crico arytenoid

(d) Oblique arytenoid

Ans.: (b)

36. Which foramen transmits olfactory nerves?

(a) Foramen spinosum

(b) Jugular foramen

(c) Cribriform

(d) Foramen ovale

Ans.: (c)

37. Which muscle is not supplied by hypoglossal nerve?

(a) Styloglossus (b) Stylopharyngeus

(c) Hyoglossus (d) Genioglossus

Ans.: (b)

38. Spinal root of accessory nerve innervates:

(a) Sternocleido mastoid (b) Styloglossus

(c) Digastric (d) Stylohyoid

Ans.: (a)

39. Posterior 1/3 of tongue supplied by glossopharyngeal nerve develops from:

(a) Mandibular arch (b) Hyoid arch

(c) Hypobranchial eminence

(d) Tuberculum impar

Ans.: (c)

40. Which is the first branch of facial nerve?

(a) Chorda tympani (b) Posterior auricular

(c) Greater petrosal (d) Nerve to stapedius

Ans.: (c)

41. All the three germ layers are present in:

(a) Tympanic membrane (b) Cornea

(c) Heart (d) Urachus

Ans.: (a)

42. Parotid gland is which type of gland?

(a) Salivary (b) Endocrine

(c) None (d) Sweat

Ans.: (a)

43. Waldeyer's ring is formed by all except:

(a) Tubal tonsil

(b) Retro pharyngeal nodes

(c) Palatine tonsil

(d) Pharyngeal tonsils

Ans.: (b)

44. Internal auditory meatus transmits:
(a) Facial nerve (b) Auditory nerve
(c) Both (a) and (b) (d) None of the above
Ans.: (c)

45. Ophthalmic artery is a branch of:
(a) Maxillary artery
(b) External carotid artery
(c) Internal carotid artery
(d) Subclavian artery
Ans.: (c)

46. CSF composition resembles with
(a) Lymph (b) Blood
(c) Plasma (d) Bile
Ans.: (a)

47. Thyrohyoid membrane is pierced by which artery:
(a) Superior laryngeal (b) Inferior thyroid
(c) Inferior laryngeal (d) Superior thyroid
Ans.: (d)

48. Which type of joint is median atlantoaxial:
(a) Pivot (b) Hinge
(c) Saddle (d) Ellipsoid
Ans.: (a)

49. Klinefelter's syndrome is associated with chromosome complement:
(a) 47, XXX (b) 47, XXY
(c) 47, XYY (d) 47, YYY
Ans.: (b)

50. Which nerve supplies lower 1/3rd of auricle?
(a) Great auricular nerve
(b) Auriculotemporal
(c) Lesser occipital (d) 3rd occipital
Ans.: (a)

51. All of the following are the branches of external carotid except:
(a) Posterior auricular (b) Occipital
(c) Ophthalmic (d) Facial
Ans.: (c)

52. Which of the gland is not provided secretory fibers by facial nerve?
(a) Parotid (b) Lacrimal
(c) Submandibular (d) Sublingual
Ans.: (a)

53. Only one muscle depresses the mandible. Which one is it?
(a) Medial pterygoid (b) Temporalis
(c) Lateral pterygold (d) Masseter
Ans.: (c)

54. Which muscles may elevate the larynx?
(a) Sternothyroid (b) Thyrohyoid
(c) Sternohyoid (d) Omohyoid
Ans.: (b)

55. Which of the following nerve supplies the cornea?
(a) Supraorbital (b) Infraorbital
(c) Lacrimal (d) Nasociliary
Ans.: (d)

56. By how many openings do the semicircular canals open into the vestibule?
(a) 2 (b) 3
(c) 4 (d) 5
Ans.: (d)

57. The vocal folds are abducted by:
(a) Posterior cricoarytenoid muscle
(b) Aryepiglottic
(c) Cricothyroid muscle
(d) Lateral cricoarytenoid muscle
Ans.: (b)

58. Stylopharyngeus muscle is supplied by nerve:
(a) IX (b) X
(c) XI (d) XII
Ans.: (a)

59. Lower end of filum terminate is attached to the dorsum of:
(a) First coccygeal vertebral
(b) Second lumbar vertebra
(c) Fifth lumbar vertebra
(d) Last sacral vertebra
Ans.: (a)

60. Which is not the branch of maxillary artery?
(a) Anterior tympanic (b) Middle meningeal
(c) Inferior alveolar (d) Facial artery
Ans.: (d)

61. The grey appearance of spinal grey matter is due to the presence of:

(a) Neuronal body (b) Neuroglia
(c) Neurites (d) Blood vessels

Ans.: (a)

62. In the tegmentum of midbrain, the lemnisci are arranged from medial to lateral side as

(a) Medial, spinal, trigeminal, lateral
(b) Medial, lateral, spinal, trigeminal
(c) Lateral, trigeminal, spinal, medial
(d) Medial, trigeminal, spinal, lateral

Ans.: (d)

63. Tela choroides is defined as:

(a) Double fold of pia mater
(b) Double fold of ependyma with vascular fringes
(c) Single layer of pia mater with ependyma
(d) Double fold of ependyma

Ans.: (a)

64. Which of the following sulcus of cerebral cortes is a limiting sulcus?

(a) Central (b) Calcarine
(c) Precentral (d) Parieto-occipital

Ans.: (a)

65. Which cranial nerve is attached to dorsal aspect of brain?

(a) Facial (b) Glossopharyngeal
(c) Hypoglossal (d) Trochlear

Ans.: (d)

IN EACH OF THE FOLLOWING QUESTIONS, ANSWER

(a) If (1) is correct only.
(b) If (2) is correct only.
(c) If both (1) and (2) are correct.
(d) If neither (1) nor (2) are correct.

1. Which of the following statements is (are) correct?

(1) Coronal planes in the body are vertical planes that lie parallel to the median plane.
(2) The dorsal surface of the big toe is the upper surface of the toe.

Ans.: (b)

2. Which of the following statements is(are) correct?

(1) A joint is where two or more bones come together and there is always movement between the bones.
(2) In a primary cartilaginous joint the bones are united by plate of fibrocartilage and the ends of the bones are covered with hyaline cartilage.

Ans.: (b)

3. Which of the following statements is (are) correct?

(1) A synapse is site where two neurons come into close proximity but not into anatomical continuity.
(2) Preganglionic nerve fibres pass to spinal nerves in the grey rami communicates.

Ans.: (a)

4. Which of the following statements is (are) correct?

(1) The articular surfaces of all synovial joints are covered with fibrocartilage.
(2) The cavity of a bursa occasionally communicates with the cavity of a synovial joint.

Ans.: (a)

5. Which of the following statements is (are) correct?

(1) The long bones of the limbs are developed by endochondral ossification.
(2) A sesamoid bone is a small nodule of bone found in a tendon.

Ans.: (a)

6. Which of the following statement is (are) correct?

(1) The epiphysis is the center of ossification found in the shaft of a long bone.
(2) Growth that takes place in an epiphyseal plate is largely responsible for increasing the diameter of a long bone.

Ans.: (a)

7. Which of the following statements is (are) correct?

(1) By definition the origin and insertion of a skeletal muscle can never be interchanged.
(2) The strength of a skeletal muscle is directly proportional to the length of the muscle fibres.

Ans.: (d)

8. Which of the following statements is (are) correct?

(1) The superficial fascia in the eyelids and penis has no adipose tissue.
(2) The deep fascia is often thickened in front of joints to form retinacula.

Ans.: (c)

9. Which of the following statements is (are) correct?

(1) The stability of a joint depends on the shape of the articular surfaces, the strength of the ligaments and the tone of the muscles around the joint.

(2) The capsule and ligaments of a joint are devoid of a sensory nerve supply.

Ans.: (a)

10. Which of the following statements is (are) correct?

(1) The skin creases found in the front of joints are sites where the skin is firmly attached to underlying structures by bones of fibrous tissue.

(2) The surface of the skin covered by the nail is called the nail bed.

Ans.: (c)

In questions 11 to 15, contains four suggested answers out of which one or more are correct. Choose the answer:

(a) If 1, 2, 3 are correct
(b) If 1 and 3 are correct
(c) If 2 and 4 are correct
(d) If only 4 is correct
(e) If all are correct

11. The superior colliculus of midbrain is:

(1) Visual reflex center
(2) Higher center for vision
(3) Situated in midbrain
(4) Visual relay center

Ans.: (a)

12. The lateral geniculate body receives:

(1) Contralateral temporal retinal fibres
(2) Ipsilateral temporal retinal fibres
(3) Ipsilateral nasal retinal fibres
(4) Contralateral nasal retinal fibres

Ans.: (c)

13. The lesion of oculomotor nerve leads to:

(1) Diplopia
(2) Ptosis
(3) Dilatation of pupil
(4) Lateral squint

Ans.: (e)

14. The optic nerve is considered a tract because:

(1) The sheaths covering the optic nerve are derived from the three meninges
(2) Its fibres have no neurilemma sheath
(3) It is attached to forebrain
(4) It cannot regenerate

Ans.: (e)

15. A fracture of cranial cavity passing through jugular foramen will cause paralysis of:

(1) Accessory nerve
(2) Vagus nerve
(3) Glossopharyngeal nerve
(4) Facial nerve

Ans.: (a)

FILL IN THE BLANKS

1. Adduction means movement __________ central axis.

Ans.: Towards

2. Belly is the __________ contractile part of a ________.

Ans.: Fleshy, muscle

3. Barr bodies are found in all cells of __________.

Ans.: Females

4. Blood brain barrier exists at the __________ level between __________ and __________ cells.

Ans.: Capillary, blood and nerve

5. Body is studied region wise is called as __________ anatomy.

Ans.: Regional

6. Cadaveric anatomy is studied on __________.

Ans.: Dead bodies

7. Connective tissue is made up of __________, __________ and __________.

Ans.: Cells, Fibres and Matrix

8. Contralateral means __________ side.

Ans.: Opposite

9. Embryology deals with __________ and __________ changes of an individual.

Ans.: Prenatal and postnatal

10. In histology we study the structures of different type of tissues with the help of __________.

Ans.: Microscope

11. Internal ear known as ____________.

Ans.: Labyrinth

12. Loss of motor power in a muscle is called as ___________.

Ans.: Paralysis

13. Long process of neuron is called __________.

Ans.: Axon

14. Most of the skull bones ossifies in _________.

Ans.: Membranes

15. Main structural and functional unit of nervous system is _____________ which is _________ in origin.

Ans.: Neuron, Ectodermal

16. Nails are _________ appendages.

Ans.: Skin

17. Plasma cells produce ___________.

Ans.: Antibodies

18. Simple squamous epithelium is meant for _________ of substances.

Ans.: Exchange

19. Sebaceous glands produce ________ secretion.

Ans.: Oily

20. Skull is formed by ________ bones and _________ pairs of __________ ossicles.

Ans.: 22, 3, ear

21. Synovial type of joints have _________ and are _________ mobile.

Ans.: Cavity, freely

22. Skin is formed by two layers __________ and __________.

Ans.: Epidermis and dermis

23. Sinus aids are __________ spaces.

Ans.: Dilated

24. Sibsons fascia is also known as ___________.

Ans.: Supra pleural membrane

25. Tumours of muscles are known as ____________.

Ans.: Sarcoma

Index

A

A.S.O.M. (Acute Suppurative Otitis Media) 237
Abducent nerve 106, 264
Abduction 7
Accessory lacrimal glands 103
Accessory nerve 270
Accessory thyroid 207
Adduction 7
Adenohypohysis 254
Adenoid nodes 170
Adipocytes 13
Agenesis of tongue 168
Agueusia 168
Amphiarthrosis (cartilaginous joint) 32
Anastomoses 24
Anastomosis 8
Anatomical features of neck 113
Anatomical nomenclature 5
Anatomical planes 6
Anatomical position 6, 40
Anatomical position of skull 45
Anatomy
- history 3
- introduction 3
- subdivision 4

Angular artery 84
Ankyloglossia or tongue tie 168
Anosmia 177
Anterior ethmoidal sinuses 180
Anthropometry 41
Apical abscess 159
Apocrine glands 37
Aponeurosis 7
Appendicular skeleton 28
Aqueous humour 111
Arborvitae 293
Arcus senilis 108
Areolar connective tissue 38
Arrangement of structures in the body 8
Arrectores pilorum 37
Arterial supply of face 84
Arteries 7, 23
Arteriosclerosis 25
Arytenoid cartilage 219
Ascending pharyngeal artery 195
Asterion 274
Asthenia 295
Asynergia 295
Ataxia 295
Atitude 295
Atonia 295
Auditory tube 237
Auricle 228
Auscultation 5
Autonomic Nervous System (A.N.S.) 19, 22, 280
Avulsion of scalp 77
Axial skeleton 28
Axon 20, 280

B

Barr body 10
Basilar sulcus 296
Basle Nomina Anatomica (BNA) 5
Belly 7
Bifid tongue 168
Blepharitis 99
Blind spot 111
Blood and nerve supply of peripheral nerves 22
Blood brain barrier 21
Blood circulation 25
Blood pressure 25
Blood supply of
- blood vessels 24
- bones 29
- cerebellum 294
- duramater 248
- face 85
- larynx 223
- long bone 30
- medulla oblongata 300
- middle ear 233
- palate 163
- pharynx 215
- pons 297
- scalp 75
- skeletal muscles 17
- spinal cord 305
- teeth 158
- thyroid gland 206
- tongue 167
- trachea 225

Blood supply to the brain 287
Blood vessels 23-24, 99
Blue sclera 109
Bone growth 30

Bones 28
 blood supply 29
 classification 29
 functions 28
 nerve supply 30
Bony framework 182
Bony labyrinth 239
Bony landmarks of the back 87
Bony orbit 96
Bony ossicles of middle ear 232
Boundaries of parotid bed 129
Brachial plexus 187
Brain 279, 281, 290
Bregma 59, 274
Buccinator (muscle of cheek) 80
Bucco-pharyngeal fascia 115

C

Cadaveric anatomy 4
Cald well 179
Canal of schlemn 108
Capacitance vessels 24
Capillaries 8, 23
Capillary structure 24
Capsular or satellite cells 20
Capsule of submandibular gland 137
Capsule of the parotid gland 131
Capsule of thyroid gland 205
Caput succedanum 77, 274
Carcinoma of oesophagus 227
Cardiac muscle 16
Cardiovascular system 23-27
Carotid artery 193
Carotid body 193
Carotid canal 245
Carotid sheath 115
Carotid sinus 193
Carotid triangle 124
Cartilage 30
Cartilages of the larynx 217
Cartilaginous joints 32
Cavernous sinus 249
Cavernous sinus thrombosis 251
Cavities 8
Cell 9, 13
Cell and its components 9-10
Cell membrane 9
Central Nervous System (C.N.S.) 19, 279
Central sulcus 281
Central vein of retina 105
Cephal haematoma 77
Cerebellar hemisphere 293
Cerebellum 293
Cerebro-Spinal Fluid (C.S.F.) 300
Cerebrospinal nerves 279
Cerebrospinal part (somatic) 19
Cerebrum 281
Cervical sympathetic trunk 201
Chalazion 99, 275
Chochlear part of VIIIth nerve 240
Chorda tympani nerve 145
Choroid 109
Chyle 26
Ciliary body 109
Ciliary ganglion 106
Circle of willis 287
Circular sinus 251
Circulation of blood 25
Classification of
 blood vessels 23
 bones 29
 connective tissue 14
 joints 32
 muscles of back 88
 paranasal sinuses 178
Cleft palate 163
Clubbing 36
Cochlea 239
Codont 21
Collagen fibres 14
Collateral circulation 24
Colliculi 290
Colliculi of mid brain 290
Comparative anatomy 5
Congestive heart failure 201
Conjunctiva 99
Connections of cerebellum 295
Connections of the mid brain 292
Connective tissue 13, 14, 16, 38
Cornea 108
Corniculate cartilages 219
Coronal plane 6
Cranial cavity 242
Cranial fossae 242
Cranial nerves 257, 272
Cranio-sacral outflow 22
Cranium 45
Cribriform plate 70, 243
Cricoid cartilage 218
Cricothyroid muscle 220
Crista galli 243
Cuneiform cartilage 219
Cupped disc 109
Cyanosis 36
Cyclitis 110
Cytoplasm 9

D

Dangerous area of face 85
Dangerous area of the nose 177
Dangerous layer of scalp 274
Decalcification of enamel and dentin 159
Deep cervical muscles 182
Deep cervical nodes 169
Deep fascia 38
Deep lingual artery 196
Deep muscles – erector spinae muscle 91
Deep muscles – semispinalis muscle 92
Deep muscles – splenius muscle 91
Dental caries 159
Dental curve 159
Denticle 159
Depressions 8
Dermatome 21
Dermis 35
Dermoid cyst 77
Descriptive terms 6
Diaphragma sellae 247
Diaphysis 29
Diathroses (synovial joint) 32
Diencephalon 287
Digastric muscle 121
Digastric triangle 123
Diphtheria 216
Diphydont 157
Discolouration of tooth 159
Distal 6

Distributing vessels 23
Disused atrophy and hypertrophy 18
Dorsal surface 164
Dorsal surface of pons 297
Dorsum of the tongue 164
Dubois formula 34
Duct of cochlea 240
Dural venous sinuses 249
Duramater or patchy meninx 246
Dysarthria 295
Dysdiadochokinesis 295

E

Ear 228
Ear drum 234
Ear ossicles 233
Ear wax 235
Eccrine glands 37
Ectopic thyroid tissue 207
Ectropion 99
Elastic cartilage 31
Elastic fibres 14
Electromyography 5
Elevations 8
Embryology or developmental anatomy 5
Emissary sphenoidal foramen of vesalius 245
Emissary veins 253
End arteries 25
Endocrine glands 40
Endolymph 239
Endoscopy 5
Endosteal layer 246
Entropeon 99
Ependymal cells 20
Epidermis 35
Epiglottis 219
Epiphyseal plate of cartilage 29
Epiphysis 29
Epistaxis 175, 177
Epithelial tissue 11
Epi-tympanum 230
Erector spinae (sacro-spinalis) 91
Eruption of teeth 157
Ethmoid bone 70
Ethmoidal air cells 70
Ethmoidal foramina 243
Ethmoidal spine 67
Eustachian tube 237
Exchange vessels 24
Experimental anatomy 5
Exposure keratitis 108
Extension 7
Extensor surface 6
External auditory meatus 229
External carotid artery 131, 194
External ear 228
External features of the skull 45
External nose 174
External occipital crest 87
External occipital protuberance (inion) 87
Extra ocular muscles 100
Extrinsic muscles of the tongue 165
Eyeball 99, 107
Eyelids 98

F

Face 78
Facial artery 196
Facial muscles 79
Facial muscles and its nerve supply 83
Facial nerve 131, 265
Facial nerve testing 82
Facial skeleton 45
Falx cerebri 247
Fascia 14
Fascicular architecture of muscle 16
Fibres 14
Fibroblast 13
Fibrochondroma of the palate 163
Fibrocyte 13
Fibrous joints 32
Fibular 6
Filiform papillae 165
Fissured tongue 168
Flat bone 29
Flexion 7
Flexor surface 6
Foliate papillae 165
Fontanelles of skull 51
Fontenelles 51
Foramen caecum 243
Foramen lacerum 245
Foramen magnum 61
Foramen ovale 245
Foramen rotundum 245
Foramen spinosum 245
Forebrain 281
Foreign bodies 235
Forensic dentistry 159
Framework of nose 174
Frontal air sinus 179
Frontal bone 58
Frontal lobe 283
Function of neuron 307
Functions of
- bones 28
- cerebellum 294
- connective tissue 14
- deep fascia 39
- frontal lobe 283
- glial and ependymal cells 21
- larynx 223
- lymphoid system 26
- middle ear 232
- occipital lobe 284
- paranasal air sinuses 178
- parietal lobe 284
- skin 36
- skull 50
- substantia nigra 292
- superficial fascia 38
- tears 103
- temporal lobe 284

Fungal infections of nail 36
Fungiform papillae 165

G

Glial and ependymal cells 21
Glossopharyngeal nerve (IXth cranial nerve) 267

Grey matter 280
Gross anatomy 4

H

Haemorrhage 25
Haemotympanum 237
Hair 36
Hair follicle 37
Hard palate 161
Head injury 77
Headache 84
Heart 23
Heart muscle cell 16
Hemiglossia 168
Heterodont 157
Highest point of the iliac crest 87
Hind brain 293
Histology (microscopic anatomy) 5
Horizontal plane 6
Hutchinson's tooth 159
Hyaline cartilage 31
Hyoglossus 122
Hyoid bone 126
Hyper acousia 237
Hypertrophy of conchae 177
Hypoglossal nerve (motor cranial nerve) 271
Hypoparathyroidism 209
Hypopharyngeal pouch 216
Hypophysis cerebri (pituitary gland) 253
Hypo-tympanum 230

I

Iliac crest 87
Incisor crest 58
Inferior angle of scapula 87
Inferior colliculi 291
Inferior nuchal line 87
Inferior sagittal sinus 252
Inferior surface of the cerebrum 285
Inferior thyroid artery 206
Inferior thyroid vein 206
Inflammatory stenosis 235
Infra temporal fossa 140
Infrahyoid muscles 128
Inlet of larynx 222
Insertion 7
Inspection 5
Inter peduncular fossa 286
Inter transversari 93
Internal carotid artery 198, 254
Internal carotid artery and its branches 200
Internal ear 239
Internal jugular vein 199
Interspinalis 93
Investing layer of deep fascia of neck 113
Iridodialysis 110
Iris 110
Iritis 110
Irregular bone 29
Irregular connective tissue 14
Irregular dentition 159
Isthmus 204

J

Joints 31
Joints of middle ear 233
Jugular foramen 63
Jugum sphenoidale 243

K

Keratinized stratified squamous epithelium 12
Keratitis 108

L

Labyrinth 239
Labyrinthine part 70
Lacrimal apparatus 102
Lacrimal canaliculi 103
Lacrimal circulation 103
Lacrimal fossa 59
Lacrimal gland 102
Lacrimal punctum 98
Lacrimal sac 103
Lambda 274
Laryngeal inlet 212
Laryngo pharynx 212
Laryngocele 223
Larynx 217
Lateral lobe of thyroid 204
Lateral pterygoid 142
Lateral rotation 7
Lateral sulcus (sylvian sulcus) 282
Lateral wall of nose 176
Latissimus dorsi 89
Layers of eyelids 98
Layers of the scalp 74
Layngoscopy 223
Lens 112
Levator labii superioris 71, 81
Levator palati 162
Levator scapulae 89
Levators costarum 91
Ligaments 7
Ligaments of auricle 229
Ligamentum nuchae 87
Lingual artery 195
Lingual nodes 168, 170
Lingual thyroid 168
Lingual tonsil 172
Lithotomy position 6
Living anatomy 5
Lobulation of the cerebrum 282
Long bone 29
Longus capitis 183
Longus colli 183
Loose areolar tissue 77
Lymph nodes 26
Lymph nodes draining 169
Lymphatic system 26
Lymphatics 17
Lymphatics of the orbit 105

M

Macroglia 20
Macroglossia 168
Macrophages 13
Macroscopic anatomy 4
Malignant tumours 216
Mandible 52
Mandibular canal 55
Mandibular nerve 147, 264

Masseter muscle 141
Mast cells 14
Master of endocrine orchestra 253
Mastoid antrum 236
Mastoid process 235
Matrix 14
Maxillae 56
Maxillary air sinus 56, 178
Maxillary artery 146
Maxillary artery (internal maxillary artery) 197
Maxillary nerve (sensory) 264
Maxillary nerve (V_2) 154
Meatus 176
Medial border of scapula 87
Medial pterygoid 143
Medial rotation 7
Medial surface of the brain 285
Medial surface of the cerebrum 285
Median or midsagittal plane 6
Medulla 257
Medulla oblongata 299
Meibomian glands 98
Membranes and ligaments of larynx 221
Membranous labyrinth 239
Mesencephalon 292
Mesenchymal stem cell 13
Meso-tympanum 230
Metaphysis 29
Microglia 21
Microglossia 168
Microscopic structure of
  lymph node 26
  parotid gland 133
  submandibular gland 138
  thyroid gland 207
Mid brain 290
Middle constrictor of phyarnx 122
Middle cranial fossa 244
Middle ear cavity 230
Middle thyroid vein 206
Migrant cells 13
Movements of rima glottids 223
Mucous membrane of the larynx 222
Muller's muscle 79
Mumps 134
Muscle fibre 16
Muscle in the anterior triangle of neck 127
Muscle of neck 82
Muscles 15
Muscles lateral to plexus 185
Muscles medial to plexus 183
Muscles of
  auricle 229
  back 88
  mastication 141, 144
  middle ear 233
  mouth 80
  nose – nasalis 81
  orbit 79
  pharynx 213
  soft palate 163
  the larynx 219
  the orbit 100
  tongue 165
Muscular spasm 18
Muscular system 15-18
Muscular tissue 11
Muscular triangle 126
Musculus uvulae 162
Mylohyoid muscle 122
Myoepithelial cells 16
Myringitis 235
Myringotomy 235

N

Nails 36
Nasal cavity 175
Nasal crest 58
Nasal muscles 174
Naso lacrimal duct 103
Naso pharynx 212
Nasociliary nerve 106
Neck 113
Neonatal skull 51
Nerve supply of bones 30
Nerve supply of parotid gland 132
Nerve supply of scalp 74
Nerve supply of submandibular gland 137
Nerves 21
Nerves of the orbit 105
Nervous system 19-22, 279
Nervous tissue 11, 19, 280
Neuroglia 20, 280
Neuroglial cells 20
Neurohypophysis 254
Neuron 19, 280
Neurovascular hilum 17
Nomenclature of muscles 17
Norma frontalis 46
Norma lateralis 47
Norma occipitalis 46
Norma verticalis 45
Nostrils 174
Nuclei 262
Nuclei of cranial nerves 257
Nucleus 10
Nuroglial cells 20
Nystagmus 295

O

Oblique – fasciculi 17
Oblique plane 6
Occipital artery 197
Occipital bone 61
Occipital lobe 284
Oculomotor nerve 106, 260
Oesophageal varices 227
Oesophagitis 227
Oesophagus 226
Olfactory nerve 257
Omohyoid 118
Ontogeny 5
Openings 8
Ophthalmic artery 104
Ophthalmic division of trigeminal nerve 106
Ophthalmic nerve 262
Ophthalmic veins 105
Optic foramen 244
Optic nerve 105, 258
Orbicularis oris 80
Orbit and eyeball 96
Orbital fascia 104
Orbital fascia (tenon's capsule) 97
Orbital plate of frontal bone 243
Orbital septum 98, 99
Orbit-bony features 96

Organ of corti 240
Origin 7
Oro-pharynx 212
Ossification 55
Osteomyelitis 77
Otic ganglion 144
Otorrhoea 235
Oto-sclerosis 237
Otoscope 235
Outer fibrous coat 108

P

Paired cartilages 219
palate 161
Palatine bone 72
Palatine tonsils 171
Palatoglossus 162
Palatopharyngeus 162
Palmar 6
Palpation 5
Palpebrae 98
Palpebral fissure 98
Papillae 165
papilloedema 275
Parallel – fasciculi 16
Paralysis 18
Paralysis of soft palate 163
Paranasal air sinuses 178
Parasympathetic Nervous System (PNS) 22
Parathyroid glands 207
Para-vertebral muscles 182
Parietal bones 60
Parietal lobe 283
Parotid duct (stensen's duct) 132
Parotid gland 129
Parts of pons 297
Peduncles of cerebellum 294
Percussion 5
Perforation of tympanic membrane 235
Pericervical collar 169
Perilymph 239
Peripheral nerves 280
Peripheral Nervous System (P.N.S.) 19, 279
Perpendicular plate 70
pharyngeal diverticulum 214
Pharyngeal keratosis 216
Pharyngeal tonsil 172
Pharyngitis 215
Pharyngo tympanic tube 237
Pharyngoscopy 216
Pharynx 211
Phylogeny 5
Physical anthropology 5
Pigmentation of skin 34
Pinna 228
Piriform fossa 213
Plantar 6
Plasma cells 13
Polyphydent dentition 159
Pons 257, 296
Portal blood circulation 25
Portal vein 25
Postaxial border 6
Posterior auricular artery 197
Posterior belly 121
Praecoxdentia 159
Preaxial border 6
Preganglionic fibres 22
Pre-tracheal fascia 114
Pre-vertebral muscles 182
Pre-vertebral region 182
Pronation 7
Prone position 6
Prosencephalon 281
Protraction 7
Proximal 6
Pseudostratified epithelium 12
Pterion 274
Pterygo palatine fossa 153
components 154
Pterygo palatine ganglion 154
Ptosis 99
Pulmonary blood circulation 25
Pulse pressure 25
Pyorrhoea alveolaris 159

R

Radial 6
Radiographic anatomy 5
Radiography 5
Ramus of the mandible 54
Raphe 7
Rectus capitis anterior 184
Rectus capitis lateralis 185
Reflex arc 21
Regeneration of skeletal muscle 18
Regional anatomy 4
Regular connective tissue 14
Relationship of lymph system to the blood system 26
Resident cells 13
Resistance vessels 23
Reticular fibres 14
Retina 110
Retraction 7
Retro mandibular vein 131
Retropharyngeal abscess 215
Retropharyngeal space 215
Rhomboidei 90
Rhomboidei muscles 90
Ribs 28
Rima glottids 223
Root of neck 182
Rule of nine 34

S

Saccule 240
Sacrum 87
Sagittal plane 6
Scala media 240
Scaleno vertebral triangle 183
Scalenus anterior 184
Scalenus medius 185
Scalenus minimus 185
Scalenus posterior 185
Scalp 74
Scalp wound bleed profusely 77
Scalp wounds-heal quickly 77
Schwann cells 20
Sclera 108
Scleritis 109
Sebaceous cyst 77
Sebaceous glands 37
Secretions of the gland 207
Segments and chambers of eyeball 111
Semi spinalis 92
Semicircular canals 239

Semicircular ducts 240
Semispinalis capitis and longissimus capitis 92
Sensory or cutaneous nerves of face 82
Septal deviation 177
Septal haematoma 177
Sequestrum dermoid 163
Serratus posterior inferior 90
Serratus posterior superior 90
Seventh cervical spine (C7) 87
Sex chromatin or barr bodies 10
Shaft of hair 37
Shunts 24
Sibson's Fascia 188
Side of the neck (quadrilateral space) 116
Sigmoid sinus 252
Simple columnar epithelium 11
Simple cuboidal epithelium 11
Simple epithelium 11
Simple squamous epithelium 11
Singer's nodes 223
Sinus venosus sclerae 108
Sinusoids 24
Skeletal muscle 15, 16
Skeletal system 28-33
Skin 98
Skin and fasciae 34
Skin appendages 36
Skull 28, 45
Skull cap 242
Smooth articular areas 8
Smooth muscles 15
Soft palate 161
Soma or cell body 19
Sphenoid bone 67
Sphenoidal air sinus 181
Spinal nerves 21
Spiral or twisted fasciculi 17
Splenius 90
Sprain 18
Stapedius 233
Staphyloma 109
Static tremor 295
Sternocleidomastoid 118
Straight sinus 252
Stratified columnar epithelium 13
Stratified cuboidal epithelium 12
Stratified epithelium 12
Stratified squamous epithelium 12
Structure of skin 34
Structure of submandibular gland 138
Stye (hardeolum externum) 99
Styloglossus 139
Stylohyoid ligament 139
Stylohyoid muscle 122, 139
Styloid process 139
Stylomandibular ligament 139
Stylopharyngeus 139
Subclavian artery 189
Subdivision of anterior triangle of neck 123
Sublingual salivary gland 138
Subluxation of mandible 152
Submandibular duct 137
Submandibular gland 135
Submental triangle 123
Sub-occipital muscles 93
Substantia nigra 291
Sulci 281
Superficial fascia 37, 98
Superficial nodes 169
Superficial temporal Artery 197
Superior angle of scapula 87
Superior colliculi 290
Superior nuchal line 87
Superior orbital fissure 244
Superior sagittal sinus 252
Superior thyroid artery 195, 206
Superior thyroid vein 206
Supination 7
Supine position 6
Supporting cells 20
Supporting tissue 16
Suprahyoid muscles 127
Surface anatomy (topograhic anatomy) 5
Surface irregularities of the skin 35
Sweat glands (sudoriferous) 37
Sympathetic nervous system 22
Synapse 20, 280
Synarthroses (fibrous joint) 32
Synechiae 110
Synergists 18
Synovial joints 33
Systemic anatomy 4
Systemic blood circulation 25

T

Tardadentia 159
Taste buds 165
Tears 103
Tectorial membrane 240
Teeth 157
Temporal bone 64
Temporal fossa 76, 140
Temporal lobe 284
Temporalis muscle 142
Temporo mandibular joint 150
Temporo mandibular joint syndrome 152
Tendon 7
Tensor palati 162
Tensor tympani 233
Tentorium cerebelli 247
Thickness of skin 34
Thoracolumbar outflow 22
Thymus gland 209
Thyroid cartilage 217
Thyroid gland 204
Thyroidea ima artery 206
Tibial 6
Tissues 11-14
Tongue 164
Tonsil 173
Tonsillar bed 171
Tonsillar node 170
Torus palatinus 163
Trachea 224
Tracheaitis 226
Tracheostomy 226
Transitional epithelium 12
Transverse plane 6
Transverse sinus 252
Transverso spinalis 93
Trapezius 88

Tributaries of internal jugular vein 201
Tributaries or incoming channels 250
Trigeminal ganglion 255
Trigeminal nerve 262
Trigeminal neuralgia 84
Trochlear nerve 106, 261
Trochlear spine 59
Tubal tonsils 172
Tumours 18
Tumours of parathyroid glands 208
Tunica adventitia 24
Tunica intima 24
Tunica media 24
Tunnel of corti 240
Twinning of tooth 159
Tympanic cavity proper 230
Tympanic membrane 234
Tympano sclerosis 237
Tympanoplasty 235

U

Ulcers of tongue 168
Ulnar 6
Utricle 240
Uvula 162

V

Vagus Nerve (Xth cranial nerve) 268
Vallate papillae 165
Vascular catastrophies 25
Vascular pigmented coat (uveal tract) 109
Vein of kocker 206
Veins 7, 23
Veins of cerebrum 287
Venous drainage 75
Venous sinuses 249
Ventral surface of pons 296
Vermis 293
Vertebrae 28
Vertebral artery 190
Vertigo 295
Vestibular part of VIIIth nerve 240
Vestibule 239
Vestibulitis 177
Vestibulo cochlear nerve 266
Vibrissae 174
Vidian's nerve 154
Viscera 8
Vitreous body 112
Vomer bone 73

W

Waldeyer's lymphatic ring 173
Waldeyer's ring 171
Wharton's duct 137
White fibro cartilage 31
White fibrous tissue 14
White matter 280

Z

Zygomatic bone 71
Zygomaticus major 81
Zygomaticus minor 81

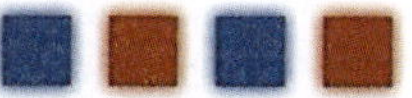

Notes

Notes 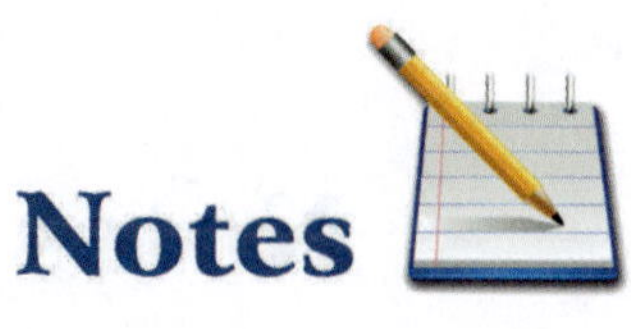

Notes